Y0-EGI-576

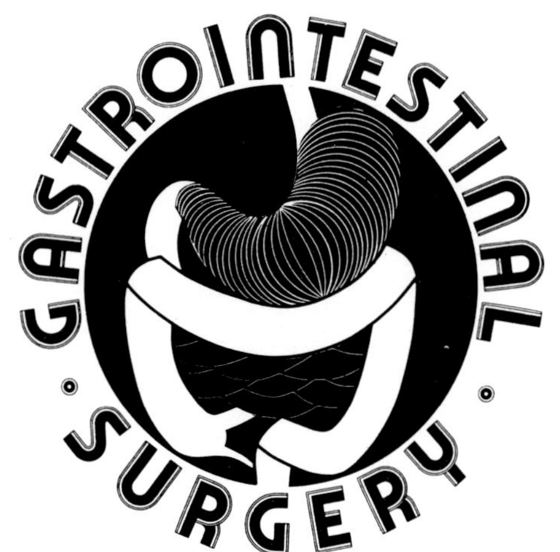
GASTROINTESTINAL
SURGERY

From the Annual Continuation Course in Surgery, University of Minnesota, Department of Surgery, Minneapolis, Minnesota

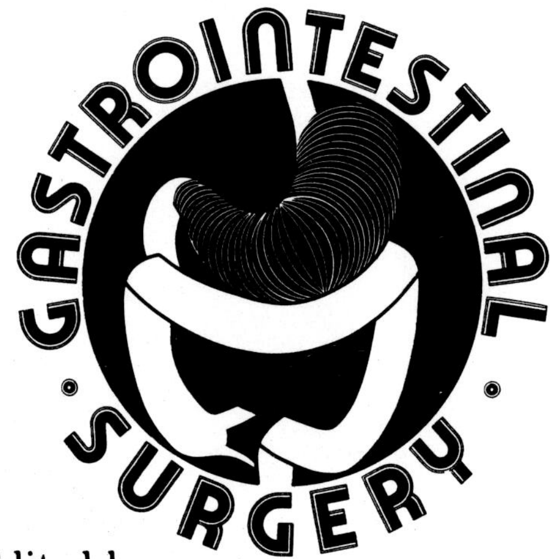

Edited by

JOHN S. NAJARIAN, M.D.

Professor and Chairman,
Department of Surgery,
University of Minnesota Medical School,
Minneapolis, Minnesota

and

JOHN P. DELANEY, M.D.

Associate Professor,
Department of Surgery,
University of Minnesota Medical School,
Minneapolis, Minnesota

Published by

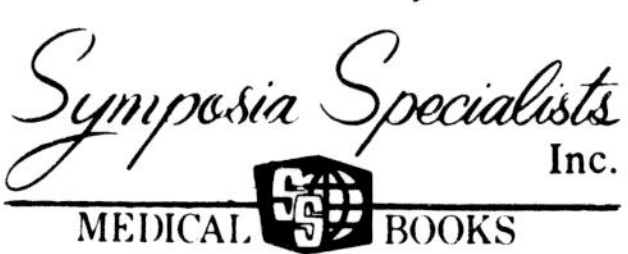

Distributed by

YEAR BOOK
MEDICAL PUBLISHERS
CHICAGO • LONDON

A HOME STUDY TEXTBOOK PROGRAM

This book approved for
Category I Accreditation

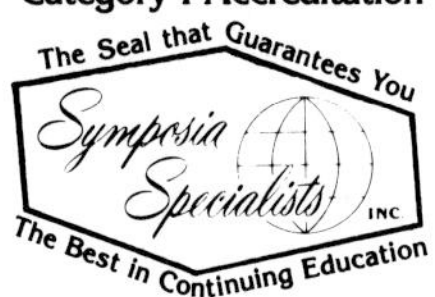

As an organization accredited for Continuing Medical Education the University of Minnesota designates that this continuing medical education activity meets the criteria for **30 CREDIT HOURS IN CATEGORY I FOR THE PHYSICIAN'S RECOGNITION AWARD** of the American Medical Association *provided it is used and completed according to the instructions.*

To obtain the final examination, see colored insert at inside back cover.

Symposia Specialists, Inc.
1460 N.E. 129th Street
Miami, FL 33161

Distributed by
Year Book Medical Publishers
35 E. Wacker Drive
Chicago, IL 60601

Library of Congress Catalog Number 79-63657
International Standard Book Number 0-8151-6326-6

Printed in the United States of America

Contents

INTESTINE

MISCELLANEOUS

Preface

Each year the surgical faculty at the University of Minnesota, with the help of a group of distinguished scholars from around the world, presents a continuation course. This book emanates from one of these courses, on gastrointestinal surgery. Some of the chapters approximate what was presented verbally during the course while others represent considerable expansions of the original talks.

Anatomically, the topics range up and down the alimentary canal from Zenker's diverticulum in the upper esophagus to carcinoma at the anal verge. Intellectually, the subjects range from gastric cellular physiology to the mechanics of constructing an anastomosis. The body of knowledge required of the modern gastrointestinal surgeon extends far beyond operative aspects of disease management. Much of the material is not strictly surgical in character but relates rather to the pathology, pathophysiology and nonoperative management of a variety of gastrointestinal diseases.

No claim is made that this volume represents a comprehensive coverage of all of gastrointestinal surgery; rather, we have attempted to emphasize recent advances and controversial topics.

The chapters are organized into anatomic regions — esophagus, stomach and intestine. A number of the topics are more general, not lending themselves to any particular anatomic designation, and are therefore grouped in a fourth section labeled miscellaneous.

One of the more popular features of previous books has been the panel discussions. The statements of the panelists are reproduced essentially as presented at the time of the course, with minimal alterations for the sake of written clarity.

The editors consider this volume to represent an up-to-date survey of progress in gastrointestinal surgery — a relatively compact compendium of what's new. While it is particularly useful to surgeons working in this field, much of the material should also be of value to physicians engaged in nonoperative care of patients with gastrointestinal disorders.

John S. Najarian

John P. Delaney

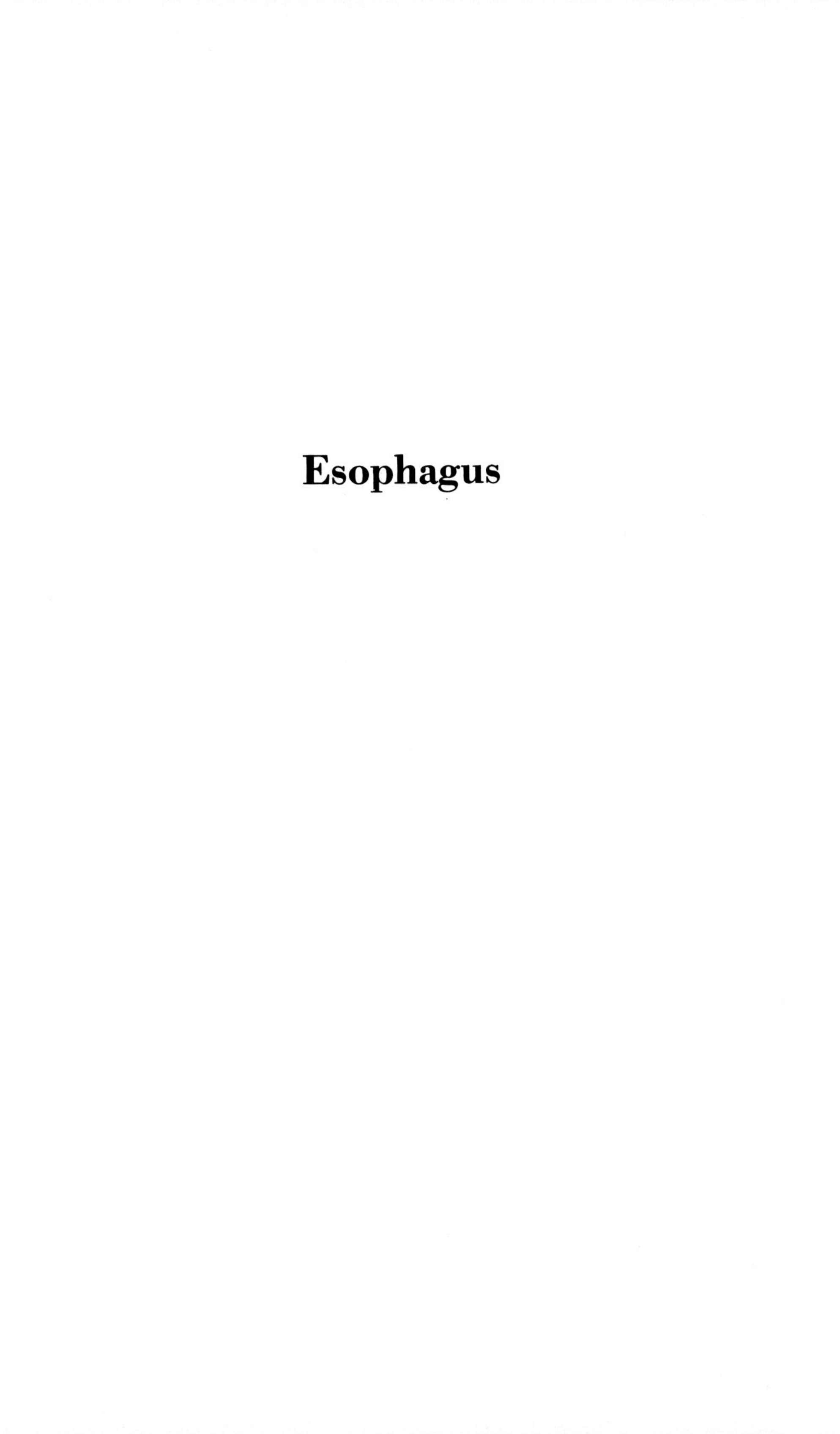

Esophagus

Medical Therapy in Reflux Esophagitis and Stricture: Some Ruminations

Howard M. Spiro, M.D.

Objectives

At the conclusion of this paper the reader will be able to realize that esophagitis, a relatively new disorder, proposes many unanswerable questions. The reader will be able to identify the factors that create difficulties in the diagnosis and management of the disease process.

The general concepts of esophagitis are in flux, hard-won and much-studied physiological certainty being replaced by a recognition that techniques for studying esophageal physiology have been less reliable than once hoped. Esophagitis is a relatively "new" disorder and, in the excitement of discovery, the idea that symptoms do not necessarily correlate with the presence of disease is only now beginning to permeate the physician's views of esophagitis. It is hard for clinicians to accept the idea, for example, that not everyone with a raging esophagitis endoscopically has symptoms or, conversely, that we cannot always find in the patient with heartburn all the morphological witnesses of esophagitis. With this in mind, I will review some of the problems in the diagnosis and management of esophagitis as it appears to the gastroenterologist in 1978 and will comment on our ignorance about the natural history of reflux esophagitis.

The role of mechanical and hormonal factors in controlling lower esophageal function is not as certain as it was. Several

---

Howard M. Spiro, M.D., Professor, Department of Medicine, Yale University School of Medicine, New Haven, Conn.

years ago it seemed likely that circulating gastrin prevented reflux by tightening the lower esophageal sphincter and that other postprandial hormones, somewhat antagonistic in nature, relaxed the lower esophageal sphincter and that reflux would likely respond to hormonal manipulations of the lower esophageal sphincter. Surgeons generally ignored these attractive medical concepts and went about their business creating a barrier between the esophagus and the stomach, and they were not far wrong! The role of mechanical factors, which have been so long ignored by the internists because they are hard to study, is returning to primacy as the accuracy and reproducibility of motility tracings have come under judgment. Indeed, the indications and selections of diagnostic procedures and the very definitions of esophagitis are under review. We have to ask whether esophagitis is important if it is seen endoscopically and not felt by the patient or whether only symptomatic esophagitis counts. Many physicians feel that the acid infusion test of Bernstein, or any fluid such as orange juice, which leads to heartburn, gives information of clinical value, whereas others feel that the most meaningful clinical studies are those which actually measure for how long and how often acid regurgitates back into the esophagus. The basic question which the physician must ask himself, at a time when costs are paramount, is how his diagnostic procedures change therapy.

Generally speaking, the therapy of reflux esophagitis still involves the classical, mechanical and dietary manipulations which range from raising the head of the bed after meals, through advising the patient to walk around after meals, to the various mechanically modified regular bland diets which the physician has prescribed for so long. Modern therapy of reflux esophagitis considers the role of three types of drugs: (1) antacids and "floaters," (2) H_2 blockers such as cimetidine [1] and (3) metaclopramide [2]. From the surgical standpoint, the role and timing of operations is crucial [3], but as this is well discussed by others, I will refrain from further comments.

From the therapeutic standpoint the clinician does well to regard reflux esophagitis as part of the whole peptic ulcer disease syndrome in that whenever acid overflows into areas contiguous to the stomach, it raises havoc, whether a duodenal ulcer or reflux esophagitis. This may be an oversimplification, since the heartburn induced by relatively nonacid fluids such as orange juice may give rise to heartburn from a mechanism different from that induced by 0.1 N hydrochloric acid. Nevertheless, from a clinical standpoint it is easiest to think of reflux esophagitis and the substernal postprandial persistent heartburn which it engenders as the result of too much acid in the esophagus.

Other physiological factors may be important, but in general, for symptomatic esophagitis we can conclude that there must be (1) some irritant like acid, pepsin or bile regurgitating from the stomach, (2) factors which weaken the mechanical barrier at the gastro-esophageal junction, whether this is simply an intrinsic incompetence of the lower esophageal sphincter or the presence of a tube which puts the sphincter at a mechanical disadvantage and (3) much neglected, the secondary changes in motility which lead to delayed acid clearance [4]. Obviously, all of these can play a role in the vicious circle of reflux esophagitis; when vomiting is also present, this contributes. Whether alcohol leads to exogenous esophagitis is under judgment.

The diagnosis of reflux esophagitis divides into (1) tests which demonstrate esophagitis, which are really of more importance to the clinician, such as the acid infusion tests and esophagoscopy and biopsy and (2) tests which evaluate sphincter competence, largely manometry and the measurement of intra-esophageal pH.

The medical management of esophagitis involves measures to reduce reflux, acid levels, and the level of other irritants. These measures have not changed very much in the past five years, but a number of drugs now on the horizon may prove helpful. Although four or five years ago bethanechol seemed to be a drug which would tighten the lower esophageal sphincter to prevent reflux, not many subsequent studies have suggested that it has a place in clinical medicine and bethanechol still seems to be a drug whose time has not arrived. On the other hand, metaclopramide, the dopamine depleter, which tightens the lower esophageal sphincter and causes the stomach to contract and empty itself, should theoretically be an ideal drug in the management of reflux esophagitis because these actions enhance acid clearing from the esophagus. Unfortunately, the

FDA has not yet approved this drug for distribution, largely because of evidence that it is no more effective than a placebo. Metaclopramide is available "over the counter" in Europe, by prescription in Canada and the United Kingdom; but in the United States its use has been approved only to move tubes into the small intestines.

The role of the H_2 blocker, cimetidine, will no doubt much enlarge in the management of reflux esophagitis. Cimetidine reduces acid secretion, and since all the measures to relieve the pain of reflux esophagitis have to do with reducing acid that refluxes into the esophagus, it seems likely that the H_2 blockers will have a role in therapy. So far, studies in the United States have not demonstrated a statistically significant benefit over placebo for cimetidine. Nevertheless, this may simply be because the right patients have not been chosen. It seems reasonable for the physician to try the effect of cimetidine in his patient with persistent heartburn at night. Indeed, currently I believe that in any person with persistent reflux esophagitis, a six to eight week course of cimetidine should be suggested before turning to operative repair. As for other agents, cholestyramine for bile reflux esophagitis has turned out neither anecdotally nor in controlled studies to be very useful. Gaviscon and other demulcent agents seem to be useful in reducing symptoms and several controlled studies suggest that they have a place in the management of patients with reflux esophagitis. They are certainly much liked by patients, and this alone is something to say for them.

As I try to find the data, I am convinced that the natural history of esophagitis is more talked about than understood. Conventional wisdom has it that heartburn means acid reflux and that acid reflux leads to esophagitis and that esophagitis long continued and untreated is followed after a time by stricture. Sometimes, it is now recognized, reflux of acid seems not to lead to esophagitis but to the appearance of a columnar epithelium lining the lower end of the esophagus, the so-called Barrett's esophagus. Most of us believe that in some patients esophagitis may predispose to an epidermoid carcinoma in the original squamous epithelium and, sometimes, to adenocarcinoma when the esophagus has been lined by columnar epithelium. Most of us generally also hold that esophageal stricture in esophagitis results from failure of medical therapy, or patient neglect. Surgeons, more than gastroenterologists, believe that repeat bougienage injures the esophagus and spreads fibrosis to all its layers, indeed that bougienage encourages more reflux and ultimately, therefore, worsens the stricture. A number of patients with stricture do benefit from operation, but I am convinced from looking over the literature and trying to find the long-term histories that prove the sequence of esophagitis-to-stricture that more observations of the natural history of unoperated esophagitis and stricture are needed.

For example, when a patient presents with a benign stricture after a very short history of heartburn, too short to permit the conclusion that reflux was persistent, we talk about "silent esophagitis." There is, after all, quite a variable relation between the symptoms of esophagitis, the morphology which accompanies it, and the physiological derangements which seem so reasonable. In general, 10% to 20% of patients with endoscopic esophagitis seem to have had no complaints as far as their esophagus is concerned. On the other hand, we all have seen patients with many years of impressive gastro-esophageal reflux in whom stricture never develops, so that the development of a stricture seems to be unpredictable. Although the data are not very firm, I think that strictures in reflux esophagitis develop every early in about half the observed patients in published reports having had symptoms for only two or three months before discovery of the stricture. In about half the patients, strictures develop late, only after many years of reflux esophagitis. It is surprising how few gastroenterologists, however, can quickly cite patients whom they have followed for years over the entire sequence of postulated events from esophagitis to stricture. I am not suggesting that this sequence is not a real one, but simply emphasize how difficult it is to find the evidence. Certainly I have not found firm figures published in this regard. While many believe that once begun, bougienage needs to be repeated often, even after the esophagus has been dilated to a "forty-french" and maintained at that diameter for a few weeks, there is very little evidence for this. Even in surgical surveys the reported response to bougienage seems to be quite long lasting.

In summary, there seems little correlation between the severity and duration of heartburn, the development of esophagitis, or the subsequent appearance of a stricture. We need to know much more about the incidence and prevalence of reflux, about the natural history of esophagitis and why most patients with reflux esophagitis, no matter how they are defined, go happily about their business, taking occasional burning in their chests as a sign that they are still alive. We need to know whether the sequence we all believe in so fervently represents stages of reflux esophagitis with an equilibrium between the increased turnover of cells in the papillae which are the defense against surface erosion or whether, as could be the case, reflux esophagitis and "peptic stricture" represent different kinds of responses to esophageal irritation. Even more important, we need to understand why about 10% of patients with persistent reflux develop a Barrett's epithelium and why others with equally persistent reflux stubbornly maintain an eroded but squamous epithelium.

Another basic problem is to define a stricture, at first sight a rather obvious decision. Yet sometimes what looks on radiological examination like a stricture is a fibrotic ring, and sometimes, I suspect more often, it turns out simply to be an edematous stiffening, sometimes only spasm and sometimes a combination of both. Most strictures described by surgeons seem to be low and annular with much edema and spasm above them; to the gastroenterologist or radiologist they often appear as long esophageal strictures on x-ray but, in fact, the surgeon finds only a short segment of fibrosis. It seems probable that edematous stiffening and secondary spasm account for the disappearance after bougienage of many supposed strictures and that the true stricture is either a short ring of fibrotic squamous epithelium or the result of a deep penetrating columnar epithelium with "gastric" ulceration. Now that the surgeons are turning their efforts largely to antireflux operations and less often resecting esophageal strictures, it will be much more difficult to look at the entire spectrum of pathology and we will have to return to the remarkably good older pathological studies. Looking at those studies, I accept the classification of stricture as (1) chronic superficial erosion in squamous epithelium with varying degrees of damage, the muscle coats usually being spared, (2) a localized penetrating ulcer often of columnar epithelium with chronic involvement of all layers of the esophagus, or (3) a combination of the two. I recognize that one of the current real problems of evaluating strictures is the difference between a biopsy "nibble," which we clinicians take as evidence of esophagitis, but which show only the very superficial layers of the squamous epithelium and through-and-through resections so triumphantly waved at the gastroenterologist by surgeons of past years. The definitions of esophagitis in these two circumstances certainly must be different.

Another problem of course is that the histology of a stricture depends to some extent upon its cause. Reflux usually produces a short annular stricture, except when it is associated with vomiting, or an inlying tube, when it is long and narrow. Congenital strictures may represent webs, rings or columnar epithelium, sometimes with parietal cells. Systemic disorders such as scleroderma or epidermolysis bullosa lead to very nasty and refractory strictures. Finally, exogenous noxious agents such as lye and even excessive alcohol are also thought to be the cause of some esophageal strictures [5]. I suspect that the rapid appearing true stricture may often represent simply healing of a gastric ulcer of Barrett's esophagus.

Still, other factors remain undefined. Individual susceptibility to damage from acid reflux must depend upon the degree of basal hyperplastic reparative response and the nature of other reparative processes. We are at a loss to know why columnar epithelium ever develops. We need to know more about the balance between individual susceptibility and the aggravating factors we love to study, such as the weak lower esophageal sphincter, high acid levels and excessive bile. Postoperative strictures certainly seem to depend upon individual susceptibility. Studies in New Haven suggest that the role of the inlying tube is to put the lower esophageal sphincter at a mechanical disadvantage so that it cannot contract as well as normally. Yet, if that were the only important factor, esophageal stricture should be much more common after nasogastric tubes and experience suggests that it is quite rare. The rare occurrence of such strictures suggests that individual susceptibility must play a role, but I do not know what that means! Most of the time postoperative strictures occur very rapidly after nasogastric intubation, but sometimes their recognition is delayed for many years when as it is generally agreed they are long and hard to dilate.

It should be clear from the foregoing that we do not have answers to many questions and I will close simply by repeating some questions. Why do most patients with reflux not go on to serious trouble? Are there stages of reflux esophagitis or does an esophageal stricture represent a different disorder from superficial reflux? What are the long-term effects of therapy on columnar epithelium, on reflux esophagitis, on stricture? Finally, since about 10% of the patients seem to develop a Barrett's esophagus, is the increased frequency of carcinoma in such patients a true phenomenon or simply the result of increasing reliance on endoscopy? Are we really seeing this lesion with its malignant potential more frequently or just recognizing it more frequently? This is really the most important problem for the esophagologist of the next decade, for if antireflux operations prevent the development of Barrett's epithelium or if they get rid of it, then we will see in the repair of hiatus hernia or in the development of antireflux operations a new industry which will rival that of coronary bypass.

References

1. Wesdorp, E., Bartelsman, J., Pape, K. et al: Oral cimetidine in reflux esophagitis. Gastroenterology 74:821-824, 1978.
2. McCallum, R.W., Ippoliti, A.F., Cooney, C. and Sturdevant, R.A.: A controlled trial of metaclopramide in symptomatic gastro esophageal reflux. N. Engl. J. Med. 296:354-357, 1977.
3. Behar, J., Sheahan, D., Biancani, P. et al: Medical and surgical management of reflux esophagitis. N. Engl. J. Med. 293:263-268, 1975.
4. Stanciu, C., Heare, R.C. and Bennet, J.R.: Correlation between manometric and pH testing for gastro esophageal reflux. Gut 18:536-540, 1970.
5. Kaufman, S.E. and Kaye, M.D.: Induction of gastroesophageal reflux by alcohol. Gut 19:336-338, 1978.

Self-Evaluation Quiz

1. Clinically, it is easiest to think of reflux esophagitis and the substernal postprandial persistent heartburn which it causes as the result of too much gastrin in the esophagus.
   a) True
   b) False
2. Two tests which evaluate sphincter competence are:
   a) Acid infusion and manometry

b) Esophagoscopy and manometry
c) Manometry and intra-esophageal pH
d) Biopsy and intra-esophageal pH

3. H_2 blockers:
a) Are represented by cimetidine and benelux
b) Increase acid secretion
c) Are being phased out
d) Decrease acid secretion

4. Metaclopramide:
a) Increases acid secretion
b) Increases insulin production
c) Depletes dopamine
d) Increases dopamine

5. A patient with persistent reflux esophagitis should receive:
a) Immediate surgery
b) Six to eight weeks of cimetidine
c) Three to six weeks of cimetidine
d) Two weeks of cimetidine followed immediately by surgery

6. In general, what percentage of patients with endoscopic esophagitis seem to have no complaints re their esophagus?
a) 5%–10%
b) 10%–20%
c) 20%–30%
d) 30%–40%

7. Correlation between severity and duration of heartburn, the development of esophagitis, or the subsequent appearance of a stricture is:
a) Nil
b) 25%
c) 50%
d) 100%

Answers on page 721.

Surgical Treatment of Reflux Peptic Esophagitis

E. R. Woodward, M.D., F.A.C.S.

Objectives

1. To relate pathogenesis of reflux peptic esophagitis to incompetence of the lower esophageal sphincter.
2. To review principles, method and results of three operations used to restore LES competence: (a) Belsey cardioplasty, (b) Nissen fundoplication and (c) Hill posterior gastropexy.

Modern surgery for peptic esophagitis dates from the classic presentation of the late Phillip Allison [1] in 1951. Allison provided a clear description of the clinical syndrome and emphasized the crucial importance of esophagoscopy in confirming the presence of esophagitis. He also correctly attributed the syndrome to abnormal reflux of gastric juice containing hydrochloric acid and pepsin. In addition, he reported an operative procedure designed to correct this reflux. Subsequent experience has demonstrated that his method has a relatively high failure rate, but the basic concept remains valid, ie, the objective of the surgeon is to prevent abnormal gastroesophageal reflux.

The importance of a competent, reliable closure mechanism between stomach and esophagus is apparent. The unfavorable pressure relationships, with negative endothoracic pressure affecting the esophagus and positive intra-abdominal pressure

---

E. R. Woodward, M.D., F.A.C.S., Professor and Chairman, Department of Surgery, College of Medicine, University of Florida; Chief of Surgery, Shands Teaching Hospital and Clinics, Gainesville, Fla.

This work was performed at the University of Florida, Gainesville, and was supported by NIH grant AM-13544.

affecting the stomach, tend to promote gastroesophageal reflux. Added to this is the well-known exquisite sensitivity of the stratified squamous mucosa of the esophagus to the destructive digestant activity of acid-pepsin [2]. An anatomically distinct sphincter is readily demonstrated in all mammals except primates. Because of this, the factors producing closure of the esophagogastric junction in the primate until recently have been conjectural. A pinchcock action has been attributed to the crural structures of the diaphragm. It has been theorized that the acuteness of the angle of His between the esophagus and the gastric fundus has a valvular effect. However, with the development of image intensification and cineradiography, Gould and Barnhard [3] demonstrated an anatomically distinct lower esophageal sphincter (LES) in the normal human subject.

The physiologic characteristics of the LES were demonstrated in the 1950s by the classic work of Code [4] and Ingelfinger [5], along with their many co-workers. Using very sensitive pressure transducers and recording polygraphs, a resting "high pressure zone" was found at the esophagogastric junction. That this represented, at least in large measure, an intrinsic LES was indicated by receptive relaxation in this zone following deglutition and its accompanying peristaltic wave. Further, it was found that in patients with a sliding hiatal hernia the characteristics of the pressure profile in the sphincteric zone were abnormal, and in patients with reflux peptic esophagitis the resting pressure in the LES was distinctly lower than in normal subjects [6].

Most patients with reflux peptic esophagitis have the sliding or concentric type of esophageal hiatus hernia. The distal esophagus is tethered within the esophageal hiatus of the diaphragm by the phrenoesophageal membrane. This specialized portion of the transversalis fascia contains elastic tissue that permits the esophagogastric junction to move in the accommodation of peristaltic activity of the esophagus. The normal degeneration of elastic tissue with aging probably accounts for the higher incidence of sliding hiatal hernia with increasing age. However, only a small minority of the very large number of human subjects who have a sliding hiatal hernia proceed to develop reflux peptic esophagitis. The difference between the two groups can be readily identified by manometric study of the LES. In the large number of subjects without symptoms or endoscopic findings of esophagitis, manometry identifies a high pressure zone in the reclining subject with a resting pressure higher than 15 cm water. The sphincter relaxes with deglutition and contracts following completion of the peristaltic wave. Because of mediastinal translocation of the sphincter the tracing is often abnormal as described by Code et al [7], demonstrating double respiratory reversal, dual pressure peaks and other abnormalities. In the individual with symptomatic and endoscopically confirmed esophagitis, the resting pressure in the LES is usually less than 15 cm water. In other words, it is a loss of strength to the point of ineffective sphincteric action that is the basic pathogenic mechanism leading to reflux peptic esophagitis. The reasons why this should develop in a minority of subjects with sliding hiatal hernias are unknown. However, it is clear that the thoracic location of the sphincter does not necessarily interfere with its function. In patients with congenital or acquired short esophagus, the fundus of the stomach can be wrapped around the distal esophagus in a Nissen fundoplication and can be left entirely within the thorax by suturing the diaphragm circumferentially to the gastric fundus. This procedure not only provides clinical relief from reflux, but also restores resting pressure in the LES to the normal range despite the supradiaphragmatic location of the repair.

A small, but significant number of patients present with reflux peptic esophagitis in the absence of a sliding hiatal hernia. Failure to demonstrate a hernia radiographically can be confirmed by manometry, endoscopy and surgical exploration. Again, these patients can be distinguished from normal individuals by a manometric study of the LES. The resting pressure in the reclining subject will nearly always be less than 15 cm water. Therefore, the LES can fail even when in its normal location within or just below the esophageal hiatus. Again, the cause for sphincter failure is unknown.

Allison believed that restoration of normal anatomy would result in restoration of a functionally normal closure mechanism between stomach and esophagus. His operation consisted of exposure of the esophageal hiatus by a left transthoracic approach, reduction of the hernia into the abdomen by traction through a counter incision in the diaphragm and suture of the splayed out phrenoesophageal membrane to the under surface of the diaphragm. His procedure was widely adopted, but many observers found that recurrence of the hernia and persistence or recurrence of reflux peptic esophagitis were discouragingly frequent. It became apparent that the phrenoesophageal membrane was not strong enough to have reparative value and that the most important part of the procedure was snug closure of the esophageal hiatus posterior to the esophagus. Because the crural structures slant progressively more and more caudad as one extends posteriorly, this area is exposed more readily through an abdominal approach. Therefore, in the late 1950s and early 1960s, operation through the abdomen became the most commonly used technique. Again, recurrence of hernia and persistence or recurrence of reflux peptic esophagitis were seen in a significant number of patients. We reported 22 instances of recurrent esophagitis in 127 patients so treated, an incidence of 17% [8]. It is interesting that radiographic study readily demonstrated recurrence of sliding hiatal hernia, indicating the relative ineffectiveness of the procedure in the restoration of normal anatomy. However, in those patients in whom the repair remained intact, esophagitis regularly healed and remained healed. Clearly, moving the sphincteric zone into the abdomen had a favorable effect, and this was confirmed by manometric study; the weak resting pressure nearly always observed preoperatively was at least doubled in successful cases after operation.

Since the mucosal injury in reflux esophagitis is due to the HCl and pepsin content of gastric secretion, it is not surprising that methods to suppress gastric secretion were widely advocated in conjunction with esophageal hiatal herniorrhaphy. We reported our experience in 62 patients operated on between 1958 and 1965 in whom vagotomy and pyloroplasty were added to transabdominal crural repair [8]. When studied five or more years later, nine of the 62 patients, or 15%, had persistent or recurrent esophagitis. Statistical analysis indicated that the recurrence rate was no different from that following crural repair alone in a similar number of patients. It is clear that the exquisite sensitivity of the esophageal mucosa is such that only small amounts of acid-pepsin are necessary to produce esophagitis, and, as long as reflux is present, only complete suppression of gastric secretion is effective. Furthermore, the additive surgery not only failed to improve clinical results significantly, but also there was a sharp increase in chronic morbidity. The dumping syndrome was observed in 26% of the patients, and 13% had postvagotomy diarrhea. Both were self-limited in duration in most cases but, nonetheless, it is obvious that vagotomy and pyloroplasty are contraindicated as a part of the surgical treatment of reflux peptic esophagitis. Since duodenal ulcer may coexist with reflux peptic esophagitis, the added surgery may be considered in such patients, providing the severity of their duodenal ulcer justifies the risk of the associated morbidity. Unless pyloric stenosis is present, proximal gastric or parietal cell vagotomy can be considered in such cases. A Nissen fundoplication can easily be performed following this procedure, and since a gastric drainage procedure is not required, the dumping syndrome and diarrhea do not occur.

It became apparent that esophageal hiatal herniorrhaphy alone was not an adequate operation and that the objective of the surgeon should be reinforcement of the LES and restoration of its sphincteric function to prevent further gastroesophageal reflux. The first such procedure was introduced by Belsey in 1955 and consisted of transthoracic reconstruction of the cardia. Results of Belsey's "Mark IV cardioplasty" in 632 patients were reported in 1967 [9]. Follow-up for more than five years of 219 cases had shown a recurrence rate of 11%. More recently Orringer, Skinner and Belsey [10] reported results in 892 patients who were operated on through 1965. There were nine operative deaths (1%). Follow-up evaluation was available in 848 patients (95%). Among 776 patients followed up for more than three years, 12% had a documented hiatal hernia or recurrent reflux. Of 513 patients followed up for more than seven years, the recurrence rate remained 12%. Only nine of 98 patients with recurrent hernia and/or reflux remained asymptomatic.

The Belsey cardioplasty begins with thorough mobilization of the distal esophagus and esophagogastric junction through a left thoracotomy. The sliding hernia is reduced and the fundus is approximated to the distal esophagus in beltlike fashion using three layers of sutures and surrounding approximately two thirds of the distal esophagus. The operation thrusts the esophagogastric junction into an infradiaphragmatic location and at the same time applies positive intrafundic pressure against the lower esophagus. Thus, an increase in intragastric pressure tends to compress the lower esophagus. The operation is usually effective in restoring LES competence, but has the disadvantage that it can be accomplished with ease only by the thoracic approach.

In 1956 Nissen [6] described fundoplication to correct gastroesophageal reflux and reported his early results in 1963 [11]. In 1973 Rossetti and Allgower [12] reported on 1,231 patients operated on in the same clinic. In patients with uncomplicated reflux esophagitis the operative mortality was 0.6% (seven of 845 cases). They presented results in 590 patients observed between 3 and 12 years after surgery. The "post-fundoplication syndrome" occurred in 62 patients or 10%. We have referred to this as the "gas-bloat syndrome" and have found it to be present in 20% of our patients one year postoperatively [8]. Rossetti and Allgower had seven patients who required reoperation because of the development of gastric or duodenal ulcers and five patients with recurrence of hernia and reflux esophagitis (1%). Of the 590 patients, 516 (87%) were free of symptoms. Our long-term experience is similar in that we have seen gastric ulcer in six patients, five of whom had the "gas-bloat syndrome" [13]. We have recently reviewed 165 patients treated by Nissen fundoplication [14]. Sixty-five had been operated on by the transthoracic approach. Thirteen (8%) had symptoms of gastroesophageal reflux, but this was confirmed endoscopically in only seven (4%). Even with longer follow-up, 18 (11%) still had moderate symptoms of the "gas-bloat syndrome," which was completely disabling in 3 (2%). In two patients the repair had to be taken down to provide relief.

Nissen described his fundoplication as a "valvuloplasty." The fundus of the stomach is wrapped completely around the distal esophagus and sutured on the right or lesser curvature side of the esophagus. The positive intragastric pressure is transmitted to this "jacket" surrounding the lower esophagus and compresses it. When intragastric pressure increases from whatever cause, the pressure within the fundus increases and the esophagus is more firmly compressed. This functions as a one-way valve permitting antegrade emptying into the stomach and preventing gastroesophageal reflux. The post-fundoplication syndrome results from aerophagia with inability of the subject to eructate the excess air. The resultant distention produces a feeling of pressure in the left upper quadrant or epigastrium, particularly postprandially, often to the point of overt pain.

The Nissen fundoplication is performed by the transabdominal approach in the uncomplicated case. It can also be easily performed by a left transthoracic approach, which is useful in cases of extreme obesity or in patients who have had previously unsuccessful transabdominal hiatal herniorrhaphy, and is especially useful in patients with brachyesophagus or acquired short esophagus due to extensive scarring and subsequent contracture. In addition to ease of dissection in the presence of the frequently observed periesophagitis, the fundus can be brought through the esophageal hiatus which is enlarged by a short radial incision, and the fundoplication can be left above the diaphragm with no tension on the repair or the esophagus. Clinical, cineradiographic, manometric and pH studies indicate that the endothoracic fundoplication exerts an equally effective valvuloplastic effect and also restores resting pressures in the LES to the normal range.

A third concept in esophageal hiatal herniorrhaphy designed to strengthen the LES was proposed by Hill et al in 1961 [15], and the results of an eight-year experience were presented in 1967 [16]. Hill and co-workers reported 149 cases with no mortality. In no case could anatomic recurrence of the hernia be demonstrated radiographically. While three patients had gastroesophageal reflux demonstrated by pH measurements, only four (3%) had symptoms suggestive of persistent or recurrent esophagitis. Side effects of surgery were negligible and manometric study revealed return of LES resting pressure to normal or near normal levels in most cases. Our own results using the Hill method are good, but not quite as outstanding.

The Hill technique is performed through a transabdominal approach. The hernia is reduced and the distal esophagus is mobilized. The crural structures are approximated posterior to the esophagus and the esophagogastric junction at the lesser curvature is sutured to the median arcuate ligament. Hill refers to this as "posterior gastropexy." This maneuver maintains a long segment of intra-abdominal esophagus, thus exposing the LES to the positive intra-abdominal pressure. In addition, the medial border of the gastric fundus is plicated to the left wall of the abdominal esophagus, although it is not belted around the esophagus to the extent described in the Belsey procedure.

The most frequent indication for surgical intervention in reflux peptic esophagitis is failure to adequately control symptoms by medical therapy. Precise figures are lacking, but since the amount of acid-pepsin secretion needed to activate and perpetuate esophagitis is so slight, it is probable that medical therapy is less successful than in peptic ulcer of the stomach and duodenum. In the absence of complications it is important that the patient have an adequate trial of medical therapy. The onset of complications will frequently point the patient toward surgical intervention. By far the most common complication is stricture secondary to peptic esophagitis. This is a special problem since the surgeon must overcome both gastroesophageal reflux and the mechanical problem introduced by esophageal stenosis. Much less frequent is the complication of hemorrhage. Acute hemorrhage from reflux peptic esophagitis is rare and can almost always be brought under control by medical means so that elective surgery can be undertaken at a later date. Anemia from chronic blood loss secondary to esophagitis is more common. In such patients it may be difficult or impossible to elicit a history of characteristic symptoms of reflux, and endoscopy will often play a decisive role. An adequate antireflux operation has a very high success rate in such patients.

The selection of the appropriate operation should be individualized and should never be decided on the basis of whether the consulting surgeon is a general or a thoracic surgeon. In the absence of stricture, the three operative procedures discussed above have certain advantages and disadvantages. The most certain operation for correction of reflux esophagitis and prevention of recurrent sliding hiatal hernia is Nissen fundoplication. Manometric study indicates that this procedure produces normal resting pressures in the LES in a much higher percentage of cases and to a much more physiologic range than either of the other procedures [17]. The Nissen fundoplication has the theoretical advantage that serosa-to-serosa approximation is accomplished with prompt fibrinous binding followed rapidly by fibrous binding. On the other hand, the Belsey procedure applies the serosa of the fundus to the non-serosa covered longitudinal musculature of the esophageal wall. Theoretically, one would expect a higher recurrence rate with the Belsey procedure and there are suggestive data that this is in fact the case. Another advantage of the Nissen operation is that it can be accomplished with equal ease through either the abdominal or the left transthoracic approach, depending upon circumstances presented by the individual patient.

On the other hand, the side effects of the Nissen procedure are a significant factor. The post-fundoplication syndrome or, in more descriptive terms, "gas-bloat syndrome" contributes significantly to the morbidity of the Nissen procedure. It appears that fundoplication interrupts the normal homeostatic device by which ingested air and the consequent fundic air bubble are regulated by conscious or unconscious eructation. In the presence of a fundoplication, compression of the esophagus by ingested air prevents or diminishes adequate eructation. Fortunately, this is self-limited in most cases. It is present in 50% of patients in the immediate postoperative period, but the incidence falls to 20% at one year [8]. In patients with severe symptoms of reflux a minor degree of this syndrome is considered a favorable exchange. On the other hand, the syndrome can be so severe that the patient requests that the repair be taken down in order to gain relief from the symptoms.

We have found the Belsey operation to be particularly useful in patients who have had a previous partial or subtotal gastrectomy. It requires a minimum of tissue to accomplish an adequate partial wrap around the distal esophagus by the fundus and establishment of an intra-abdominal segment of esophagus including the LES. Except for this specific indication, the surgeon who is equally accomplished in transabdominal and transthoracic surgery of the esophagogastric junction will usually consider the Belsey procedure to be a third choice.

The Hill posterior gastropexy has the very important advantage that early and late iatrogenic symptoms are rare. As in all esophagogastric surgery, temporary dysphagia may occur. Reestablishment of an adequate LES can be accomplished, but less frequently than with the Nissen procedure. We consider it the procedure of choice in the patient in whom an abdominal approach is feasible, no prior esophagogastric surgery has been performed and the indication for surgery is medical intractability rather than a complication of reflux esophagitis. We believe that the minimal incidence of side effects more than counterbalances the somewhat less effective results of the procedure in terms of prevention of recurrent hernia and restoration of normal LES pressure profiles. The Hill procedure also has the disadvantage that it can be accomplished only by the transabdominal route.

References

1. Allison, P.R.: Reflux esophagitis, sliding hiatal hernia, and the anatomy of repair. Surg. Gynecol. Obstet. 92:419-431, 1951.
2. Plzak, L.F., Fried, W. and Woodward, E.R.: Relative susceptibility of the gastrointestinal tract to experimental acute peptic ulceration. Surg. Forum 7:389-393, 1957.
3. Gould, D.M. and Barnhard, H.J.: Changing concepts in the structure, function and disease of the lower esophagus. Am. J. Med. Sci. 233:581-595, 1957.
4. Code, C.F., Creamer, B., Schlegel, J.F. et al: An Atlas of Esophageal Motility in Health and Disease. Springfield, Illinois:Charles C Thomas Publishers, 1958.
5. Ingelfinger, F.J.: Esophageal motility. Physiol. Rev. 38:533-584, 1958.
6. Nissen, R.: Eine einfache operation zur beeinflussung der refluxoesophagitis. Schweiz. Med. Wochenschr. 86:590-593, 1956.
7. Code, C.F., Kelley, M.L., Schlegel, J.F. et al: Detection of hiatal hernia during esophageal motility tests. Gastroenterology 43:521-531, 1962.
8. Woodward, E.R., Thomas, H.F. and McAlhany, J.C.: Comparison of crural repair and Nissen fundoplication in the treatment of esophageal hiatus hernia with peptic esophagitis. Ann. Surg. 173:782-792, 1971.
9. Skinner, D.B. and Belsey, R.H.R.: Surgical management of esophageal reflux and hiatus hernia — long-term results with 1,030 patients. J. Thorac. Cardiovasc. Surg. 52:33-54, 1967.
10. Orringer, M.B., Skinner, D.B. and Belsey, R.H.R.: Long-term results of the Mark IV operation for hiatal hernia and analyses of recurrences and their treatment. J. Thorac. Cardiovasc. Surg. 63:25-33, 1972.
11. Nissen, R. and Rosetti, M.: Surgery of the cardia ventriculi. Ciba-Symp. 11:195-223, 1963.
12. Rossetti, M. and Allgower, M.: Fundoplication for treatment of hiatal hernia. Prog. Surg. 12:1-21, 1973.
13. Bushkin, F.L., O'Leary, J.P. and Woodward, E.R.: Occurrence of gastric ulcer after Nissen fundoplication. Am. Surg. 42:821-826, 1976.

14. Bushkin, F.L., Neustein, C.L., Woodward, E.R. et al: Nissen fundoplication for reflux peptic esophagitis. Ann. Surg. 185:672-677, 1977.
15. Hill, L.D., Chapmen, K.W. and Morgan, E.H.: Objective evaluation of surgery for hiatus hernia and esophagitis. J. Thorac. Cardiovasc. Surg. 41:60-74, 1971.
16. Hill, L.D.: An effective operation for hiatal hernia: An eight year appraisal. Ann. Surg. 166:681-692, 1967.
17. DeMeester, T.R., Johnson, L.F. and Kent, A.H.: Evaluation of current operations for the prevention of gastroesophageal reflux. Ann. Surg. 180:511-525, 1974.

Self-Evaluation Quiz

1. The objective of surgery for reflux peptic esophagitis is repair of the sliding esophageal hiatus hernia.
   a) True
   b) False
2. Despite absence of an anatomically distinct lower esophageal sphincter, present evidence favors the presence of an intrinsic sphincter in the human.
   a) True
   b) False
3. The most common cause of reflux peptic esophagitis is presence of a sliding esophageal hiatus hernia and most subjects with such a hernia will eventually develop esophagitis.
   a) True
   b) False
4. The Allison operation:
   a) Is performed by the thoracic approach
   b) Reduces the sliding hiatus hernia
   c) Sutures the phrenoesophageal membrane to the under surface of the diaphragm
   d) Approximates the crural structures of the diaphragm posterior to the esophagus
   e) All of the above
5. Incidence of recurrent esophagitis after diaphragmatic crural repair is:
   a) 5%
   b) 20%
   c) 40%
   d) 60%
   e) 80%

6. Operations to reduce gastric acid secretion such as vagotomy are very useful as a part of operative control of reflux peptic esophagitis.
   a) True
   b) False
7. The Belsey cardioplasty:
   a) Is performed through an abdominal approach
   b) Results in a significant transabdominal segment of esophagus
   c) Closes the diaphragmatic crural structures
   d) Divides the vagus nerves
   e) Adds a Finney pyloroplasty
8. The Nissen fundoplication:
   a) Can be performed through either a thoracic or an abdominal approach
   b) Wraps the fundus of the stomach around the lower esophagus approximating the fundus on the lesser curvature side
   c) Reduces the sliding hiatus hernia
   d) May or may not involve closure of the diaphragmatic crural structures
   e) All of the above
9. The major disadvantage of the Nissen fundoplication is:
   a) A high rate of recurrent esophagitis
   b) Frequent recurrence of sliding hiatus hernia
   c) Development of the "post-fundoplication syndrome"
   d) Development of peptic ulcer in the fundic wrap
   e) Dysphagia for solid food
10. Clinically successful antireflux surgery is usually accompanied by an increase of lower esophageal sphincter pressure into the normal range.
    a) True
    b) False

Answers on page 721.

Reflux Esophagitis

David B. Skinner, M.D., F.A.C.S.

Objectives

1. To review current knowledge about relationships among hiatal hernia, gastroesophageal reflux, and esophagitis.
2. To review methods employed to diagnose and quantitate reflux.
3. To present indications for anti-reflux surgery.
4. To discuss normal mechanisms for the control of reflux.
5. To present principles for successful anti-reflux surgery.

Gastroesophageal reflux, hiatal hernia and reflux esophagitis have been topics of great interest, not only because of their frequency, but also because they have been identified and treated only in recent years. Hiatal hernia was not diagnosed in a living human being prior to the introduction of barium swallow radiography at the beginning of this century. During the first half of the 20th century hiatal hernia was thought to be similar to other types of body cavity hernias and treated as such. Operations were uncommon, and successful surgical treatment of hiatal hernia was even less frequent. The concept of gastroesophageal reflux causing esophagitis and symptoms and being associated with hiatal hernia was first introduced by Allison in 1951 [1]. Since that time there has been great development in this field. Reflux and hiatal hernia have become among the most common conditions of the upper alimentary tract. Methods have been evolved for the diagnosis of these conditions, indications for medical and surgical treatment established, and new techniques for management developed.

Twenty-seven years after Allison's classical paper, several statements can be made with certainty. It is gastroesophageal

---

David B. Skinner, M.D., F.A.C.S., Professor and Chairman, Department of Surgery, University of Chicago/Division of Biological Sciences and the Pritzker School of Medicine, Chicago, Ill.

reflux and not hiatal hernia which causes the symptoms of heartburn and regurgitation. These symptoms are aggravated by and related to postural change. The complications of esophagitis, stricture, bleeding esophagitis and aspiration are all related to gastroesophageal reflux and not hiatal hernia. Reflux is the most common cause of ulcerative esophagitis.

Hiatal hernia is extremely common and is estimated to occur in about 10% of the adult American population. It is divided into two principal types. More than 95% of diagnosed hiatal hernias are of the Type I, sliding, or axial variety. They are clinically irrelevant unless associated with abnormal gastroesophageal reflux. Hiatal hernia and reflux may occur together but are separate and distinct clinical entities. In my practice, about 80% of adult patients with advanced degrees of abnormal reflux have a hiatal hernia identifiable by radiography or operative resection. However, it is estimated that only about 5% of patients with a Type I hiatal hernia have abnormal and clinically significant reflux. Therefore, in clinical practice, radiographic diagnosis of hiatal hernia is of no significance and should be ignored. It is only when symptomatic gastroesophageal reflux can be documented objectively that therapy is considered.

The exception to this rule about hiatal hernia is the presence of the rare Type II or paraesophageal hernia. When this true anatomical hernia is seen, its natural history is to enlarge progressively until the entire stomach is in the chest. At this point the cardia and the pylorus are adjacent and the remainder of the stomach is lying free in a huge hernia sac. This stomach is subject to volvulus, gastric obstruction, strangulation and development of gastric ulcers. For these reasons the Type II hiatal hernia should be repaired whenever it is seen even if it is asymptomatic. In the only prospective study of this condition which has been done, Belsey observed 21 patients with large Type II hiatal hernias which were asymptomatic [2]. Within a period of several years six of these patients succumbed to serious complications of the hernia. The remaining 15 were admitted for surgical repair.

Hiatal hernia is a radiographic diagnosis but clinically irrelevant. In less than half of the patients with abnormal gastroesophageal reflux does the radiologist demonstrate reflux spontaneously. Other tests have been developed to diagnose reflux. The first of these was esophageal manometry which dates back to Walter Cannon in the early part of this century. In 1956 Code and associates described a distal esophageal high pressure zone which they believed represented a lower esophageal sphincter and the primary mechanism for control of reflux [3]. Modification of manometric techniques by Winans and Harris led to semiquantitative manometric studies of the distal esophageal high pressure zone [4]. While the amplitude and length of this high pressure zone did have a statistical correlation with the presence or absence of abnormal reflux, the overlap was so great that manometry alone was not a useful test to diagnose reflux in the individual patient.

In 1958 Tuttle and Grossman introduced the long gastrointestinal pH electrode and employed it for the diagnosis of reflux by withdrawing the electrode tip slowly from the stomach into the esophagus [5]. Since acid-mucous tended to stick to the pH probe tip, the Tuttle test has had an unacceptable incidence of false-positive results. In 1964 Kantrowitz, my associates and I modified the technique to develop a standardized acid reflux test [6]. This involved challenging the cardia with respiratory and postural maneuvers while the patient was in four different body positions. A semiquantitative score for reflux defined as a drop in pH in the esophagus 5 cm above the high pressure zone was obtained. The standard acid reflux test has received fairly wide application as a method for diagnosing reflux and has been more sensitive and accurate than the Tuttle test or manometry. Nevertheless, this test has approximately a 20% incidence of false-negative results.

At present a battery of esophageal function tests is often performed at one sitting including manometry, the standard acid reflux test, acid clearing and the acid perfusion (Berstein) test [8]. After completion of manometry and the standard acid reflux test a 15 cc bolus of acid is placed in the midesophagus to measure clearing. Acid is emptied from the esophagus in the supine position only by swallowing. Normal individuals clear acid with ten swallows or less. Those patients with esophagitis have both frequent reflux and prolonged contact of regurgitated gastric juices with the esophageal mucosa. The acid clearing test detects such patients with risk of esophagitis. Finally, symptoms of reflux overlap with complaints caused by a number of other chest and upper abdominal conditions. The perfusion of acid alternately with saline into the esophagus provides a method for detecting those patients whose symptoms are reproduced by acid perfusion of the esophagus. These tests provide all the basic information necessary to assess the motor and functional disorders of the esophagus and to diagnose gastroesophageal reflux objectively. Such tests take about one hour and can be done in the outpatient setting.

In the last several years, the 24-hour pH monitoring of the esophagus has become available using the technique developed by DeMeester and Johnson [8]. The test is performed in a hospitalized patient with an indwelling esophageal pH meter on a long electrode which permits the patient to be up out of bed for a portion of the 24 hours and resting in the supine position for the balance of the time. A pH-regulated diet is provided. From observations made in normal control subjects, it is clear that everyone refluxes at times. This normal physiological reflux generally occurs after meals. Reflux in the supine position at night is rare in normal people. From analyzing the patterns of reflux seen in a variety of patients with symptomatic reflux and its complications, several subsets of abnormal reflux are identified [9]. There are a few patients who reflux only in the upright position throughout the course of the day. They have normal postprandial reflux but this continues and is of increased frequency. Often they are highly symptomatic. Because of repeated swallowing and ingestion of food and antacids, the pH does not remain low in the esophagus for any length of time so they are not at risk to develop esophagitis.

A second subset has reflux predominantly at night. When asleep, swallowing is infrequent but acid is normally cleared from the esophagus only in conjunction with a swallow. Nocturnal supine reflux may lead to prolonged periods of low pH in the esophagus. These patients may be completely unaware of reflux since they are asleep throughout the event and may present with advanced esophagitis or stricture without severe symptoms during the daytime.

The third group of abnormal reflux patients are those who reflux both in the upright and supine position. This is the most common pattern and is generally associated both with symptoms and with risk of esophagitis.

Based on this type of analysis it is possible to redefine indications for treatment by knowing which patients are most at risk to develop esophagitis and who are most likely to have aerophagia with postoperative gaseous distention. Those who reflux in the supine position have the greater risk of esophagitis. Patients with pure upright reflux have little risk of esophagitis but, because of their habit of air swallowing, do appear to be at risk for developing a postoperative gas bloat syndrome due to continuing aerophagia. Surgery has been avoided in patients with pure upright reflux in recent years. Most recently, our group has become interested in the problem of alkaline gastroesophageal reflux [10]. This has been identified by 24-hour pH reflux testing and has been associated with an increased incidence of esophagitis and stricture. Such findings suggest that acid reducing operations which promote duodenal gastric reflux of biliary-pancreatic secretions do not protect the patients from the consequences of unrelieved gastroesophageal reflux. The 24-hour esophageal pH monitoring is generally well accepted by patients and combines the advantages of the standard acid reflux test, acid clearing test and acid perfusion test. It is currently the most accurate and physiological method available for assessing patients with suspected reflux.

When symptomatic gastroesophageal reflux is diagnosed, a decision must be made as to whether the patient should have medical or surgical treatment. To a large degree this is based upon the findings of esophagoscopy. Endoscopy represents the only satisfactory method for diagnosing esophagitis, since this condition cannot be judged from specific symptoms or from the results of esophageal function tests. By endoscopy, esophagitis may be graded as none, Grade I in which there is mucosal erythema only, Grade II in which there are frank visible ulcerations of the esophagus, Grade III in which there are ulcerations and fibrosis of the wall and Grade IV in which there is a full blown stricture which prevents passage of the endoscope. Biopsy of the esophagus is not particularly helpful, since the changes of Grade I esophagitis represent a completely reversible condition and do not demonstrate any frank inflammation in the wall of the esophagus [11]. The finding of increased activity in the basal layer and proximity of the rete pegs to the surface accounts for the erythema seen but does not indicate an advanced degree of esophagitis requiring treatment.

With the results of the workup complete including careful history, radiographic studies of the entire upper gastrointestinal tract, esophageal function tests, 24 hour pH monitoring if available and endoscopy, the clinician is now able to assess the indications for treatment. The principal indications for surgical treatment are the complications of reflux including ulcerative esophagitis, stricture, bleeding esophagitis or ulcer, or aspiration. Anti-reflux surgery may occasionally be done to relieve symptoms but only if reflux is carefully documented as the cause of the symptoms, the symptoms are not controllable by intensive medical therapy over several months and the reflux pattern is not purely upright. As mentioned above, the presence of the Type II paraesophageal hiatal hernia or the large combined type of hiatal hernia is an indication for operation even if asymptomatic because of the risk of mechanical complications from these true intrathoracic hernias.

Once indications for antireflux surgery are present, the operation selected should be one which restores the normal mechanisms at the cardia which prevent reflux in well human beings. An anatomically identifiable sphincter in the distal esophagus has never been demonstrated in human beings. However, many have accepted the evidence of esophageal manometry demonstrating a high pressure zone in the distal esophagus to indicate that there was an intrinsic muscular sphincter in the distal esophagus. Specific neuro and hormonal control have been attributed to this sphincter muscle.

Based upon the early postoperative findings after antireflux surgery which demonstrated that this distal esophageal high pressure zone was increased in amplitude immediately after surgery, and based upon the absence of an identifiable sphincter, factors other than an intrinsic sphincter seemed likely to explain the barrier to reflux. The distal esophageal segment has been shown to have the properties of preventing reflux, relaxing with swallow, and responding to hormones such as gastrin. Any theory offering an alternative explanation other than a sphincter as a barrier to reflux must account for these findings.

An important bit of evidence about the distal esophagus was presented in the observations of Bombeck, Nyhus and Dillard who studied the relationship of esophagitis in cadavers to the insertion of the phrenoesophageal membrane [12]. Regardless of the presence or absence of hiatal hernia, a low insertion of the phrenoesophageal membrane just at the junction of the tubular esophagus with the gastric pouch was associated with an increased incidence of esophagitis. An insertion of the phrenoesophageal membrane into the submucosa of the esophagus 3 cm or more above the junction of esophageal tube with gastric pouch was associated with the absence of esophagitis whether or not a hiatal hernia was present. This called attention to the phrenoesophageal membrane as determining the level at which the esophagus entered the true abdominal cavity, and the importance of an intra-abdominal segment of esophagus.

Henderson presented experiments in which the anatomical sphincter in the distal esophagus of the dog was resected and replaced with a gastric tube [13]. If the gastric tube entered the large gastric pouch 6 cm or more below the diaphragm there was no reflux esophagitis even when the animal was stimulated with histamine. Insertion of the new swallowing tube into the gastric pouch at the level of the diaphragm led to the development of esophagitis.

Rhesus monkeys have anatomical and physiological characteristics of the distal esophagus similar to humans and are an upright species. They have no identifiable distal esophageal sphincter. If the distal esophagus of Rhesus monkeys is resected and replaced with a gastric tube which enters the abdomen for several centimeters prior to entering into the gastric pouch, there is no change in the amplitude of the distal esophageal high pressure zone even though the so-called sphincter segment is resected [14]. Furthermore, the high pressure zone in the gastric tube shows a drop in pressure coincident with swallowing. These gastric tubes used to replace the esophagus respond to gastrin, cholecystokinin, secretin and glucagon in a manner similar in amplitude to that of the normal distal esophagus of the monkey prior to resection.

Our current theory to explain the normal barrier to reflux is that a swallowing tube of small diameter entering the large gastric pouch within a common pressure chamber of the abdomen maintains intraluminal resting pressure higher than the gastric pouch as would be expected from the Law of LaPlace. Furthermore, alterations in muscle tone of the foregut caused by any of the hormones cause a response of greater amplitude in the smaller diameter tube as would be predicted from the laws of physics. In other experiments we have replaced the distal esophagus of monkeys with jejunal segments or colon segments. As long as these are brought into the stomach several centimeters below the diaphragm and sutured in a way to prevent distention, they remain a small tube entering a large pouch. A high pressure zone can be identified in these other segments of bowel, and drop in high pressure zone amplitude coincident with swallowing has been shown in both jejunal and colon segments. The evidence accumulated suggests that the properties of the distal esophageal high pressure zone are nonspecific and can be duplicated with any segment of gut of small diameter passing from the esophagus into the gastric pouch within the common pressure chamber of the abdomen.

Most recently an in vitro model has been developed in which the properties of a distal esophageal high pressure zone are duplicated using cadaver human esophagi in a model system [15]. The quantitative data obtained indicate that a 3 to 4 cm segment of intra-abdominal esophagus represents an ideal length for maintaining competency of the cardia when the abdominal thoracic pressure difference is approximately 10 cm of water in amplitude. This model system duplicates to a surprising degree the actual numbers and measurements found in normal human beings.

From these experimental and clinical observations, a successful operation for the control of reflux should restore 3 to 4 cm of distal esophagus within the common pressure chamber of the abdomen and permit application of increased abdominal pressure to the intra-abdominal segment. Several antireflux operations have been demonstrated to be successful in 85% or more of patients in long-term follow-up and share these common principles. These include the techniques introduced by Belsey [16], Hill [17] and Nissen [18]. In each of these procedures plication of the stomach to the intra-abdominal esophagus is employed to help in retaining the esophagus within the abdomen. The plication of stomach around the esophagus prevents distention of the intra-abdominal swallowing tube and allows direct transmission of abdominal pressures to the intra-abdominal segment of esophagus. These several operations differ principally in technical details. Which of these will prove to be the operation of choice in the long run will depend upon such factors as ease in teaching, long-term recurrence rates, which are not yet available, specific complications associated with each operation and the incidence of side effects such as the gas bloat syndrome and dysphagia. It is clear from the early postoperative results presented for each of these procedures that they do share common principles for the successful control of reflux [19,20].

References

1. Allison, P.R.: Reflux esophagitis, sliding hiatal hernia, and the anatomy of repair. Surg. Gynecol. Obstet. 92:149, 1951.
2. Belsey, R.: Peptic ulcer of the esophagus. Ann. R. Coll. Surg. (England) 14:303, 1954.
3. Fyke, F.E., Code, C.F. and Schlegel, J.F.: The gastroesophageal sphincter in healthy human beings. Gastroenterologia 86:135, 1956.
4. Winans, C.S. and Harris, L.D.: Quantitation of lower esophageal sphincter competence. Gastroenterology 52:779, 1967.
5. Tuttle, S.G. and Grossman, M.I.: Detection of gastroesophageal reflux by simultaneous measurement of intraluminal pressures and pH. Proc. Soc. Exp. Biol. Med. 98:225, 1958.
6. Kantrowitz, P.A., Corson, J.G., Fleischli, D.L. and Skinner, D.B.: Measurement of gastroesophageal reflux. Gastroenterology 56:666, 1969.
7. Skinner, D.B. and Booth, D.J.: Assessment of distal esophageal function in patients with hiatal hernia and/or gastroesophageal reflux. Ann. Surg. 172:627, 1970.
8. Johnson, L.F. and DeMeester, T.R.: Twenty-four hour pH monitoring of the distal esophagus: A quantitative measure of gastroesophageal reflux. Am. J. Gastroenterol. 62:325, 1974.
9. DeMeester, T.R., Johnson, L.F., Joseph, G.J. et al: Patterns of gastroesophageal reflux in health and disease. Ann. Surg. 184:459-470, 1976.
10. Pellegrini, C.A., DeMeester, T.R., Wernly, J.A. et al: Alkaline gastroesophageal reflux. Am. J. Surg. 135:177-183, 1978.
11. Ismail-Beigi, F., Horton, P.F. and Pope, C.E., II: Histological consequences of gastroesophageal reflux in man. Gastroenterology 56:163, 1970.
12. Bombeck, C.T., Dillard, D.H. and Nyhus, L.M.: Muscular anatomy of the gastroesophageal junction and role of phrenoesophageal legament. Autopsy study of sphincter mechanism. Ann. Surg. 164:643, 1966.
13. Henderson, R.D.: Gastroesophageal junction in hiatus hernia. Can. J. Surg. 15:63, 1972.

14. Moossa, A.R., Cooley, G.R. and Skinner, D.B.: Intraluminal and intraperitoneal pressures at the cardia: Effect of hormones and surgical intervention. Surg. Forum 24:370, 1973.
15. DeMeester, T.R., Wernly, J.A., Bryant, G.H. et al: Clinical and in vitro analysis of determinants of gastroesophageal competence: A study of the principles of antireflux surgery. Am. J. Surg. (Accepted for publication.)
16. Skinner, D.B. and Belsey, R.H.R.: Surgical management of esophageal reflux and hiatus hernia. J. Thorac. Cardiovasc. Surg. 53:33, 1967.
17. Hill, L.D.: An effective operation for hiatal hernia: An eight-year appraisal. Ann. Surg. 166:681, 1967.
18. Nissen, R.: Gastropexy and "fundoplication" in surgical treatment of hiatal hernia. Am. J. Dig. Dis. 6:954, 1961.
19. Skinner, D.B. and DeMeester, T.R.: Gastroesophageal reflux. Current Problems in Surgery, Volume XIII, No. 1, January, 1976.
20. DeMeester, T.R., Johnson, L.F. and Kent, A.: Evaluation of current operations for the prevention of gastroesophageal reflux. Ann. Surg. 180:511, 1974.

Self-Evaluation Quiz

1. Allison first introduced the concept of reflux-induced esophagitis.
   a) True
   b) False
2. Hiatal hernia causes the symptoms of heartburn and regurgitation.
   a) True
   b) False
3. Which is not a complication of gastroesophageal reflux?
   a) Esophagitis
   b) Obesity
   c) Stricture
   d) Bleeding
   e) Aspiration
4. Type I is more common than type II hiatal hernia.
   a) True
   b) False
5. Patients having a Type I hiatal hernia should undergo anatomical repair to avoid mechanical complications of the hernia.
   a) True
   b) False

6. Hiatal hernia is best diagnosed by:
   a) Symptoms
   b) Radiography
   c) pH reflux testing
7. The acid perfusion test determines the presence or absence of esophagitis.
   a) True
   b) False
8. Which of the following is *not* best diagnosed by esophageal manometry?
   a) Achalasia
   b) Scleroderma
   c) Esophageal reflux
   d) Esophageal spasm
9. Which of the following is *not* a clear indication for antireflux operations?
   a) Severe symptoms of heartburn
   b) Ulcerative esophagitis
   c) Recurrent aspiration pneumonia
   d) Esophageal stricture
10. Grade I esophagitis (erythema) inevitably proceeds to esophageal ulceration.
    a) True
    b) False
11. The point at which the esophagus enters the abdomen is marked by:
    a) The level of the diaphragm
    b) The insertion of the phrenoesophageal membrane
    c) The junction of squamous and columnar epithelium
12. The distal esophageal high pressure zone is caused by intrinsic specialized muscle function of the distal esophagus.
    a) True
    b) False

Answers on page 721.

The Role of X-Ray Therapy in the Treatment of Carcinoma of the Esophagus

Seymour H. Levitt, M.D.

Objectives

The objectives are to acquaint the physician with the role of radiation therapy in the treatment of carcinoma of the esophagus. This is to include all aspects of radiation therapy and the treatment of carcinoma of the esophagus including palliative and curative, pre- and postoperative. At the end of this paper, the reader should have knowledge of the appropriate utilization of radiation therapy in the treatment of cancer of the esophagus.

Introduction

This paper will deal with the role of radiation therapy in the treatment of carcinoma of the esophagus, a relatively rare disease in this country. It has been estimated that with the present methods of treatment and diagnosis, even in the best circumstances, only 20% of the patients will be cured. Actually, the number of patients cured of this disease is quite low, regardless of whether radiation alone, surgery alone, or combinations are used.

Because the number of cases in most institutions is low and because the treatments vary from one to the next, even the larger institutions in this country do not have large series of patients treated in a consistent manner. In order to find a series

Seymour H. Levitt, M.D., Professor and Head, Department of Therapeutic Radiology, University of Minnesota Medical School, Minneapolis.

of patients treated with either radiation or surgery in a consistent manner, one must turn to the European literature.

Radiation Therapy Alone

Probably the best results and the best documented series on the treatment of carcinoma of the esophagus with radiation therapy alone is that of Pearson [1-3] who reported in a number of papers on a series of patients treated for carcinoma of the esophagus between the years 1931 and 1969 in Edinburgh, Scotland. He reported that the percentage of radical treatments, including both surgery and radiation therapy, increased during that period and the percentage of patients treated palliatively decreased. This was due to improvements in surgical and radiotherapeutic equipment, techniques and the physicians performing the procedures. He also noted that in the Edinburgh series, the one-year and five-year survival rates increased with the percentage of patients treated radically. Pearson also observed that in the most recent period, radical radiotherapy became the more prevalent type of treatment; whereas, in the middle years between 1948 and 1964, surgery was the predominant treatment technique.

In his group of patients, there was a consistent increase in survival in those treated by radiation, compared to the patients treated by surgery, except for lesions of the lower third of the esophagus. Pearson related this improvement, not to a superiority of radiation over surgery, but to the postoperative morbidity that developed in the group of patients treated surgically.

Of some 800 patients treated at Edinburgh, the difference in survival, comparing radical radiation therapy to radical surgery, at both one and five years was statistically significant at the 0.05 level (20% and 11% at five years, respectively).

Preoperative Irradiation

There are a number of reports in the literature on preoperative irradiation including those of Akakura, Marx and Nakayama [4-6]. The total radiation dose is similar, except for Nakayama, who developed a technique in which he used 500 rads daily for four or five days, followed immediately by surgery. Akakura used 150 to 200 rads daily to a total dose of 5,000 to 6,000 rads followed in two to four weeks by operation. Marks used 250 rads daily × 18 followed in four to eight weeks by surgery.

In evaluating the results, it is important to note that these were not randomized studies. In Akakura's study, preoperative radiation plus operation gave a 25% five-year survival. Operation alone gave a 15.6% survival. Marx et al, preoperative radiotherapy plus resection, gave a 13.9% five-year survival; operation only, 6.1% survival. Nakayama reported the best results: 37.5% five-year survival; operation only, 19%. Nakayama's results were on a very small number of patients and have not been verified in other studies. Pearson's five-year results again were 20%, radical radiation therapy alone and 11%, radical surgery alone, respectively.

Postoperative Irradiation

Postoperative irradiation has been used in only a limited manner to treat known residual areas of disease. The doses used have been 5,000 to 6,000 rads delivered to limited fields. Recent reports show results with this treatment have been good, especially when used immediately post surgery [7, 8].

At the Medical College of Virginia at Richmond, we analyzed the data on the patients that were treated at that institution over a number of years [7]. There were some 90 patients in this study; only one of the 90 survived five years. Seventy-nine of these 90 were treated with radiation only. There were 11 patients treated with surgery and radiation therapy. Five of these were treated preoperatively and six postoperatively. The median survival in the combined treatment group was fairly similar. The one patient surviving five years was treated postoperatively. In all patients who were treated with radiation alone or in combination with surgery, the length of the lesion affected the median survival. As the lesions became larger, regardless of the method of treatment, the results of treatment worsened. Patients with lesions 0 to 5 cm in length had a median survival of seven and six months, respectively. In patients treated with radiation alone or with combined radiation and surgery, patients with lesions greater than 6 cm had a median survival of three and four months, respectively.

Palliative Radiotherapy

Radiation therapy, in addition to being used as a curative agent, is also extremely effective as a palliative agent. At MCV 39 patients did not achieve relief of symptoms and the median survival was two months; 40 patients who experienced relief, particularly those who received relief early, had a median survival of seven months.

Radiation dose had an effect on the response to treatment and survival. The patients who tolerated and received higher doses of radiation had a longer median survival. It is important to note when reading the literature that one should evaluate the amount of radiation the patient has received. If they have not or cannot receive adequate irradiation, the tumor will not be controlled.

One of the problems that radiation therapists have in caring for patients with carcinoma of the esophagus is determination of indications for not treating. Our feeling has been that patients who have had a gastrostomy because of obstruction or who have a tracheo-esophageal fistula at presentation do not benefit from radiation treatment and should receive some other form of palliation. In the study at the Medical College of Virginia, there were ten patients with tracheo-esophageal fistulas; three of these patients had T-E fistulas before radiation therapy started and radiation therapy was begun in the hope of palliation. The median survival was one month, which is barely enough time and may be not even enough to complete irradiation treatment. If the fistulas developed between the time radiation started and ended, the patient had a median survival of 3.5 months. Patients with T-E fistulas developing after radiation therapy had a median survival of 7.0 months. Our conclusions are that patients with a tracheo-eosphageal fistula prior to therapy should not have treatment started. Patients who develop T-E fistulas during treatment should have treatment stopped immediately. These data also demonstrated the need for very careful evaluation of patients with barium swallows, bronchoscopy, esophagoscopy, even in palliative situations to make sure that they are candidates for radiation therapy.

Patients who require a gastrostomy prior to radiation therapy because of obstruction do not respond well. Of the seven such patients, the median survival was one month. Some patients did require a gastrostomy after the radiation therapy had been started or completed. These patients had a median survival of 3.0 months. From our data, we conclude that (1) a patient with a tracheo-esophageal fistula should not be treated with radiation therapy and (2) those patients who have had a gastrostomy because of the obstruction of the esophagus are not good candidates for radiation therapy and do not benefit from that procedure.

Discussion

Generally speaking, the results of treatment of carcinoma of the esophagus with any treatment are quite dismal. There have been some reports of improvement recently. Although some series report improved survival with surgery and preoperative radiotherapy, or postoperative radiotherapy combined, the overall results of such treatment do not appear better than those of irradiation alone. Insofar as radiation is concerned, the results are better today because of improved treatment, improved equipment, better means of localizing the tumor, the use of computers and advanced physics and more experienced physicists and radiation therapists.

Megavoltage radiotherapy should be used because it provides a more penetrating beam with a better depth dose, better cutoff of dose at the beam margin, less irradiation of the normal tissue and better patient tolerance of treatment. There is also less differential absorption of radiation by bone and less underdosage of tumor lying behind the bone in the treatment beam. Many physicians have never had patients treated with anything other than cobalt or linear accelerators, but there were many patients treated in the past with orthovoltage irradiation. It was impossible to deliver an adequate dose to the tumor because of a differential absorption of that type of radiation by bone plus a very severe skin reaction in many cases.

There are a number of nonradiation factors which enter into the improved survival rate, such as better diagnostic methods, the use of CAT scanners and the use of better methods of esophagoscopy all of which help us to better define the tumor and determine those patients that can benefit from treatment, as opposed to those who cannot.

The reasons for failure: (1) in most cases the disease is widely disseminated at presentation; (2) we deal with debilitated patients; and (3) the tumor or treatment volume is too large to deliver a tumorcidal dose.

What are the possibilities for further improvement?

1. Prevention. We know that the disease does develop in certain locales. We know that there are factors which may lead to the development of carcinoma of the esophagus. For instance, we know that in certain provinces of China, the higher incidence of carcinoma of the esophagus has definitely been traced to the mineral constituents in the soil and the food. So these are important factors, which may help to prevent the disease.

2. Earlier diagnosis is important. A major problem is that most of these patients have advanced disease by the time we see them.

3. The development of systemic treatment. At the present time, there are no chemotherapeutic agents or any other agent for systemic treatment which has proven to be effective in this disease.

4. Better radiotherapy. This means that we have better trained radiotherapists, that we have better centers, that we have the use of many of the diagnostic and therapeutic treatment planning and localizing tools that are available in larger centers but which are not available in some of the smaller community hospitals.

Summary

Radiation therapy with megavoltage equipment appears to be the treatment of choice for cure in carcinoma of the upper two thirds of the esophagus. Surgery is recommended for lesions of the lower one-third T-E fistulas or obstruction requiring gastrostomy are contraindications to initiating radiotherapy. Much improvement in prevention, diagnosis and treatment is needed in this disease.

References

1. Pearson, J.G.: The value of radiotherapy in the management of squamous oesophageal cancer. Br. J. Surg. 58:794-798, 1971.

2. Pearson, J.G.: Carcinoma of the oesophagus — operation or radiation. Langenbecks Arch. Chir. 337:739-743, 1974.
3. Pearson, J.G.: The present status and future potential of radiotherapy in the management of esophageal cancer. Cancer 39:882-890, 1977.
4. Akakura, I., Nakamura, Y., Kakegawa, T. et al: Surgery of carcinoma of the esophagus with preoperative radiation. Chest 57:47-57, 1970.
5. Marks, R.D., Jr., Scruggs, H.J. and Wallace, K.M.: Postoperative radiation therapy for carcinoma of the esophagus. Cancer 38:84-89, 1976.
6. Nakayama, K.: Pre-operative irradiation in the treatment of patients with carcinoma of the oesophagus and of some other sites. Clin. Radiol. 15:232-241, 1964.
7. Frazier, A.B., Levitt, S.H. and DeGiorgi, L.S.: Effectiveness of radiation therapy in the treatment of carcinoma of the esophagus. A retrospective study. Am. J. Roentgenol. Radium Ther. Nucl. Med. 108:830-834, 1970.
8. Fraser, R.W., Wara, W.M., Thomas, A.N. et al: Combined treatment methods for carcinoma of the esophagus. Radiology 128:461-465, 1978.

Self-Evaluation Quiz

1. A constant increase in survival of patients treated by all methods in the past 30 years is due to the improved surgical techniques.
   a) True
   b) False
2. In a series of patients treated in Edinburgh, the difference in survival comparing radical radiation therapy to radical surgery is not statistically significant.
   a) True
   b) False
3. The studies of preoperative radiation which have been reported in the literature show improved results over surgery alone are not randomized studies.
   a) True
   b) False
4. The best results reported with preoperative radiation are those of Nakayama.
   a) True
   b) False
5. Nakayama's results with preoperative radiation and radical surgery have been verified in other studies.
   a) True
   b) False

6. The length of the lesion in the esophagus is directly correlated with prognosis, ie, the larger the lesion, the worse the prognosis.
   a) True
   b) False
7. Generally, patients with lesions larger than 6 cm have a very poor prognosis.
   a) True
   b) False

Answers on page 721.

Carcinoma of the Esophagus

David B. Skinner, M.D., F.A.C.S.

Objectives

1. To review the symptoms and diagnosis for carcinoma of the esophagus.
2. To stress the importance of early case finding.
3. To present the preoperative evaluation of a patient.
4. To describe different types of surgery for palliation and cure.

Difficulty in swallowing or dysphagia is the most common presenting symptom of carcinoma of the esophagus. Dysphagia can be caused by many conditions including reflux induced strictures, lye strictures, rings and webs, diffuse esophageal spasm, achalasia and idiopathic strictures. As a symptom of dysphagia, carcinoma is more common than all of these combined by a ratio of two to one. Any patient complaining of difficulty in swallowing should be suspected of having carcinoma until proved otherwise and should be evaluated by barium swallow radiographic studies and esophagoscopy.

Unfortunately, dysphagia is a late symptom of esophageal neoplasm. Because of the remarkable ability of esophageal smooth muscle to stretch without raising intraluminal tension, the carcinoma must involve 90% or more of the esophageal circumference before the patient experiences dysphagia [1]. When obstruction to swallowing develops, the disease is already advanced and chances for cure are poor. Taking all patients presenting with symptomatic esophageal carcinoma, only about 5% to 10% can be expected to survive five years even if they all receive optimal treatment.

David B. Skinner, M.D., F.A.C.S., Professor and Chairman, Department of Surgery, University of Chicago/The Division of Biological Sciences and The Pritzker School of Medicine, Chicago, Ill.

There are no specific early symptoms of esophageal carcinoma although vague chest pain may be recalled by some patients. If improvement in the dismal statistics for patients with esophageal carcinoma is to be achieved, the best hope depends upon earlier diagnosis. Since there are no early symptoms, this requires the identification of high-risk groups of patients and the development of techniques adaptable for use in mass screening of populations. These techniques must have a high diagnostic accuracy. High-risk population groups include patients who are both heavy drinkers and smokers, patients living in known high incidence regions, those with achalasia or other causes of long-term esophageal obstruction such as lye stricture and those with dietary habits associated with a high incidence of this disease. Screening techniques currently being evaluated are based upon esophageal cytology. Specimens may be obtained by aspirating ingested balanced electrolyte solution, brushing of the esophageal lumen, or the inflation of a balloon with abrasion of the esophageal mucosa. At present, Leven and I at the University of Chicago are consulting for a collaborative study sponsored by the National Iranian Cancer Society to use per oral brush cytology of the esophagus in a high-risk population identified in remote villages on the shores of the Caspian Sea [2]. Preliminary results in obtaining diagnosis of early asymptomatic carcinoma are encouraging. Based upon cases in my own practice, early cancer of the esophagus with a primary tumor diameter of 2 cm or less has a highly favorable prognosis following radical surgical resection. Further validation of cytology techniques and assessment of their use in population screening may lead to earlier diagnosis and more favorable outcome.

When cancer of the esophagus is suspected, the patient is admitted to the hospital for an extensive workup. Treatment to prepare the patient for possible surgery is carried out in parallel with diagnostic studies. Such patients are often in poor nutritional state and have extensive weight loss. If so, parenteral hyperalimentation is given during the diagnostic workup. Pulmonary complications of esophageal obstruction are common, so pulmonary physical therapy and postural drainage are used frequently.

The initial diagnostic study is barium swallow radiographic examination. Although the diagnosis of carcinoma may be highly suspected based upon the radiographic findings of an irregular ulcerated mass obliterating the lumen, radiographic diagnosis can never be accepted as definitive. There are many examples of esophageal strictures which appear benign to the examining radiologist, but which prove to be malignant upon biopsy or exploration, and examples of deep ulcerative lesions in the midesophagus interpreted as malignant which prove to be a nonmalignant condition such as a Barrett's ulcer of the esophagus when a tissue diagnosis is established. Unless great care is taken by the radiologist and double-contrast studies are employed, early lesions of the esophagus may be easily missed. This is particularly true in a patient with achalasia where the esophagus is greatly dilated and the large amount of barium required to distend the esophagus may obscure detail.

If a patient has the symptom of dysphagia or a lesion is identified by barium swallow, esophagoscopy is performed. Initially the flexible fiberoptic esophagoscope may be used as the optical system improves visualization of mucosal detail. Biopsies and cytology are obtained. If a specific tissue diagnosis is not made, the rigid open lumen esophagoscope is employed. With this instrument a stricture may be dilated with bougies during endoscopy to facilitate biopsy further into the narrowing. A larger size biopsy forceps may be employed to obtain deeper biopsies of the esophageal wall. It is not uncommon for esophageal carcinoma to undermine normal mucosa and for negative biopsies to be obtained from the shelving edge of the tumor.

Once the tissue diagnosis is established, the evaluation continues to determine the patient's general condition and to determine the extent of the disease. Further radiographic studies of the entire upper gastrointestinal and lower gastrointestinal tract are obtained to ascertain the availability of the stomach or colon for possible esophageal reconstruction. If there is any question of an additional underlying esophageal disorder such as achalasia or spasm, esophageal motor function tests may be useful in determining the suitability of the remaining esophagus for reconstruction. Pulmonary function tests are routinely used since many of these patients have chronic pulmonary aspiration. Careful examination of the oral cavity is made prior to endoscopy to insure that dental caries and abscesses do not lead to complications of the surgical procedures. Since chest pain is a common complaint in these patients and since the surgical procedures to be employed are extensive, thorough cardiological evaluation is essential. If indicated by symptoms and electrocardiographic evaluation, cardiographic stress testing and even coronary angiography may be necessary to determine the extent of possible coronary artery disease which in turn may influence therapeutic decisions.

In evaluating the extent of the tumor, the use of the gallium^{67} total body scan is particularly helpful. This isotope localizes in squamous carcinomas of the esophagus and has detected previously unsuspected metastases. If indicated by biochemical tests or physical findings, the liver-spleen scan may be useful in pointing to the need for a preliminary liver biopsy. Bone scan may be indicated by symptoms or physical findings. If suspected metastases are identified, they are biopsied to establish the systemic spread of the disease before therapeutic decisions are made. For lesions of the middle or upper third of the esophagus, bronchoscopy is routinely performed to detect impingement or invasion upon the membranous portion of the trachea or left mainstem bronchus.

In rare cases, carcinoma may be highly suspected but undiagnosed by all of the aforementioned diagnostic studies. In such cases diagnosis must depend upon thoracotomy and operative exploration and biopsies. If a stricture is difficult to dilate, is suspicious of carcinoma and yet all endoscopic biopsies are negative, a blind resection of the stricture as if it were carcinoma is justified.

Based upon preoperative findings, including the patient's overall condition and evidence of local or systemic spread, decisions are made about treatment. Whenever possible, surgical resection of the primary tumor and one-stage esophageal reconstruction are done. This offers the best palliative technique available as well as the best hope for long-term cure. Resectability of esophageal neoplasms depends more upon their location than cell type. If carcinoma of the cardia involving the distal esophagus is included as an esophageal neoplasm, the resectability rate for squamous carcinoma or adenocarcinoma involving the distal esophagus is identical and approximately twice that for the resectability of middle third carcinoma, which is almost always of the squamous cell variety. The difference in resectability rates is caused by the early invasion of adjacent structures such as trachea and aorta in the middle third of the esophagus, whereas these vital structures are not commonly involved at an early stage for lower third lesions. In my series, the overall resectability rate including all patients presenting with carcinoma of the esophagus has been 55%, with approximately 70% resectable in the lower third, 40% in the middle third and 30% in the upper third [3].

Resection is the palliative as well as curative procedure of choice compared to radiation therapy, intubation or bypass. Each therapeutic technique carries its own mortality. While the operative mortality of esophagectomy is recognized and varies in reported series from 5% to 30%, it is not commonly appreciated that radiation therapy also involves therapeutic mortality. In our experience at the University of Chicago the mortality rate from the direct effects of radiation therapy during treatment has been 10%. The mortality rate for radical resection of the thoracic esophagus has been 7%. Both in our series and in the experience reported by Wilson, Plested and Carey, surgical resection has given superior results for palliation [4]. In patients who eventually died of the disease, survival from the time of presentation until death averaged approximately five months longer following resection than radiation therapy in both series. Patients treated by resection rarely had recurrent dysphagia and did not develop tracheoesophageal fistulas or mediastinal abscesses, which occurred frequently after radiation therapy. For these reasons resection is preferred whenever it is possible.

In earlier times, leakage from the esophageal anastomosis was a major cause of operative mortality. In a personal experience using techniques as taught by Sweet and Belsey, operative mortality with standard esophagectomy was 34% in 35 consecutive cases. Of the 12 deaths, seven were caused by esophagogastric anastomotic leaks, and the remainder were caused by myocardial infarction or respiratory complications. This unhappy experience led to a change of anastomotic technique.

At present, esophagogastrostomy anastomosis is performed end-to-side. The transected stomach is closed and advanced in the posterior mediastinum to a level above the point of anastomosis. The stomach is anchored with multiple sutures to the prevertebral fascia. The end of the esophagus is anastomosed with a single layer of running 5-0 wire suture to a newly made opening in the anterior aspect of the stomach. In this way the posterior portion of the anastomosis is buttressed by gastric serosa. The stomach can be partially folded over the anterior anastomosis to complete protection of the single layer anastomosis. Employing this technique, there has been one localized but fatal leak from an esophagogastric anastomosis in the last 44 consecutive cases. The use of a running 5-0 monofilament wire anastomosis for direct esophago-colon or esophago-jejunal anastomoses has also been highly successful and has led to no fatal leaks in 53 such interposition operations performed for benign or malignant disease.

With the problem of anastomotic leakage resolved, surgery can be planned as a method of choice in most patients either for palliation or possible cure. When the resection can encompass all of the apparent disease, a radical en bloc resection is performed employing the surgical philosophy originally advanced by Logan [5]. For lower third lesions at least 10 cm distal to the aortic arch and carcinomas at the gastric cardia, this resection includes proximal stomach, omentum, spleen, retroperitoneal nodes, a muscle cuff of the esophageal hiatus and all posterior mediastinal tissues lying between the myocardium and vertebral bodies up to the level 10 cm above the tumor. The anastomosis is done at this point. The mediastinal resection includes removal of the thoracic duct and azygos vein as well as all posterior mediastinal fat and lymphatics. Windows of pericardium and pleura overlying the esophagus are removed. This operation is done through a left thoracotomy with division of the diaphragm around its periphery from the chest wall and later reattachment during closure.

For middle third carcinoma, posterior mediastinectomy is done through a right thoracotomy in the fifth interspace. Again, an en bloc resection of the posterior mediastinum from the membranous portion of the trachea or myocardium back to the vertebral bodies is performed throughout the entire intrathoracic course of the esophagus. In patients who are not obese and have not had previous abdominal surgery or duodenal ulcer disease, it is often feasible to advance the entire stomach through the hiatus as described by Belsey and Hiebert [6]. If this cannot be done, a separate abdominal incision is made to mobilize the stomach, or colon if the stomach is not suitable. The esophageal anastomosis is done through a separate neck incision. To date, 41 radical resections for neoplasms of the distal or midesophagus have been performed with an operative mortality of 7%. Among 25 patients operated upon three or more years ago, six (24%) have survived at least three years. Follow-up continues.

For cervical carcinoma a radical resection of the cervical esophagus with bilateral modified neck dissection is performed. If the tumor is at the level of the cricopharyngeus, laryngectomy is included and transection is made at the base of the tongue and hypopharynx. In such cases, the intrathoracic esophagus is removed by blunt dissection through the cervical and abdominal incision. The stomach, by preference, or left colon is mobilized through the abdominal incision and advanced through the posterior mediastinum for anastomosis to the hypopharynx. These radical operations are reserved for patients in whom the entire extent of disease appears to be encompassed by the surgical resection.

When local extension or unsuspected systemic metastases are encountered at surgery, a less extensive resection of surrounding tissues is done for palliation if possible. Nevertheless, a 10 cm or more margin should be taken from the primary tumor to avoid local anastomotic recurrence and return of dysphagia. When systemic metastases are known preoperatively, and the patient is not totally obstructed, radiation therapy is given for palliation. Life expectancy in such cases is less than one year. In such patients endoluminal intubation using a Mousseau-Barbin or Celestin tube may provide helpful terminal palliation for total esophageal obstruction.

Some patients with advanced local disease including tracheo-esophageal fistulas may be inoperable but without systemic spread. Such individuals may benefit from the creation of an end cervical esophagostomy and gastrostomy and the use of the extracorporeal esophagogastrostomy tube [7].

While current outlook for long-term cure of patients with esophageal carcinoma is dismal, most patients benefit at least temporarily from one of the aforementioned surgical procedures. The choice of procedures is made based upon extensive preoperative evaluations. Results from the radical en bloc resections now employed will be determined by further long-term follow-up, but these operations can be performed with an acceptable mortality rate. Overall significant improvement in the management of this disease depends upon further successful application of early case finding techniques.

References

1. Sweet, R.H.: Carcinoma of the esophagus and stomach. JAMA 137:1213-1219, 1948.
2. Dowlatshahi, K. et al: Early detection of cancer of oesophagus along Caspian Littoral. Lancet, January 21, 1978, pp. 125-126.
3. Skinner, D.B.: Esophageal malignancies: Experience with 110 cases. Surg. Clin. North Am. 56:137-147, 1976.
4. Wilson, S.E., Plested, W.G. and Carey, J.S.: Esophagogastrectomy versus radiation therapy for midesophgeal carcinoma. Ann. Thorac. Surg. 10:195-202, 1970.
5. Logan, A.: The surgical treatment of carcinoma of the esophagus and cardia. J. Thorac. Cardiovasc. Surg. 46:151, 1963.
6. Belsey, R. and Hiebert, C.A.: An exclusive right thoracic approach for cancer of the middle third of the esophagus. Ann. Thorac. Surg. 18:1-15, 1974.
7. Skinner, D.B. and DeMeester, T.R.: Permanent extracorporeal esophagogastric tube for esophageal replacement. Ann. Thorac. Surg. 22:107-111, 1976.

Self-Evaluation Quiz

1. Dysphagia is the most common presenting symptom for carcinoma of the esophagus.
   a) True
   b) False
2. Diffuse esophageal spasm and achalasia are two motor abnormalities of the esophagus causing dysphagia.
   a) True
   b) False
3. There are early specific symptoms of esophageal carcinoma.
   a) True
   b) False
4. Which of the following is *not* associated with an increased incidence of carcinoma of the esophagus?

a) Achalasia
b) Lye stricture
c) Hot tea drinking
d) Heavy tobacco use
e) Heavy alcohol ingestion

5. Barium swallow is the diagnostic study that should be done in any patient complaining of dysphagia.
   a) True
   b) False
6. A negative biopsy obtained by flexible fiberoptic esophagoscope rules out carcinoma of the esophagus.
   a) True
   b) False
7. Of the techniques available including surgical resection, radiation therapy, intubation and bypass, surgical resection provides the longest average increase in patient survival.
   a) True
   b) False
8. Are carcinomas of the lower, middle or upper esophagus more likely to be resectable?
   a) Lower
   b) Middle
   c) Upper
9. What should be the minimal margin proximally and distally for resection for carcinoma of the esophagus?
   a) 5 cm
   b) 10 cm
   c) 20 cm
10. Treatment is not available for patients with malignant tracheoesophageal fistula.
    a) True
    b) False

Answers on page 721.

Replacement of the Esophagus for Carcinoma of the Esophagus

Edward W. Humphrey, M.D.

Objectives

1. To identify the principles of therapy as they apply to the reconstruction of a conduit for swallowing.
2. To identify the four types of reconstructions discussed and the advantages and disadvantages of each of the procedures.
3. To discuss palliation with reference to irradiation, gastrostomy, repeated dilatation and colon bypass.

Introduction

The operative approach to reconstruction of a conduit for swallowing varies greatly and the evidence supporting any one approach as superior is not convincing. However, certain principles of therapy can be formulated: (1) extent of the resection should not be limited by the method of reconstruction; (2) risk of the operation should be at a minimum; and (3) reconstruction should provide the patient with an adequate conduit for swallowing that not only is relatively free of long-term complications but also will not obstruct early in the course of the disease in those patients who are not cured of their carcinoma.

The type of reconstruction used depends greatly upon the extent of the resection performed. If a significant portion of the proximal stomach is removed, advisable for carcinoma of the cardioesophageal junction or lower third of the esophagus, the Gavriliu tube cannot be used, and the remaining stomach, even

---

Edward W. Humphrey, M.D., Department of Surgery, Minneapolis Veterans Administration Hospital and the University of Minnesota Hospital, Minneapolis.

when completely mobilized, will reach only slightly above the azygos vein. Figure 1 shows the usual gastric resection line for a carcinoma of the lower third of the esophagus. Of the other methods of reconstruction, the use of a jejunal interposition seems to have little advantage over a direct esophagogastrostomy. The length that can be obtained is usually no more than and often less than that of the stomach itself. It requires two additional anastomoses and the blood supply is less reliable. For these reasons it will not be discussed in more detail.

Mobilized Stomach

The use of the completely mobilized stomach placed in the posterior mediastinum with an intrathoracic esophagogastrostomy is probably the most commonly used method for restoring esophagogastric continuity. In performing this operation, the duodenum and head of the pancreas are extensively mobilized. The left gastric and short gastric arteries are divided. The greater omentum is separated from the stomach, preserving the gastroepiploic arcade, the right gastroepiploic artery, and the right gastric artery as detailed in Figure 1. Although most patients do not have a problem with gastric emptying following an esophagectomy, about 20% do. For this reason, it is my practice to make a pyloroplasty routinely. Through a right lateral thoracotomy, the stomach is placed posterior to the pulmonary hilus and an end-to-side esophagogastrostomy performed as shown in Figure 2. A valve is created by intussuscepting the esophagus into the stomach in an attempt to alleviate the reflux esophagitis that often occurs following this operation.

The advantage of this procedure is it requires only one anastomosis and is done as part of the esophagectomy, thus requiring only one operation. The disadvantages are that regurgitation and esophagitis may be a problem, the length of residual stomach may be insufficient to permit the removal of an adequate margin of esophagus above the cancer, and, most importantly, there is an intrathoracic anastomosis which has a high leak rate. Hankins et al [2] reported that five of 17 patients undergoing an operation for carcinoma of the esophagus developed a fatal anastomotic leak. Magill and Simmons [3] found a 21% anastomotic leak incidence after esophago-

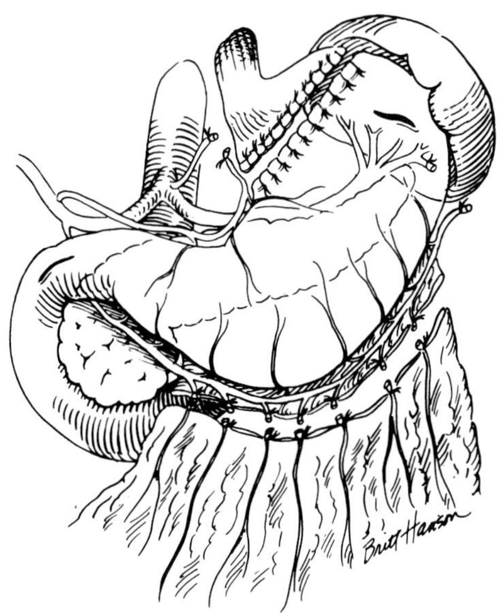

FIG. 1. Preparation of the stomach for esophagogastrostomy. Figure illustrates the usual level of transection of the stomach for a carcinoma of the lower third of the esophagus, and the arterial supply to the gastric pouch.

gastrostomy or esophagojejunostomy. Fifty-six percent of these patients died within three months.

Reversed Gastric Tube

A reversed gastric tube fashioned from the greater curvature of the stomach was originally described by Gavriliu [1] and then independently by Heimlich [4]. This reconstruction is usually done as a second operation two or three weeks after the esophageal resection, but may be done prior to or at the same time as the resection. Figure 3 illustrates the preparation of the stomach for this type of reconstruction. The omentum is separated from the stomach, taking care to preserve the vascular arcade of the gastroepiploic vessels by dividing the omentum near the transverse colon. The spleen is removed, but the left gastroepiploic artery, which provides the blood supply, is preserved by dividing the splenic vessels at the hilus of the spleen. The tail of the pancreas must then be mobilized to

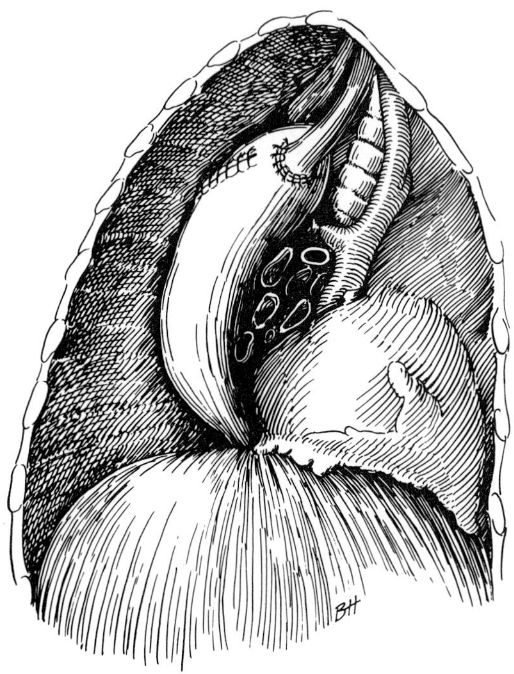

FIG. 2. Completed esophagogastrostomy. View from a right thoracotomy.

provide enough length of the vasculature. The construction of the tube is begun by making an incision on the greater curvature of the stomach 5 to 6 cm from the pylorus. A #48 esophageal dilator is inserted into the stomach and held along the greater curvature by the assistant. The GIA surgical stapler is used to construct the tube, dividing the stomach adjacent to the dilator as far proximally as necessary to obtain an adequate length. The staple line on both the stomach and the gastric tube should be inverted using interrupted sutures and the omentum wrapped around the tube. The tube may be placed either retrosternally or subcutaneously as shown in Figure 4. The antral end of the tube is anastomosed to the cervical esophagus end to end, being particularly careful of the three cornered junction area.

The advantages of this procedure are that it may be quicker to perform than a colon interposition and the length is usually adequate to reach the neck so no intrathoracic esophageal

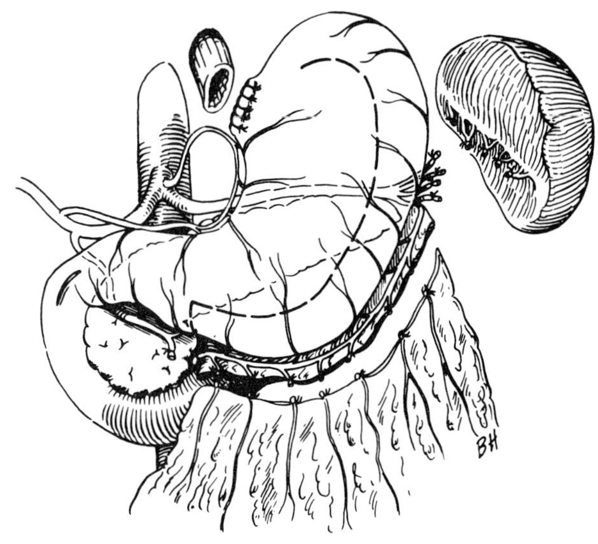

GAVRILIU - HEIMLICH TUBE

FIG. 3. Dashed line shows the stapled line of division on the greater curvature for construction of the tube.

anastomosis is made. The disadvantages are that it cannot be used if the proximal portion of the stomach has been resected; it requires a splenectomy and mobilization of the pancreas; the blood supply may be inadequate and there is a long gastric suture line in the chest. Table 1 lists the complications reported for this procedure from three centers.

Isoperistaltic Gastric Tube

A similar tube, the Beck tube, constructed in an isoperistaltic manner has been advocated by Postlethwait. An extensive mobilization of the duodenum and head of the pancreas is performed that permits the pylorus to ascend almost to the esophageal hiatus. The greater curvature of the stomach is freed from the omentum in a fashion similar to the Gavriliu tube, except that the right gastroepiploic vessels are preserved and the left gastroepiploic vessels are divided as illustrated in Figure 5. An incision is made on the greater curvature of the fundus just to the left of the cardioesophageal junction and a #48

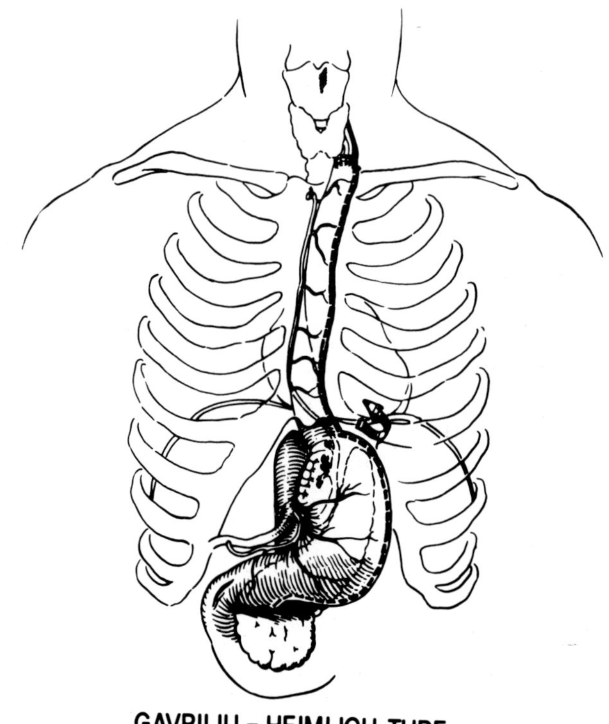

FIG. 4. Completed reversed gastric tube with the pancreas mobilized.

Table 1. Reversed Gastric Tube

Author	*Number of Patients*	*Postoperative Mortality*	*Leak Rate*
Gavriliu	526	3.6%	7.6%
Heimlich	53	5.7%	15%
Griffen	10	20%	60%

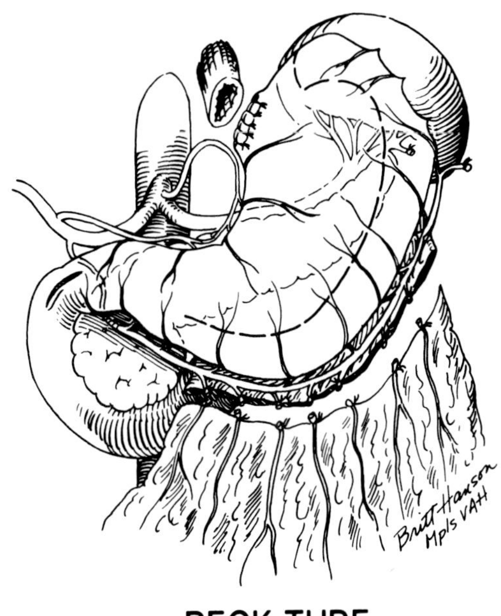

FIG. 5. Dashed line shows the stapled line of division on the greater curvature for construction of the tube.

esophageal dilator inserted. The tube is fashioned with the GIA stapler, in the manner previously described, to a point about 5 cm proximal to the pylorus. After a pyloroplasty has been made, the proximal end of this tube is brought into the neck either retrosternally or subcutaneously and anastomosed to the cervical esophagus.

The advantages of this operation are (1) it does not require a splenectomy or mobilization of the pancreas and so may be performed more quickly than can the Gavriliu operation and (2) it is usually long enough to reach the neck and it is isoperistaltic, although it is unlikely that either this tube or the reversed gastric tube exhibits any coordinated peristalsis.

The disadvantages are (1) it leaves a deformed gastric pouch (Fig. 6) which may be prone to ulceration; (2) the blood supply may be inadequate, and the length may be inadequate if the proximal portion of the stomach is resected; and (3) there is also a long gastric suture line in the chest.

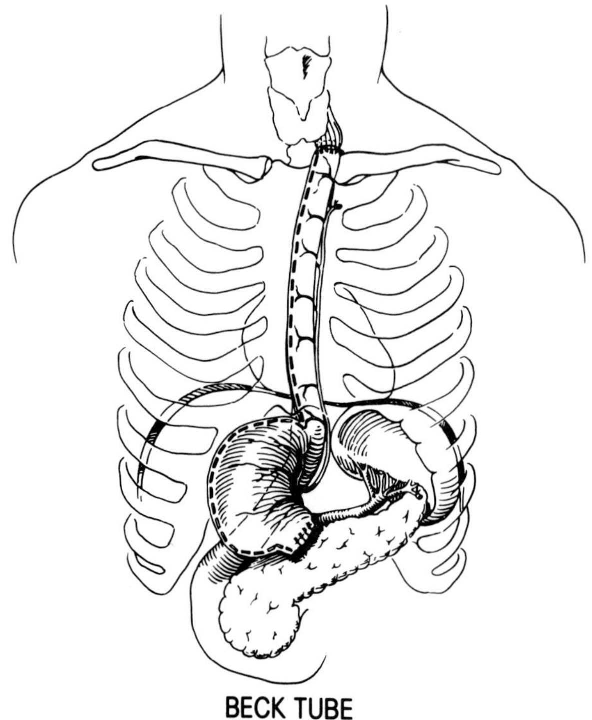

FIG. 6. Completed isoperistaltic gastric tube.

Colon Interposition

Over the past 15 years I have found a colon interposition to be the most versatile and routinely successful method of replacing the esophagus. I now do a total thoracic esophagectomy for all patients with a squamous cell carcinoma that is resected. The colon interposition is done at a second stage, two or three weeks after the esophagectomy. The use of the right colon results in fewer postoperative swallowing problems, but it has the more inconstant blood supply. Figure 7 illustrates the usual pattern of the arterial supply for the colon and the lines of division. Prior to doing a colon interposition an arteriogram is obtained to determine the adequacy of the collateral vessels between the middle colic and the right colic artery. This is the

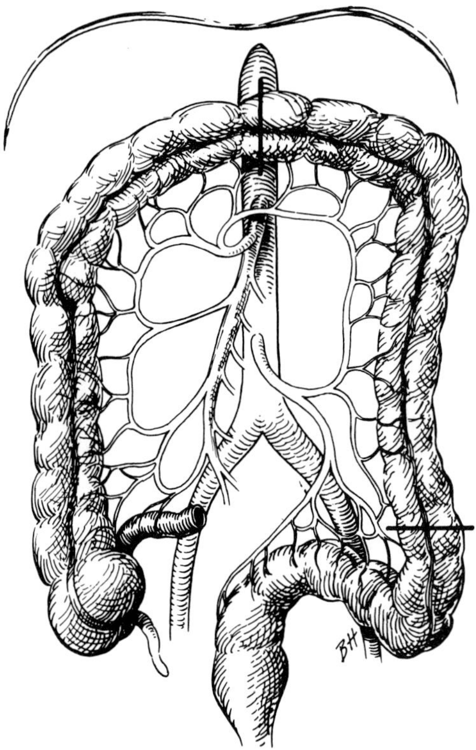

FIG. 7. Usual arterial pattern of the colon. Solid lines indicate division levels for a left colon interposition. The division of the transverse colon is the same for a right colon interposition.

usual point of a deficiency, if one exists. If there is an uncertainty, I use the left colon.

To interpose the right colon, it is freed of its lateral attachments and of its attachments to the omentum. The mesenteries of the right colon, cecum and the distal ileum are mobilized to the superior mesenteric vessels and divided, still preserving all the vascular supply. Using an umbilical tape, the distance from the origin of the middle colic artery to the esophageal stoma in the neck is measured. This distance is then laid off along the vascular arcade in the mesentery, not along the colon itself, and the site of proposed division is marked. This usually requires the inclusion of a variable length of terminal ileum. A bulldog-type clamp is placed on the ileocolic artery and on the right colic artery near its origin from the superior mesenteric artery. The collateral connections between the two branches of the right colic artery are usually deficient so unless the bifurcation of this vessel is intact and included with the colon, the blood supply to the cecum and terminal ileum is often deficient.

While temporarily occluding the two arteries to the right colon, the thoracic tunnel is constructed large enough for the surgeon to insert his hand, so as not to compromise the venous drainage of the colon. This tunnel may be either retrosternal or subcutaneous. The retrosternal position is shorter, somewhat quicker to make and cosmetically more acceptable. However, it cannot be used if there has been a previous sternotomy or if the patient has a permanent tracheostomy. Often the sternal head of one sternocleidomastoid muscle must be divided. I have very rarely ever found it necessary to remove a portion of the clavicle or sternum to obtain enough room. The subcutaneous position is safer, for if necrosis of the interposed organ occurs, the patient does not develop a mediastinitis. If the patient survives for more than one to two years, he will routinely develop an upper abdominal ventral hernia through the defect in the fascia created for the entrance of the colon or stomach from the subcutaneous position.

After a thoracic tunnel has been constructed, if the blood supply to the colon appears adequate, the right colic and marginal branch of the ileocolic arteries are divided. The ileum is divided at the site marked and the distal end temporarily closed with sutures. An umbilical tape is drawn through the tunnel, tied to the ileal sutures and used to guide the passing of the colon through the tunnel, not to pull it through. When the colon is positioned with the terminal ileum in the neck as shown in Figure 8, the site for the cologastrostomy is chosen and the colon carefully divided so as to preserve the vascular supply. The cologastrostomy, then an ileotransverse colostomy are constructed. After the abdomen is closed, I perform the esophagogastrostomy immediately rather than several days later as advocated by some.

A left colon interposition is performed in a similar manner and is illustrated in Figure 9. After detaching the omentum and

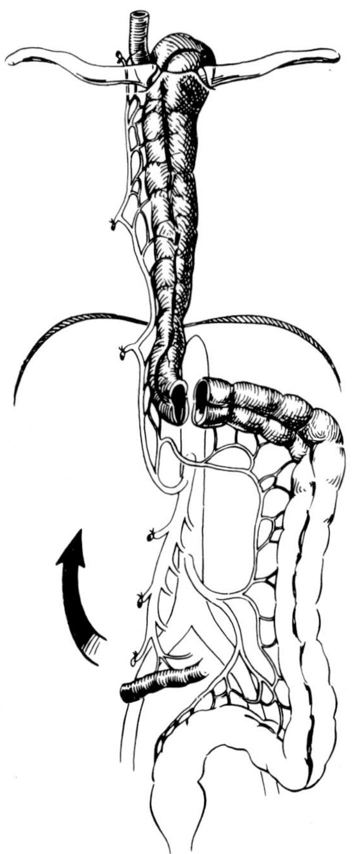

FIG. 8. Completed preparation of the right colon for interposition.

mobilizing the left colon and sigmoid, the mesentery of the left colon and sigmoid are freed and the left colic artery is divided at its junction with the inferior mesenteric artery so as to preserve the superior hemorrhoidal artery. The inferior mesenteric vein must be ligated and divided. The distance from the origin of the middle colic artery to the esophageal stoma is measured and this distance laid out along the vascular arcade of the middle colic and left colic arteries. The marginal vascular connections between the superior hemorrhoidal and the left colic artery are divided at this point which is usually in the mid-sigmoid colon.

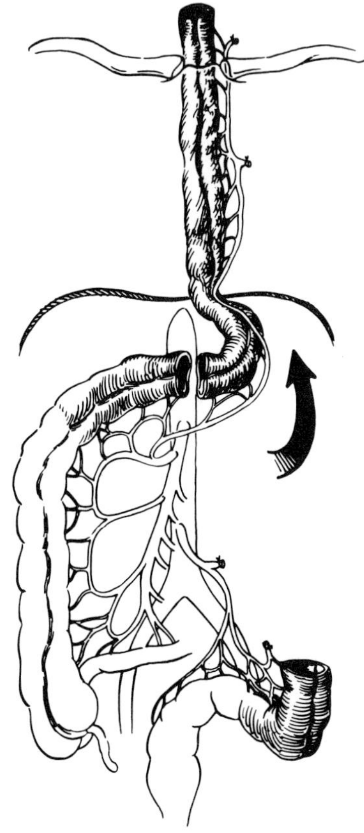

FIG. 9. Completed preparation of the left colon for interposition.

The thoracic tunnel is constructed, the sigmoid colon is divided and the proximal end oversewn. This end is passed into the neck through the thoracic tunnel; the cologastrostomy and transverse-sigmoid colocolostomy performed and the operation completed by constructing a cervical esophagocolostomy. In all 20 left colon interpositions performed at this institution, the blood supply has been adequate.

Palliation

If it is accepted that no local therapeutic maneuver directed at the cancer will prolong the life of a patient not cured, then palliation in the context of the present discussion can be defined as restoration of the pleasure of eating and drinking, plus control of such symptoms as those from a tracheo-esophageal fistula. Although irradiation is a valuable method for restoring deglutition in patients with a squamous cell carcinoma of the esophagus, it is of little value to those with an adenocarcinoma and if a T-E fistula is present will increase the severity of symptoms. A gastrostomy does little except to make home care easier. Repeated dilatation may improve swallowing for a short period, but has not been very satisfactory. It also carries a risk of tearing the esophagus, the cancer and, occasionally, the aorta.

If the patient has a predicted survival of at least six months, we have found the most useful treatment to be a colon bypass of the esophagus. The esophagus is divided in the neck, the distal end is closed and remains in the chest. A subcutaneous colon transplant is performed with an anastomosis in the neck. If a tracheo-esophageal fistula is present, the esophagus is also ligated in the abdomen. I have not encountered problems from this proximal and distal closure of the esophagus.

If the patient has a predicted survival of less than 6 months, I have found the Herring esophageal tube helpful, although not without problems. The placement of this tube requires a gastrotomy. A nasogastric tube is passed through the esophagus into the stomach by the anesthesiologist, the Herring tube is fastened to it and then pulled into the stomach until the flange is at the superior margin of the carcinoma. The lower cuff is put on the Herring tube and moved superiorly until it is at the inferior margin of the carcinoma. One 2-0 nonabsorbable suture is used to fasten the lower end of the tube to the stomach wall.

References

1. Gavriliu, D.: Aspects of Esophageal Surgery. Current Problems in Surgery, Vol. 12, No. 10, 1975.
2. Hankins, J.R., Cole, F.N., Attar, S. et al: Adenocarcinoma involving the esophagus. J. Thorac. Cardiovasc. Surg. 68:148, 1974.
3. Magill, T.G. and Simmons, R.L.: Resection of cardio-esophageal carcinoma. Arch. Surg. 94:865, 1967.
4. Heimlich, H.J.: Esophagoplasty with reversed gastric tube. Am. J. Surg. 123:80, 1972.

Self-Evaluation Quiz

1. The most commonly used way of restoring esophagogastric continuity is:
   a) Gavriliu tube
   b) Jejunal interposition
   c) Completely mobilized stomach placed in anterior mediastinum with intrathoracic esophagogastrostomy
   d) Completely mobilized stomach placed in posterior mediastinum with intrathoracic esophagogastrostomy
2. What percentage of patients have a problem with gastric emptying following esophagectomy?
   a) 5%
   b) 10%
   c) 20%
   d) 28%
3. According to Hankins, how many patients who underwent surgery for carcinoma of the esophagus developed fatal anastomotic leaks?
   a) 3 of 12
   b) 5 of 17
   c) 6 of 20
   d) 20 of 72
4. What procedure requires only one anastomosis done as part of esophagectomy?
   a) Mobilized stomach
   b) Reversed gastric tube
   c) Isoperistaltic gastric tube
   d) Colon interposition
5. What procedure leaves a long suture line, is quicker than colon interposition, provides adequate length for intrathoracic esophageal anastomosis and requires splenectomy?
   a) Mobilized stomach
   b) Reversed gastric tube
   c) Isoperistaltic gastric tube
   d) None of the above
6. What procedure does not require splenectomy, leaves a deformed gastric pouch and possibly inadequate blood supply along with inadequate length?
   a) Mobilized stomach
   b) Reversed gastric tube

c) Isoperistaltic gastric tube
d) Colon interposition

7. The author found colon interposition to be the most versatile and routinely successful procedure for replacing the esophagus.
a) True
b) False

8. Irradiation is good palliative treatment for patients with:
a) Squamous cell carcinoma
b) Adenocarcinoma
c) T.E. fistula
d) All of the above

Answers on page 721.

Zenker's Diverticulum

F. Henry Ellis, Jr., M.D., Ph.D.

Objectives

1. To describe the anatomic defect known as Zenker's diverticulum.
2. To discuss the etiology of the disease as it relates to an abnormality of function of the upper esophageal sphincter mechanism.
3. To review the various methods of surgical treatment emphasizing the technique and results of cricopharyngeal myotomy in appropriate cases.

Protrusion of the pharyngeal mucosa posteriorly between the oblique fibers of the inferior constrictor muscle of the pharynx and the transverse fibers of the cricopharyngeus muscle is known as a pharyngo-esophageal diverticulum. First described by Ludlow in 1767 [1], the condition has been well recognized for many years. With increased longevity of the population, it is being encountered more commonly now than in the past. Following Ludlow's description, Zenker's name became associated with this condition, and in 1875 he and von Zeimssen collected 22 cases from the literature and added 5 of their own [2]. They were the first to describe the nature of these diverticula in detail, accurately identifying their anatomic location and theorizing their etiology.

In the next 100 years, remarkably little was added to these original contributions until recently. Uncertainty regarding the nature of upper esophageal dysphagia primarily because of a lack of understanding of the normal and abnormal function of

---

F. Henry Ellis, Jr., M.D., Ph.D., Chairman, Department of Thoracic and Cardiovascular Surgery, Lahey Clinic Foundation and New England Deaconess Hospital; Associate Clinical Professor of Surgery, Harvard Medical School, Boston, Mass.

the pharynx and upper esophagus contributed to this time lag. An understanding of the normal anatomy and physiology of this area is, therefore, essential before discussing the nature of disease processes that may affect it.

Anatomy and Physiology

The cricopharyngeus muscle runs transversely across the posterior wall of the esophagus connecting the two lateral borders of the cricoid cartilage (Fig. 1). This muscle is bordered superiorly by the oblique fibers of the inferior pharyngeal constrictor muscle that pass upward and backward from their

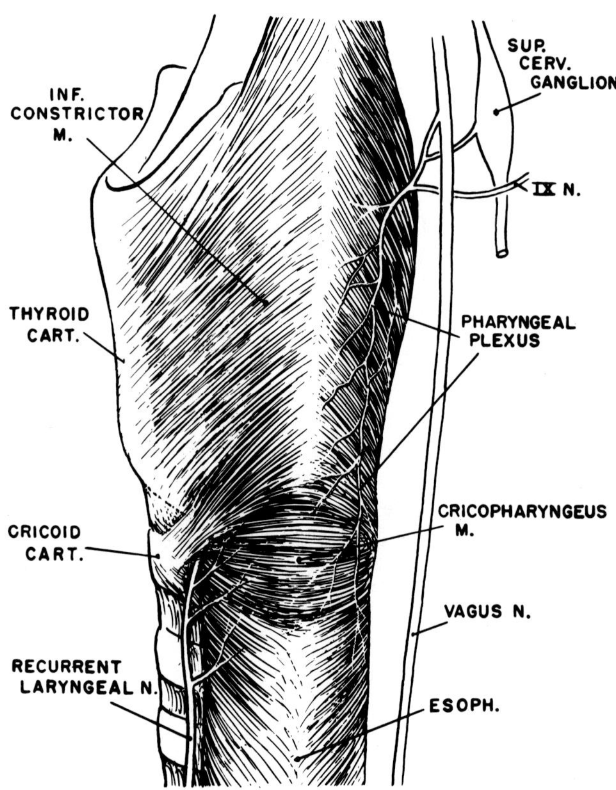

FIG. 1. Anatomy of pharynx and upper esophagus. Posterolateral view. (From Ellis [6].)

origin on the thyroid cartilage to insert into a median raphé. Inferiorly, the cricopharyngeus muscle blends into the circular and longitudinal muscle fibers of the upper esophagus. It is sometimes difficult at the operating table to define precisely the limits of these various muscle groups although it is usually easier to separate the cricopharyngeus muscle from the oblique constrictor fibers of the pharynx than from the circular muscle of the esophagus. The transverse fibers of the cricopharyngeus muscle have shown sufficient anatomic differentiation to justify their being called a true sphincter.

Whether or not the cricopharyngeus muscle can be seen in contrast roentgenography of the upper swallowing passages in the normal individual remains controversial. A posterior indentation of the barium column at the junction of the hypopharynx and esophagus in the lateral projection has been termed the "hypopharyngeal bar." While some have considered this to be a normal finding, others maintain that demonstration of such an indentation is always abnormal [3], representing cricopharyngeal disease. Whether abnormal or not, the x-ray location of the hypopharyngeal bar provides added information about the normal anatomic location of the cricopharyngeus muscle.

The innervation of the upper esophageal sphincter remains a subject of controversy. While the motor supply of the cricopharyngeus muscle in the dog is from a single nerve derived from the vagus by its pharyngeal branch [4], no such nerve has been identified in man. There is no convincing evidence that the recurrent laryngeal nerve is concerned with cricopharyngeal function, since this muscle functions normally in patients with bilateral vocal cord palsy. On the other hand, some patients with pharyngeal palsy show abnormal function of the upper esophageal sphincter leading to the supposition that the nerve of the sphincter may be derived from pharyngeal branches of the vagus through the pharyngeal plexus.

Whatever its innervation may be, the normal function of the upper esophageal sphincter has recently been well studied [5]. A zone of elevated pressure is regularly detected in man between the upper esophagus and the pharynx varying from 2.5 to 6.5 cm in length with an average of 3.0 cm (Fig. 2). Since the width of the band of maximum pressure is about 1 cm and

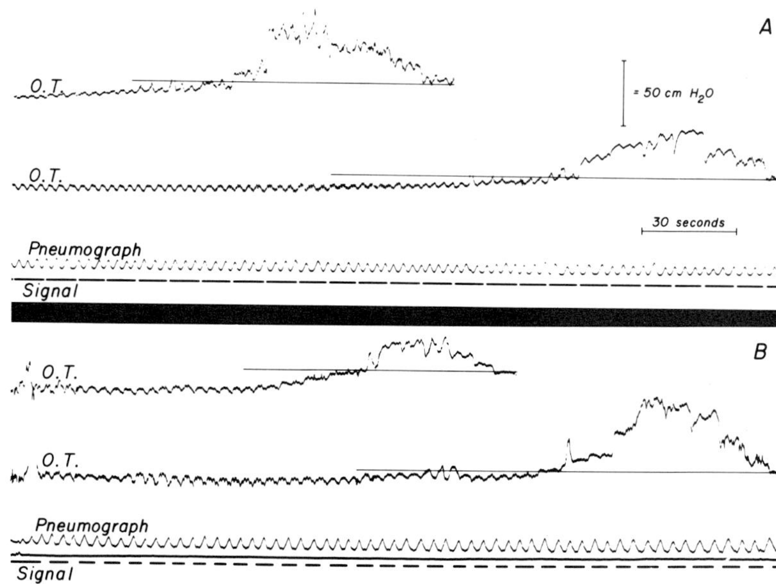

FIG. 2. Resting pressure profile of pharyngo-esophageal sphincter in two healthy individuals (A and B) during successive withdrawals of two open-tipped recording tubes (O.T.) spaced 5.0 cm apart. (From Code and Schlegel [5].)

corresponds to the location of the cricopharyngeus muscle, the adjacent pharyngeal and esophageal muscles must contribute to the total width of the zone of elevated pressure, as defined manometrically. The maximum resting pressure ranges from 18 to 60 cm above atmospheric pressure and consecutive determinations in any one individual over a period of time often register widely differing values. The sphincter relaxes with swallowing and then contracts (Fig. 3). Relaxation occurs early in the deglutitive sequence simultaneously with or just after the contractions of the tongue and upper part of the pharynx. Normally, the sphincter always opens before pharyngeal contraction, and the period of sphincteric relaxation is brief, less than 1 second in duration. After pharyngeal contraction, the sphincter contracts, producing pressures of 70 to 100 cm of water lasting 2 to 4 seconds. As the contraction subsides, sphincteric pressure returns to resting levels.

The act of swallowing is thus a complex phenomenon in which the muscles of the tongue, larynx, pharynx and upper

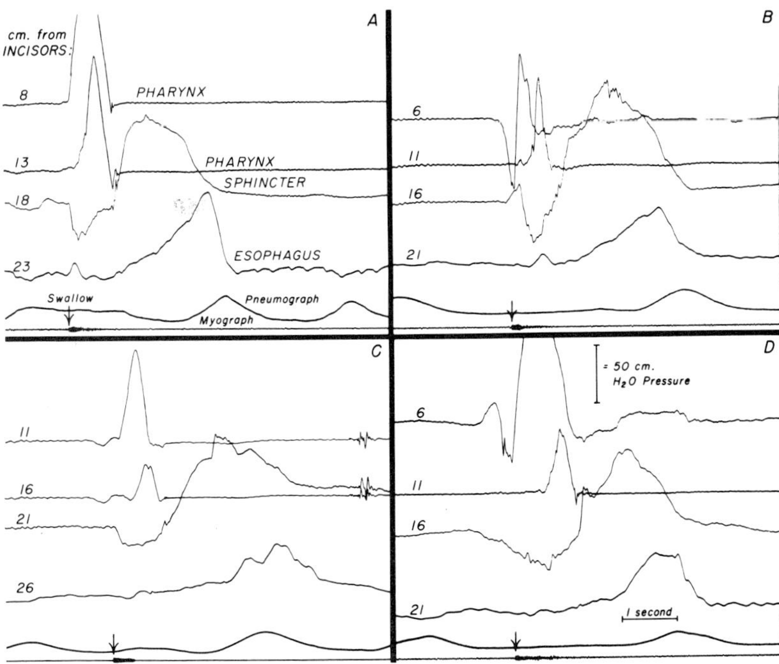

FIG. 3. Four tracings of the deglutitory response of the pharynx, upper esophageal sphincter and the esophagus. (From Code and Schlegel [5].)

esophagus are precisely coordinated. It is clear that if anything disturbs this coordinated sequence of events, the ingested bolus may have difficulty in reaching the esophagus. Such a disturbance could result either from ineffective contraction of the pharyngeal muscle or from some abnormality of function of the cricopharyngeus muscle such as premature contraction or incomplete relaxation. Any of these disturbances could lead to symptoms of dysphagia. Unfortunately, little objective data are available to explain the precise mechanism that is responsible for upper esophageal dysphagia in many of the diseases that affect this area.

Classification of Disorders of Upper Esophageal Sphincter Function [6]

Lack of objective data makes the subject of derangement of pharyngo-esophageal function a confused one. Accordingly, the classification of these disorders presented in Table 1 must be considered as tentative. However, it does serve to place the condition under discussion ie., pharyngo-esophageal diverticulum, in proper perspective in relation to the many other conditions that are known to affect this region. Cricopharyngeal myotomy has been reported as helpful in relieving dysphagia in up to 50% of patients suffering from neuromuscular disorders [7] and it is widely used in conjunction with certain major oropharyngeal resections, including laryngectomy [8]. Esophageal manometry is an essential determinant in identifying those individuals who may be helped by cricopharyngeal myotomy.

Pharyngo-esophageal Diverticulum

Etiology

Ever since the suggestion by Kelly [9] in 1919 that there was "spasm" at the entrance to the esophagus in patients with the disease that later became known in Great Britain as the Paterson-Kelly syndrome and in this country as the Plummer-Vinson syndrome, a variety of proposals have been offered to explain abnormalities of function of this portion of the gullet. In addition to Kelly, a number of others have emphasized the

Table 1. Abnormalities of Pharyngo-esophageal Function

Central nervous system disease
Bulbar poliomyelitis
Cerebrovascular accident
Amyotrophic lateral sclerosis
Supranuclear ophthalmoplegia
Multiple sclerosis
Muscular diseases
Muscular dystrophy
Myasthenia gravis
Thyrotoxic myopathy
Dermatomyositis
Postsurgical dysphagia
Radical oropharyngeal surgery
Idiopathic incoordination
Pharyngo-esophageal diverticulum

role of cricopharyngeal spasm in certain swallowing disorders. In 1946, Lahey directed attention to the cricopharyngeal muscle, implicating it in the etiology of esophageal diverticula, and advised forceful dilation of the muscle as well as surgical excision [10]. Negus also advised dilation in patients with pharyngo-esophageal diverticula, although he considered crico-pharyngeal incoordination rather than spasm as the cause of the pouch [11, 12]. Delayed relaxation of the sphincter was considered an important mechanism by Cross and associates [13].

A related concept is that of cricopharyngeal "achalasia" in which theoretically the sphincter fails to relax. As early as 1926 Jackson and Shallow postulated such a mechanism as being the cause of pharyngo-esophageal diverticula [14]. Asherton is usually given credit for introducing the term achalasia in 1950 as applied to various neuromuscular disorders affecting the cricopharyngeus muscle [15]. Sutherland revived the term in 1962 and implicated this mechanism in the development of pharyngo-esophageal diverticula [16]. Belsey also used the term in explaining the development of diverticula although he seems to use the term achalasia and spasm synonymously [17].

Another possible mechanism for which there is recent physiologic support is that of premature contraction of the sphincter. In 1961 Ardran and Kemp, basing their findings on radiography of the upper food passages, described partial or incomplete closure of the cricopharyngeal sphincter before all of the ingested bolus had been displaced from the pharynx into the esophagus [18]. Lund has also described similar findings in instances of pharyngo-esophageal diverticulum [4]. Esophageal manometric studies carried out on patients with pharyngo-esophageal diverticula by myself and my colleagues have supported this concept of premature contraction of the upper sphincter in patients with upper esophageal pouches [19]. Recently, Smiley and associates [20] suggested that gastro-esophageal reflux leads to cricopharyngeal muscular spasm and that this is the primary cause of upper esophageal pouches. Support for this concept is lacking [21].

Controversy persists regarding the etiology of upper esophageal pouches. It is compounded by the unhappy introduction of the term "cricopharyngeal achalasia" into the dispute, for as far as I am aware, there is no documentation in any disease state of failure of relaxation of the upper esophageal sphincter and certainly not in cases of pharyngo-esophageal diverticulum.

Diagnosis

Pharyngo-esophageal diverticula rarely occur under the age of 30, most developing in people over the age of 50, belying an earlier popular notion that the disease is congenital in origin due to a weak point in muscle layers posteriorly permitting an outpouching of mucosa at that point. The symptoms are characteristic and consist of difficulty in swallowing, noisy gurgling in the throat accompanying swallowing and regurgitation of ingested material after eating. Sometimes when the pouch is large, regurgitation can lead to coughing and choking spells if regurgitated contents are aspirated. Such episodes are prone to occur at night when the patient is recumbent. Ultimately if symptoms are ignored, fatigue, weight loss, malnutrition and suppurative lung complications may develop.

The diagnosis can be established only by roentgenographic examination of the esophagus, which clearly identifies the posteriorly directed pharyngeal pouch (Fig. 4). Esophagoscopy is not necessary and in fact may be contraindicated because of the danger of accidental perforation. Esophageal manometry is difficult to perform because the recording catheters tend to enter the pouch rather than the true lumen of the esophagus. Records, when obtained, however, reveal the incoordination previously referred to whereby the sphincter is in the process of contracting or has completed its contraction phase during the moment of maximal pharyngeal contraction (Fig. 5). Such abnormalities of coordination have never been seen in normal individuals but are common in patients with upper esophageal pouches.

Surgical Treatment

Early surgical efforts initiated before the turn of the century included extirpation, invagination of the diverticulum into the esophagus and diverticulopexy, not all of which were successful. The first successful operation was a two-staged pharyngo-esophageal diverticulectomy carried out by Goldmann in 1909 [22], although Mayo is generally credited with its

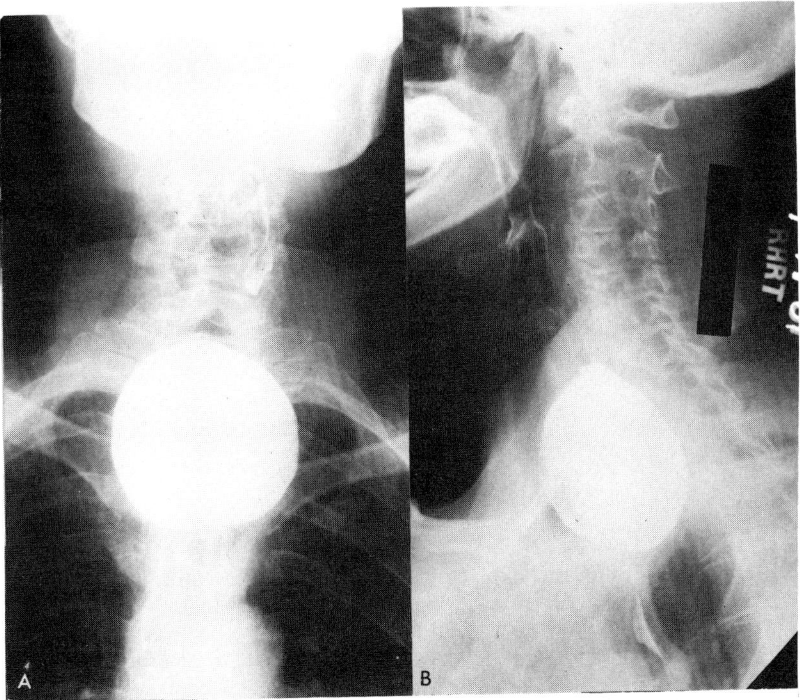

FIG. 4. Roentgenographic appearance of a pharyngo-esophageal diverticulum: A, postero-anterior view; B, lateral view. (From Ellis, F.H., Jr.: Disorders of the esophagus in the adult. *In* Sabiston, D.C. and Spencer, F.C.: *Gibbons Surgery of the Chest.* Philadelphia:W.B. Saunders Co., 1976, p. 691.)

development in this country. This procedure was championed for many years, most recently by Lahey and Warren [23]. The one-stage operation favored earlier by Harrington [24] has gradually superseded the two-stage procedure and is now the most commonly employed surgical technique. The largest reported series of one-stage pharyngo-esophageal diverticulectomy is that by Welsh and Payne from the Mayo Clinic in which 809 patients are reported between the years 1944 and 1972 [25]. There was a 1.4% mortality rate, and residual or recurrent diverticula were later detected in 3.3% of patients. Cricopharyngeal myotomy was not done in any of these individuals although now these surgeons suggest its addition to

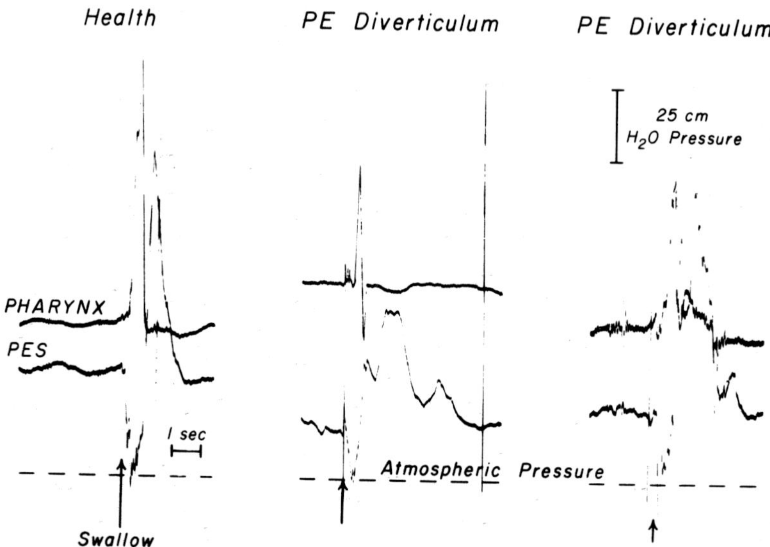

FIG. 5. Deglutition pressures at pharyngo-esophageal junction in a normal person and in two patients with pharyngo-esophageal diverticula. Note that in health (left panel) the pharyngo-esophageal sphincter (PES) is open during the entire period of pharyngeal contraction. In the two patients with diverticula, part or all of the period of pharyngeal contraction occurs after closure of the sphincter (middle and right panels). (From Ellis et al [19].)

diverticulectomy in an effort to reduce the already low incidence of recurrence.

The concept of purposely weakening the sphincter in managing patients with pharyngo-esophageal diverticula is not new. Negus [11] advocated peroral dilation of the sphincter while Dohlman and Mattsson among others have used endoscopic diathermy division of the septum, or common wall, between the esophagus and the diverticulum [26]. Sutherland's revival of the term "cricopharyngeal achalasia" in 1962 [16] led to the use of cricopharyngeal myotomy in patients with pharyngeal pouches not only by him but by others [27, 28]. I have found this procedure to be a simple, safe alternative to diverticulectomy for patients with small to moderate sized pouches and use it in preference to diverticulectomy when the pouch is less than 4 cm in diameter (Fig. 6). When diverticulec-

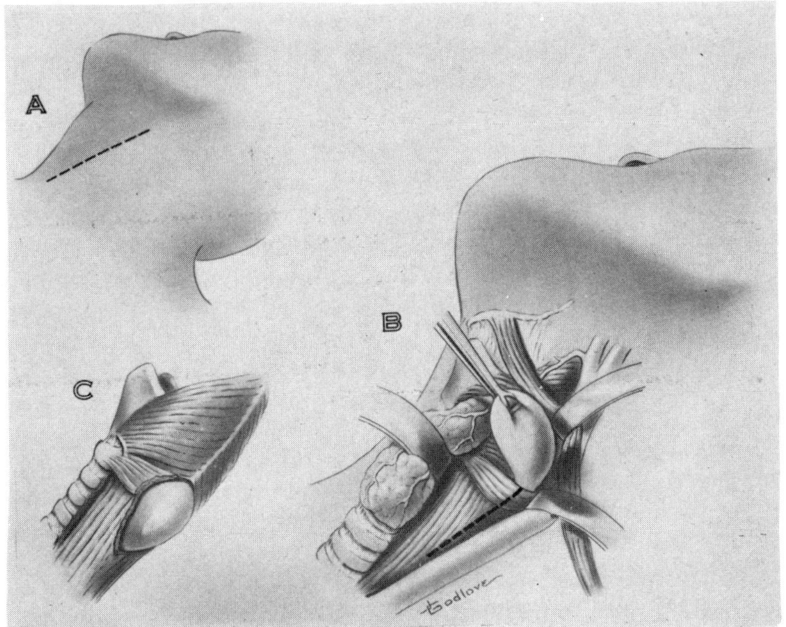

FIG. 6. Technique of esophagomyotomy: A, site of skin incision; B, exposure of diverticulum. Dotted line indicates proposed myotomy site; C, completed operation. (From Ellis et al [19].)

tomy is employed, cricopharyngeal myotomy should always accompany the procedure, since recurrent diverticula are seen from time to time, more frequently in the hands of surgeons less skillful than Welsh and Payne in the management of this disease.

Surgical Technique

Surgical exposure of the cricopharyngeal muscle for myotomy is through a vertical or curved transverse left cervical incision. The incision is deepened between the sternocleidomastoid muscle laterally and the larynx medially, ultimately retracting the carotid sheath and its contents laterally and the thyroid gland and larynx medially. The area of the diverticulum can be promptly recognized arising from the posterior wall of the pharyngo-esophageal junction at a point a little above the level of the omohyoid muscle. The diverticulum is freed to its neck, thus exposing the transverse fibers of the cricopharyngeal muscle bordering the inferior margin of the neck of the diverticulum. A longitudinal incision through the muscle is made, carried down to the mucosa and extended distally onto the esophagus, the length of the incision averaging about 3 cm. After myotomy, the esophageal and cricopharyngeal muscles are dissected from the underlying mucosa for about half the circumference of the mucosal tube to allow the mucosa to protrude freely through the incision. The cervical incision is closed in the usual way without drainage and the patient is allowed free oral feedings and is discharged from the hospital in a few days.

Conclusions

Zenker's diverticulum, long recognized as a cause of upper esophageal dysphagia, is now better understood than ever before. While its etiology remains in dispute, an underlying motility disturbance characterized by incoordination of the upper esophageal sphincter appears to be its most likely cause. Section of the cricopharyngeus muscle should be an integral part of the surgical management of the disease whether or not diverticulectomy is also performed.

References

1. Ludlow, A.: Obstructed deglutition, from a preternatural dilatation of, and bag formed in, the pharynx. Med. Soc. Phys. 3:85, 1762-1767.
2. Zenker, F.A. and von Ziemssen, H.: Krankheiten des Oesophagus. *In* von Ziemssen, H.: Handbuch der Speciellen Pathologie und Therapie, Vol. 1. Leipzig:F.C.W. Vogel, 1875, p. 1.
3. Brunner, H.: X-ray examination of cricopharyngeal sphincter: "Hypopharyngeal bar." J. Laryngol. Otol. 66:276-282, 1952.
4. Lund, W.S.: A study of the cricopharyngeal sphincter in man and in the dog. Ann. R. Coll. Surg. Engl. 37:225-246, 1965.
5. Code, C.F. and Schlegel, J.F.: Motor action of the esophagus and its sphincters. *In* Handbook of Physiology — Alimentary Canal, Section 6, Chapter 90. Bethesda, Maryland:American Physiologic Society, 1967, pp. 1821-1839.
6. Ellis, F.H., Jr.: Upper esophageal sphincter in health and disease. Surg. Clin. North Am. 51:553-565, 1971.
7. Mills, C.P.: Dysphagia in pharyngeal paralysis treated by cricopharyngeal myotomy. Lancet 1:455-457, 1973.
8. Mladick, R.A., Horton, C.E. and Adamson, J.E.: Cricopharyngeal myotomy: Application and technique in major oral-pharyngeal resections. Arch. Surg. 102:1-5, 1971.

9. Kelly, A.B.: Spasm at entrance to oesophagus. J. Laryngol. Otol. 34:285-289, 1919.
10. Lahey, F.H.: Pharyngo-esophageal diverticulum: Its management and complications. Ann. Surg. 124:617-636, 1946.
11. Negus, V.E.: Pharyngeal diverticula: Observations on their evolution and treatment. Br. J. Surg. 38:129-146, 1950.
12. Negus, V.E.: The etiology of pharyngeal diverticula. Bull. Johns Hopkins Hosp. 101:209-223, 1957.
13. Cross, F.S., Johnson, G.F. and Gerein, A.N.: Esophageal diverticula. Associated neuromuscular changes in the esophagus. Arch. Surg. 83:525-533, 1961.
14. Jackson, C. and Shallow, T.A.: Diverticula of oesophagus; pulsion, traction, malignant and congenital. Ann. Surg. 83:1-19, 1926.
15. Asherton, N.: Achalasia of cricopharyngeal sphincter: Record of cases, with profile pharyngograms. J. Laryngol. Otol. 64:747-758, 1950.
16. Sutherland, H.D.: Cricopharyngeal achalasia. J. Thorac. Cardiovasc. Surg. 43:114-126, 1962.
17. Belsey, R.: Functional disease of the esophagus. J. Thorac. Cardiovasc. Surg. 52:164-188, 1966.
18. Ardran, G.M. and Kemp, F.H.: The radiography of the lower lateral food channels. J. Laryngol. Otol. 75:358-370, 1961.
19. Ellis, F.H., Jr., Schlegel, J.F., Lynch, V.P. et al: Cricopharyngeal myotomy for pharyngo-esophageal diverticulum. Ann. Surg. 170:340-349, 1969.
20. Smiley, T.B., Carer, T.B. and Porter, D.C.: Relationship between posterior pharyngeal pouch and hiatus hernia. Thorax 25:725-731, 1970.
21. Stanciu, C. and Bennett, J.R.: Upper esophageal sphincter yield pressure in normal subjects and in patients with gastroesophageal reflux. Thorax 29:459-462, 1974.
22. Goldmann, E.E.: Die zweizeitige Operation von Pulsionsdivertikeln der Speiseröhre. Beitr. Klin. Chir. 61:741, 1909.
23. Lahey, F.H. and Warren, K.W.: Esophageal diverticula. Surg. Gynecol. Obstet. 98:1, 1954.
24. Harrington, S.W.: Pulsion diverticula of the hypopharynx: A review of forty-one cases in which operation was performed and a report of two cases. Surg. Gynecol. Obstet. 69:364, 1939.
25. Welsh, G.F. and Payne, W.S.: The present status of one-stage pharyngo-esophageal diverticulectomy. Surg. Clin. North Am. 53:953-958, 1973.
26. Dohlman, G. and Mattsson, O.: Endoscopic operation for hypopharyngeal diverticula: A roentgencinematographic study. Arch. Otolaryngol. 71:744, 1960.
27. Akl, B.F. and Blakeley, W.R.: Late assessment of results of cricopharyngeal myotomy for cervical dysphagia. Am. J. Surg. 128:818-822, 1974.
28. Hiebert, C.A.: Surgery for cricopharyngeal dysfunction under local anesthesia. Am. J. Surg. 131:423-426, 1976.

Self-Evaluation Quiz

1. Which of the following describes the sites of protrusion of the pharyngeal mucosa in a case of pharyngoesophageal diverticulum?
   a) Between the fibers of the cricopharyngeus muscle
   b) Distal to the cricopharyngeus muscle
   c) Between the oblique fibers of the inferior constrictor muscle of the pharynx and the transverse fibers of the cricopharyngeus muscle
   d) Between the middle and inferior constrictor muscles of the pharynx
   e) Through the longitudinal muscle of the cervical esophagus
2. Which of the following characterizes the motility pattern of a Zenker's diverticulum?
   a) "Spasm" of the upper esophageal sphincter (UES)
   b) Achalasia of the UES
   c) Failure of pharyngeal contraction
   d) Premature contraction of the UES
   e) Motor loss in the body of the esophagus
3. Symptoms of a Zenker's diverticulum may include all of the following except:
   a) Dysphagia
   b) Odynophagia (painful swallowing)
   c) Regurgitation
   d) Aspiration pneumonitis
   e) Noisy deglutition
4. A pharyngoesophageal diverticulum frequently develops in young individuals supporting a congenital origin of the disease.
   a) True
   b) False
5. The primary cause of an upper esophageal pouch is gastroesophageal reflux with secondary spasm of the cricopharyngeus muscle.
   a) True
   b) False
6. The diagnosis of an upper esophageal pouch can be made by roentgenography and endoscopy is not necessary.

a) True
b) False

7. Methods of treatment have included all of the following except:
   a) Invagination of the pouch
   b) Colon bypass
   c) One stage resection
   d) Diverticulopexy
   e) Cricopharyngeal myotomy
8. Cricopharyngeal myotomy alone is successful in treating upper esophageal pouches larger than 5 cm in diameter.
   a) True
   b) False

Answers on page 721.

Achalasia of the Esophagus

F. Henry Ellis, Jr., M.D., Ph.D.

Objectives

The diagnosis of esophageal achalasia is based on the clinical symptoms of obstruction to swallowing in an otherwise healthy individual in the middle age group of 30 to 50 years of age. Roentgenographic and manometric findings are diagnostic and demonstrate lack of peristalsis in the body of the esophagus and distal esophageal obstruction due to failure of the lower esophageal sphincter to relax.

Treatment may be by forceful dilation or by esophagomyotomy. The latter procedure is preferred because it produces lasting relief of symptoms in over 90% of patients with minimal complications and should be performed early in the course of the disease.

Introduction

Esophageal achalasia is a disease of unknown etiology characterized by absence of peristalsis in the body of the esophagus, failure of the lower esophageal sphincter (LES) to relax in response to swallowing and a higher than normal resting LES pressure. While the development of sophisticated manometric techniques was required to elucidate the details of the abnormal motility pattern of this disease, the term "achalasia" preceded these developments. It was first used in 1913 by Sir Cooper Perry at the request of Sir Arthur Hurst [1] who was searching for a word to describe his concept of the disorder. Thus, failure of relaxation of achalasia describes only one aspect of this disorder, for the term fails to describe the motility

---

F. Henry Ellis, Jr., M.D., Ph.D., Chairman, Department of Thoracic and Cardiovascular Surgery, Lahey Clinic Foundation and New England Deaconess Hospital; Associate Clinical Professor of Surgery, Harvard Medical School, Boston, Mass.

abnormality in the body of the esophagus and the elevated resting LES pressure.

Pathogenesis

Many etiologic theories have been advanced over the years, but it is now generally agreed that achalasia has a neurogenic basis. Degenerative changes and a reduction in number of the ganglion cells of Auerbach's plexus were first described by Rake [2] in 1926 in a presumed case of esophageal achalasia. Similar observations have been reported by many others since then. One of the more detailed studies was that of Cassella and associates [3] who conducted ganglion cell counts on the postmortem esophagi of nine patients with achalasia and compared them with the counts from 45 specimens of patients who died from nonesophageal causes. They found that alterations in ganglion cells are usually, but not always, present in the esophagi of patients with esophageal achalasia, a finding others have also noted.

The inconsistency in ganglion cell changes led Cassella and associates [3, 4] to postulate an extraesophageal neurogenic basis for the disease, and they included in their study an examination of the vagus nerve and of its central nuclei. Consistent ultrastructural changes were found in biopsy specimens of branches of the vagus nerve taken at the time of esophagomyotomy from patients with achalasia while no such changes were seen in similar specimens from patients without esophageal disease. The study of Kimura [5] was confirmed by the finding of a nearly 50% bilateral reduction in neurones from the dorsal motor nucleus of the vagus nerve of two patients with achalasia as compared to cell counts from the same region of an individual whose death was not related to esophageal disease.

These pathologic findings are consistent with the concept of a central origin of the disease perhaps by a neurotropic virus with primary involvement of the dorsal motor nucleus of the vagus nerve with secondary degeneration of the vagus and transynaptic degeneration of the ganglion cells of Auerbach's plexus. However, not all would agree that transynaptic degeneration can occur. Nonetheless, support for the concept has recently been provided by Lise and associates [6] who included histochemical techniques in their studies. Smith [7] suggested that a neurotropic virus of marked specificity may be involved, attacking both the neurones in the brain and in the esophagcal wall traveling along the vagi between these two points.

There is other evidence for an extraesophageal site of denervation in achalasia. In vitro [8] and in vivo [9] studies using cholinesterase inhibitor have shown a normal response of the sphincter indicating local release of acetylcholine, which supports preganglionic and not postganglionic denervation. The recent finding of supersensitivity of the lower sphincter to endogenous and exogenous gastrin provides further suggestive evidence in favor of denervation [10]. If the vagus nerve is involved in the disease, one might expect to find other evidences of vagal nerve dysfunction, and such is indeed the case. Woolam and associates [11] demonstrated abnormal vagal nerve function in 14 of 32 patients with achalasia as evidenced by negative or abnormal results with Hollander tests and by reduction of maximal gastric acid response to betazole (histalog). These abnormalities in gastric secretions have been confirmed by others [12, 13].

Clinical Features

Symptomatology

Whatever the cause of the disease may be, its clinical manifestations are well recognized. Obstruction to swallowing is the most common and usually the earliest symptom of esophageal achalasia. It occurs in nearly all patients, and while it may be intermittent in the early phase of the disease, it soon becomes constant. Regurgitation is the second most common symptom, occurring in 70% of patients, being particularly noticeable in some patients during sleep. Nocturnal regurgitation may give rise to respiratory symptoms. In fact, chronic cough and repeated pulmonary infections are occasionally the presenting symptoms of patients with esophageal achalasia. Andersen and colleagues [14] found that aspiration pneumonitis was by far the most common respiratory complication of achalasia. Others included lung abscess, bronchiectasis and pulmonary fibrosis.

Pain is infrequent, occurring in little more than a fourth of the cases. When present, it is usually an early symptom, and it may be difficult in such patients to distinguish this symptom from the pain of diffuse esophageal spasm. The pain is usually located substernally, but may be epigastric and not infrequently is referred to the neck and occasionally to the back, shoulders or arms. Ultimately, with long-standing achalasia of the esophagus, loss of weight almost invariably occurs. The incidence of carcinoma of the esophagus in untreated cases is seven times as high as in the normal population [15].

Differential Diagnosis

Diffuse spasm of the esophagus. It is important that esophageal achalasia be differentiated from diffuse esophageal spasm, for they are different diseases. The differentiation is most difficult during the early stages of achalasia when pain may be a prominent feature. Clinical and radiographic findings at this stage may not differentiate the two. Patients who present features of both achalasia and diffuse spasm have been designated as having vigorous achalasia on the basis of manometric studies that demonstrate simultaneous deglutitive contractions of considerable amplitude, but never as massive or high peaked or prolonged as in diffuse spasm [16]. Sphincteric relaxation is rarely seen whereas the sphincter relaxes normally in diffuse spasm.

Tumors and strictures. Before esophageal dilatation has become marked, distal esophageal obstruction, whether by tumor or stricture, can give rise to clinical and radiographic features indistinguishable from esophageal achalasia. In such cases, endoscopic examination of the distal esophagus is essential before making a diagnosis of esophageal achalasia. Manometry provides final confirmation.

Organic obstructive lesions are rarely capable of producing the degree of esophageal dilation seen in long-standing cases of esophageal achalasia. An exception is the fibrolipoma, which usually arises in the upper part of the esophagus and presents as an elongated intraluminal mass [17]. It may reach a large size so as to distend the esophagus markedly. Radiographically, the distended esophagus may appear to contain ingested food and secretions, and endoscopy may be confusing because the mucosa overlying the tumor is intact.

Chagas disease. Chagas is a disease indistinguishable from esophageal achalasia as seen in the rest of the world. It is encountered in South America, particularly in Brazil and Chile, where it has been recognized for some time. Infestation by Trypanasomi cruzi organisms may result in "mega-esophagus" as well as megacolon, megaduodenum and mega-ureter [18, 19]. The complement fixation test for Chagas disease is usually positive in these patients. Not only have the ganglion cells of Auerbach's plexus been shown to be destroyed in such cases, but also esophageal motility studies have revealed the characteristic pattern of esophageal achalasia [20].

Miscellaneous. There are a number of unclassified esophageal motor disorders that may simulate achalasia [21]. While such patients resemble those with achalasia, in some respects they exhibit evidence of normal motor function of the esophagus. Perhaps they represent incomplete forms of the disease. Occasionally, vagotomy will reproduce a syndrome similar to esophageal achalasia [22, 23]. In a study of 15 patients with postvagotomy dysphagia, Andersen and associates [22] found five with roentgenographic and manometric findings similar to those of achalasia. A similar mechanism may be involved in the few instances of malignant involvement of the vagus nerve resulting in esophageal achalasia [24].

Diagnosis

While careful attention to the patient's symptoms may suggest a diagnosis of esophageal achalasia, a definitive diagnosis rests primarily on two diagnostic techniques, radiography and esophageal manometry, endoscopy being of chief value in excluding an organic lesion at the esophagogastric junction.

Roentgenologic Manifestations

Although occasionally the existence of esophageal achalasia may be suggested by the findings on a plain thoracic roentgenogram, particularly in the advanced stages of the disease, fluoroscopic observation of swallowed contrast medium is of decisive importance in the diagnosis. All the observed changes reflect two basic abnormalities — the absence of organized peristaltic contractions throughout the body of the esophagus and failure of the lower esophageal sphincter to relax in response to swallowing. These two abnormalities combined lead to retention and ultimately to dilatation of the esophagus, which may conveniently be classified into three stages: mild, moderate and severe (Fig. 1).

Esophageal Manometry

While the diagnosis of esophageal achalasia can usually be made with some competence by roentgenographic techniques in the advanced stages of the disease, this is not so easily done when the disease is mild and of short duration. It is in this stage of the disease that the use of esophageal manometry is of special use to confirm the diagnosis. It was originally stated that the resting pressures at the gastroesophageal sphincter in most patients with achalasia were the same as those in health [25]. The findings supporting this statement were based on studies using balloon-covered transducers and open-tipped, nonperfused catheters. The recent introduction of constantly perfused catheters has demonstrated that there indeed is "spasm" in cardiospasm, for the resting pressures at the lower sphincter have been found by these techniques to be elevated to two or more times the level found in normal individuals [26]. This elevated sphincteric pressure has been related to supersensitivity of the lower sphincter to endogenous gastrin in patients with achalasia. In the body of the esophagus, resting pressures are generally elevated over that of fundic pressure due to dilatation and retention, while pressures in the upper sphincter are usually in the normal range.

Abnormal function of the LES is responsible for the patient's symptoms. The upper segment of the sphincter nearly always fails to relax with swallowing. Relaxation often does occur with swallowing in the lower portion of the sphincter though the relaxation is of limited duration, being terminated by a premature restoration of tone (Fig. 2). In addition to failure of relaxation of the upper portion of the sphincter, premature contraction is observed in this region early in the deglutition sequence. All of these abnormalities combined limit the period during which the esophagus may empty to a few seconds. Thus, both relaxation and contraction of the achalasic sphincter are abnormal.

There is no peristalsis in the body of the esophagus in patients with achalasia (Fig. 2). Swallowing is followed by

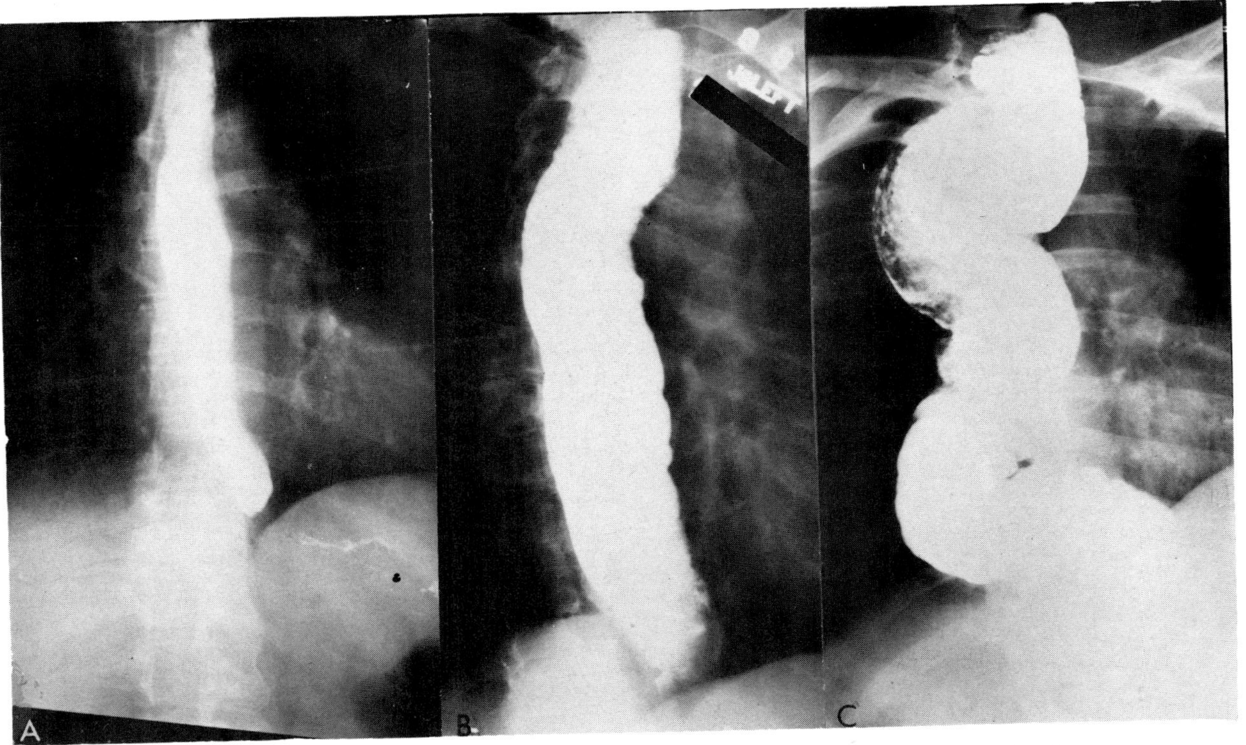

FIG. 1. Roentgenographic appearance of three stages of achalasia: A, mild; B, moderate; C, severe.

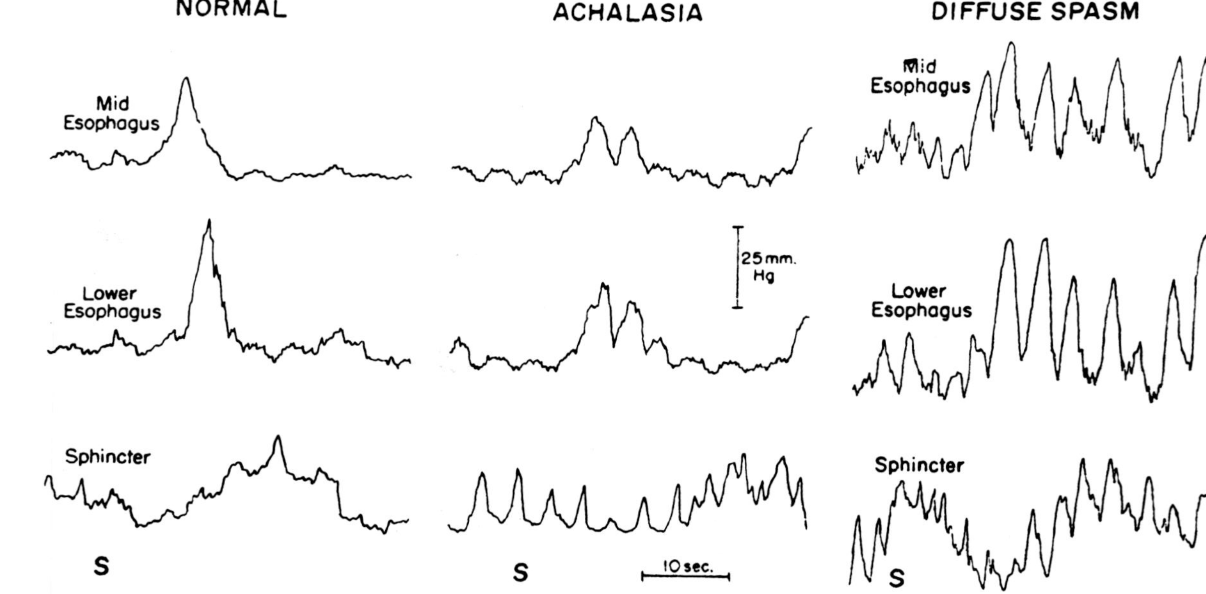

FIG. 2. Response to deglutition in the esophagus and LES of a healthy person (*left*), a patient with achalasia (*middle*) and a patient with diffuse spasm of the esophagus (*right*). Note lack of peristalsis in the esophagus and failure of adequate relaxation of the sphincter in the patient with achalasia. (S = swallow.)

modest elevations of pressure, which are simultaneous throughout the organ. Their amplitude is usually less than in health, and in advanced achalasia it may be difficult to detect any response to swallowing at all, the esophagus being completely paralyzed. As indicated earlier, the term "vigorous achalasia" has been applied to patients who have an abnormal achalasic pattern of contractions, but in whom the strength of the contraction is equal to or exceeds that seen in health. These contractions are nearly always repetitive [16].

Treatment

In the past, medical efforts to relieve the symptoms of patients with achalasia by reducing or eliminating the distal esophageal obstruction have been unsuccessful. Pharmacologic agents may be developed in the future that will be effective in reducing or eliminating the hypersensitivity of the achalasic sphincter to gastrin and thus relieve the distal esophageal obstruction. Current therapeutic efforts are designed to weaken the sphincter by mechanical or surgical methods.

Forceful Dilation

The use of dilation in the treatment of esophageal achalasia is as old as the history of the disease itself. While simple bougienage continued to enjoy favor for many years, it is not currently a preferred method of therapy because its effects are evanescent. Only by employing forceful dilation, which can effectively disrupt the distal esophageal musculature, is it possible to relieve permanently the patient's symptoms of dysphagia. A variety of methods of accomplishing forceful dilation are available, including mechanical [27], pneumatic [28] and hydrostatic dilators [29]. The results seem to be comparable regardless of the instrument used, provided the procedure is technically successful.

The technique of hydrostatic dilatation, as first proposed by Plummer [30], is illustrated in Figure 3. Sanderson and associates [29] have reported the results of treatment using this technique. Follow-up data were available for 313 patients who had had this treatment, the mean follow-up period being 9½ years. Nearly 20% of the patients required repeated treatments. Eighty-one percent of the patients were improved, 65% having

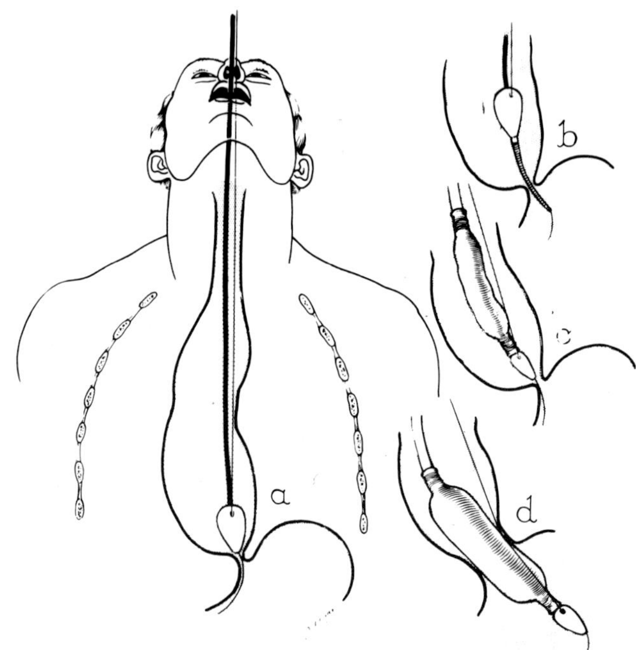

FIG. 3. Method of performing dilations. A, Passage of no. 41 French, olive-tipped bougie to stomach. B, Sound (50 or 60 French) guided by a flexible wire spiral is passed into stomach. C, Hydrostatic dilator is passed to cardia. D, Distention of hydrostatic dilator across cardia. (From Olsen, A.M., Harrington, S.W., Moersch, H.J., et al: J. Thorac. Cardiovasc. Surg. 22:168, 1951.)

excellent or good results while 16% had only fair results. Poor results were noted in 19% of the patients. Although there were no deaths in this series, 5% experienced significant complications. Ten patients required surgical intervention for rupture of the distal part of the esophagus. The other patients with complications who did not require operation in all likelihood had esophageal rupture of minor degrees and were treated successfully with antibiotics and intravenous fluids.

Forceful dilation, therefore, is a valuable form of therapy for esophageal achalasia, but it is not without complications and often must be repeated to be effective. Since the results of surgical treatment with a modified Heller myotomy have proved to be superior, it should be the treatment of choice for this disease in all but patients in whom operation is contraindicated.

Surgical Treatment

The surgical treatment of esophageal achalasia is basically a 20th century development, having been initiated by Mikulicz who reported performing retrograde dilation of the esophago-gastric junction through a gastrostomy in 1903 [31]. Since then, a variety of other surgical techniques have been proposed. Those involving surgical destruction of the esophagogastric junction [32-34] became extremely popular for a number of years until it was shown by Barrett and Franklin [35] that severe reflux esophagitis almost invariably developed thereafter. Fortunately, operations of this type are rarely performed for symptomatic achalasia.

Modern surgery for the disease was first initiated on April 14, 1913, when Heller [36] performed a double cardio-myotomy on a 49-year-old woman who had suffered from dysphagia for approximately 30 years. This technique later underwent many modifications, the most important of which was restriction of the procedure to one myotomy [37]. It gradually became the treatment of choice, first on the Continent and later in Great Britain. Surgeons in the United States were slow to adopt it, and not until the late 1940s did they use it to any great extent. Even today in the United States there are some who prefer forceful dilation as the primary form of treatment in this disease. The results of a properly performed esophagomyotomy as outlined later indicate why operation is preferable to dilation.

Technique of esophagomyotomy. Since the results of surgery are so closely dependent upon the technique of its performance, particularly as regards the avoidance of postoperative reflux esophagitis, the method described by Ellis and associates [38] in 1967 will be presented in some detail.

A thoracotomy is the preferred approach, for it provides the most direct access to the distal esophagus. An incision through the bed of the nonresected eighth rib has proved satisfactory. The mediastinal pleura is opened, the inferior pulmonary ligament is divided and the lung is retracted cephalad. The esophagus is then carefully mobilized and encircled with a Penrose drain (Fig. 4A). In so doing, the vagi must be preserved carefully. The esophagus is then gently elevated by the encircling Penrose drain so that the esophagogastric junction is

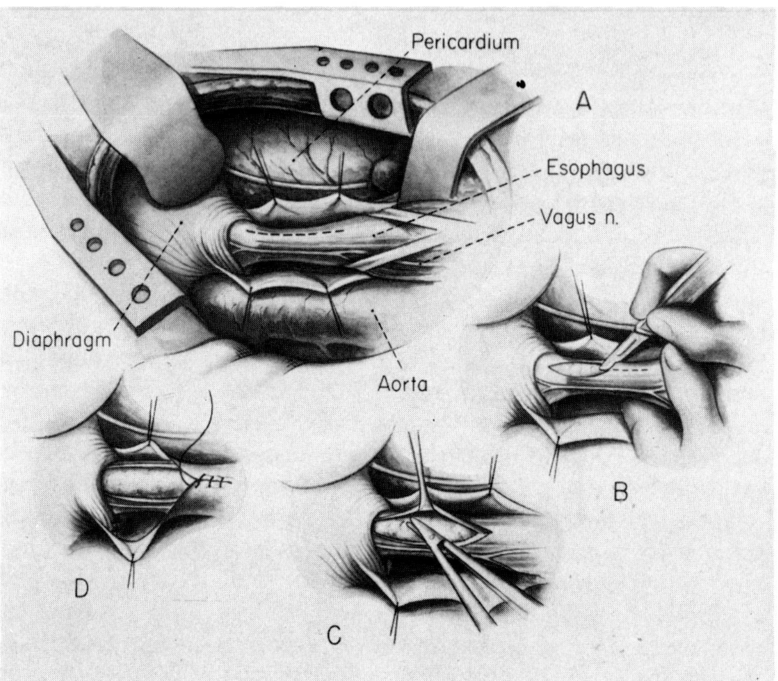

FIG. 4. Transthoracic exposure of distal esophagus for esophagomyotomy. A, The esophagus has been mobilized and elevated from its bed by a Penrose drain. The intended line of incision is indicated by the dotted line. B, Beginning the incision. C, Dissection of mucosa from muscularis. D, Restoration of esophagogastric junction to intra-abdominal position with suture narrowing of esophageal hiatus if necessary. (From Ellis et al [38].)

delivered for a short distance into the chest without necessitating division of any of the hiatal attachments to the esophagogastric junction. Any deliberate incisions into the diaphragm or the phreno-esophageal membrane are avoided.

With the esophagus under tension and compressed by the supporting fingers of the left hand, a longitudinal myotomy is begun on the left anterolateral surface of the esophagus (Fig. 4B). The incision is deepened through the encircling muscles of the lower end of the esophagus down to the mucosa and is then extended distally just across the esophagogastric junction to insure complete division of the distal esophageal musculature. External identification of the esophagogastric junction is difficult, but the presence of a few small veins traversing the organ serves as a reasonably satisfactory landmark and helps to identify the stomach margin. The incision through the gastric musculature is limited to less than 1 cm and usually only a few millimeters in length. The incision is then extended proximally over the dilated thick walled portion of the esophagus. The proximal extension of the incision insures total division of the circular muscle in the area of the obstruction and nothing more. The incision then varies in length depending upon the anatomic circumstances of the particular patient, but it is usually between 5 and 8 cm long.

After the myotomy is completed, the muscle wall is dissected laterally from the mucosa so that approximately half or more of the circumference of the esophageal mucosa is freed, permitting it to pout freely through the incision (Fig. 4C). This maneuver is performed to minimize the possibility of reapproximation of the incised esophageal wall by scar in the postoperative period. Concomitant fundoplication of either the Nissen or Belsey type is currently widely advocated to avoid postoperative reflux [39, 40]. If the myotomy is properly done, these ancillary maneuvers are unnecessary and may lead to postoperative obstruction particularly if a complete wrap is done.

When the incision has been completed, the esophagus is allowed to return to its position in the mediastinum, which restores the esophagogastric junction to its normal intra-abdominal position. Rarely, a small diaphragmatic hernia coexists and should be repaired concurrently. If the operative manipulations have inadvertently disturbed the supporting structures of the esophagogastric junction, normal anatomy should be restored by fixing the esophagogastric junction in position with interrupted sutures and the phreno-esophageal membrane by narrowing the hiatus by suture approximation of the diaphragmatic crus posteriorly (Fig. 4D). The mediastinal pleura is then closed, and the thoracic incision is closed in layers with catheter drainage in the usual fashion.

Oral fluids may be permitted the night of operation if mucosal integrity has not been impaired, and a normal diet is resumed as rapidly as possible. The drainage tube is removed on the day after operation, and the patient should be ready for dismissal five or six days after operation.

Results. An analysis of the results of esophagomyotomy done without antireflux surgery as reported in the literature from 1968 to 1978 is presented in Table 1. Only reports involving a sizable number of carefully followed cases were included. It revealed that 84% of patients were improved even when all patients lost to follow-up were considered as failures of treatment.

A short summary of my own experience lends support to the view that this operation is the preferred method of treatment. There was only one death among the 368 operations performed at the Mayo Clinic between 1950 and 1970 and none in an additional 58 cases operated on at the Lahey Clinic between 1970 and 1978. The results in 256 of the early cases available for follow-up were analyzed in detail during a follow-up period of 1 to 17½ years, averaging 5½ years [42]. Ninety-four percent of the patients experienced definite improvement; only 6% had poor results. Poor results were due to a number of avoidable factors, including postoperative hiatal hernia and operation on patients with marked esophageal

Table 1. Esophagomyotomy for Esophageal Achalasia 1968-1978

		Improved		*Unimproved*		
Author	*Total*	*No.*	*Per-cent*	*No.*	*Hospital Deaths*	*Lost*
Tala et al [41]	43	32	74	3	0	8
Ellis and Olsen [42]	269	240	89	16	1	12
Lortat-Jacob and Fekete [43]	345	286	83	2	7	50
Rapant and Kralik [44]	129	122	95	7	0	0
Rees et al [45]	59	43	73	9	0	7
Lagache et al [46]	48	42	88	1	3	2
Grimes et al [47]	50	47	94	3	0	0
Borgeskov and Nilsson [48]	52	43	83	9	0	0
Akuamoa [49]	101	74	73	11	0	16
Barker and Franklin [50]	30	28	93	2	0	0
Effler et al [51]	100	90	90	5	0	5
Wingfield and Karwowski [52]	27	20	74	5	0	2
Maillet et al [53]	72	70	96	2	0	0
Black et al [54]	108	71	66	37	0	0
Pinotti et al [55]	118	112	95	6	0	0
Chaib et al [56]	200	152	76	48	0	0
Total	1751	1972	84	166 (9.4%)	11 (.07%)	102 (6%)

fibrosis resulting from multiple previous dilations and rehealing of the myotomy. Reflux esophagitis as an isolated event followed esophagomyotomy in only 3 of 256 cases (1.1%). This is in contrast to other reports with incidences varying as high as 40% [40, 57]. Results in 53 of 58 patients recently undergoing esophagomyotomy and evaluated 6 to 97 months (average, 42 months) postoperatively confirm these findings. Fifty patients (94.3%) were improved by surgery, and only one (1.8%) had significant reflux. It is suggested that the surgical technique described may be partly responsible for this low incidence. Postoperative manometry supports this view, for the findings are strikingly consistent, including a reduction in length of the sphincteric zone and abolition of its suprahiatal portion. The subhiatal segment of increased pressure is partially retained, and this undoubtedly accounts for the fact that reflux is so rarely a problem [38]. While postoperative esophageal roentgenography is of interest, persistent esophageal dilation does not necessarily imply a poor result. Approximately 75% of patients will show a reduction in esophageal caliber after operation but it does not necessarily return to normal.

Indications for Esophagomyotomy

Some consider resorting to surgery only after failure of forceful dilation. Others believe it to be ineffective in the late stages of the disease in the presence of a large, dilated, tortuous, sigmoid-shaped esophagus; we have been advised by still others to avoid its use early in the disease, reserving its application to patients in the later stages. In my experience, esophagomyotomy has had a high success rate nearly independent of age, sex, previous treatment, duration of symptoms and stage of disease. It has produced good results even in advanced stages of so-called megaesophagus, though to be sure the results in such cases are more likely to be good than excellent because the atonic esophageal sac must drain by gravity in the absence of effective esophageal contractions. Operation at an earlier stage of the disease would seem preferable, for there were no failures among patients whose disease was classified as mild. Because of the excellence of the results, esophagomyotomy should now be considered the primary treatment of choice for the symptomatic patient with esophageal achalasia and should be performed early in the course of the disease.

References

1. Hertz, A.F.: The bismuth meal. Br. Med. J. 1:13, 1913.
2. Rake, G.W.: Annular muscular hypertrophy of the oesophagus: Achalasia of the cardia without oesophageal dilation. Guys Hosp. Rep. 76:145-152, 1926.
3. Cassella, R.R., Brown, A.L., Jr., Sayre, G.P. et al: Achalasia of the esophagus: Pathologic and etiologic considerations. Ann. Surg. 160:474-487, 1964.
4. Cassella, R.R., Ellis, F.H., Jr. and Brown, A.L., Jr.: Fine-structure changes in achalasia of the esophagus. I. Vagus nerves. Am. J. Pathol. 46:279-288, 1965.
5. Kimura, K.: The nature of idiopathic esophagus dilation. Jpn. J. Gastroenterol. 1:199-207, 1929.
6. Lise, M., Perrino, G., Cordioli, G.P. and Cagol, P.P.: The autonomic nervous system in esophageal achalasia. Chir. Gastroenterol. 6:103-110, 1972.
7. Smith, B.: The neurological lesion in achalasia of the cardia. Gut 11:388-391, 1970.
8. Misiewicz, J.J., Walter, S.L., Anthony, P.P. et al: Achalasia of the cardia: Pharmacology and histopathology of isolated cardiac sphincteric muscle from patients with and without achalasia. Q. J. Med. 38:17-30, 1969.
9. Cohen, S., Fischer, R. and Tuch, A.: The site of denervation in achalasia. Gut 13:556-558, 1972.
10. Cohen, S., Lipshutz, W. and Hughes, W.: Role of gastrin supersensitivity in the pathogenesis of lower esophageal sphincter hypertension in achalasia. J. Clin. Invest. 50:1241-1247, 1971.
11. Woolam, G.L., Maher, F.T. and Ellis, F.H., Jr.: Vagal nerve function in achalasia of the esophagus. Surg. Forum 18:362-365, 1967.
12. Iordanskaia, N.I.: (Functional disorders of the vagus nerves in cardiospasm.) Vestn. Khir. 88:24-28, 1962.
13. Reding, R., Petermann, J. and Rosenbaum, K.D.: Die Prüfung der Erregungsleitung der Nn. vagi bei der Achalasia cardiae durch den Hollandertest. Chirurg. 39:3510-3513, 1968.
14. Andersen, H.A., Holman, C.B. and Olsen, A.M.: Pulmonary complications of cardiospasm. JAMA 151:608-612, 1953.
15. Wychulis, A.R., Woolam, G.L., Anderson, H.A. et al: Achalasia and carcinoma of the esophagus. JAMA 215:1638-1641, 1971.
16. Sanderson, D.R., Ellis, F.H., Jr., Schlegel, J.F. et al: Syndrome of vigorous achalasia: Clinical and physiologic observations. Dis. Chest 52:508-517, 1967.
17. Bernatz, P.E., Smith, J.L., Ellis, F.H., Jr. and Andersen, H.A.: Benign, pedunculated, intraluminal tumors of the esophagus. J. Thorac. Cardiovasc. Surg. 35:503-512, 1958.
18. Köberle, F.: Enteromegaly and cardiomegaly in Chagas disease. Gut 4:399-405, 1963.

19. Atias, A., Neghme, A., Aguirre MacKay, L. and Jarpa, S.: Megaesophagus, megacolon and Chagas' disease in Chile. Gastroenterology 44:433-437, 1963.
20. Pinotti, H.W.: Contribuicao para o estudo da fisiopatologia do megaesofago. Thesis, University of Sao Paulo, Brazil, 1964.
21. Hogan, W.J., Caflisch, C.R. and Winship, D.H.: Unclassified oesophageal motor disorders simulating achalasia. Gut 10:234-240, 1969.
22. Andersen, H.A., Schlegel, J.F. and Olsen, A.M.: Postvagotomy dysphagia. Gastrointest. Endosc. 12:13-18, 1966.
23. Dahm, K.: Le cardiospasm: Une complication rare après vagotomie sélective. Acta Gastroenterol. Belg. 31:883-888, 1968.
24. Kolodny, M., Schrader, Z.R., Rubin, W. et al: Esophageal achalasia probably due to gastric carcinoma. Ann. Intern. Med. 69:569-573, 1968.
25. Butin, J.W., Olsen, A.M., Moersch, H.J. and Code, C.F.: A study of esophageal pressures in normal persons and patients with cardiospasm. Gastroenterology 23:278-293, 1953.
26. Cohen, B.R. and Guelrud, M.: "Cardiospasm" in achalasia: Demonstration of supersensitivity of the lower esophageal sphincter. Gastroenterology 60:769, 1971.
27. Schindler, R.: Observations on cardiospasm and its treatment by brusque dilatation. Ann. Intern. Med. 45:207-215, 1956.
28. Vantrappen, G., Hellemans, J., Deloof, W. et al: Treatment of achalasia with pneumatic dilatations. Gut 12:268-275, 1971.
29. Sanderson, D.R., Ellis, F.H., Jr. and Olsen, A.M.: Achalasia of the esophagus: Results of therapy by dilation, 1950-1967. Chest 58:116-121, 1970.
30. Plummer, H.S.: Cardiospasm with report of cases. Minn. State Med. Assoc. Northwestern Lancet 26:419-424, 1906.
31. von Mickulicz, J.: Small contributions to the surgery of the intestinal tract. 1. Cardiospasm and its treatment. 2. Peptic ulcer of the jejunum. 3. Operative treatment of severe forms of invagination of the intestine. 4. Operation on malignant growths of the large intestine. Boston Med. Surg. J. 148:608-611, 1903.
32. Wendel, W.: Zur Chirurgie des Oesophagus. Arch. Klin. Chir. 93:311-329, 1910.
33. Heyrovsky, H.: Casuistik und Therapie der idiopathischen Dilatation der Speiseröhre: Oesophagogastroanastomose. Arch. Klin. Chir. 100:703-715, 1913.
34. Backer-Gröndahl, N.: Cardiaplastik ved Cardiospasmus. Forhandlingar vid Nordise Kirurgisk Forenings 11:236-242, 1916.
35. Barrett, N.R. and Franklin, R.H.: Concerning unfavourable late results of certain operations performed in treatment of cardiospasm. Br. J. Surg. 37:194-202, 1949.
36. Heller, E.: Extramuköse Cardiaplastik beim chronischen Cardiospasmus mit Dilatation des Oesophagus. Mitt. Grenzgeb. Med. Chir. 27:141-149, 1913.
37. De Brune-Groenveldt, J.R.: Over cardiospasmus. Ned. Tijdschr. Geneeskd. 54 (Sect. 2):1281-1282, 1918.

38. Ellis, F.H., Jr., Kiser, J.C., Schlegel, J.F. et al: Esophagomyotomy for esophageal achalasia: Experimental, clinical and manometric aspects. Ann. Surg. 166:640-656, 1967.
39. Peyton, M.D., Greenfield, L.J. and Elkins, R.C.: Combined myotomy and hiatal herniorrhaphy: A new approach to achalasia. Am. J. Surg. 128:786-790, 1974.
40. Monsour, K.A., Symbas, P.H., Jones, E.L. et al: A combined surgical approach in the management of achalasia of the esophagus. Am. Surg. 42:192, 1976.
41. Tala, P., Luosto, R. and Mamies, T.: Achalasia cardiae. Ann. Chir. Gynaecol. Fenn. 57:281-286, 1968.
42. Ellis, F.H., Jr. and Olsen, A.M.: Achalasia of the esophagus. Philadelphia:W.B. Saunders Co., 1969, p. 196.
43. Lortat-Jacob, J.L. and Fekete, F.: Traitement chirurgical du méga-oesophage idiopathique. Aropos de 345 interventions chirurgicales. Actual. Hepatogastroent. 5:A197-214, 1969.
44. Rapant, V. and Králik, J.: Die Problematik der Therapie der Achalasie der Speiseröhre. Bruns Beitr. Klin. Chir. 218:12-22, 1970.
45. Rees, J.R., Thorbjarnarson, B. and Barnes, W.H.: Achalasia: Results of operation in 84 patients. Ann. Surg. 171:195-201, 1970.
46. Lagache, G., Combemale, B. and el-Hassan, S.: Une statistique de 53 opérations de Heller pour mégaoesophage idiopathique. Lille Med. 15:647-651, 1970.
47. Grimes, O.F., Stephens, H.B. and Margulis, A.R.: Achalasia of the esophagus. Am. J. Surg. 120:198-202, 1970.
48. Borgeskov, S. and Nilsson, T.: A follow-up study with pH pressure measurements in patients treated for cardiospasm by Heller's operation. Scand. J. Thorac. Cardiovasc. Surg. 4:83-86, 1970.
49. Akuamoa, G.: Achalasia oesophagi. Results of the Heller operation. Acta Chir. Scand. 137:782-788, 1971.
50. Barker, J.R. and Franklin, R.H.: Heller's operation for achalasia of the cardia. A study of the early and late results. Br. J. Surg. 58:466-468, 1971.
51. Effler, D.B., Loop, F.D., Groves, L.K. et al: Primary surgical treatment for esophageal achalasia. Surg. Gynecol. Obstet. 132:1057-1063, 1971.
52. Wingfield, H.V. and Karwowski, A.: The treatment of achalasia by cardiomyotomy. Br. J. Surg. 59:281-284, 1972.
53. Maillet, P., Micol, P., Parasal, J.P. et al: Les resultats du traitement chirurgical du megaoesophage (72 observations). Ann. de Chirurgica 27:579-586, 1973.
54. Black, J., Vorbach, A.N. and Collis, J.L.: Results of Heller's operation for achalasia of the oesophagus. The importance of hiatal repair. Br. J. Surg. 63:949-953, 1976.
55. Pinotti, H.W., Ellenbogen, G., Rodrigues, J.G. et al: Surgical treatment of the megaesophagus. Chir. Gastroent. 11:7-14, 1977.
56. Chaib, S.A., Lopasso, F.P., Parra, O.M. et al: Tratamento do megaesofogo pela tecnica de Heller-Vasconcelos. Experiencia de 200 casos. Rev. Hosp. Clin. Fac. Med. Sao Paulo 32:178-183, 1977.

57. Jekler, J., Lhotka, J. and Borek, Z.: Surgery for achalasia of the esophagus. Ann. Surg. 160:793-800, 1964.

Self-Evaluation Quiz

1. Which of the following symptoms is *not* a feature of esophageal achalasia?
   a) Dysphagia
   b) Regurgitation
   c) Aspiration
   d) Heartburn
   e) Weight loss
2. Pathologic findings in this disease include all but which of the following:
   a) Esophageal dilatation
   b) Loss of cells in Auerbach's plexus
   c) Electron microscopic changes in the vagus trunk
   d) Fibrous stricture of distal esophagus
   e) Loss of cells from dorsal motor nucleus of vagus
3. Which of the following is the most definitive in diagnosing achalasia?
   a) Endoscopy
   b) Roentgenography
   c) Esophageal manometry
   d) Cinefluorography
   e) History
4. Which of the following is *not* a feature of the motility pattern of esophageal achalasia?
   a) Lack of peristalsis in body of esophagus
   b) Elevated resting pressures at LES
   c) Abnormality of function of cricopharyngeal sphincter
   d) Resting pressures in body of esophagus are higher than fundic pressure
   e) Failure of relaxation of LES
5. The LES in patients with esophageal achalasia is hypersensitive to gastrin.
   a) True
   b) False
6. Simple bougienage is a satisfactory form of therapy for achalasia.

a) True
b) False

7. Cardioplasty should never be used to treat achalasia because it leads to reflux esophagitis.
   a) True
   b) False
8. A properly performed esophagomyotomy (modified Heller's procedure) includes all but which of the following maneuvers?
   a) Transthoracic approach
   b) Performance of an antireflux operation
   c) Short myotomy of distal 5 to 6 cm of esophagus with minimal extension into stomach
   d) Preservation of vagus nerves
   e) Esophageal hiatus is not incised

Answers on page 721.

Chemical Injury to the Esophagus

Robert W. Anderson, M.D.

Objectives

1. To differentiate corrosive chemical injuries caused by liquids versus solids.
2. To enumerate differences in the pathology of burns of the esophagus.
3. To note cautions to be observed in diagnosis and to consider the possibility of long-term sequelae.

Introduction

Chemical injury to the esophagus is an uncommon but serious problem that usually results from either the accidental or suicidal ingestion of a caustic substance or acid. Due to the widespread use by certain socioeconomic groups of household lye as an ingredient in homemade soap or cleaning agents, this caustic is often easily available to children. The unfortunate habit of storing it in used soft drink bottles has contributed to the frequency of accidental injuries in children. Prior to 1965, most lye injuries were the result of the ingestion of household lye in the form of flakes or solid pellets, and the most common result was burns of the oropharyngeal area and upper digestive tract. Late sequelae were usually related to the development of segmental strictures in the esophagus, which occurred in 10% to 25% of patients who ingested the material.

Since 1965, liquid and solid drain cleaners which contain highly concentrated forms of either sodium or potassium hydroxide have been produced commercially. The liquid agents produce a far more extensive esophageal injury and may also

Robert W. Anderson, M.D., Associate Professor of Surgery, University of Minnesota Medical School, Minneapolis.

damage the stomach. There has been legislation in the form of the Federal Hazardous Substance Act which has modified the concentration of the liquid corrosives and also required child-proof packaging. Nonetheless, there are still numerous reports of accidental ingestion of substances such as Draino, Liquid-Plumr, or Easy-Off. There have also been numerous instances reported of caustic injury to the esophagus by Clinitest tablets which are alkaline-reducing agents used to test for sugar content in the urine of diabetics. Household bleaches contain sodium hydroxide, but the concentration is low enough that serious injury to the esophagus following ingestion is quite uncommon. Acid from batteries or in other forms is another agent responsible for corrosive injuries to the esophagus. Highly concentrated solutions of household ammonia are known to produce serious injuries. Chemical injury has been reported following the ingestion of miscellaneous substances with a high concentration of potassium, ascorbic acid, chloral hydrate, nonphosphate detergents and various chemotherapeutic agents. We have recently treated several patients who developed severe acute chemical injuries to the esophagus following oral chemotherapy for malignancy. In most instances these patients had been treated with mediastinal radiation therapy several years earlier; it may be that the irradiated esophagus is particularly susceptible to chemical injury, and it is possible that the incidence of such injuries will rise as chemotherapy becomes more aggressive and survival improves in treated patients.

It is unfortunate that most corrosive esophageal injuries will occur in children and the majority are seen in patients younger than the age of 5 [1]. Those injuries which are seen in adults are frequently the result of suicide attempts, although there have been reports of caustic injury of the upper gastrointestinal tract as the result of ingesting illegal whiskey to which lye has been added to produce the taste of a higher alcohol content [2], and alcoholics often mistake caustic liquids for alcoholic beverages. Although the incidence of corrosive esophageal injuries in children has decreased in the past decade, approximately 5,000 per year occur in children under the age of 5. It is unfortunate that these injuries ever occur since they are all totally preventable. Increasing publicity and education could conceivably eliminate the problem.

Pathology of Corrosive Injury

The histologic changes in the esophagus following corrosive injury will depend upon the nature, concentration and amount of the agent swallowed. Injuries of the esophagus due to chemical burns may be classified in a manner similar to that used to describe thermal burns of the skin [3]. A minimal or first degree burn involves only the superficial mucosa and results in superficial mucosal hyperemia, mucosal edema and superficial sloughing. Second degree burns involve all layers of the esophagus with exudate, superficial ulceration, loss of mucosa and erosion transmucosally into the periesophageal tissues. Third degree burns involve the entire esophageal wall and have eroded through the esophagus into the periesophageal tissues, including the mediastinum and the pleural or peritoneal cavity. The third degree type of injury frequently results in acute systemic illness and shock, and those who survive develop numerous complications including abscesses and the formation of fistulae.

The pathology of corrosive esophagitis has been described extensively in previous publications [4-7]. Solid alkalis tend to adhere to the oropharynx and esophagus and produce injuries in these areas, whereas, liquid alkalis and acids have a high specific gravity and therefore tend to pass rapidly through the esophagus and enter the stomach. The liquid caustics induce severe pylorospasm upon entering the stomach and result in violent regurgitation of material and a continuing exposure of both the stomach and the esophagus to the caustic. For these reasons most patients who ingest granular forms of lye have segmental injuries which are confined to the esophagus, whereas, those who are exposed to liquid caustics usually have damage to the entire esophagus and 10% to 30% sustain damage to the stomach which may lead to late fibrosis or symptoms of gastric outlet obstruction [8].

Acid ingestion may occur accidentally in children, but is also a frequently used method in attempted suicide by adults. Most often, tissue damage rather than death is the result. Acid ingestion causes a coagulative necrosis of the surface epithelium of the stomach and usually spares or only minimally damages the esophagus, since the rapidly occurring superficial coagulation that occurs during transit of the acid through the esophagus prevents deeper penetration of the tissue. The pathology produced by acid ingestion is modified by the amount of food or liquid in the stomach at the time of exposure, the amount and concentration of the acid and the contact time with the gastric mucosa. Severe full thickness injury with perforation of the stomach and peritonitis is not uncommon with acid injuries, may occur with liquid alkali, but is uncommon with solid alkali. Conversely, esophageal perforation with mediastinitis is most often the result of liquid or solid alkali ingestion and is rare following acid injury.

Clinical Management of Corrosive Injuries

The first step in the management of any patient with suspected chemical injury of the esophagus is to confirm whether ingestion has taken place and to identify the ingested agent. In some instances this may be a relatively simple matter, but in the case of a young child or depressed adult who is found in the proximity of a container of some potentially injurious agent, this may not be an easy matter to resolve. The patient who has ingested a corrosive agent may have minimal or no symptoms, may complain of severe pain related to oral burns, may experience dysphagia and an inability to swallow secretions, or may present in shock because of esophageal or gastric perforation with secondary mediastinitis or peritonitis.

All patients in whom a chemical injury of the esophagus is suspected should be admitted to the hospital for evaluation, be allowed to ingest nothing by mouth and have intravenous fluids started. Further management should be guided by the extent of injury demonstrated and by the patient's clinical course.

Careful examination of the lips, tongue, buccal and pharyngeal mucosa must be correlated with the history and may provide sufficient evidence to document chemical ingestion. Severe burns of the oral passage may be associated with hoarseness, stridor or dyspnea which suggest either associated laryngeal edema or actual epiglottic and laryngeal damage due to aspiration of the corrosive agent. Such patients may require immediate intubation or tracheostomy for respiratory support and must be carefully observed for respiratory dysfunction.

Patients who ingest liquid alkali, acids or large amounts of solid caustic agents may present with severe substernal, back or abdominal pain. The presence of these symptoms or the presence of shock or abdominal rigidity is indicative of mediastinal or peritoneal extension. Because of the high mortality observed with such injuries, recent reports have stressed the importance of early exploratory surgery as both a diagnostic and therapeutic tool [8, 9]. If necrosis of the stomach or stomach and esophagus is found, a resection should be performed and reconstruction carried out at a later date.

All patients in whom esophageal injury is suspected should be esophagoscoped shortly after admission unless there is evidence of perforation or severe laryngeal edema which precludes safe passage of the instrument. Esophagoscopy is done solely for diagnosis and since the injured esophagus is quite weak and friable, no attempt should be made to pass the instrument beyond the site where injury is first observed in order to avert perforation. The severity of the injury can be well assessed endoscopically and we have relied on this method to guide further therapy.

Patients with oral burns have approximately a 50% incidence of esophageal injury, conversely, the absence of oral burns does not preclude esophageal injury and every patient in whom there is suspicion of chemical ingestion should be evaluated endoscopically.

Patients in whom no evidence of esophageal injury is noted endoscopically should be observed for a brief period of time and have a radiologic examination of the esophagus as an outpatient in about two weeks to be sure that no injury was missed and that there is no evidence of stricture formation.

The classification of esophageal burns into "superficial," "intermediate" or "deep," depending upon the degree of penetration of the caustic liquid, is important since it determines the late changes associated with the healing process which results in subsequent stricture formation.

Any patient who is documented to have an esophageal burn by endoscopy is at risk for developing a stricture and the early treatment of these patients is aimed at the prevention of this complication. The treatment consists of intravenous fluid therapy, broad spectrum antibiotics, sedation and steroids. Both experimental [10] and clinical [11-13] work has confirmed the efficacy of adequate steroid and antibiotic therapy in reducing the incidence of late complications related to corrosive injury of the esophagus.

Radiologic study of the esophagus during the acute stage is of limited value unless perforation is suspected, in which case it is indicated. After 48 hours the characteristic features of injury most frequently observed are gaseous dilatation of the esophagus due to air trapping and intramural retention of the contrast material [14]. Additional radiologic findings that may be observed are blurring of the mucosal margins, linear streaking and abnormal displacement of the pleural reflection. The stomach and duodenum should also be evaluated at 48 hours for evidence of injury.

After the acute reaction has subsided, usually two weeks following injury, serial barium contrast studies are necessary to demonstrate the presence or absence of stricture. This study should be repeated at three-month intervals if any suspicion exists as to the continued progression of the injury or at any time that symptoms of dysphagia develop.

Any patient in whom ulcerating lesions of the esophagus develop following corrosive injury is at risk for developing a stricture, and ulcerations will almost invariably progress to stricture. Earlier forms of management recommended the institution of bougienage early after chemical injury, but the ability of antibiotics and steroids to modify healing has decreased the incidence of stricture formation. In a collected series of reports since 1960 by Postlethwait, totaling 2109 patients, 28.9% had ulcerative esophagitis and of these 17.9% developed a stricture [15].

Early dilatation of patients who are administered steroids as part of their treatment is contraindicated because of the impaired healing and weakness in the esophagus. There is also evidence to suggest that dilatation during the early stages of chemical injury may intensify the damage to the esophagus. The approach advocated by Haller et al [12] appears to be logical. If evidence of stricturing appears, the steroid should be tapered and dilatation begun. In children or uncooperative adults, the safest form of chronic dilatation appears to be the use of retrograde Tucker-type dilators which are guided by a string placed through a previously performed gastrostomy. If an adequate lumen can be obtained by this method, the gastrostomy and string can be removed and patency of the lumen maintained by antegrade dilatations. For minimal stricturing in cooperative patients the use of antegrade dilatations may be acceptable from the outset.

The length of time that the surgeon should persist in dilation before a more radical method of treatment should be considered must be carefully individualized. The indications for surgical intervention for stricture formation that we have observed are those advocated by Cardona and Daly [13] and include the development of complete stenosis of the esophagus, marked irregularity of pocketing on barium swallow, the development of fistula or perforation, postdilatation inflammatory reaction characterized by recurrent fever or pain, or the inability to maintain a lumen which will support the patient's nutritional requirements. Repetitive dilatation may become an onerous task for both the patient and the physician if it is required at frequent intervals. On occasions the use of intralesional steroid therapy has been recommended to soften localized strictures and to permit more effective dilation, but long diffuse strictures are probably best managed surgically.

The decreasing morbidity and mortality after reconstructive surgical procedures has caused most surgeons to be more liberal in recommending reconstructive procedures rather than persisting in dilation if a satisfactory result does not appear forthcoming. In the Duke University series 16% of patients required surgery within two years following the initial injury [15].

The choice of operation cannot be stated dogmatically and several equally satisfactory procedures are currently used. Local resection of short strictures has been performed in a number of instances, but generally this has not been successful due to the fact that the extent of damage to the wall of the esophagus is greater than can be appreciated and the anastomosis is invariably performed in a diseased area. The currently employed operations utilize the stomach, jejunum or colon as an esophageal substitute. The arguments favoring one or the other organs in the various locations are stated with equal fervor by their various proponents. The proponents of the jejunum or colon transplant feel that the viable tube-like structure more nearly approximates the normal esophagus and permits reconstruction with decreased morbidity and mortality. The stomach remains in place, thereby retaining its normal function with regard to capacity and digestion. Because of occasional difficulties which were encountered with impaired nutrition and slow emptying following stomach transplantation by the transthoracic route, my personal preference is either the use of the right or left colon substernally or a gastric tube, if the stomach is suitable. The colon has been utilized in preference to the jejunum because it is felt that one can more regularly obtain a segment with a better blood supply when the colon is used.

One question which remains unanswered is whether the damaged esophagus should be removed. If the esophagus is left in place, complications due to secretions or infection in the segment might occur and also the possibility of carcinoma arising on the basis of injured tissue must be considered. It is widely acknowledged that patients with corrosive injuries to the esophagus are at higher risk to develop esophageal cancer [15] and those in whom the esophagus is in place, whether functional or nonfunctional, must be carefully observed for many years since the reported latency period is between 20 and 40 years [16]. It appears prudent to remove the injured esophagus unless extensive periesophagitis has caused dense adherence to contiguous vital structures which increases the surgical risk of the procedure.

References

1. Leape, L.L., Ashcraft, K.W., Scarpelli, D.G. and Holder, T.M.: Hazard to health — liquid lye. N. Engl. J. Med. 284:578, 1971.
2. Kiviranta, U.K.: Liquor adulterated with lye as a cause of dysphagia and stricture of the esophagus. N. Engl. J. Med. 234:220, 1950.
3. Hollinger, P.H.: Management of esophageal lesions caused by chemical burns. Ann. Otol. Rhinol. Laryngol. 77:819, 1968.
4. Jackovich, L.: Essay on the histo-pathology of lye poisonings (Bietrage zur Histo-Pathologie der Laugen-vergiftungen). Dtsch. Z. Ges. Gerichtl. Med. 16:352, 1931.
5. Stumboff, A.V.: Chemical burns of the oral cavity and esophagus. Arch. Otolaryngol. 52:419, 1950.
6. Kirsh, M.M. and Ritter, F.: Caustic ingestion and subsequent damage to the oropharyngeal and digestive passages. Ann. Thorac. Surg. 21:74, 1976.

7. Dafoe, C.S. and Ross, C.A.: Acute corrosive oesophagitis. Thorax 24:291, 1969.
8. Gryboski, W., Page, R. and Rush, B.F., Jr.: Management of total gastric necrosis following lye ingestion. Ann. Surg. 161469, 1965.
9. Gago, O., Ritter, F.N., Martel, W. et al: Aggressive surgical treatment for caustic injury of the esophagus and stomach. Ann. Thorac. Surg. 13:243, 1972.
10. Weisskopf, A.: Effects of cortisone on experimental lye burn of the esophagus. Ann. Otol. Rhinol. Laryngol. 61:681, 1952.
11. Viscomi, G.J., Beekhuis, G.J. and Whitten, C.F.: An evaluation of early esophagoscopy and corticosteroid therapy in the management of corrosive injury of the esophagus. J. Pediatr. 59:356, 1961.
12. Haller, J.A., Jr., Andrews, H.G., White, J.J. et al: Pathology and management of acute corrosive burns of the esophagus: Results of treatment in 285 children. J. Pediatr. Surg. 6:578, 1971.
13. Cardona, J.C. and Daly, J.F.: Current management of corrosive esophagitis: An evaluation of results in 239 cases. Ann. Otol. 80:521, 1971.
14. Martel, W.: Radiologic features of esophagogastritis secondary to extremely caustic agent. Radiology 103:31, 1972.
15. Postlethwait, R.W.: Chemical burns of the esophagus. *In* Surgery of the Esophagus. Charles C Thomas & Co. (In press).
16. Kiviranta, U.K.: Corrosion carcinoma of the esophagus; 381 cases of corrosion and 9 cases of corrosion carcinoma. Acta Otolaryngol. 4289, 1952.

Self-Evaluation Quiz

1. Segmental strictures in the esophagus due to corrosives occur in ______ of victims:
   a) 5% – 15%
   b) 10% – 25%
   c) 15% – 35%
   d) 12% – 16%
2. Most corrosive esophageal injuries occur in victims under 5 years of age.
   a) True
   b) False
3. First degree esophageal burns involve:
   a) Hyperemia, and edema and sloughing
   b) Abscesses
   c) Shock
   d) Fistulae
4. Victims who ingest liquid alkali, acids or large amounts of solid caustic agents may experience severe substernal, back or abdominal pain.

a) True
b) False

5. The author's preference is to use the right or left colon substernally, or else use a:
   a) Gastric tube
   b) Jejunum
   c) Synthetic tube
   d) None of the above
6. Clinitest tablets:
   a) Are always harmless
   b) React dangerously with sugar water
   c) Can locate strictures
   d) Can be corrosive
7. Corrosive injuries can be associated with:
   a) Clinitest tablets
   b) Ascorbic acid
   c) Susceptibility of irradiated mediastinal tissue
   d) All of the above
   e) None of the above
8. Solid alkalis do not tend to adhere to the oropharynx and esophagus.
   a) True
   b) False

Answers on page 721.

Discussion

Moderator: Richard L. Varco, M.D.

Moderator: Dr. Feinberg, I have inquiries from the audience about whether you routinely recommend use of the CAT scanner for people who are thought to have an esophageal lesion, perhaps malignant. Can you comment briefly on how you decide when to use it and when you do not?

Dr. Feinberg: The experience with CAT scan and the low volume of carcinoma of the esophagus makes it probably statistically not too valid yet. But I think it is probably the best noninvasive approach to gross delineation of extension of the esophageal lesion into the mediastinum with the least trauma to the patient. It should help the surgeon in early lesions and certainly the radiotherapist in planning. Even though I do not spend too great a percentage of my time on CAT, I have been trying to sell it to our staff.

Moderator: We do not want to dwell too long on this, but let us take a case of carcinoma of the esophagus with perforation, not a free perforation, but a contained one, and there is an associated inflammatory reaction. How does the scanner distinguish between tumor and inflammatory reaction?

Dr. Feinberg: It merely gives you the extent. So it does not distinguish between the two.

Moderator: Dr. Spiro, there are a number of questions here centering around several issues which relate to drug therapy in the management of esophagitis. You mentioned Gaviscon, but you did not talk much about it. Would you also please relate any experience that you have regarding the need to interrupt cimetidine therapy. If you do interrupt it, do you expect rebound of acid production? Do you do anything when you get rebound?

Dr. Spiro: Let us take those questions one at a time. Just like a surgeon: too much, too fast, too often!

Let me take the Gaviscon issue. Gaviscon, for anybody who does not know, is a drug that is a combination of agents which supposedly bubble up into the esophagus to protect the mucosa. It has enormous patient acceptance at the present time. There are several physiological studies to suggest that it is as good as an antacid. There are none to suggest it is better than antacid. Tom Hendrix, at Johns Hopkins, feels that it is a very useful drug. Dr. Bennett in Great Britain is certainly one of the physicians who has also commented that it is a useful drug. Since I regard most therapy of the upper GI tract as largely either sacramental or placebo in nature, I would say that Gaviscon, if you watch out for the amount of sodium in it, is as good as anything else at the present time. My wife says it makes an excellent mouthwash too because it bubbles in your mouth!

Turning to cimetidine, at the moment there is no statistical evidence that cimetidine or Tagamet is clearly useful in the patient with reflux esophagitis although some quasianecdotal series from Europe suggest that it is in fact useful. A most recent study showed that oral cimetidine in reflux esophagitis improved (1) the histological features of esophagitis and (2) the endoscopic features of esophagitis, but did not change the response to the Bernstein test. It was no different from the placebo in terms of symptom response. What one can say is this: Tagamet makes the esophagoscopist feel better when he looks down the patient's throat but the patient with reflux esophagitis does not necessarily feel any better. We keep coming back to this issue of who we are trying to make feel better, the patient or the physician!

How much acid or symptomatic rebound there is we do not know. In duodenal ulcer, it is reasonable to wean the patient off cimetidine, but I am not yet sure what we should be doing for reflux esophagitis after the approved period of six to eight weeks which the Food & Drug Administration gives us for duodenal ulcer. I simply express a clinical prejudice that says one should use cimetidine in the patient with refractory reflux esophagitis, particularly at bedtime, but I cannot prove it at the moment.

Moderator: I have a number of questions that relate to different methods which attempt, by operative means, to prevent reflux. I would like to lump them, by asking several of the panel members — Dr. Ellis, Dr. Skinner, Dr. Woodward, and Dr. Humphrey — please pick the particular antireflux operation you prefer and give us a brief but workable set of directions for doing that operation. Several members of the audience have asked how long a segment of the esophagus is brought into the Nissen. Does it make any difference if you have some of it above or below the diaphragm? So I would like each of you to pick one operation and tell us briefly why it is your favorite and a brief description of the salient features of the operation. Let us begin with Dr. Ellis.

Dr. Ellis: I have been using the Nissen fundoplication now for about ten years and for several reasons: First, it is the most successful operation, in terms of raising sphincter pressure. There is experimental evidence that supports its superior antireflux capabilities, in contrast to the Hill operation which is really just a modified fundoplication, and the Belsey procedure, which is a 260 degree wrap instead of a 360 degree wrap. I have not encountered "gas bloat" problems to the extent that Dr. Woodward has, probably because we do the fundoplication over a 38 or a 40 French Maloney dilator.

How long a segment of the esophagus should be wrapped? I think this is important and it probably explains the fact that this procedure is more successful than the Hill procedure, because it wraps more of the esophagus. In the experimental laboratory we found that, if you wrap a segment of the esophagus similar in length to the length of the normal high pressure zone, you achieve the best results. Anything more does no good and may lead to more obstructive symptoms or difficulties in belching and anything less leads to a higher incidence of gastroesophageal reflux. So a wrap that includes a length of esophagus comparable to the high pressure zone, which is about 3 or 4 cm in length, is ideal.

The advantages of the Nissen fundoplication are that you can leave the fundoplication in the chest and, provided the hiatus is widened to prevent obstruction at that level, equally good results in terms of the antireflux properties are achieved. I am not obsessed, as Dr. Skinner is, with the necessity for an intraabdominal segment of the esophagus. If it were so important, then every patient with a sliding hernia would reflux, which of course they do not do.

Moderator: Dr. Skinner, would you comment?

Dr. Skinner: We have been evaluating the Nissen, Belsey and Hill operations to get some comparative results. I shall talk about the Belsey, since Dr. Ellis has discussed the Nissen. I think the key with any of these repairs is getting the esophagus mobilized sufficiently so that you can restore an intraabdominal segment. The Belsey procedure is a transthoracic operation. We select it, particularly in patients with recurrences, because we believe that inadequate mobilization is a principal cause of recurrence in people with severe esophagitis, where dissection of the mediastinum from the abdominal approach may be difficult, and in obese patients where exposure is difficult. Otherwise, we would use the transabdominal approach. Once the esophagus is fully mobilized, the placement of the sutures between the stomach and esophagus and in the second row, diaphragm, stomach and esophagus is critical. Particularly important is the bite in the muscle of the esophagus. This is clearly the weak point in the Belsey operation, since the esophageal muscle does not hold sutures well. There is no collagen there to grasp hold. As we looked at a large series of patients we have followed for ten years or longer, most of the recurrences clearly came from the esophageal sutures tearing out. This operation does give 85% documented success rate at ten years. At the present time, there are no ten-year comparative data available for the other types of repairs, so I do not think at this time we can say which is the best repair in the long run. These operations each employ similar principles.

Just a comment about Dr. Ellis' intrathoracic Nissen: If you widen the hiatus, so that the stomach is not indented by the hiatus as it goes up through, then the wrap is still intraabdominal. In other words, when the abdominal pressure rises, it is transmitted through the cavity of the stomach to the intragastric wrap of esophagus. I believe the same principle still applies, that it is a small tube entering a large pouch, where the transmission of raised intraabdominal pressure can be applied equally both to the swallowing tube and to the gastric pouch. I think the principle is still consistent. We do not like the intrathoracic Nissen because of the incidence of gastric ulcers, perforation and bleeding that have been seen with it.

Moderator: Dr. Woodward, would you please comment?

Dr. Woodward: We use the Belsey repair only when we do not have enough stomach left from a previous subtotal gastrectomy to do a good Nissen fundoplication. We use the Nissen about three to one over the Hill, because in the complicated case, the results are clearly better. Since the other two operations have been discussed, I shall promote the Hill. We are extremely pleased with the results in intractable but otherwise uncomplicated cases of reflux esophagitis. The operation is exceedingly well tolerated by the patient. Using the Upper Hand Retractor, which I am sure Dr. Goligher will enlarge upon, the exposure of the perihiatal area is absolutely outstanding. Although technically more demanding for the surgeon, the operation is certainly exceedingly well tolerated by the patient. I do not see why all the big fuss is made about locating the median arcuate ligament. It is very easy to expose. Dr. Hill does it the hard way. He locates it from below, starting at the celiac axis. We do it the easy way. We come from above through the V that forms as the crura approach the aortic hiatus. I think the key to the operation is getting adequate bites of both the posterior and the anterior layers of the structures that are on the lesser curvature and at the esophagogastric junction. This is a combination of coiled up phrenoesophageal membrane and hepatogastric ligament. Using this method, we have been able to get as good an elevation of pressure as with the Nissen fundoplication, provided that we are not dealing with a Barrett's esophagus or an acquired short esophagus.

Moderator: As I understand it, Dr. Woodward, the results that you get with the Hill procedure in the more complicated cases are better than the results you are getting with the Nissen, is that correct?

Dr. Woodward: Are you talking about the patient with advanced esophagitis?

Moderator: No, I am not talking about that. Let me put it in a different way: Was there a difference in your failure rate between the two, that favored one or the other?

Dr. Woodward: Yes, in the complicated case, the failure rate was initially much lower with the Nissen. We agree with Dr. Ellis that leaving the repair above the diaphragm leaves one with a fully functional sphincter action.

Moderator: Dr. Humphrey, would you comment?

Dr. Humphrey: We are using the Nissen almost routinely now. For a period of three years, we used a combination of the Hill and Belsey repairs. Dr. Eisenberg said the only thing we did not do was to drive a stick through the stomach. However, we found that we had a 15% recurrence rate in those three years. The reason that these Belsey repairs failed is, as Dr. Skinner said, that the sutures pulled out of the esophageal muscle. I should not imply, however, that the Nissen is without problems and without failures. Each year brings us an additional number of so-called slipped Nissens, in which the stomach moves up into the chest through the wrap around. This has been a particular problem in patients who gain a great deal of weight after repair. Because of this, I have started putting sutures in both the right and the left part of the esophagus when doing the repair. Whether or not that will help, I do not know yet. But it may slow down the movement of the stomach up through the rent.

Moderator: Dr. Spiro, when do you send a patient to a surgeon for management of reflux esophagitis?

Dr. Spiro: We published a paper in *The New England Journal of Medicine* about three years ago that pleased the surgeons very much. I wish I had the data with me here today so I could tell you about the follow-up four or five years down the line. It is important to recognize that we were dealing with United States veterans because veterans are a different population from most other people; Dr. Woodward is laughing at that. It is true that you must have a little calcification in the pancreas to get into our Veterans Administration Hospital. But in that group of patients we found that if they had grade three or four esophagitis, and they went through what I would call a modified Belsey repair, three quarters of the patients three years later were very satisfied with their operations and had done very well. Only about one fifth of the patients who had been treated medically did very well in that same period of time. Now, as a gastroenterologist, who is a member of the union, I have to say there is one thing wrong with that study: the patients were originally selected as medical failures to begin with. Therefore, using the kind of standard therapy that we had available back then, we had already cast the die against medical therapy because they were failures. In that sense, I now recommend surgery for patients who have intractable strictures. But I think much of the data about when you operate on strictures, when you resect them, etc., is a little uncertain. I was very happy to hear Dr. Skinner say that many strictures should be dilated. Certainly, patients who have intractable esophagitis who have to live upright lives or who do not respond to cimetidine deserve operation.

The remarkable thing is, however, that we do not send ten patients a year for hiatus herniorrhaphy. Most gastroenterologists tend to wonder why the surgeons are always seeing these patients and we are not. So the long answer to the question is that patients with refractory symptoms with recurrent trouble who do not respond to medication deserve operation. Our study needs reproduction in a non-veteran setting, simply to find out whether the data are as good and as impressive as our Veterans Administration study suggests.

Moderator: Dr. Levitt, I have two questions and I would like to combine your answers. First, with regard to using hyperalimentation in individuals, even when they can take a modest but not a high caloric volume by mouth, in the course of receiving radiation therapy for carcinoma of the esophagus, what is your practice at the present time? Second, I would like you to comment on the statistics presented by Dr. Skinner with regard to the apparently more favorable results currently being obtained with surgical management of carcinoma of the esophagus, as contrasted with radiation. Would you please comment on those two questions?

Dr. Levitt: We have not personally handled any patients with carcinoma of the esophagus with hyperalimentation. We have in most instances been able to keep the patients reasonably well nourished and in reasonably good condition with routine radiotherapy and with symptomatic treatment. I think it is an interesting approach, though, and it might be something to consider in patients who are extremely debilitated prior to instituting radiotherapy.

Moderator: Do you ever have to stop or to interrupt their therapy because of impaired nutrition?

Dr. Levitt: It is very infrequent. I might point out, and I am not trying to contrast this with anybody else, that we treat our patients in a different manner from many other institutions. We watch patients very closely. Our daily doses are usually somewhat lower. The patients have in my experience tolerated treatment better. We do not treat everybody with 200 rads a day, come hell or high water. Most of our patients are treated with 150 to 175 rads per day and they are watched closely. If they are having problems, we will treat them symptomatically. If they become quite ill, then we stop treatment. But usually if you will titrate your treatment this way and observe your patients closely, if they are in good condition when you start, then you are going to do all right.

The other side of that coin is that one has to select patients who are going to be appropriate candidates for radiotherapy, just as one does for surgery. I do not think one should treat every patient who is sent to you regardless of his condition. So I think patients have to be in reasonable condition in order to tolerate therapy.

If I may, to answer a comment that Dr. Skinner made, I want to make it very clear that I did not say that patients with tracheoesophageal fistulas should not be treated. I think they should not be treated with radiation therapy. Anybody who wants to operate on a patient with a tracheoesophageal fistula with whatever palliative procedure is contemplated, I think that is fine. But I do not think these patients are candidates for radiation therapy.

Dr. Spiro: I am surprised that none of the speakers who talked about cancer of the esophagus mentioned bougienage during radiation. This is something we have been doing for the past several years and it seems to me that it does prevent the scarring that one runs into after the radiation is over. Do you have any comments about that?

Dr. Levitt: No, I really do not. A situation we do not like is to have patients being treated with bougienage during radiation therapy treatment.

Dr. Spiro: That is all right. Our radiation therapy people thought so, too. Since we have started doing it, there does not seem to be any problem.

Dr. Levitt: How many patients have you treated in this way?

Dr. Spiro: I do not have the figures with me today.

Dr. Levitt: All treatments, when you begin, are outstanding except that when we go along we find out they are not quite that good. I personally believe you are looking for trouble to use bougienage in a patient who is getting radiation therapy, with all the trauma that is going on in that area. However, I am certainly open to suggestion and would be most interested in the results.

The next question was, Why is Dr. Skinner reporting such good results with surgery, in contrast to the figures I gave?

There are probably a number of reasons for that. First, the results that Dr. Skinner reported are really not any better than those that are reported from centers where there are large numbers of patients treated with radiation that are comparable to patients treated with surgery. Second, I do not know what the selection was in his choice of patients for the surgical procedure. But I am sure there was some selection and that these are the most capable candidates because that is usually the situation one finds when a patient is being treated surgically. If you look at any series that compares radiation to surgery, if you look at it very closely you will find patients treated with surgery are usually surgical candidates. They are in better condition. The lesions are smaller and so forth. Other than that, I cannot explain why the radiation therapy at the University of Chicago was not as effective as it might be any more than I could explain why the surgery in a series reported by Dr. Pearson was worse than radiation therapy. I guess that is an individual situation.

Moderator: Dr. Ellis, a member of the audience would like some additional comments from you on the management of the Zenker's diverticulum, specifically, when would you operate upon an individual? On the diagnosis alone or does the individual have to be symptomatic? After the individual is operated upon, when can he start on clear liquids? When can he start a general diet?

Dr. Ellis: I think the patient should have symptoms before having surgery. I am not apt to see a patient unless he is referred because of upper esophageal dysphagia which leads to an x-ray which shows a pouch. The size of the pouch really does not determine whether or not he should be operated upon. Once the diagnosis is made, I think he should have surgery, not only to relieve symptoms but also to prevent the pouch from getting larger and to avoid the complications, which are primarily those of aspiration.

To answer the second question, if one does just a cricopharyngeal myotomy, the patient can eat the evening of the same day. If a diverticulectomy is done, oral feedings are delayed for a few days, although I am not really sure it is necessary because he is swallowing saliva all the time. By custom I guess we tend to avoid all liquids and solids for a few days if we have a suture line in the GI tract. One of the advantages of doing a myotomy is that patients can be fed immediately and can be out of the hospital in a few days.

May I say a word or two about the radiation problem, because I have always been concerned about the data frequently quoted, Pearson's data. Every discussion always brings up his data and as far as I know he is the only radiotherapist in the world who ever achieved those types of results. No one seems to quite understand why. Certainly, our radiotherapists do not understand why. In talking to him, and in looking over the data, I think there are some clues which I would like to air to get reactions from the rest of the group.

In the first place, he does not note in any of his articles the fact that less than half of the patients who enter the protocol ever complete it and therefore are not even included in the final statistics. He is also comparing his results with those of Andrew Logan, who in those days had a 25% or 30% surgical mortality. All of those cases are included in the end results of the surgical treatment. So I think there is a difference in the composition of the surgical and radiotherapy groups that are being compared. I would like to hear the opinions of the others on this. Is there any evidence, other than Pearson's, that x-ray therapy alone can produce such good results? Am I right in assuming there is a bizarre case selection which skews the results?

Dr. Levitt: I think, in all fairness to Dr. Pearson, if you read his articles carefully, he does point out that he feels the difference in survival is due to morbidity at surgery rather than to superiority of the method and that the cases that he reports are those cases that are selected for a radical procedure. If you will read his latest article, you will see that the patients whom he reports on, both for surgery and radiotherapy, are those that are selected for radical treatment. I do not think anybody has that many patients to report in the literature, because most patients with carcinoma of the esophagus are treated with surgery. Again, these are the selected patients, these are the best patients, these are the most favorable patients, with the smallest lesion and in the best condition. So unless you get into a place like England, Edinburgh or some of the Scandinavian countries, you will not find them, not in this country, that is for sure.

Moderator: I have a series of questions for Dr. Spiro. Why did you come down on the side of liquid antacids rather than tablet form, because it is easier to carry tablets rather than a bottle around.

Dr. Spiro: Liquids have been shown in most studies, probably not double-blind, to be more symptomatically effective than tablets. Empirically, one finds that the patients who take Tums, Rolaids or the equivalent just do not seem to have the same kind of relief as with liquids.

Moderator: Dr. Woodward, this question relates to the recent publicity about placing a collar of plastic about the esophagus as a means of preventing migration of the stomach into the chest as well as reflux esophagitis. Would you comment about the general procedure?

Dr. Woodward: I think this question arises from an exhibit at the college meeting in Dallas last fall. Of course, I just shudder at the thought of a solid foreign body being placed next to a hollow viscus, because the hollow viscus does not like it. I would expect there would be a fair number of fistulas as a result. I would think it would be a disastrous approach. Second, in order to function properly, the esophagogastric junction has to have pliability and flexibility. A completely solid and inflexible foreign body is certainly not going to be conducive to this end. I just do not think it has any place at all in the surgical therapy of reflux esophagitis.

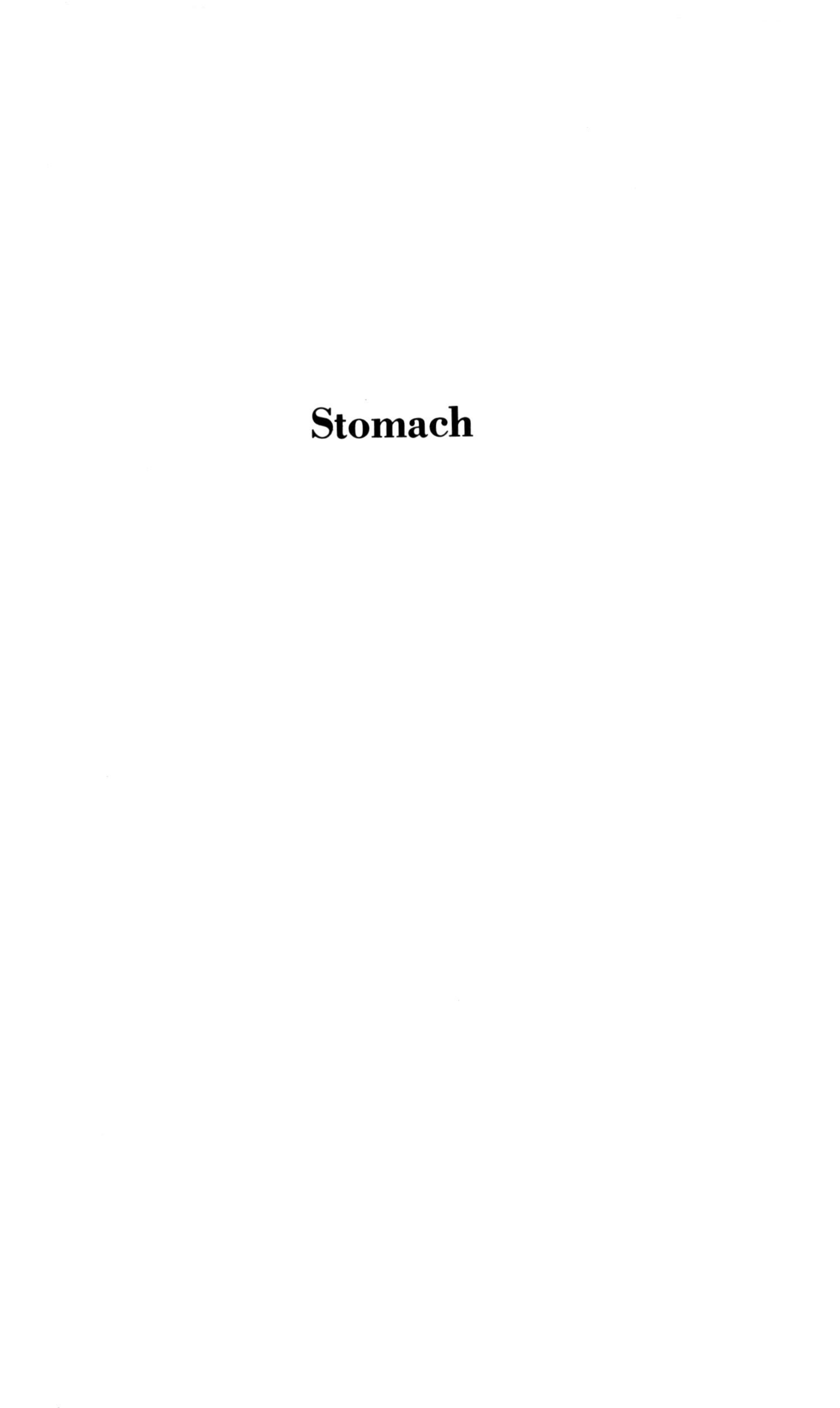

Stomach

Role of Gastrointestinal Hormones in Gastric Secretion

James C. Thompson, M.D.

Objectives

At the conclusion of this paper the reader will be able to identify the experimenters who advanced the theories of the role of hormones in gastric secretion; the mechanisms that control gastric secretion; the properties and actions of gastrin, acetylcholine and secretin; the agents that suppress acid secretion from any form of gastric secretory stimulation; and eight new candidate hormones.

Introduction

The entire field of endocrinology began in one sense on the afternoon of January 16, 1902, when Bayliss and Starling demonstrated that the introduction of hydrochloric acid into a denervated loop of small intestine elicited the brisk secretion of pancreatic juice. Unlike most such discoveries, the two principals, Bayliss and Starling, understood the significance of this observation immediately. They suggested that some unidentified blood-borne chemical messenger was released from the acidified intestine to mediate this response. Starling, in fact, coined the very word "hormone," which is from a Greek word that means to set in motion, spur on, arouse to activity.

Three years later, in 1905, J.S. Edkins, working at St. Bartholomew's Hospital in London, prepared extracts of antral mucosa which, when injected into cats, stimulated gastric secretion. Edkins called this activity "gastrin" and he reported his findings in the *Proceedings of the Royal Society*. This

James C. Thompson, M.D., Professor and Chairman, Department of Surgery, The University of Texas Medical Branch, Galveston.

immediately launched a long and bitter dispute which centered about whether or not the active material from the antrum was a new hormone or whether it was histamine. We now know that the basis for this dispute is one of Nature's dire tricks, that is, the antral mucosa contains large amounts of both agents.

The man who put us back on the right track was Simon Komorov, who was one of Pavlov's last students. Komorov came to Montreal to work with Babkin at McGill University and later came to Philadelphia to work with Harry Shay at Temple University. Komorov decided that gastrin was probably a polypeptide, as was secretin, and that it should be studied by methods applicable to polypeptide chemistry. Komorov described the isolation of a crude gastrin preparation in the *Revue Canadienne de Biologie* in 1942. The extraction was difficult and the results capricious.

The physiologic evidence that gastrin was released on distention of the antrum was provided by Dragstedt and Woodward. They showed that the release of gastrin was suppressed by acidification of the antrum and suggested that this was a biologic feedback mechanism.

In 1960, R.A. Gregory, in Liverpool, England, set about preparing some gastrin from the then-existing recipe. He and his colleague, Hilda Tracy, found that they were in fact unable to produce gastrin by any of the then-published methods. They began a major effort which culminated four years later in the isolation, chemical characterization and synthesis of pure hog gastrin.

Our knowledge of the mechanisms that control gastric secretion and our current state of knowledge of the various gastrointestinal (GI) hormones will be discussed here. I would like to start with the events that occur when we eat a meal. Pavlov, in 1892, divided gastric secretion into three so-called phases. He said that when we see or chew food or swallow it, the vagal nuclei on the medulla are stimulated and they send out peripheral impulses along the vagi. Some of these end up in the gastric mucosa and they liberate acetylcholine. Acetylcholine has the capacity to directly stimulate the parietal cell to secrete acid. When food gets into the stomach, that stimulates the gastric phase. In the gastric phase, distention of the stomach stimulates the vagi and distention of the distal stomach, the antrum, stimulates the release of the hormone, gastrin.

The major mechanisms for release of gastrin are distention of the antrum, contact of the antral mucosa with certain amino acids and contact of the antral mucosa with alcohol or with calcium. A minor mechanism is direct vagal release of gastrin, an important mechanism in some animals, but not in man. Gastrin has the capacity to stimulate acid secretion directly.

One of the most important aspects of gastrin release is that it is pH sensitive. When gastrin and acetylcholine are liberated, acid is secreted by the parietal cells. When acid flows distally and the antral pH falls to about 3.5, gastrin output is diminished. When the pH reaches 1.5, gastrin output is completely blocked. That means that gastrin, in common with other hormones, has a typical endocrine closed-loop relationship with its product, that is, gastrin stimulates the release of hydrochloric acid. When sufficient concentration of hydrogen ion develops, it blocks further release of gastrin.

Acid secreted by the stomach eventually flows into the duodenum. When a sufficiently low pH is reached, about 4.5, secretin is released. Secretin flows through the blood to the pancreas, where it stimulates release of bicarbonate. Bicarbonate flows into the duodenum, raises the pH and blocks the output of secretin so that secretin has a typical endocrine closed-loop relationship with bicarbonate.

I would like for a moment to return to the actual mechanism of stimulation of acid secretion by the parietal cell. There is recent evidence to show that parietal cells have membrane receptors for acetylcholine, gastrin, histamine and probably for the intestinal phase hormone as well. Most importantly, the parietal cell does not secrete with any great efficiency until all receptor sites are occupied. That is the current theory. If that theory is correct, it certainly ties up a lot of loose ends. It explains why vagotomy works and it explains why the H_2 blocking agents work. When vagotomy is performed, acetylcholine stimulation is removed and this tremendously desensitizes the reactivity of the parietal cell to stimulation, so that acid output from the stomach is diminished, even though gastrin levels rise after vagotomy.

We have recently learned that the histamine$_2$ blocking agents greatly suppress acid secretion from any form of gastric secretory stimulation. These agents, metiamide, or cimetidine, which is called Tagamet by Smith, Kline & French Laboratories, prevent histamine from occupying its receptor site on a parietal cell and they greatly desensitize the parietal cell to stimulation. It is clear that the H_2 receptor site is far more important than all of the others because, when it is blocked, acid secretion is diminished far more than when any other single site is blocked.

We know that gastrin and probably all peptide hormones exist in several different molecular sizes. These always seem to include a smaller active form and one or more larger forms which contain a smaller molecule plus extra peptides whose function is unknown. They probably act to protect the smaller active form from rapid catabolic destruction.

There are at least four forms of gastrin. The first form isolated had 17 amino acids and is called G-17. It is also now called little gastrin. There is minigastrin with 14 amino acids, a big gastrin with 34 amino acids, a larger form called Component I by Rehfeld and a compound about the size of albumin, which is referred to as big-big gastrin.

The tumor of one of our patients with the Zollinger-Ellison (Z-E) syndrome showed an actual gel filtration separation of different forms of gastrin. The apparent importance of these findings of different molecular forms is that, although all molecular species are recognized equally by radioimmunoassay methods, the larger forms, that is, in this instance, big-big gastrin and Component I, are biologically inactive. They are, however, equally recognized on a molar basis, so that their presence introduces an inactive variable into the equation.

Gastrin

Gastrin was first described in 1905, but it was not until 1964 that the hormone was purified. This purification initiated the biochemical era of gastrointestinal endocrinology. Gastrin is apparently synthesized and it is certainly stored in specific gastrin cells located in the mucosa of the antrum and of the upper small bowel. Although almost three dozen actions have been described, certainly the most important action is stimulation of acid secretion from the parietal cell. It also causes release of pepsin, it enhances gastric mucosal blood flow and has an important action as a growth hormone on the stomach, proximal small bowel and pancreas.

As clinicians, we are interested in gastrin because it is a major stimulant of normal acid secretion and because it is the etiologic agent in the Z-E syndrome. Since gastrin stimulates acid secretion, and since the duodenal ulcer diathesis is associated with an increased output of acid, it has been tempting for those of us particularly who spend our lives in this field to relate changes in gastrin metabolism to ulcer formation. So far, however, that idea has not been fruitful.

To come now to a practical point, when should one obtain a measurement of serum gastrin? I think that this should be ordered for any patient who has a duodenal ulcer that recurs after operation, in any patient who seems to have a particularly virulent form of ulcer disease, a form associated with a great hypersecretion of acid with basal secretory levels of greater than 15 mEq/hr, or who develops ulcers in the postbulbar area of the duodenum or in the proximal small bowel. Patients who have chronic diarrhea associated with acid hypersecretion should have measurements of serum gastrin. Patients with duodenal ulcer and hypercalcemia should be studied to rule out the possibility of an associated hypergastrinemia, the so-called multiple endocrine adenoma I syndrome.

Cholecystokinin

In 1928 Andrew Ivy reported that fat in the small intestine stimulated the release of a substance that caused contraction of the gallbladder. He named this material cholecystokinin. Later, Harper and Raper at Newcastle-on-Tyne, England, found that a hormone released from the duodenal mucosa would stimulate enzyme secretion from the pancreas. They named this activity pancreozymin. Mutt and Jorpes later found that the two agents were identical and we now call it cholecystokinin, or CCK, because that was the first name given.

CCK is present in special cells in the proximal small bowel which are called "I" cells in the Wiesbaden classification. It is released by contact of these cells with amino acids, fatty acids and acids. CCK is a strong stimulant of contraction of the gallbladder and of release of digestive enzymes by the pancreas. It has been shown recently to be a powerful stimulant of small intestinal motility. In addition, CCK elicits the release of bicarbonate and insulin from the pancreas. It stimulates the flow of hepatic bile and stimulates pancreatic growth. Acting alone, it is a fairly strong stimulant of gastric acid secretion.

Clinically, CCK is used as a standard radiologic assay of gallbladder function. It has been used to evaluate pancreatic function in patients with chronic pancreatitis. Because it is a strong peristaltic stimulant, we have been experimenting with its use in the treatment of postoperative ileus. Our early results are encouraging. The mucosa of the upper gastrointestinal tract is a vast pharmacopoiea of endocrine-producing cells.

Secretin

Secretin arises from the "S" cells and they are located throughout the distal stomach, duodenum, jejunum and upper ileum. The "S" cells reside in the transitional zone between the villae and the intestinal crypts. Secretin is a strongly basic peptide which at neutral pH is bound in place by tissue protein. When hydrochloric acid enters the duodenum, secretin is set free from its electrostatic binding to proteins and it is discharged into tissue fluid and then into the circulation in a highly ionized state.

Although secretin activity was discovered in 1902, it was not until 1966 that Mutt and Jorpes at the Karolinska Institute in Stockholm described the amino acid sequence.

The most important action of secretin is stimulation of secretion of water and bicarbonate by the pancreas. Bicarbonate secretion is equivalent to the secretion of acid by the stomach. Stoichiometric neutralization occurs in the crucible of the duodenum. Secretin stimulates bile secretion. It diminishes gut motility. It diminishes secretion of acid by the stomach. It inhibits the food-stimulated release of gastrin. Clinically, secretin is used as one of the standard tests of pancreatic function. Also, it is used as a discriminatory test for the Z-E syndrome, since it causes rapid release of gastrin from Z-E tumors, but it either suppresses release or causes no change of gastrin levels in control individuals or in patients with duodenal ulcers.

To summarize the events in the duodenum: (a) acid enters the duodenum and causes release of secretin; (b) secretin goes to the pancreatic acinar cells and releases bicarbonate; (c) amino acids from food, particularly phenylalanine and tryptophane, fatty acids, particularly those with chain lengths of greater than CCK and hydrochloric acid all have the capacity to stimulate CCK; and (d) CCK stimulates the pancreatic acinar cells.

There are actually two different kinds of juices elaborated by the pancreas. One of them is high in enzymes but low in bicarbonate and water. It comes from the acinus and it is stimulated by CCK and somewhat by acetylcholine and by gastrin. There is recent evidence to show that a specific hormone may be released from the duodenum called chymodenin. It seems to bring about specific release of chymotrypsin. If this is true, the enzyme secretion of the pancreas is under much more exquisite control than we formerly thought.

The stimulation of the ductal cells to secrete water and bicarbonate is mainly the province of secretin, although vasoactive intestinal peptide, another peptide from the duodenal mucosa, also has that capacity.

I would like now to discuss briefly some of the other gastrointestinal hormones and then to summarize their effects on the parietal cell. Pancreatic glucagon is the hormone of energy release and insulin is the hormone of energy storage. There is a material in the intestinal tract of man which is identical with pancreatic glucagon. In addition, there is another peptide with a smaller molecular weight (2,700 as opposed to 3,100) which cross-reacts identically with specific glucagon antisera. Unger has proposed that this hormone be called GLI for glucagon-like immunoreactivity. Glucagon is a powerful inhibitor of bowel motility and is used clinically in x-ray studies for hypotonic duodenography. Glucagon is also released by a rare gut tumor (glucagonoma).

Gastric inhibitory polypeptide (GIP) (isolated by John Brown and Viktor Mutt in 1969) comes from small bowel mucosa. The amino acid sequence was determined and it was found to have many similarities with the structure of glucagon and secretin. Circulating levels of GIP show a biphasic response to food with an initial peak release stimulated by glucose and a late plateau in response to fat. GIP inhibits secretion of gastric acid and pepsin. It suppresses the food-stimulated release of gastrin. GIP stimulates the release of insulin. In fact, studies on the time course of release of GIP after oral glucose indicate that

GIP may be the insulin-releasing factor. This now appears to be its most important role.

Vasoactive intestinal polypeptide (VIP) was first isolated from the mucosa of the small bowel by Sami Said and Viktor Mutt in 1972. It has many important and potent metabolic effects, but its physiologic role is a complete mystery. The mechanisms for its release, for example, are unknown. Many believe that its chief function is that of a neurotransmitter. VIP may be the agent responsible for the Verner-Morrison syndrome of watery diarrhea in some patients. This is a condition caused by a nonbeta cell tumor of the pancreas associated with diarrhea and hypochlorhydria or achlorhydria of the stomach. It has been cured by excision of the tumor. The incidence of malignancy and the biologic growth potential of these tumors are identical with those of the Z-E tumors.

The new candidate hormones, some of which will surely be granted full membership and some of which will probably be discarded, are bombesin, chymodenin, intestinal phase hormone, motilin, pancreatic polypeptide, serotonin, enkephalins and prostaglandins.

Bombesin is a 14-amino acid peptide isolated by Erspamer in Rome from the skin of certain European frogs. That sounds like it is just a bit of esoterica, but Erspamer predicted that this material, which has the property of releasing gastrin on infusion, would be found to be present in mammalian mucosa, a fact now known to be true.

Chymodenin is a basic polypeptide with a molecular weight of around 5000 secreted from duodenal mucosa which has the ability to release chymotrypsin.

Madame LeBedinskaya, working in Pavlov's laboratory, showed a secretagogue released from the intestine. Gregory and Ivy in 1941 introduced protein into the small bowel of dogs which resulted in the secretion of acid by the stomach. Orloff, in San Diego, has worked for the last several years on attempts at characterization of the *intestinal phase hormone*. It seems to be released from the small bowel by protein and it does not seem to be gastrin.

Motilin is a 22-amino acid peptide, isolated by Brown, which has the capacity to stimulate motility in the stomach and small bowel. There is good evidence that this hormone is involved in normal physiologic control of gastrointestinal secretion.

Pancreatic polypeptide, a 36-amino acid peptide extracted from the pancreas, seems to have both stimulatory and inhibitory actions on gastric and pancreatic secretions. It is present in high concentrations in patients with pancreatic tumors, particularly in the Z-E tumor. It has been suggested that it might be used as a marker for this disease.

Serotonin, or 5-hydroxytryptamine, differs from all of the previous compounds in that it is not a peptide but a vasoactive amine secreted into the portal circulation from duodenal mucosa after duodenal acidification. Jaffe has suggested that it may be one of the physiologic messengers for duodenal inhibition of gastric secretion.

Somatostatin is a 14-amino acid peptide originally isolated from the hypothalamus by Schally in New Orleans and Guillemin in La Jolla, for which they shared the Nobel Prize in 1978. It suppresses the release of pituitary growth hormone. It has also been shown to suppress the release of gastrin and of secretin. We have just shown that it does suppress release of CCK. It also directly inhibits gastric and pancreatic secretion.

Enkephalins and *endorphins* are widely distributed peptides which seem to function as neurotransmitters. Enkephalins have been isolated from the GI tract by Konturek and colleagues in Poland. Endorphins have been demonstrated in the central nervous system where they function in a manner similar to morphine.

Prostaglandins are 20-carbon fatty acids with molecular weights of around 340. There are at least three groups: PGE, PGA and PGF. Within each group there are a number of subdivisions which are named depending upon the number of double bonds in the side chains. For example, PGE_2 is a member of the E group of prostaglandins with two double bonds in the side chain. The prostaglandins inhibit as well as stimulate basal gastric secretion. They may stimulate or inhibit GI motility. There is abundant evidence which has been recently summarized by Jaffe that the prostaglandins may be involved in at least two endocrine diarrheagenic syndromes originally thought to be caused by other agents. The first of these is the Verner-Morrison syndrome, which is believed to be caused by VIP. The other is the carcinoid syndrome, which is associated with excess quantities of serotonin.

Ultrastructural studies show that the parietal cell contains masses of intracellular canaliculi. On stimulation, these canaliculi open so that they communicate directly with the lumen of the fundic gland. Those agents which stimulate the cell's activity are acetylcholine, gastrin, histamine and the intestinal phase hormone. We also must now add bombesin and insulin which probably operate by the vagi. I should note that CCK acting alone is a stimulant of parietal cell secretion, but in the presence of gastrin, which is almost always the case under physiologic conditions, it is in fact a competitive inhibitor.

Self-Evaluation Quiz

1. The antral mucosa contains:
   a) Gastrin
   b) Histamine
   c) Both of the above
   d) Neither one
2. Dragstedt and Woodward showed that histamine was released on distention of the antrum.
   a) True
   b) False
3. Pavlov partitioned gastric secretion into:
   a) Two phases
   b) Three phases
   c) Four phases
   d) Five phases
4. A major mechanism of the release of gastrin is not:
   a) Cardial distention
   b) Amino acids on antral mucosa
   c) Alcohol on antral mucosa
   d) Calcium on antral mucosa
5. The parietal cell does not secrete efficiently until:
   a) One quarter of the receptor sites are filled
   b) One half of the receptor sites are filled
   c) All the receptor sites are free
   d) All the receptor sites are filled
6. A tumor of one of the author's patients with the Zollinger-Ellison syndrome showed:

a) A theoretical gel filtration separation of gastrin forms
b) An actual gel filtration separation of gastrin forms
c) Alkaline reaction
d) Huysen's lines

7. Gastrin was first described in:
a) 1898
b) 1905
c) 1920
d) 1931

Answers on page 721.

Gastric Motility, Applied Physiology

Keith A. Kelly, M.D.

Objectives

The objectives of this paper are to describe the changes in gastric motility that result from gastric operations and to show how such changes result in troublesome postoperative symptoms.

The goal of this article is to describe how gastric operations produce changes in gastric motility that lead to unpleasant symptoms, such as bloating with meals, dumping, diarrhea or bilious vomiting. A better understanding of these disorders may help surgeons to design operations in the future that will avoid such symptoms.

Two Gastric Regions

First of all, surgeons should be aware, as Cannon was years ago [1], that the stomach has two distinct motor regions, a proximal region and a distal region, and each has its own unique motor function. The proximal stomach acts as the gastric reservoir, receiving and storing food. Its slow, sustained contractions regulate intragastric pressure and thereby control gastric emptying of liquids [2]. In contrast, the distal stomach acts as the gastric mixer and grinder. It has a pacemaker which generates electrical cycles, called pacesetter potentials, which in turn phase the onset of peristaltic contractions [3]. These peristaltic contractions regulate gastric emptying of solids [4].

Keith A. Kelly, M.D., Associate Professor of Surgery, Mayo Medical School, Rochester, Minn.

Supported by USPHS, NIH Grant AM18278.

It follows, then, that operations on the proximal stomach should disturb gastric emptying in a different way than operations on the distal stomach. Our hypothesis is that operations on the proximal stomach disturb gastric emptying of liquids, while operations on the distal stomach disturb gastric emptying of solids. In the remainder of this paper evidence will be presented that supports this hypothesis.

Proximal Stomach

Motor physiology. Turning first to the proximal stomach, its contractile pattern is nicely studied using an isolated pouch of gastric fundus and orad corpus that is completely separated from the main stomach, but retains its extrinsic innervation [5]. The motor events of such a pouch are still subject to neural and hormonal control and yet can be recorded without interference from the contractions of the main stomach.

Two types of phasic contractions are recorded from such an isolated, separated, gastric fundal pouch — slow and more rapid phasic contractions (Fig. 1). The slow phasic contractions have a frequency of about one every three minutes and an amplitude of about 40 cm H_2O. In contrast, the more rapid phasic contractions occur at a frequency of five per minute and an amplitude of 10 to 15 cm H_2O. Both types of phasic contractions are superimposed on a sustained or tonic contraction of about 10 cm H_2O. These proximal contractions exert a

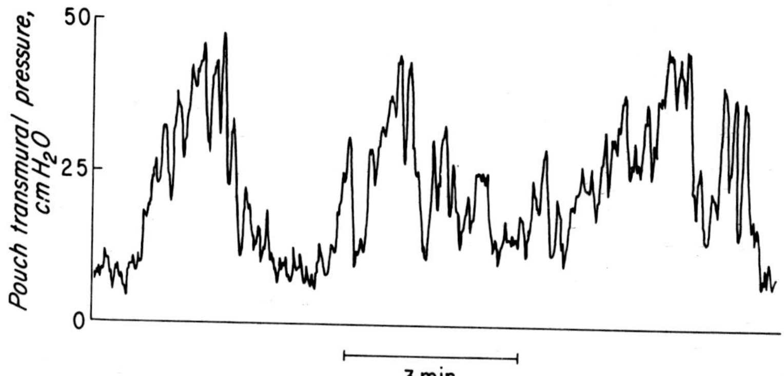

FIG. 1. Contractions of a vagally innervated gastric fundal pouch. (From Kelly, K.A.: Canine gastric motility. Proc. Fourth International Symposium on Gastrointestinal Motility. Vancouver:Mitchell Press, 1973.)

steady pressure on the gastric content gradually forcing it toward the distal stomach and duodenum.

Proximal gastric contractions are regulated by neural and hormonal controls which adjust the strength of these contractions as the stomach fills [6, 7]. This process is called gastric adaptation. As the volume in a bag positioned in the proximal stomach is increased by instilling water into the bag, the pressure across the wall of the stomach gradually increases to about 10 cm H_2O. Then with further expansion of the intragastric volume, no further increase in intragastric pressure occurs (Fig. 2). The stomach adapts or accommodates to increasing distention without increasing pressure [2].

This adjustment of intragastric pressure by the proximal stomach is important, because the rate of gastric emptying (dv/dt) depends upon the difference in pressure between the stomach (P_S) and the duodenum (P_D) and varies with the resistance at the pylorus (R_P).

$$dv/dt = \frac{P_S - P_D}{R_p}$$

Pyloric resistance to the passage of solids is usually so great that they are retained in the stomach and not allowed to pass into the duodenum. However, the pylorus offers little resistance to the passage of liquids, so that they readily flow around the

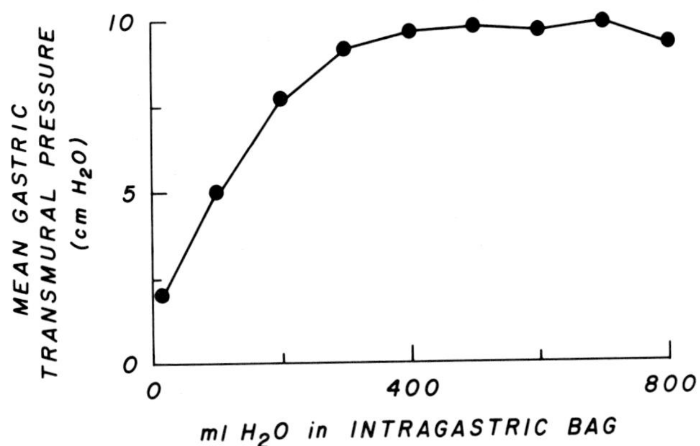

FIG. 2. The stomach adapts to distention, keeping intragastric pressure low as intragastric volume expands greatly. (From Kelly, K.A.: Gastric motility after gastric operations. Surg. Ann. 6:103-123, 1974.)

gastric solids, through the pylorus and into the duodenum. The rate at which liquids empty into the duodenum, therefore, depends mainly upon the gradient in pressure between the stomach and duodenum. Because the slow, sustained contractions of the proximal stomach are the main determinant of intragastric pressure, they have a major influence on the rate of liquid emptying.

To summarize, the proximal stomach acts as the gastric reservoir. Its slow, sustained contractions regulate intragastric pressure and thereby control gastric emptying of liquids.

Proximal gastrectomy. Resections of the proximal stomach disturb gastric accommodation and speed gastric emptying of liquids. This can be illustrated by the operation, gastric fundectomy. In this operation done in dogs, only the gastric fundus was removed, leaving the pacemaker and the entire distal stomach intact [2].

Before fundectomy the stomach accommodated to distention beautifully in each of the four dogs studied. After fundectomy, accommodation was impaired, and much greater increases in intragastric pressure occurred with gastric distention. The greater increases in pressure after fundectomy led to more rapid gastric emptying of liquids in all four animals (Fig. 3). Fundectomy impaired accommodation, so that increased intragastric pressure resulted. When rapid gastric emptying of

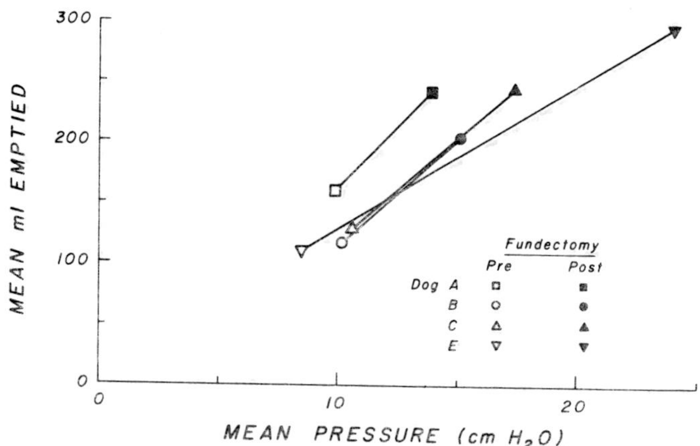

FIG. 3. Fundectomy increases gastric transmural pressure and speeds gastric emptying of 400 ml of 154 mM NaCl. (From Wilbur, B.G. et al [2].)

liquids occurs in patients after gastric fundectomy, it can lead to dumping and diarrhea.

Proximal gastric vagotomy. The new operation, proximal gastric vagotomy, also disturbs gastric accommodation to some extent. In proximal gastric vagotomy, the vagal nerves to the fundus and corpus of the stomach are divided, but those to the antrum are left intact. The vagal fibers to the proximal stomach help to inhibit proximal gastric contractions during distention and thereby enhance accommodation. Thus, vagal denervation of the proximal stomach might be expected to impair accommodation and lead to rapid gastric emptying of liquids.

In dogs, gastric accommodation to distention was impaired after proximal gastric vagotomy compared to before vagotomy [7]. The mean pressure in the stomach increased to greater heights during distention after proximal gastric vagotomy than it did before vagotomy. Such greater increases in pressure with gastric distention after vagotomy may cause patients to experience easy-filling or bloating after the operation.

Again, as with fundectomy, the increased intragastric pressure after proximal gastric vagotomy led to more rapid gastric emptying of liquids [7], and this was true for both isotonic NaCl solutions and hypertonic glucose solutions. Fortunately, the accelerated gastric emptying that occurs in patients after proximal gastric vagotomy is seldom great enough to result in dumping and diarrhea.

In contrast to its effect on liquids, proximal gastric vagotomy did not alter gastric emptying of solid spheres, because it does not greatly disturb the distal stomach and gastric peristalsis. Whereas, complete gastric vagotomy and truncal vagotomy, both of which denervate the distal stomach, markedly slowed gastric emptying of spheres.

But before turning to the distal stomach, let me summarize the consequences of operations on the proximal stomach. Resection or vagotomy of the proximal stomach decreases the reservoir capacity of the stomach and impairs gastric accommodation. Greater increases in intragastric pressure occur with distention, and gastric emptying of liquids is faster.

Distal Stomach

Motor physiology. Let us turn now to operations on the distal stomach. Distal gastric operations disturb gastric emptying of solids. Such disturbances can be effectively studied using small, radiopaque plastic spheres that have a specific gravity similar to that of gastric content. The spheres can be swallowed or placed via a tube into the stomach, and their motions in the stomach and rate of emptying can be followed fluoroscopically [8].

Once the spheres are in the stomach, they are picked up by the antral peristaltic waves which propel them toward the pylorus (Fig. 4). The spheres, however, are not allowed to pass through the pylorus because of their large size, and so they are trapped in the distal antrum, where the advancing peristaltic wave grinds them together. Finally, because they cannot pass through into the duodenum, they are retropelled forcefully toward the more proximal stomach as the peristaltic wave passes over them. This sequence of propulsion, grinding and retropulsion occurs over and over thoroughly triturating the spheres in an attempt to break them down into tiny particles that will be allowed to pass into the duodenum [9]. Once content is emptied into the duodenum, the distal antrum and pylorus prevent its reflux back into the stomach.

The plastic spheres, however, are indigestible and cannot be broken down. They are retained in the stomach for long periods lasting one to two hours or more, until a powerful burst of contractions finally appears and sweeps the spheres rapidly

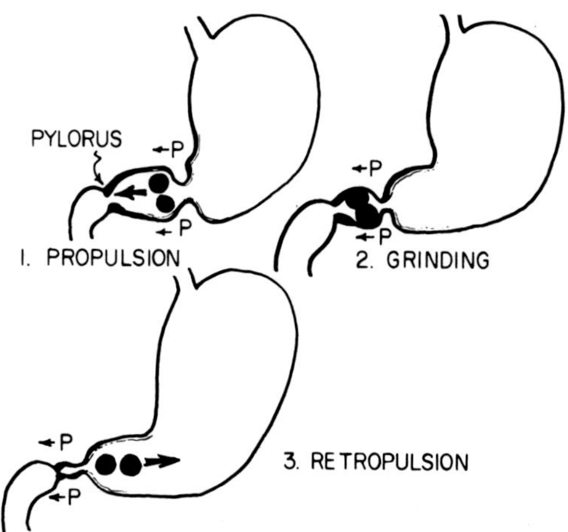

FIG. 4. Consequences of antral peristalsis [4].

out of the stomach. This burst of contractions is called the "activity front." The "activity front" acts as the interdigestive housekeeper of the gastrointestinal tract, because it sweeps intraluminal debris distally during fasting [10].

To summarize, the distal stomach provides continence for gastric solids. It triturates or grinds digestible solids into small pieces and mixes them with gastric juice. Its powerful bursts of interdigestive contractions expel indigestible solids during fasting. Lastly, it provides a barricade against the reflux of duodenal content into the stomach.

Distal gastrectomy. Resections of the antrum and pylorus markedly interfere with the pattern of emptying of solids. To study this point, the distal antrum and pylorus were excised in a series of dogs and gastroduodenostomy performed. The pattern of emptying of spheres was studied before and after the operation [4]. Before operation, the rate of gastric emptying of spheres was slow in each of four dogs studied. Two to four hours were required to empty 50% or more of the spheres. However, after operation, the ability of the stomach to retain the spheres was lost, gastric trituration was abolished, and the spheres were rapidly emptied, usually in 20 to 30 minutes (Fig. 5). Distal gastrectomy made the stomach incontinent for solids, destroyed gastric mixing and grinding and speeded emptying of solids. Such disturbances can lead to dumping and diarrhea.

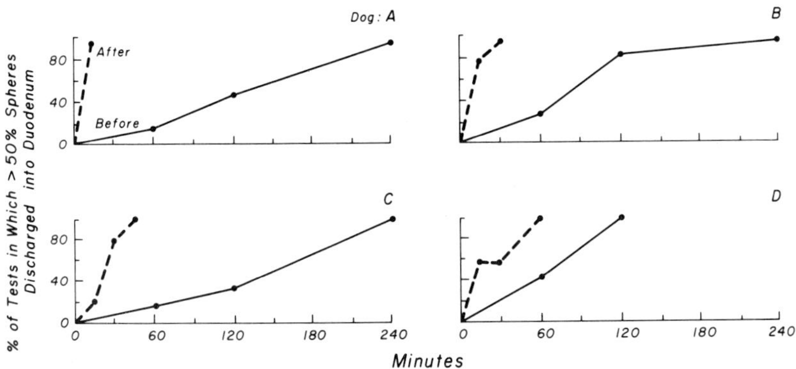

FIG. 5. Distal antrectomy destroys gastric continence for solids and speeds their emptying. (From Kelly, K.A.: Gastric motility after gastric operations. Surg. Ann. 6:103-123, 1974.)

Distal gastric vagotomy. Vagotomy of the distal stomach also markedly alters gastric emptying of solids, as shown in a study of dogs before and after division of all of the extrinsic nerves to the antrum and pylorus, a kind of distal highly selective vagotomy [10]. Before denervation, the spheres were emptied by the powerful bursts of fasting antral contractions, usually in two to four hours. However, after denervation, these fasting bursts did not appear, antral peristalsis was greatly weakened, and the spheres emptied from the stomach very slowly in five of six dogs studied (Fig. 6). Why one of the dogs was not affected by antral denervation is unknown. Antral denervation abolished the powerful periodic bursts of fasting antral contractions in the other animals, thereby weakening the force which expels the spheres, and so slowing their rate of emptying.

In contrast to the slow rate of gastric emptying of solids after extrinsic denervation of the distal stomach, gastric emptying of liquids was unaltered. This finding emphasizes the minor role of the distal stomach in gastric emptying of liquids. The rate of emptying of liquids is controlled mainly by the proximal stomach.

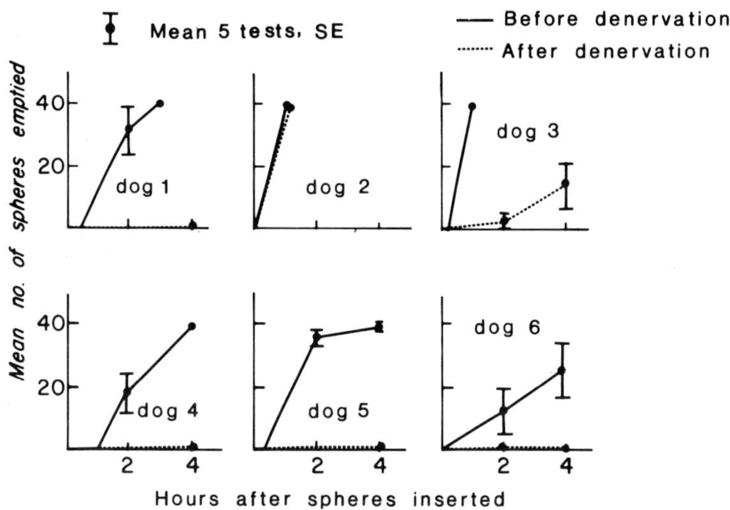

FIG. 6. Antral denervation slows gastric emptying of spheres during fasting. (From Mroz and Kelly [10].)

Gastric "drainage" operations. The rate of gastric emptying of solids is so slow after vagotomy of the distal stomach that gastric "drainage" procedures, like gastroenterostomy, are usually required. However, although such operations do speed gastric emptying of solids when such emptying is sluggish, they also allow for reflux of duodenal content back into the stomach through the artificial opening. Such reflux can damage the gastric mucosa and lead to adverse sequelae such as bile vomiting, alkaline gastritis, pain and anemia.

The production of bile-reflux after gastrojejunostomy is illustrated by comparing gastric aspirates in animals before and after antral gastrojejunostomy. The aspirate before gastrojejunostomy was nearly clear. However, after antral gastrojejunostomy, the aspirate was deeply stained with bile that had refluxed from the jejunum into the stomach through the stoma [11].

To summarize, resection or bypass of the distal stomach impairs gastric continence for solids, speeds gastric emptying of solids and results in duodenal-gastric reflux. Vagotomy of the distal stomach impairs gastric grinding and slows gastric emptying of solids.

References

1. Cannon, W.B.: The movements of the stomach studied by means of the roentgen rays. Am. J. Physiol. 1:359-382, 1898.
2. Wilbur, B.G., Kelly, K.A. and Code, C.F.: Effect of gastric fundectomy on canine gastric electrical and motor activity. Am. J. Physiol. 226:1445-1449, 1974.
3. Code, C.F., Szurszewski, J.H., Kelly, K.A. and Smith, I.B.: A concept of control of gastrointestinal motility. *In* Code, C.F. and Heidel, W. (eds.): Handbook of Physiology. 1968, vol. 5, chapter 139, pp. 2881-2896.
4. Dozois, R.R., Kelly, K.A. and Code, C.F.: Effect of distal antrectomy on gastric emptying of liquids and solids. Gastroenterology 61:675-681, 1971.
5. Okike, N. and Kelly, K.A.: Vagotomy impairs pentagastrin-induced relaxation of the canine gastric fundus. Am. J. Physiol. 1:E504-E509, 1977.
6. Wilbur, B.G. and Kelly, K.A.: Gastrin pentapeptide decreases canine gastric transmural pressure. Gastroenterology 67:1139-1142, 1974.
7. Wilbur, B.G. and Kelly, K.A.: Effect of proximal gastric, complete gastric and truncal vagotomy on canine gastric electrical activity, motility, and emptying. Ann. Surg. 178:295-302, 1973.

8. Schlegel, J.F., Coburn, W., Jr., and Code, C.F.: Gastric emptying of solid and compliant spheres in dogs. Physiologist 9:283, 1966.
9. Hinder, R.A. and Kelly, K.A.: Canine gastric emptying of solids and liquids. Am. J. Physiol. 233:E335-E340, 1977.
10. Mroz, C.T. and Kelly, K.A.: The role of the extrinsic antral nerves in the regulation of gastric emptying. Surg. Gynecol. Obstet. 145:369-377, 1977.
11. Kelly, K.A., Morley, K.D. and Wilbur, B.G.: Effect of corporal and antral gastrojejunostomy on canine gastric emptying of solid spheres and liquids. Br. J. Surg. 60:880-884, 1973.

Self-Evaluation Quiz

1. The proximal stomach regulates gastric emptying of liquids, and the distal stomach regulates gastric emptying of solids.
   a) True
   b) False
2. Intragastric pressure is a major determinant of gastric emptying of solids.
   a) True
   b) False
3. The proximal stomach has peristaltic contractions.
   a) True
   b) False
4. The distal stomach:
   a) Grinds gastric content
   b) Provides continence for solids
   c) Mixes gastric content with gastric juice
   d) Prevents duodenal-gastric reflux
   e) All of the above
5. Vagotomy of the proximal stomach:
   a) Speeds gastric emptying of liquids
   b) Speeds gastric emptying of solids
   c) Results in duodenal-gastric reflux
   d) Often results in dumping
   e) Is commonly followed by diarrhea
6. Gastroenterostomy results in small intestinal-gastric reflux.
   a) True
   b) False
7. Vagotomy of the distal stomach slows emptying of liquids.
   a) True
   b) False

8. In proximal gastric vagotomy:
   a) All gastric vagal branches are divided
   b) Only the vagal trunks are divided
   c) The vagal nerves to the antrum are cut
   d) The vagal nerves to the fundus and corpus are cut
   e) None of the above

Answers on page 721.

The Importance of Gastroscopy to the Surgeon

Robert R. M. Gifford, Sr., M.D., Thomas D. Dressel, M.D. and Robert L. Goodale, Jr., M.D., Ph.D.

Objectives

1. To consider combined x-ray and endoscopy for gastric ulcer, multiple abnormalities, active bleeding and unclear diagnoses.
2. To consider endoscopic techniques for esophageal lesions, gastric malignancies, ulcers, procedures in debilitated patients, and for certain procedures involving the stomach, bile duct and the duodenum.

Today fiberoptic gastroscopy is widely accepted in community hospitals as well as in teaching centers because its diagnostic accuracy is very high. The technique is safe and well tolerated. When x-ray and endoscopic procedures are combined, a correct diagnosis is obtained in around 95% of the cases. The two techniques are ideally complementary. If radiographic studies are normal and no malignancy or bleeding is suspected, endoscopy is not required. When there is a gastric ulcer, multiple abnormalities, active bleeding, or when the diagnosis is unclear, the two procedures have been enormously helpful in combination. The few minutes required for endoscopic diagnosis, the ability to obtain biopsy confirmation of gross lesions, the location of the exact bleeding site to the exclusion of nonbleeding lesions are all incontestable advantages of endoscopy.

Robert R. M. Gifford, Sr., M.D., Thomas D. Dressel, M.D. and Robert L. Goodale, Jr., M.D., Ph.D., Department of Surgery, University of Minnesota Medical School, Minneapolis.

This work was supported by a grant from the Ralph and Marian Falk Surgical Research Foundation.

When comparing the results of emergency endoscopy versus x-ray study for upper GI hemorrhage, endoscopy is clearly superior. The fact that bleeding lesions are often superficial is the explanation. In the Allan and Dykes [1] study (Table 1), endoscopy altered management in 40% of the cases of upper GI hemorrhage. Superficial esophageal and gastric erosions, Mallory Weiss tears and the presence of blood clots or food were the usual causes for failure of the radiologist to make the diagnosis. Bleeding too massive to allow adequate irrigation, strictures, poor cooperation and occasional observer incompetence were the causes of endoscopic failures. The small sample of experience seen in Table 2 from several centers shows what is currently achieved by endoscopy.

We evaluated the accuracy of endoscopy for diagnosing nonbleeding lesions at this hospital over the past ten years. Table 3 summarizes our experience. The endoscopist's initial visual written impression and endoscopic biopsy were compared to the final discharge diagnosis. One hundred patients with esophageal lesions were reviewed. The initial endoscopic visual impression was correct in 85% of the malignancies and 92% of benign lesions.

Three hundred fourteen patients with gastric lesions were reviewed. The original visual endoscopic impression of malig-

Table 1. Fifty Cases of UGI Bleeding

8	Endosc. showed Dx. (x-rays normal)
1	Endosc. no ulcer (x-rays ulcer)
2	Endosc. showed 2nd lesion (x-rays 1 lesion)
9	Endosc. excluded lesions clinically suspected
20	(40%) Endoscopy contributed to management by providing new information or by exclusion
9	(18%) Endoscopy corrected radiological errors (Allan and Dykes [1])

Table 2. Emergency Diagnosis of Upper GI Bleeding by Fiberoptic Endoscopy

Author	*Year*	*Cases*	*Accuracy %*
University of Minnesota	1973	25	88
Katz et al [2]	1975	100	86
Villar et al [3]	1977	192	96

Table 3. Accuracy of Visual Impression and Endoscopic Biopsies in Esophageal and Gastric Lesions at the University of Minnesota Hospitals

Final Diagnosis	*Patients*	*Correct Visual Impression (%)*	*Correct Biopsy (%)*	*Combined Accuracy (%)*
Esophageal malignancy	40	34 (85)	36 (90)	38 (95)
Esophageal benign lesion	60	55 (92)	59 (98)	–
Gastric malignancy	94	80 (85)	70 (74)	85 (90)
Gastric benign lesion	220	203 (92)	220 (100)	–
Total	414			

nancy was correct in 85% of gastric cancers and 92% of benign lesions. These figures are comparable to generally published figures from other authors and represent a gradual improvement in accuracy as experience has been gained.

The endoscopic biopsy proved to be about as accurate as visual diagnosis for esophageal lesions. For gastric malignancies, biopsies were 11% less sensitive than the gross impression. By combining the two tests, one or both were positive in 90% of gastric malignancies and 95% of esophageal malignancies.

Why are gastric malignancies harder to diagnose endoscopically than esophageal malignancies? The problems are with interpretation of the ulcerating and infiltrative lesions and getting deep enough biopsies rather than with overlooking the lesion. Others have had similar results [4] (Table 4).

Table 4. Appearance of Gastric Malignancies and Accuracy of Diagnosis

	Endoscopic Gross Accuracy	*Endoscopic Biopsy*
Exophytic	100%	100%
Infiltrative	85%	70%
Ulcerating	64%	82%

Landres et al [4].

Why aren't endoscopists finding more early gastric carcinomas, since one claim for endoscopy is that it increases the accuracy? For instance, in certain centers in Japan, one third of the cases are early, whereas a survey of endoscopists in this country showed only one-tenth of identified gastric cancers to be of the early type. Part of the answer is the decreased prevalence rate in this country, as compared to Japan so our index of suspicion is lower. When we look at the 12 gastric cancers which were node negative (of 94 reviewed at our institution), eight had symptoms which led to x-rays (Table 5), but the remaining four had anemia or other signs. The lesions were seen in 10 by x-ray and in all 12 by endoscopy. Biopsies were positive in eight. All 12 patients had either symptoms, anemia, or guaiac positive stools which justified workup. There were no completely fortuitous diagnoses; it's just a question of heeding the symptoms or signs. Even the three early lesions confined to mucosa or submucosa had guaiac positive stools or symptoms. It is possible we can find more early cancer with the guaiac screening test.

Of patients with benign ulcer disease who were incorrectly thought to have cancer, gastric resection can be justified as appropriate definitive treatment.

Thus, endoscopy with biopsy confirmation greatly facilitates the preoperative diagnosis of malignancy. The diagnostic accuracy rate in this series is in keeping with results generally published.

In the field of therapeutic or operative endoscopy there are some trends of interest to the surgeon with debilitated patients. Obstructing esophageal cancers or cancers with tracheoesophageal fistulas can be palliated nonoperatively [5] by the insertion of a tube stent over an endoscope which is used as a guide (Fig. 1). The risk of perforation after blind dilation is as high as 38%.

Table 5. Twelve Gastric Carcinoma – Node Negative (In 94 Gastric Malignancies)

4	Asymptomatic when diagnosed
3	Confined to mucosa or submucosa
8	Presently alive (Includes three early cases)
4	Alive > 3 years

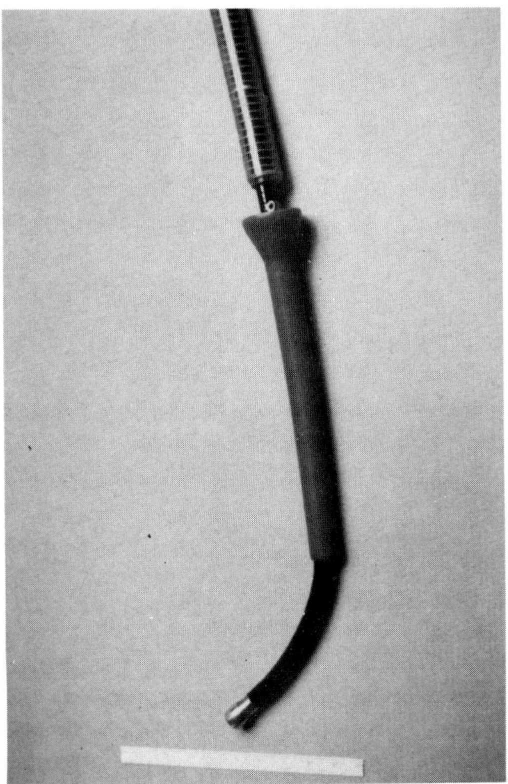

FIG. 1. Shows esophageal stent and pediatric gastroscope (7 mm dia). After scope has passed through malignant esophageal stricture, the stent is pushed into place by flexible pusher tube at top. The scope and pusher tube are withdrawn leaving stent in place.

Esophageal dilation of benign stricture does not require the usual delay of one or two days while the patient swallows a string guide. The stricture can now be safely negotiated endoscopically with a flexible guide wire and then immediately dilated. We have had no perforations in over 50 cases (Fig. 2).

Anastomotic strictures in the stomach can be dilated nonoperatively [6]. We have endoscopically dilated a gastric stricture with an instrument capable of working at right angles to the axis of the esophagus (Fig. 3).

The small intestine can be intubated nonoperatively for decompression with a long tube which is initially attached to

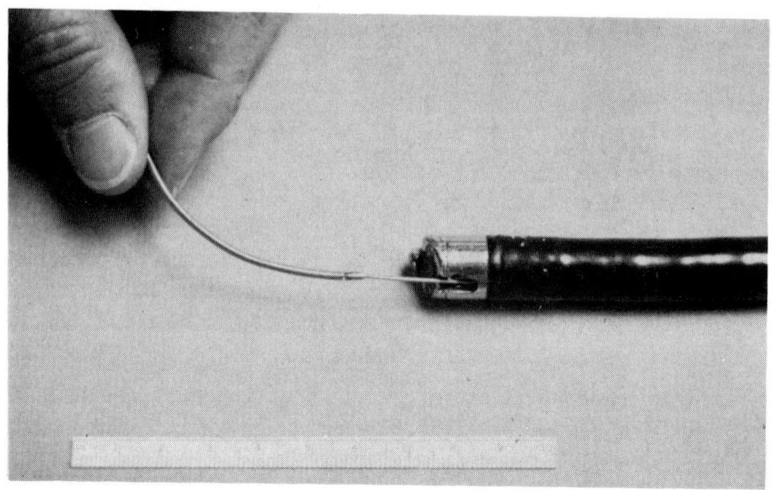

FIG. 2. Flexible guide wire for esophageal dilation. Wire passes through biopsy channel and through stricture under direct vision, preventing false passage.

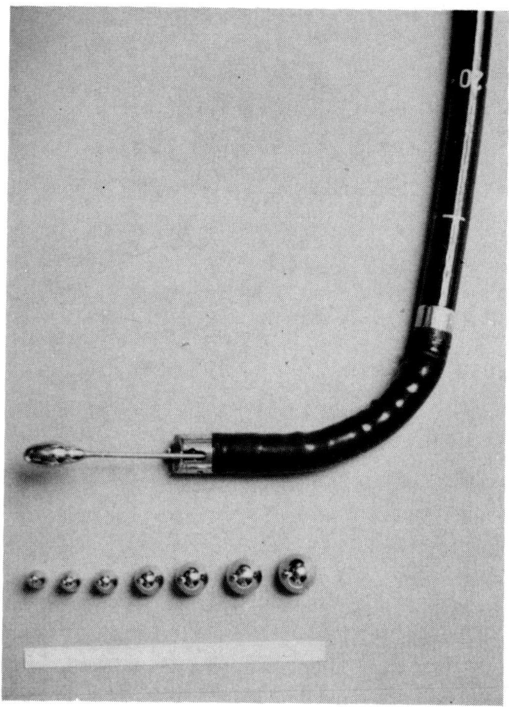

FIG. 3. Gastric anastomotic strictures can be dilated under endoscopic vision by this instrument, even when dilation force is at right angles to esophagus.

the end of the endoscope [7] (Fig. 4). We have carried out the long tube intubation in 44 patients with mechanical intestinal obstruction or ileus (Table 6). In comparison with an earlier study [8] at this institution the obstruction relented in 18% to 38% of the cases, and operation was not required. In the case of prolonged postoperative ileus it appears that about half will eventually relent without need for reoperation.

We have removed three benign pedunculated polyps in the stomach and four in the duodenum by snare and cautery wire and retrieved them in toto by suction. This technique is not recommended for sessile polyps because of bleeding risk.

The orifice of the common bile duct can be cut by cautery wire endoscopically to enlarge it and allow passage of retained common duct stores. We have done this in five such cases with the avoidance of major reoperative surgery and with reduction in hospital costs. With further development of fiberoptic endoscopy, techniques to deal with gastrointestinal problems will improve and continue to bring positive returns and reduce health care costs. Because not all endoscopists are qualified to

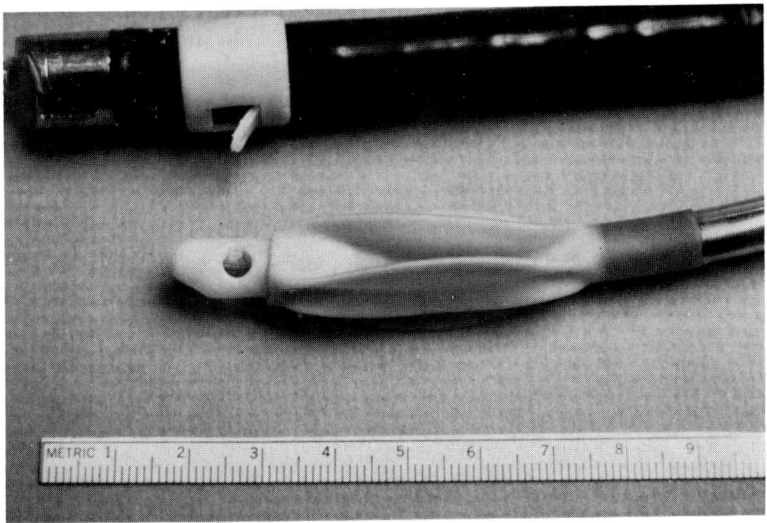

FIG. 4. Shows attachment, gastroscope and the long intestinal tube. Through the hole in the tube can be seen a stylet which attaches the tube to the scope. Tube is released by pulling the stylet, then advanced into duodenum by direct vision.

Table 6. Nonoperative Long Intestinal Tube Placement (Leonard)

Year	*1965-1967*	*1976-1978*
Technique	*Fluoroscope [8]*	*Endoscope*
Patients	31	44
Intubated duodenum	94%	94%
Intubated jejunum	94%	73%
Obst. relent without op.	18%	38%

perform all the specialized techniques, some of the therapeutic procedures may have to be done at centers by specifically trained endoscopists so that maximum benefit can be achieved with minimal risk.

Acknowledgment

The authors wish to thank Lakshmi Madireddi for her work in preparing this manuscript.

References

1. Allan, R. and Dykes, P.: A study of factors influencing mortality rates from gastrointestinal hemorrhage. Q. J. Med. 45:533-550, 1976.
2. Katz, D., Pitchumoni, C.S., Thomas, E. and Antonelle, M.A.: Endoscopy in upper gastrointestinal bleeding then and now. Gastrointest. Endosc. 21:109-111, 1975.
3. Villar, H.V., Roberts, F.H. and Watson, L.C.: Emergency diagnosis of upper gastrointestinal bleeding by fiberoptic endoscopy. Ann. Surg. 185:367-374, 1977.
4. Landres, R.T. and Strum, W.B.: Endoscopic techniques in the diagnosis of gastric adenocarcinoma. Gastrointest. Endosc. 23:203-205, 1977.
5. Tytgat, G.N., den Hartog Jager, F.C.A. and Haverkamp, H.J.: Positioning of a plastic prosthesis under fiberendoscopic control in the palliative treatment of cardioesophageal cancer. Endoscopy 8:180-185, 1976.
6. Mauer, H.G. and Goodale, R.L.: Endoscopic dilation of a gastric anastomotic stricture. Arch. Surg. 112:312-313, 1977.
7. Johnson, F.W., Goodale, R.L., Leonard, A.S. and Varco, R.L.: Rapid long tube intubation of the jejunum by a new endoscopic device. Am. J. Surg. 131:91-93, 1976.
8. Edlich, R.F., Gedgaudas, E., Leonard, A.S. and Wangensteen, O.H.: New long intestinal tube for rapid non-operative intubation. Arch. Surg. 95:443-449, 1967.

Self-Evaluation Quiz

1. When x-ray and endoscopic procedures are combined, a correct diagnosis is obtained in about:
   a) 60% of cases
   b) 75% of cases
   c) 95% of cases
   d) The same as if either procedure were used alone
2. Endoscopic biopsy proved to be about as accurate as visual diagnosis for esophageal lesions.
   a) True
   b) False
3. Minimum time required, biopsy confirmation and site of bleeding are advantages of endoscopy.
   a) True
   b) False
4. In comparing emergency endoscopy with x-ray for upper GI hemorrhage, endoscopy is:
   a) Better
   b) Worse
   c) Same
   d) Cannot be compared
5. Risk of perforation after blind dilation is as high as 38%.
   a) True
   b) False
6. Allan and Dykes showed that endoscopy altered management in ________ cases of upper GI bleeding:
   a) 28%
   b) 38%
   c) 40%
   d) 53%
7. Radiological failure to diagnose may be due to:
   a) Blood clot or food
   b) Lack of skill
   c) Patient's lack of cooperation
8. Endoscopic failures may be due to:
   a) Observer incompetence
   b) Lack of patient cooperation
   c) Strictures
   d) Massive bleeding
   e) All of the above

9. Of 100 patients with esophageal lesions, initial endoscopic visual impression was correct in what percentage of the malignancies?
   a) 48%
   b) 69%
   c) 85%
   d) 92%

Answers on page 721.

Discussion

Moderator: John P. Delaney, M.D.

Moderator: Dr. Kelly, following truncal vagotomy is there actually a pyloric spasm or is there merely a failure of the antral pump?

Dr. Kelly: Post-vagotomy gastric stasis is more a failure of the antral pump. There have been studies to show that the pylorus is really wide open after vagotomy, that it is probably more patulous than in controls. The problem is that there are very few distal peristaltic waves; so mixing and grinding is impaired and gastric emptying of solids is slow.

Moderator: Is there any place for pyloromyotomy as contrasted with pyloroplasty as a drainage procedure?

Dr. Kelly: Well, I suppose there could be, but I am not aware of a good controlled trial. The advantage of the proximal vagotomy is, of course, that it maintains the distal gastric extrinsic innervation so gastric emptying of solids is nearly normal and the general pattern of gastric emptying is not much disturbed.

Moderator: There are a number of questions for Dr. Ellis regarding the exact technique for doing the Heller procedure. How can you tell when you are 1 cm onto the stomach, since that seems to be a very critical distance? What are the landmarks for making a proper length myotomy?

Dr. Ellis: I think the best landmark is the character of the mucosa that you encounter when doing the myotomy. The gastric mucosa is more vascular than esophageal mucosa. There are some thin-walled veins that traverse the esophagogastric junction. I think those small veins are also a good landmark. There is, of course, the peritoneal reflection and the phreno-esophageal membrane, which, as you know, inserts into the last centimeter, or so, of the esophagus. The reflection of peritoneum off the esophagogastric junction is another helpful landmark.

Moderator: Your results in avoiding subsequent reflux esophagitis are clearly superior to most of the American reports. Do you think it is possible that the transthoracic approach makes a difference? Many American surgeons use the transabdominal approach.

Dr. Ellis: Yes, I am convinced it does because, in order to do a proper myotomy from the abdominal approach, you must disrupt all of the normal hiatal attachments of the cardia and lower esophagus in order to pull it down into the field to do the myotomy. Another disadvantage of the abdominal approach is that you can be deceived and do the myotomy on the stomach. I have reoperated on patients transthoracically whose original operation was by the abdominal route and have found no evidence of an esophagomyotomy having been done. The presence of intraabdominal disease necessitating a transabdominal approach is rare. Patients with achalasia do not have duodenal ulcers and I cannot recall any having gallstones. So I do not see any real indication for using the abdominal approach.

Moderator: Dr. Goodale, should not all endoscopy be limited to surgeons?

Dr. Goodale: It certainly helps the training program for the residents see the lesions that they are going to operate on. If you are a surgeon, you sometimes appreciate a prompt endoscopy of the patient better than medical colleagues, but not always.

Moderator: Dr. Goodale, is glucagon helpful in endoscopic procedures?

Dr. Goodale: Yes, just as hypotonic duodenotomy is aided tremendously by glucagon, visualization of the papilla is aided. It is almost essential in every case for retrograde ductograms.

Moderator: You do not use it routinely for gastroduodenoscopy?

Dr. Goodale: We have noticed that sometimes the motility of the stomach is a great problem, as is pylorospasm. It is quite a bit easier to intubate a tight pylorus endoscopically after glucagon.

Moderator: I have a number of questions for Dr. Anderson about the use of steroids in acute corrosive injury of the esophagus. Precisely what steroid do you use and precisely how much?

Dr. Anderson: I think prednisone is the standard. My policy has been to start off in an adult with 60 mg prednisone daily for three days, taper it to 40 mg for three days, taper it to 20 mg and then maintain the patient on that two to three weeks. The antibiotic I use is usually ampicillin given for ten days. Obviously, you do not want to give these patients anything orally initially, so you can use any of the other steroids parenterally. Solu-Cortef or any of the others can be substituted in an equivalent dose.

Moderator: There are related questions asking if there are controlled randomized studies showing the efficacy of steroids?

Dr. Anderson: The best clinical study, the one on which most people have based their use, was Alex Haller's study. He looked at 263 children at Johns Hopkins who had suspected esophageal burn. I do not recall the exact number but I think 112 were diagnosed by endoscopy to have a burn. These were placed on steroids. In that group, six strictures developed that required dilatation. They did not do resectional therapy in any of these children. There are many other series that have been reported using the old technique which was immediate dilatation and no steroids were given with less satisfactory clinical results. The experimental evidence relates to wound healing. It is difficult to reproduce this lesion in animals because they tend to starve, if it is a severe lesion. However, over a short period of time you modify the healing response by the use of steroids. There was a recent review in the *Annals of Thoracic Surgery* by the group from Michigan who say they do not use steroids. They felt that the risk of potentially spreading the mediastinal infection was high. My preference is to use steroids, but I am aware of the potential complications any time you use steroids. The most dreaded complication, of course, is a stricture and long-term dilatation. Anything that will help to avoid this is helpful. The combination of steroids and antibiotics, either one alone does not do very much, seems to be effective.

Moderator: Is there any place for mechanical stents?

Dr. Anderson: There was a report recently on mechanical stents. I am surprised that none of the questioners asked about the nasogastric tube because I specifically avoided that issue. When I initially began seeing these patients, I always put a nasogastric tube in immediately. However, as evidence began to accumulate that the nasogastric tube potentiates reflux and causes injury to the esophagus, I stopped using it. Hyperalimentation, of course, has made it perfectly feasible to stop using the nasogastric tube routinely. Unless I see a child whom I am quite convinced is going to require a gastrostomy and require a Tucker retrograde dilatation, I do not put in a nasogastric tube. If I see such a child, I use it only until a gastrostomy is inserted, then attach a string to the nasogastric tube and pull it up. It can be very difficult to catheterize the esophagus in a child to get the string through for retrograde dilatation otherwise.

Moderator: Dr. Thompson, do you have something on caustic injury?

Dr. Thompson: I wanted to ask Dr. Anderson if he saw a patient late, three or four days after injury, would you start him on steroids then?

Dr. Anderson: No, I do not think it does any good late. Steroids must be given almost immediately after the onset of the injury or they will do no good.

Moderator: Two or three questioners want to know more about your early results, Dr. Thompson, with cholecystokinin in postoperative ileus.

Dr. Thompson: Like a lot of things we study, it turns out to be a nonproblem. We wrote a big protocol to study postoperative ileus. I had the impression that this was some kind of an epidemic. When we finally got our definition written of postoperative ileus, and then set out to try to find suitable subjects, we found that ileus was not any really big problem. We have treated three people in three years. It works just fine.

Moderator: Dr. Thompson, regarding stimuli that release gastrin, you indicated that distention, vagal stimulation, amino acids and peptides released gastrin. I think you indicated that pH is merely permissive, that is, a neutral pH is conducive to release of gastrin but is not in itself a sufficient stimulus. Why should a retained antrum give trouble, since it is not distended, not stimulated by the vagus and it does see any peptides? Why should a retained antrum cause hypergastrinemia?

Dr. Thompson: Because I think several of those premises are false. Dr. Dreyfuss showed that if you give a barium meal repeatedly a good percentage of the time the food actually travels retrogradely back into the antrum. What that means is that the antrum is in fact stimulated. It is sequestered in a permanently alkaline environment so that it can never appreciate the fruits of its labors. It keeps on putting out gastrin that stimulates acid secretion at a distant site. It has been shown now by many people that the excluded antrum is in a nearly constant state of stimulation. Apparently, this must come from some changes in pressure and also just from contact with food that regurgitates. The first part of your statement is absolutely correct, that is, raising the pH above 5 does not release gastrin.

Moderator: Are there any data on retained antrums that do not cause trouble?

Dr. Thompson: There are many patients who have retained antrums but there are very little data. I know of three patients who were discovered accidentally to have retained antral mucosa. I operated upon one of them. He was complaining of bilious vomiting. We got an upper GI series which showed filling of a retained antrum. In fact, he did have slightly elevated gastrin levels, but he had no symptoms attributable to it. This was 22 years postop. We took out the antrum because it was there. I think Jack Hansky demonstrated retained antral mucosa in seven patients who were asymptomatic.

Moderator: Does the Technetium scan have a place in identifying antral mucosa?

Dr. Thompson: I do not think you need it.

Moderator: Speaking of taking out things because they are there, Dr. Leonard, when you find a Meckel's diverticulum, when you are doing an appendectomy or something else, what do you do about it?

Dr. Leonard: I do not usually take them out, unless there is a specific reason during an appendectomy where there is perforation present.

Moderator: Let us forget the question of infection. You find it incidentally when you are doing a cholecystectomy?

Dr. Leonard: When you are doing a gallbladder on an adult, I think removal is justified. If you have a small intestinal lumen in a newborn, I do not think you are justified, otherwise with normal intestinal size resection is justifiable.

Moderator: Because of your concern about potential obstruction? Do you agree with that, Dr. Foker?

Dr. Foker: No, potential obstruction should be dealt with by the type of resection, which in turn will depend upon the configuration of the diverticulum.

Moderator: The size of the neck and the relationship of the lumen of the diverticulum as compared to that of the bowel?

Dr. Foker: Yes, that is correct. In several reported series of Meckel's, most are asymptomatic. But the percentage of reported difficulty is 30% to 40% in these series and if they are, in fact, representative, there is a good chance of a problem developing. That is substantially higher than the chance of getting appendicitis, for example, and people do many incidental appendectomies.

Moderator: Dr. Thompson, would you like to comment?

Dr. Thompson: Yes, I would certainly take it out. I do not know how data on the frequency of trouble with Meckel's were secured. I do not trust those data because I think they are weighted to begin with. Nonetheless, unless it was pretty difficult, I think I would want to remove it. As a matter of fact, there are papers suggesting that it should be removed, if discovered accidentally on small bowel series.

Moderator: Dr. Foker, I have questions on colonoscopy in the pediatric age group: Is there a special scope? Do you want the information enough to give general anesthesia to do colonoscopy?

Dr. Foker: I myself do not do colonoscopy. So I am not an expert. The case I showed in which five polyps were removed from one of my patients was done by a medical colonoscopist. As far as I know, he used a regular scope in the patient, who was 4 years of age. In this age group, one does have to use general anesthesia.

Moderator: Dr. Leonard, please comment on the use of peritoneal tap and/or laparoscopy in blunt abdominal trauma. I would like you to comment also on the acute abdomen with apparent peritonitis.

Dr. Leonard: We acquired a very small scope about a year and a half ago. This has been a very interesting tool for use in the acute abdomen, especially in the infant and small child. Peritoneoscopy is a very valuable tool in infants, for instance, who have necrotizing colitis, or where you have a problem, for instance, with a tumor versus a cyst in the abdomen of a small child. In patients with multiple problems, an immune problem, for example, where you do not want to do a laparotomy because it is a high-risk patient. We have had a number of these in which the use of peritoneoscopy has helped us considerably. I think the diagnostic tap in trauma is an excellent tool. Dr. John Perry and his group had a series of some 200 children. In 97% of those individuals, the results of the tap were correct. As a matter of fact, of the children who had positive taps, there was usually a good reason for exploration. It should be utilized in children with head injuries, especially those who are unconscious with multiple trauma. In children, as you know, we are trying to save spleens. Here is where peritoneoscopy might be a very important adjunct if you found a positive tap. You watch that infant or child as long as you can. In the laboratory we are now studying means of doing partial splenectomies, tying off the splenic artery leaving the short gastric as the blood supply and actually using suture material in the spleen. We have taken out very few severely damaged spleens in the last two to three years.

Moderator: Dr. Kelly, does the Nissen fundoplication affect gastric emptying?

Dr. Kelly: I am not certain that a good study to examine this question has been done. I would suspect very strongly that it would interfere with gastric accommodation and speed gastric emptying of liquids to some extent. Perhaps Dr. Ellis could answer the question?

Dr. Ellis: The only case that I know of in our experience who developed symptoms that sounded like the dumping syndrome after a Nissen fundoplication had a vagotomy at the same time. Not only was the vagotomy unnecessary but the Nissen was too tight, so we had to reoperate and loosen it. I cannot recall any symptomatic emptying problems, unless the vagus nerve has been damaged.

Moderator: It is an interesting question because the wrap-around certainly uses up some of the fundic reservoir, as in the dogs with the fundus resection.

Dr. Kelly: Yes, but it does leave some fundus. Apparently in most people there is enough fundus left undisturbed that they do not get symptoms from the operation.

Moderator: Dr. Goodale, with multiple colonic polyps, many people propose removing most of the colon and then the endoscopist clears residual polyps. Is there any place for this type of thing in multiple gastric polyposis?

Dr. Goodale: We have been following five patients with multiple gastric polyps and I am really amazed how benign they are. Year after year, they are very small. This is in line with what a number of people are saying now, that they can be safely removed. Perhaps we have been scared a bit by the idea that gastric polyposis has a very high malignant potential. I have not seen it yet.

Moderator: Dr. Ellis, please comment on the treatment of epiphrenic diverticulum. The questioner particularly wants to know about the relationship of achalasia and epiphrenic diverticulum.

Dr. Ellis: With very few exceptions, all patients who have an epiphrenic diverticulum have symptoms not so much from the diverticulum but from the underlying motility disturbance. This is very often diffuse spasm but it can also be achalasia.

Moderator: What is the treatment of epiphrenic diverticulum? I presume surgical treatment. When is it indicated? How does one go about it?

Dr. Ellis: In treating it, I usually take the diverticulum out, although the main part of the operation is the myotomy for the underlying disturbance, which in the case of diffuse spasm would be a long myotomy encompassing that area of the esophagus in which motility has been shown to be abnormal preoperatively. By sparing the lower sphincter, which is usually normal in these people, you do not get into the problem of reflux. The symptoms are due to spasm rather than to the diverticulum. But I would take the diverticulum out.

Moderator: Dr. Thompson, what is the course of the work-up for a patient with suspected watery diarrhea syndrome?

Dr. Thompson: That is a good question. I think you want to rule out standard causes for diarrhea. You want to try to rule out the possibility of intestinal pathogens and also different kinds of food dyscrasias or intolerances, particularly to disaccharides or monosaccharides. It is the standard kind of diarrhea work-up. I think that if the patient has low acid secretion and a continued watery diarrhea of more than three months duration, then one might begin a search for the actual tumor by angiography. About one third to one half of such lesions will visualize angiographically. In addition, 20% will visualize that are not there. So you have to have that factor to subtract from your equation. Then the next thing is just to go in and explore the pancreas. By and large these tumors have been found to be larger than most insulinomas and most gastrinomas. An active GI surgeon, interested in endocrine diseases, might see one or two or perhaps three of these in a lifetime. They are really quite rare.

Moderator: Is there any biochemical test you should be looking for?

Dr. Thompson: Of course, we would do the gamut right now. We would look for VIP and prostaglandins and serotonins. I am not sure that with the current state of the art with the VIP assay that I would be very excited about it. I am sure many of you have read the article in *The New England Journal of Medicine*, in which Dr. Said reported finding high levels of VIP in some 56 patients. I believe that turned out to be a methodologic error. The assay was not any good. We have a VIP assay which we are very strong on right now, but next month I might be a little bit nervous about it. Everybody should know that in the evolution of these assays there are periods of trial and that some are much more reliable than others. The gastrin assay is the best. There are several good secretin assays now. We have one. The cholecystokinin assays are very tricky as is the VIP assay. The GIP assay is apparently quite good. I do not have any familiarity with the serotonin or the prostaglandin assay, but Dr. Jaffe says they are good and I believe him.

Moderator: Dr. Kelly, I have a question about the postoperative, postgastrectomy, postvagotomy, or postpyloroplasty gastric retention. Do any of your studies give insights into pharmacologic treatment or any other form of treatment of this problem?

Dr. Kelly: This is really a tough problem. I guess the best thing to do is to try to avoid it by not doing the operations that lead up to it. But faced with the problem, we have tried treating these patients with metaclopromide. Some of them do seem to respond, but I must say the response is often short-lived. Long-term experience with the drug has been poor. The only other substance which has been shown scientifically to speed gastric emptying is the hormone motilin, a substance not currently available. Perhaps it might be worthwhile to explore its use in this problem. Sometimes, the surgeon is forced to re-operate. The operation I have found to be most useful in this setting is to resect the distal part of the stomach and to perform a Roux-Y gastrojejunostomy so that the food goes directly from the gastric pouch into the Roux-Y limb. At a re-operation the surgeon should always make sure that a complete vagotomy has been done at the first procedure; otherwise, you might get a recurrent ulcer in the jejunal limb. I would not want to apply this operation across the board to every patient who comes along. If a problem with postoperative gastric stasis arises, the best thing to do is to wait. I try to wait at least one year. I would try all other forms of therapy, including some special drugs like metaclopromide or possibly motilin. Then, after a period of a year, if the patient is still distressed, going downhill and losing weight and you have to do something, gastric resection and gastrojejunostomy of the Roux-Y type could be considered.

Moderator: Looking at the other side of it, is there any way you can predict that a particular patient is likely to have gastric retention following vagotomy and pyloroplasty? Are there any studies you can do in advance so that you can say, "This patient had better not have that operation"?

Dr. Kelly: Not that I know of.

Dr. Thompson: People that are obstructed preoperatively are apt to be obstructed postoperatively. That is just a truism. The vast majority of people we get that extend more than 30 days with trouble emptying are those who had gastric outlet obstruction preoperatively and they have an atonic stomach to begin with. I would like to echo what Dr. Kelly just said. I think there is a great danger now of having a fad operation, not only for this but for the so-called reflux bile gastritis. I go around now seeing many people who formerly were just classified as being mildly unhappy after gastric surgery. Now they are very apt to end up getting a Roux-Y procedure. I think that is potentially a very dangerous operation, one we should withhold until our back is up against the wall. Second, I would also like to echo his reservations about the efficacy of metaclopromide. There is going to be an article coming out in the *Annals of Surgery* from a paper at the American Surgical Association on the efficacy of metaclopromide in these emptying problems. The experience of the author may be unusual because other people who have used it have not found it to be of great help.

E. Starr Judd Lecture

Studies on the Pathogenesis of Gastric Ulceration

William Silen, M.D.

Objectives

1. To identify the many factors that alter the ability of the stomach to withstand luminal acid.
2. To discuss the concept of the "gastric mucosal barrier."
3. To review the actions of bile salts on the gastric mucosa.
4. To describe the role of nutrient HCO_3 as a protective factor.
5. To discuss the importance of the mucosal circulation in the protection against ulceration.
6. To discuss the role of pepsin.

Introduction

It is a distinctive honor to be chosen as the Judd Lecturer for this year. The list of Judd Lecturers is long and illustrious. I only hope that I can approximate in some small way the measure of the men who preceded me.

I should like to discuss today the pathogenesis of experimental gastric ulceration, a subject which has occupied the attention of my laboratory for the past ten years. The aphorism that ulceration does not occur in the absence of luminal acid is an important one which is reaffirmed and strengthened by our work. However, we have discovered that many factors alter the ability of the stomach to withstand luminal acid and it is these factors which will occupy the major portion of our discussion today.

William Silen, M.D., Johnson & Johnson Professor of Surgery, Harvard Medical School; Surgeon-in-Chief, Beth Israel Hospital, Boston, Mass.

Mucosal Permeability

The normal stomach maintains a gradient of [H+] of one million to one from lumen to blood. It is the ability to maintain such a gradient without mucosal injury that has given rise to the concept of the "gastric mucosal barrier." Under normal circumstances, a small "back-diffusion" of H+ into the gastric wall occurs and the quantity of back-diffusion of H+ is directly proportional to the luminal concentration of H+. When the gastric mucosal barrier is disturbed or "broken" by agents such as aspirin, bile salts or alcohol, the permeability of the mucosa to H+ is increased, but the rate of loss of luminal H+ remains linearly related to luminal [H+]. In other words, back-diffusion is a passive diffusional phenomenon, even when the barrier is "broken." We have recently demonstrated that glucocorticoids enhance the increased passive diffusion known to occur in response to classical barrier breakers such as aspirin or bile salts (Chung et al, in press, 1978). This finding offers a new explanation for a previously elusive effect of steroids on the stomach.

It is useful to review the actions of bile salts on the gastric mucosa as a prototype for other substances which alter the mucosal barrier. In an in vitro system with amphibian gastric mucosa mounted in an Ussing chamber the application of deoxycholate to the luminal surface causes a marked decrease in: potential difference across the membrane (PD), short circuit current (Isc), resistance (R) and detectable H+ secretion [1]. These findings indicate an increase in mucosal permeability and these changes are associated with progressive disruption and loss of surface epithelial cells as observed by scanning and transmission electron microscopy [2]. Of enormous clinical importance is the fact that different bile salts have varying effects on the mucosa, ie, deconjugated and dehydroxylated bile salts have a much more profound effect on a molar basis than do conjugated bile salts (Fig. 1). This explains the inability of some investigators to demonstrate an injurious effect of bile on the gastric mucosa since under many circumstances in the intact animal, bile salts (eg, deoxycholate) are precipitated by a low pH and are no longer active. Bile salts with a relatively high pKa (eg, deoxycholate) are injurious at neutral pH, a fact which is

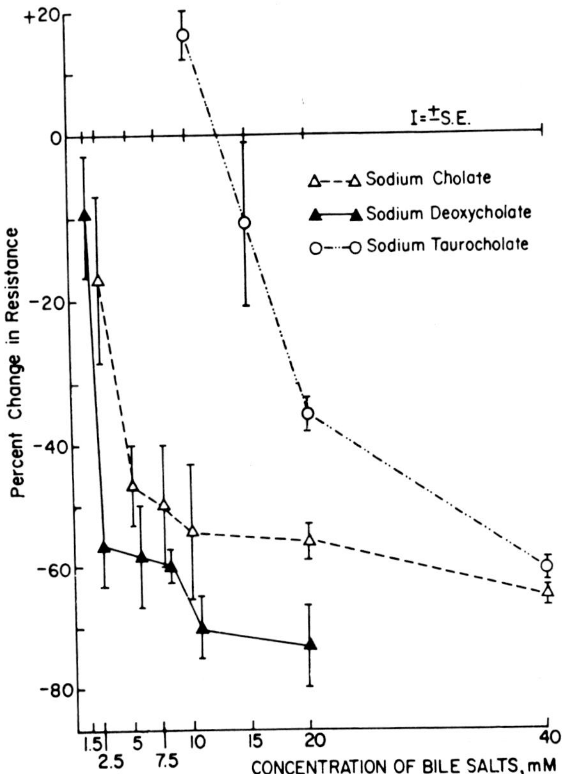

FIG. 1. Change in R after 30-minute exposure of mucosal surface of tissue to three different bile salts. (From Silen and Forte [1].)

consistent with the clinical observation that "alkaline" gastritis is usually found in the achlorhydric or hypochlorhydric stomach, a likely site for bacterial overgrowth and deconjugation of bile salts. Substances other than bile salts found in duodenal content such as lysolecithin which results from the action of pancreatic phospholipase A on biliary lecithin have an action on the mucosa similar to that of bile salts (Kivilaakso et al, in press, 1978). It is possible that a combination of lysolecithin and bile salts is more injurious to the mucosa than either agent alone.

Potent bile salts placed on the serosal side of amphibian mucosa cause an increase in resistance together with a decrease in PD, Isc and H+ secretion. Electron microscopy demonstrates a profound injury of the oxyntic cells, especially of the mitochondria. Such an effect can be observed in the oxyntic cells if the mucosal application of the bile salt is sufficiently long to allow penetration to the deeper portions of the mucosa. Similar findings have been noted in response to aspirin by other investigators [3]. Thus, the so-called barrier breakers not only cause an increase in permeability as a result of major injury to the surface epithelial cells, but also have an additional action on the oxyntic cells, which might alter the capacity of the mucosa to resist injury, as will be discussed below.

Secretory Status

It has been known for many years that for each H+ secreted into the lumen of the stomach, an equivalent HCO_3 is released into the nutrient surface of the tissue. The importance of nutrient HCO_3 as a protective factor has not been recognized until recently.

We found quite by accident during the course of other studies that the in vitro amphibian gastric mucosa, inhibited by an H_2 receptor blocking agent, is much more susceptible to injury by high concentrations of luminal H+ than the actively secreting mucosa [4] (Fig. 2).

Recent studies in our laboratory confirm this finding in rabbits in vivo (Kivilaakso et al, in press, 1978). Kivilaakso of Helsinki, working with us in Boston, has developed a method of micropuncture by which a pH microelectrode can be placed within the lamina propria of the stomach while luminal events are simultaneously investigated. In the normal resting stomach the pH in the lamina propria is $\sim$7.3 and when 100 mM HCl is placed within the lumen, the intramural pH decreases to 6.9 or below and ulceration invariably occurs. When histamine is given to the rabbit, a slight but insignificant rise in intramural pH occurs, but luminal acid fails to cause either a decrease in pH of the lamina propria or ulceration (Fig. 3). There is a highly significant correlation between loss of luminal H+ and intramural pH in these studies, strongly suggesting that the observed decreases in tissue pH are the result of back-diffusion of H+.

Thus it would appear that the actively secreting stomach with its resultant alkaline tide is more resistant to injury than the inhibited mucosa.

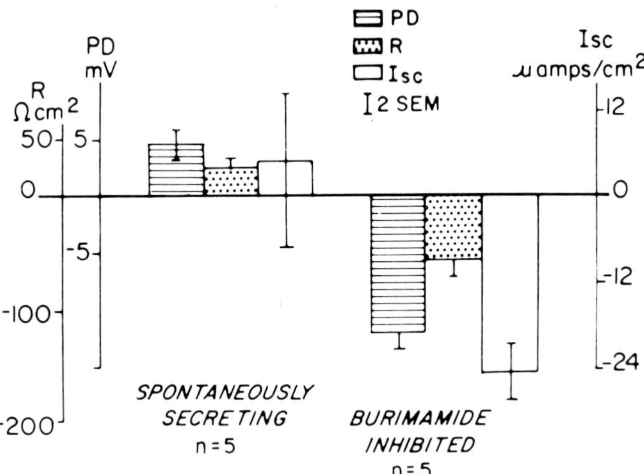

FIG. 2. Changes (Δ) in transmural electrical potential difference (PD), tissue electrical resistance (R), and short circuit current (Isc) of frog gastric mucosa after exposure to HCl, 120 mM, on the secretory surface for 30 minutes. (From Smith et al [4].)

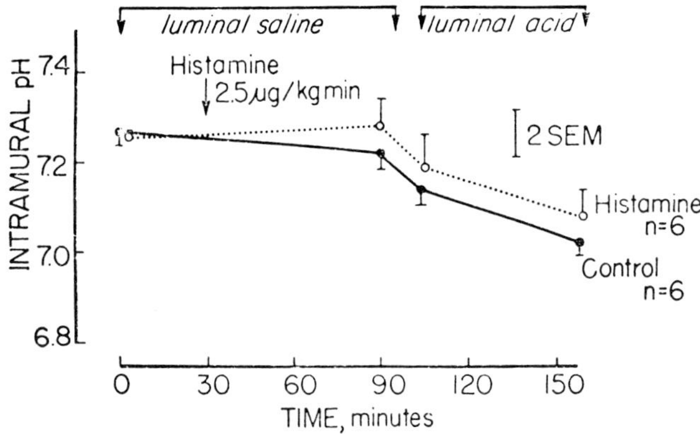

FIG. 3. Intramural pH in control and histamine treated antral pouches in response to exposure to luminal saline and acid. (From Kivilaakso et al, *Gastroenterology*, in press.)

Mucosal Circulation

The importance of the mucosal circulation in the protection against ulceration is emphasized by the almost invariable development of mucosal erosions during and after shock when luminal acid is present. Using the same preparation to determine intramural pH in the rabbit, we have shown that hemorrhagic shock causes a marked decrease in the pH of the lamina propria to below 6.9 when luminal acid is present, and under these conditions ulceration always occurs. When the luminal solution is buffered at pH 7.0 the intramural pH does not decrease significantly and ulcerations do not occur despite the shock [5] (Fig. 4). Qualitatively similar but quantitatively less striking changes are observed in the dog subjected to hemorrhage although the addition of 20 mM taurocholate to the luminal solution in the canine shock experiments caused a decrease in intramural pH and extensive ulcerations comparable to those found in the rabbit. During shock in the rabbit, focal white ischemic spots can be seen as the forerunners of ulceration.

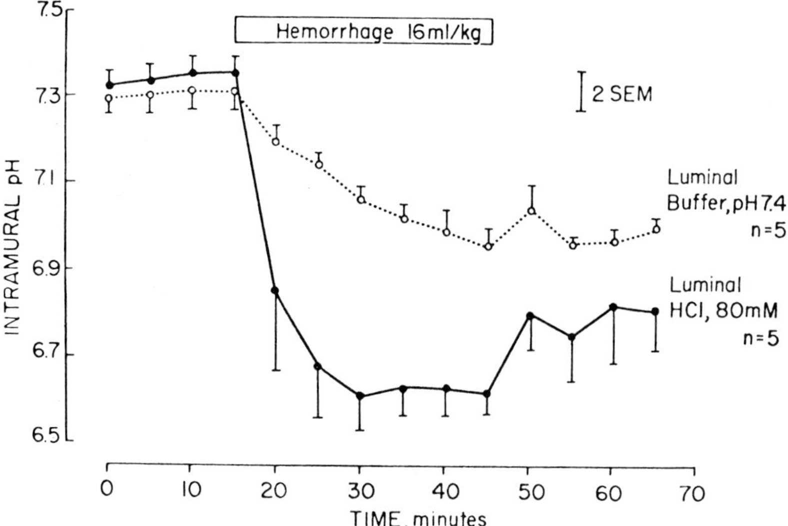

FIG. 4. Intramural pH of fundic pouches containing luminal acid (•——•) or buffer (○-----○), pH 7.4, in rabbits subjected to the standard hemorrhagic shock. (From Kivilaakso et al [5].)

Selective micropuncture shows that the intramural pH is much lower in these areas than in the surrounding more normal tissues.

Studies of the intramural pH of the antrum demonstrate that the pH of the lamina propria generally parallels the arterial pH of the animal. Although the intramural pH decreased to about 7.0 in the presence of luminal acid and only to about 7.1 when the luminal solution was buffered, no ulcers were observed. The addition of pepsin to an acid luminal solution (100 mM) causes an additional decrease in intramural pH but without the development of ulceration. Ulceration of the antrum has occurred only when extremely strong luminal acid (200 mM) is applied during shock or acetazolamide is administered. The reasons for these differences between antrum and fundus are not as yet apparent.

The mucosal circulation is therefore extraordinarily important in preventing tissue acidosis and in sweeping away excessive H+ which has diffused into the tissue.

Acid-Base Balance

Cummins, Grossman and Ivy [6] demonstrated in dogs that the gastric and duodenal ulcers which formed during the continuous intragastric infusion of 0.1 N HCl could be prevented by correction of the attendant additional acidosis with intravenous $NaHCO_3$. Davies and co-workers [7, 8] showed that ulceration uniformly occurred in sacs of amphibian gastric mucosa when CO_2 was removed from the medium. They suggested that alkalinization of the tissue occurred in the absence of exogenous CO_2 and that ulceration occurred because of the alkalinity of the tissue [7, 8].

Recent experiments in our laboratory using the gut sac preparation of Davies emphasize the importance of acid-base balance, but do not support his hypothesis. In fact, we have shown very clearly that the absence of CO_2 has nothing whatever to do with the development of the ulcers in this model. Quite the contrary, it is the absence of nutrient HCO_3 rather than the lack of CO_2 which is required for ulcers to form (Tables 1 and 2). Davies and colleagues had replaced the nutrient HCO_3 with phosphate when the CO_2 was eliminated but did not study the effect of nutrient HCO_3 when CO_2 was

Table 1. Incidence of Ulceration of Gastric Sacs in Different Incubation Mediums

Incubation Medium	pH of medium initial	pH of medium final	Gas	Number of Sacs	Ulcerated Sacs
PO_4	7.4	7.4	100% O_2	10	8
HCO_3	7.4	7.4	95% O_2 + 5% CO_2	10	1
HCO_3	8.2	8.6-8.8	100% O_2	10	1
Unbuffered	7.4	8.4-8.6	100% O_2	10	6
PO_4 + luminal buffer (pH 7)	7.4	7.4	100% O_2	4	0
HCO_3 + acetazol	8.2	8.6-8.8	100% O_2	10	5
HCO_3 + acetazol	7.4	7.4	95% O_2 + 5% CO_2	10	9
HCO_3 + SITS	7.4	7.4	95% O_2 + 5% CO_2	10	5

Table 2. Influence of the Type of Buffer and Ambient pH on the Incidence of Ulceration of Gastric Sacs

Buffer	pH	Gas	Number of Sacs	Ulcerated Sacs
TES	6.3	100% O_2	8	6
	7.4		8	5
HEPES	6.3	100% O_2	8	8
	7.4		8	5
TRIS	6.3	100% O_2	8	7
	7.4		8	8
MES	6.3	100% O_2	8	6
	7.4		8	4
TES + HCO_3	7.4	100% O_2	8	0

absent. It is evident from the data cited in Tables 1 and 2 that a high nutrient pH, even when extremely alkaline, does not protect against ulceration when HCO_3 is absent from the nutrient solution.

Role of Pepsin

Davies et al [7, 8] found, as we have, that amphibian gastric mucosa in open sheets in an Ussing chamber exposed to conditions found to be ulcerogenic in the closed sacs failed to develop ulcers. An explanation for this observation can be found in our recent experiments in which the concentration of pepsin was raised artificially in the relatively large Ussing chamber to that found in the small gut sacs. When this was done, ulceration became as frequent in the open sheets as in the closed sacs. The role of pepsin is further emphasized by our finding described above that intramural pH in the antrum of the rabbit during shock decreases to lower levels when pepsin is added to the luminal solution.

Summary

The ability of the stomach to withstand the injurious effects of luminal acid is not a static phenomenon, but is rather the result of an interplay between alterations in permeability, secretory rate, mucosal circulation, acid-base balance and luminal pepsin concentration. The availability of nutrient HCO_3 whether from alkaline tide, tissue sources, or the bloodstream has recently been shown to be of extreme importance in the protection against ulceration.

References

1. Silen, W. and Forte, J.G.: Effects of bile salts on amphibian gastric mucosa. Am. J. Physiol. 228:637-644, 1975.
2. Forte, T.M., Silen, W. and Forte, J.G.: Ultrastructural lesions in gastric mucosa exposed to deoxycholate: Implications toward the barrier concept. *In* Kasbekar, Sachs, Rehm (eds.): Gastric Hydrogen Ion Secretion. New York:Marcell Dekker, Inc., 1976, pp. 1-28.
3. Kasbekar, D.K.: Effects of salicylate and related compounds on gastric HCl secretion. Am. J. Physiol. 225:521-527, 1973.
4. Smith, P., O'Brien, P., Fromm, D. and Silen, W.: Secretory state of gastric mucosa and resistance to injury by exogenous acid. Am. J. Surg. 133:81-85, 1977.

5. Kivilaakso, E., Fromm, D. and Silen, W.: Relationship between ulceration and intramural pH of gastric mucosa during hemorrhagic shock. Surgery 84:70-78, 1978.
6. Cummins, G.M., Grossman, M.I. and Ivy, A.C.: An experimental study of the acid factor in ulceration of the gastrointestinal tract in dogs. Gastroenterology 10:714-726, 1948.
7. Davies, R.E. and Longmuir, M.: Production of ulcers in isolated frog gastric mucosa. Biochem. J. 42:621-627, 1948.
8. Davies, R.E. and Edelman, J.: The function of carbonic anhydrase in the stomach. Biochem. J. 50:190-194, 1951.

Self-Evaluation Quiz

1. The aphorism says:
   a) Ulceration can occur in any milieu
   b) Ulceration can occur in the absence of luminal acid
   c) Ulceration does not occur without luminal acid
   d) Ulceration does not occur above pH 3.5
2. From lumen to blood, the normal stomach maintains an H^+ gradient of:
   a) 500,000 : 1
   b) 1 million : 1
   c) 2 million : 1
   d) Any proportion
3. The author recently demonstrated that glucocorticoids:
   a) Enhance the decreased passive diffusion in response to classical barrier breakers
   b) Enhance the increased passive diffusion in response to classical barrier breakers
   c) Do not affect barrier breakers
   d) Do not affect the stomach
4. Deconjugated and dehydroxylated bile salts:
   a) Have a more profound effect on a molar basis than do conjugated bile salts
   b) Do not have a more profound effect on a molar basis
   c) Affect the mucosa less than do conjugated bile salts
   d) Are of no clinical significance
5. Barrier breakers:
   a) Do not injure surface epithelial cells
   b) Decrease permeability
   c) Affect oxyntic cells
   d) Increase permeability

6. Actively secreting stomach is less resistant to injury than the inhibited mucosa.
   a) True
   b) False
7. __________ ischemic spots can be seen as forerunners of ulceration in the rabbit.
   a) Incipient red
   b) Incipient white
   c) Focal red
   d) Focal white
8. The mucosal circulation is important in preventing tissue:
   a) Acidosis caused by excess H^+ diffused into the tissue
   b) Alkalosis caused by the rebound phenomenon
   c) Acidosis caused by excess H^+ injected as a bolus into the tissue
   d) Acidosis caused by excess H^+ poured over isolated seal gut

Answers on page 721.

Stomal Gastritis

John P. Delaney, M.D., Ph.D., Thomas D. Dressel, M.D. and Terrence M. Quigley, M.D.

Objectives

To define stomal gastritis by pointing out the only slight role of acidity, uncertainty of diagnosis and lack of therapeutic success with a purely medical approach. To review a surgical technique of diverting upper gastrointestinal juices away from the stomach without eliciting ulcerogenic sequelae.

Introduction

Operations for peptic ulcer disease are all too often followed by undesirable sequelae, ranging from mildly unpleasant to incapacitating. Two decades ago major emphasis was on the dumping syndrome. Only in recent years has the postoperative entity, "alkaline stomal gastritis," been widely appreciated. One of the major symptoms, bile vomiting, was previously attributed to afferent loop obstruction, despite little supporting evidence. As will be discussed, alkalinity has no pathogenic significance and "stomal gastritis" is, therefore, a more accurate term.

Case History

The patient was 30 years old when he underwent an antrectomy with vagotomy and Billroth II reconstruction in 1974 for treatment of a bleeding duodenal ulcer. Following operation, he suffered from postprandial epigastric pain and a

---

John P. Delaney, M.D., Ph.D., Thomas D. Dressel, M.D. and Terrence M. Quigley, M.D., Department of Surgery, University Hospital, Minneapolis, Minn.

Supported by a research grant from the NIH 5R01 AM 16431.

sense of fullness. Antacids provided no relief. There was spontaneous reflux of gastric contents into the esophagus at night and frequent bile vomiting. During the three years after operation, the man lost 34 pounds. A Hollander test indicated an incomplete vagotomy. X-rays showed a hiatus hernia, esophageal reflux and slow gastric emptying. No stomal ulcer could be identified. Esophageal motility studies were normal. Endoscopy confirmed the hiatus hernia and demonstrated esophagitis, with friable mucosa. There was reddening of the stomach mucosa, most marked around the anastomosis. At reoperation the vagotomy was completed, the hiatus hernia was repaired and the Billroth II refashioned as a Roux-Y anastomosis. Since then, this man has been completely free of gastrointestinal symptoms.

This case illustrates many of the important features of stomal gastritis. The first is that the pain pattern is not that of peptic ulcer. It is not relieved by antacids and is aggravated by food intake. Vomiting of bile without food is common, although not essential, to the diagnosis. Bilious vomiting is a particularly unpleasant symptom which tends to bring the patient back to the surgeon for reevaluation. Because of discomfort caused by food intake, these patients almost invariably lose weight. The major clinical features then are pain, weight loss and bile vomiting. This particular patient also had a common associated problem, namely, esophagitis.

The pylorus has been called "the second most important sphincter in the body." Normally the pylorus, in conjunction with antral peristalsis, prevents reflux of duodenal contents into the stomach. When pyloric sphincter function is destroyed by operation, be it pyloroplasty, gastroenterostomy or gastric resection, intestinal contents enter the stomach in excessive amounts. The fact that topical exposure of the gastric mucosa to intestinal juices leads to mucosal injury has long been recognized. The earliest observations came from endoscopic exam following operation in humans. Endoscopy invariably shows some degree of gastritis around gastrointestinal stomas. Changes are visible as red, friable peristomal mucosa. Mucosal biopsies reveal an inflammatory infiltrate in the lamina propria. There is a diminution of parietal and chief cell numbers and, as a consequence of this, acid secretory capacity is low or acid production may be absent.

We have studied these phenomena in the laboratory [1]. In one of the experimental models, a tube of gastric corpus was fashioned from the greater curvature, pedicled on the short gastric vessels and interposed in the jejunum [2]. Thus, the mucosa was chronically exposed to bile, pancreatic juice and whatever other substances pass through the upper intestine. Histologic changes were quite reproducible. The histology of the parent stomach was compared to that of the mucosa exposed to upper intestinal juices. Major changes were decreased numbers of acid-secreting parietal cells and pepsin-secreting chief cells. There was a disorderly "corkscrew" appearance to the glands. There was hyperplasia of mucous cells such that they penetrated into depths of the mucosa while normally the mucous cells are found mainly near the surface.

That acid plays little or no part in this process was demonstrated in another experiment [3]. The innervated vascularized antrum was interposed in the upper jejunum. Thus, the mucosa was constantly bathed in jejunal juices, but no acid was present. Here again, the mucosa developed an inflammatory infiltrate, disorderly configuration of the antral glands and mucous cell hyperplasia.

In another study we attempted to determine what constituent of jejunal contents caused the injury [4]. In one model, a tube of gastric corpus was fashioned to drain the gallbladder after ligation of the common duct. Thus, the mucosa was exposed to pure bile. In another experiment, pure pancreatic juice bathed corpus mucosa. Both developed changes comparable to the lesions induced by whole jejunal contents. The loss of parietal cells, the degree of inflammatory infiltrate and glandular disorganization was quantitatively less with exposure to pure bile or pancreatic juice than with exposure to whole intestinal contents.

In 1969, we reported observations in dogs subjected to vagotomy and pyloroplasty or to antral resection with Billroth I or Billroth II reconstructions [5]. Gastritis was most extensive after the Billroth II procedure. With Billroth I reconstruction, the changes were localized to the mucosa lying within a few centimeters of the anastomosis. After a Billroth II reconstruction, changes were found throughout the residual gastric pouch. Parietal cell numbers were markedly reduced in the gastric mucosa.

Using a different approach, Van Geetruyden studied maximal acid secretory capacity in humans who had undergone partial gastrectomy [6]. He found a progressive decrease in acid secretory capacity with passing years and postulated that this was due to a loss of parietal cells associated with gastritis caused by intestinal juice bathing the gastric mucosa. Numerous endoscopic studies have confirmed this view.

In 1967, Williams reported a clinical study on a single patient, which further defined the problem [7]. He had occasion to operate for gallstones on a patient who had previously undergone partial gastrectomy and Billroth II reconstruction. This man was afflicted with bile vomiting, pain and weight loss — the entire syndrome of stomal gastritis. At the time of cholecystectomy, a catheter was placed in the duodenum. Later, the tube was perfused with various test solutions. When saline was used, the subject experienced no symptoms. When bile was infused into the duodenum, the patient developed typical pain and subsequently vomited the bile. This stomach clearly had a specific sensitivity to bile.

The critical question is why some individuals following gastrectomy are sensitive to intestinal juices in the stomach while the majority are quite asymptomatic. All patients with an anastomosis of stomach to intestine have some degree of gastritis. Endoscopic appearance and histologic changes have little correlation with severity of symptoms. It has been estimated that from 5% to 35% of patients have symptoms secondary to gastritis following ulcer operations [8]. In one large British series, 9% of patients suffered from bile vomiting after ulcer operations [9]. Why do only a small proportion of patients with gastritis experience pain and vomit bile? An alternative question is: Why does anyone have symptoms secondary to gastritis? The inflammatory changes are confined to the mucosa which has little in the way of sensory nerve endings.

Diagnosis is uncertain. The difficulty is that intestinal contents can be found in the stomachs of all patients who have undergone an ulcer operation, with the exception of highly selective vagotomy. Histologic gastritis is found in most. Symptoms of stomal gastritis are not specific. The problem is to establish, in any particular individual, whether the symptoms are related to the mucosal inflammatory changes. If sensitivity to bile in the stomach were predictable in advance, the primary operation could be designed to eliminate reflux.

A less well-recognized association is a high frequency of esophagitis in patients with stomal gastritis, 50% in some series [8, 10-13]. One important observation in this regard is that after gastric resection there is a high incidence of esophageal reflux. This is true even in individuals not undergoing vagotomy. Reflux is probably even more frequent when vagotomy has been done and the anatomy about the gastroesophageal junction is disrupted. In one study esophageal reflux could be shown in 40% of patients after gastric resection with either Billroth I or Billroth II reconstruction [14]. A second important fact is that gastric juice containing bile is far more corrosive to the esophageal mucosa than is pure acid peptic juice [15]. A third empiric observation is that severe esophagitis in these circumstances has been completely relieved by procedures which divert intestinal juice away from the stoma, even though nothing is done to correct gastroesophageal reflux [11-13]. In many cases the pain attributed to stomal gastritis actually arises from the esophagus.

Treatment

With respect to treatment, we can largely dismiss medical measures. Metaclopramide has been used to hasten gastric emptying with little improvement in the symptoms. Another reasonable approach is oral administration of cholestyramine, which, by binding bile salts, should diminish the insult to the mucosa. As one might have predicted, clinical trials have shown little benefit. Bile is present in the upper intestine, intermittently throughout the course of the day and, therefore, cholestyramine could be effective only if given continuously. Anatacids are of little avail because acid is not the offending agent.

The only way symptoms of stomal gastritis can be relieved is by diversion of the upper gastrointestinal juices away from the stomach. Various operative rearrangements have been proposed. Examples from many series, including our own, attest to the futility of converting a Billroth II to a Billroth I anastomosis. The latter does not provide sufficient protection from reflux. Most students of the problem have come to employ a Roux-Y reconstruction as the preferred procedure, because it is simpler and more dependable than other possibilities [9, 11, 15]. As a technical point, the Roux-Y anastomosis should be made such that the efferent loop is at least 40 cm long. This will insure that no bile or pancreatic juice refluxes back into the stomach. In doing this procedure, it is very important to establish that a complete vagotomy is present. In the absence of vagotomy, the Roux-Y is an ulcerogenic arrangement, probably because the neutralizing effects of pancreatic juice are eliminated. The fact that the gastritic stomach is capable of secreting little acid does not obviate the need for vagotomy. When intestinal juices are diverted away, the gastritic mucosa reverts to histologic normity and recovers normal acid secretory capacity [16-18].

Summary

Operative loss of pyloric sphincter function allows intestinal contents to bathe the gastric mucosa. Topical bile or pancreatic juice induces peristomal gastritis. A small fraction of patients experience symptoms associated with the gastritis and/or esophagitis. The major complaints are postprandial epigastric pain, weight loss and bile vomiting. Accurate selection of patients requiring reoperation is difficult. Medical measures generally provide little relief. Complete relief of symptoms can be obtained by diversions of intestinal contents away from the stoma, which is most readily accomplished by a Roux-Y reconstruction. Complete vagotomy is essential to avoid later stomal ulcer.

References

1. Robbins, P.L., Broadie, T.A., Sosin, H. and Delaney, J.P.: Reflux gastritis: The consequences of intestinal juice in the stomach. Am. J. Surg. 131:23-29, 1976.
2. Cheng, J., Ritchie, W. and Delaney, J.: Atrophic gastritis: An experimental model. Fed. Proc. 28:513, 1969.
3. Butler, B., Cheng, J., Ritchie, W. and Delaney, J.P.: Antral gastritis and parietal cell hyperplasia. Fed. Proc. 29:255, 1970.
4. Delaney, J.P., Broadie, T.A. and Robbins, P.L.: Pyloric reflux gastritis: The offending agent. Surgery 77:764-772, 1975.

5. Ritchie, W.P., Jr. and Delaney, J.P.: Parietal cell changes in the stomach after ulcer operations. J. Surg. Res. 12:17-23, 1972.
6. Van Geetruyden, J.: Alterations de la Physiologie Gastrique Sous l'Influence de la Bile: Leur Importance pour la Pathogenie de l'Ulcere Peptique Recidivant après Gastrectomie. Bull. Acad. Med. Belg. 1:53-117, 1961.
7. Williams, J.A.: Postgastrectomy bile vomiting. Pac. Med. Surg. 75:105-107, 1967.
8. Himal, H.S.: Alkaline gastritis and alkaline esophagitis: A review. Can. J. Surg. 20:403-412, 1977.
9. Griffiths, J.M.T.: The features and course of bile vomiting following gastric surgery. Br. J. Surg. 61:617-622, 1974.
10. Coppinger, W.R., Job, H., DeLauro, J.F. et al: Surgical treatment of reflux gastritis and esophagitis. Arch. Surg. 106(4):463-468, 1973.
11. Payne, W.S.: Surgical treatment of reflux esophagitis and stricture associated with permanent incompetence of the cardia. Mayo Clin. Proc. 45:553-562, 1970.
12. Weaver, A.W., Large, A.M. and Walt, A.J.: Surgical management of severe reflux esophagitis: Eight to seventeen year follow-up study. Am. J. Surg. 119:15-20, 1970.
13. Wickbom, G., Bushkin, F.L. and Woodward, E.R.: Alkaline reflux esophagitis. Surg. Gynecol. Obstet. 139:267-271, 1974.
14. Windsor, C.W.O.: Gastro-oesophageal reflux after partial gastrectomy. Br. Med J. 2:1233-1234, 1964.
15. Gillison, E.W., DeCastro, V.A.M., Nyhus, L.M. et al: The significance of bile in reflux esophagitis. Surg. Gynecol. Obstet. 134:419-424, 1972.
16. Drapanas, T. and Bethea, M.: Reflux gastritis following gastric surgery. Ann. Surg. 179(5):618-627, 1974.
17. Herrington, J.L., Sawyers, J.L. and Whitehead, W.A.: Surgical management of reflux gastritis. Ann. Surg. 180:526-537, 1974.
18. Van Heerden, J.A., Priestley, J.T., Farrow, G.M. and Phillips, S.F.: Postoperative alkaline reflux gastritis: Surgical implications. Am. J. Surg. 118:427-433, 1969.

Self-Evaluation Quiz

1. Stomal gastritis:
   a) Involves alkalinity as a significant factor in pathology
   b) Is relieved by antacids
   c) Is not aggravated by food intake
   d) May be manifested by vomiting of bile without food
2. Major clinical features of stomal gastritis are:
   a) Weight loss, postprandial epigastric pain and bile vomiting
   b) Weight loss, postprandial epigastric pain and overacidity

c) Postprandial epigastric pain, overacidity and bile vomiting
d) Postprandial epigastric pain, alkalinity and bile vomiting

3. All patients with stomach anastomosis exhibit some degree of:
   a) Acidity
   b) Gastritis
   c) Esophagitis
   d) Hypertension
4. Endoscopy and histology:
   a) Are always correlated with symptoms
   b) Are never correlated with symptoms
   c) Do not have much correlation with symptoms
   d) Reveal stomal gastritis in 98% of cases
5. Esophagitis:
   a) Shows some correlation with stomal gastritis
   b) Shows no correlation with stomal gastritis
   c) Is more likely to be caused by pure acid peptic juice than by bile in the gastric juice
   d) Is never the cause of pain attributed to stomal gastritis

Answers on page 721.

Medical Therapy of Duodenal Ulcer

Howard M. Spiro, M.D.

Objectives

To develop a conservative approach (that is, one that does not perforce turn people into patients) for dealing with the histology, physiology and psychology involved in the therapy of duodenal ulcer.

For the clinician a major decision in the therapy of peptic ulcer is when to use H_2 blockers. Two things should be kept in mind: (1) it is very difficult to keep a peptic ulcer from healing once it has come under observation, as controlled studies of therapy of duodenal ulcer have taught us and, on the other hand, (2) for the short term at least cimetidine seems to be a harmless drug with surprisingly few side effects recognized so far. Like its H_1 blocker cousins, cimetidine has therapeutic merit without much evidence of short-term risk [1]. Whether this hubristic view will be maintained remains to be seen.

In any case, clinicians are not yet fully agreed on the role of the H_2 blockers in the acute duodenal ulcer with or without complications, nor in the chronic duodenal ulcer, nor yet even whether or how an H_2 blocker should be used to try to prevent acute ulceration.

By some the management of peptic ulcer is being compared, wrongly it seems to me, to that of hypertension. The current notion that every hydrogen ion emerging from the sea of gastric juice needs to be squashed by a combination of H_2 blockers, antacids and anticholinergic agents forgets that peptic ulcer hitherto has been for most of its owners a relatively benign

---

Howard M. Spiro, M.D., Professor, Department of Medicine, Yale University School of Medicine, New Haven, Conn.

disorder only occasionally coming to the attention of the surgeon. To insist on the perpetual eradication of ulcer pain is to make patients of persons and tells our patients that every little ache or pain needs a pill. I do not believe that the relationship between acid and ulcer pain or between ulcer crater and ulcer pain is so straightforward as to demand that acid be completely neutralized by the clinician who is not yet bent on messianic goals.

There are several drugs that the clinician will watch over the next few years. A few years ago prostaglandins looked as if they might not make it in the therapeutic race so effective and impressive were the actions of the H_2 blockers. Now that it is becoming clear that prostaglandins are "cytoprotective," that they somehow preserve the integrity of cellular membranes, their presence in the gastric mucosa in the normal state makes them seem more appealing. We may very well see the delineation of a separate role for the prostaglandins — to protect against erosive gastritis and "irritation," while the H_2 blockers are used to inhibit secretion [2]. This is the year, if not the decade, of somatostatin which seems to turn off just about every gastrointestinal function: it lowers the pressure of the esophageal sphincter, cuts out pancreatic secretion and even eliminates intestinal secretion to control the diarrhea of carcinoid syndrome. We may anticipate the use of somatostatin in some patients with duodenal ulcer [3]. Not all drugs emerging into prominence are new drugs, for bismuth has been around a long, long time. Until now its most appealing application has been on television to coat the stomach for advertisers, but now that control studies suggest a role for bismuth in the management of gastric ulcer, we may look to see this faithful old friend return to some respect.

In all his ministrations the physician will do well to keep in mind what I have already alluded to — that people should consider themselves as healthy as possible, that they should regard most illnesses as incidental to life and that they should not be made patients by well-meaning physicians. If we tell our patients that every pain needs a treatment or prevention, then we run the risk of making them neurotic. I think this problem is becoming one of the biggest considerations in the current management of patients with peptic ulcer.

The diagnosis of peptic ulcer deserves comment in any discussion of therapy. Physicians have too long been entranced by the ulcer crater simply because that was how duodenal ulcer first came to attention. Yet now that "double-blind" studies are showing the poor relationship between ulcer pain and ulcer crater, it is time to reconsider the notion of the peptic ulcer syndrome or what I have termed "Moynihan's disease" [4]. Consider for a moment the 21-year-old Jewish student with right lower quadrant pain, diarrhea, 20 lb weight loss and modest fever, all suggesting the diagnosis of regional enteritis; if on radiological examination the terminal ileum and colon appear normal, the clinical diagnosis is not discarded because of the absence of morphological proof. An appendiceal abscess may be considered, but the prudent clinician usually goes ahead to treat the patient without radiological confirmation and usually even now does not require colonoscopic glimpses into the ileum. We have not been "hung up" on the presence of a crater or even on thickening of the bowel in the patient with the clinical syndrome of Crohn's disease. In duodenal ulcer, however, because the ulcer crater was what first called attention to the peptic ulcer syndrome, clinicians have concentrated too much on that crater, even the FDA insisting on its presence as a bona fide evidence of "peptic ulcer." So much effort has been expended in watching the comings and goings of the ulcer crater that I suspect that the general welfare might have been improved had we used the term Moynihan's disease in honor of that great surgeon of Leeds who devoted so much of his life to duodenal ulcer, even if — alas — to its cure by operation. Moynihan's disease would have had the physician recognize that persons might have symptoms suggestive of duodenal ulcer without the crater, that they might have had hypersecretion, from time to time an ulcer crater, and that even duodenitis or a normal duodenum with endoscopy was still compatible with the notion of "peptic ulcer disease." All of these manifestations might have been recognized as acute or chronic stages of Moynihan's disease and the ulcer crater would not have seemed important in itself except in the presence of an acute gastrointestinal bleed. To be sure, the careless clinician might have treated a spastic colon as duodenal ulcer, but this happens so often anyway that little would be changed.

I will not comment on the role of endoscopy in the diagnosis of gastric ulcer where "mini-gastrectomy" biopsies sometimes lead us astray, but I should emphasize the endoscopic evaluation of the gastrointestinal bleeder. Surgeons know very well of the value of endoscopy in gastrointestinal bleeding, but few realize the growing skepticism of the internists. Because several studies have failed to show decreased morbidity or mortality in groups of bleeding patients, the notion is gaining respectability in medical circles that endoscopy is a little benefit for the acute GI bleeder. I think that my medical colleagues blunder on the utilitarian fallacy that the common good is all that counts and that the benefit to the individual must be weighed against the benefits to the group as a whole. In the individual patient, I like to try to find the source of the bleed, so that I can tell the patient with erosive gastritis that he need not fear another bleed if he avoids aspirin and other gastric irritants, and so that I can be more prepared to advise operation in the patient with gastric ulcer and so forth. I will not belabor this point to a convinced audience, but antipathy to endoscopy has two bases which should be distinguished: one is based on the general unpleasantness and the apparent belief in the lack of clinical utility while the other, I think, comes from the enormous cost of the procedure which seems excessive in the aggregate to many people.

Returning to the subject of medical therapy of peptic ulcer, we must consider briefly the etiology of peptic ulcer: (1) anatomical, (2) physiological and (3) psychological. Since the very name "peptic ulcer" suggests a cause which is far from known, Kothari has suggested "dyspeptic ulcer" as a much better term and he may be right! It is now generally accepted that the anatomical barriers of mucus and lipids in the cell membrane prevent the back diffusion of acid from the lumen of the stomach and, therefore, prevent autodigestion. When these barriers are weak and broken by bile, aspirin or other noxious agents, acid seeps back into the mucosa to lead to erosive gastritis, gastric ulcer and duodenal ulcer — according to these theories at least. This makes general sense, but we should recognize that most peptic ulcers occur at the boundary of acid-secreting mucosa with nonacid-secreting mucosa and that if the broken barrier was the only key to the process, ulcers created by the removal of gastric polyps or by biopsy of the duodenal mucosa in duodenal ulcer patients would not heal as readily as they do without specific reduction of the acid levels. The tendency of most ulcerations in the upper gut is to heal and we should be surprised when they do not. Not enough attention has been paid to repair and healing in the stomach and to what stimulates and retards it. I suspect that such matters may be as important as the acid-secretory levels in the duodenal ulcer patient.

All physiological studies suggest that acid is necessary to the production of an experimental ulcer: stress ulcers can be prevented by inhibition of acid. All clinical studies similarly suggest that there is increased acid in the stomach of most duodenal ulcer patients and that there is a higher than normal concentration of acid in the duodenum as a result of a rapid rate of gastric secretion and emptying and possibly also with an abnormal pancreatic bicarbonate response to the hydrochloric acid. Whatever, most duodenal ulcer patients secrete more acid in response to a given stimulant than groups of nonduodenal ulcer patients.

As acid seems like the most logical force which causes or permits peptic ulcer and as it is acid that the gastroenterologist attacks with all the forces at his command, we should ask whether the relationship between ulcer pain and acid levels is proven. Despite extensive and long-term studies in many patients, no observer so far has been able to find any difference in the pain relief of duodenal ulcer between placebo and antacids, no matter how powerful. Indeed, even in the most recent endoscopic studies of Peterson [5], which are taken to show the benefit of antacids, at the end of four weeks 69% of patients taking antacids and 63% of patients taking identical placebo were free of pain. The problem of pain relief has attended even studies of cimetidine where, overall, it may be said that the largest cooperative study in the United States found pain relief from cimetidine greater than that of placebo at three days only, when 63% of the patients taking cimetidine had no pains against 39% of patients on placebo. At all other times in the study, the relief of pain was statistically the same in both groups. It is clear that there are many factors in the pain relief of duodenal ulcer besides neutralization of acid, and such observation should keep the prudent physician from assailing every hydrogen ion so fervently [6].

There is even a poor relationship between the presence of an ulcer crater and ulcer pain, something well known to the physician who talks to his patients. Most physicians never believed that in the lawyer who had pain from Monday to Friday and was free of pain on Saturday and Sunday, the ulcer came and went during the weekend, but rather suspected that other factors influenced pain perception. Now endoscopic studies visually confirm what we have always heard; for example, in the Peterson study, one third of patients free of pain four weeks after the start of therapy still had an endoscopically visible duodenal ulcer while, equally importantly, in almost half the patients complaining of pain the duodenal ulcer could not be found endoscopically. Such observations remind us that pain has many different sources in the duodenum and it may well be that when the physician can pass a scanning electron microscope into the duodenal bulb, he will see minute junctional breaks in the barrier which account for the rapid appearance and disappearance of pain. Until that time, however, the clinician should remain wary of rigid precepts about how to treat duodenal ulcer. He should wonder whether healing the crater does more than relieve the pain and, given the data so far, whether eliminating all or most of the acid helps more than eliminating only some of it.

Still, the gastroenterologist has to do something when he is not endoscoping patients, and usually we treat duodenal ulcer in an existential manner despite the foregoing, aiming at reducing acid in the hope that decreased acid will speed healing and prevent recurrence. Fortunately, the parietal cell has three sides and as the evidence varies from time to time whether there are separate receptor sites for different stimuli or whether all agents work through histamine, we may imagine that each side of the parietal cell has a different receptor, for histamine, for acetylcholine and for gastrin. Indeed, the most recent evidence suggests that the parietal cell does have separate receptors and that the overall effect is additive, histamine and acetylcholine, for example, working together to stimulate more acid than either one separately. Blocking histamine receptors reduces the response to acetylcholine not because acetylcholine works through histamine, but rather because a combination of responses from acetylcholine and histamine receptors gives a greater response than from one alone.

In any case, medical therapy aims at acid (1) by neutralizing what is in the stomach with either food or antacids, (2) by inhibiting gastric secretion through the cell receptors already mentioned and (3) by such uncertain methods as carbenoxolone and glyptide. In this discussion I shall comment briefly on a few pertinent matters.

Milk and bland diets relieve pain even if they do not reduce acid very significantly; indeed, if anything, milk may increase the amount of acid and is now deemed harmful by the mathematically minded, even if it has had a long career in the relief of pain. I still recommend it to patients with peptic ulcer pain, even as I recognize that the benefit of most dietary therapy, such as small regular meals which I also suggest, may be as much sacramental as medical. Antacid therapy seems to be helpful in the clinic as well as in the control study, but I am not at all certain that all acid needs to be eliminated. The average antacid buffers gastric juice for 20 to 40 minutes only, antacid potency varies widely and gastric acid even more widely, the usual amount of antacid given is too low to bring about effective complete neutralization; yet, as we all know, pain is often relieved. Therefore, like many other gastroenterologists, I simply give regular amounts of liquid antacid, paying attention to the patient's bowels, not attempting to neutralize all the acid in the stomach, but simply using enough to relieve pain, recognizing the powerful placebo effect and that white liquid antacids make the logical placebos for our era. I recall that Dr. Sippy attempted to eliminate acid with diets as earnestly as some of my colleagues attempt to neutralize acids with antacids, and I choose the middle way.

The indications for the H_2 blockers change almost monthly. The publicity attendant on these new "miracle drugs" has been so great that most physicians now know that the effects of histamine that are not blocked by H_1 receptor antagonists, such as benadryl, are blocked by H_2 receptor antagonists. These include gastric acid secretion, the atrial heart rate, uterine contractility and, probably most important for long-term implications, the T-lymphocyte. We are not yet certain as to whether immunity is enhanced or suppressed by long-term use of H_2 antagonists, but sooner or later the evidence will be in. It is this effect on the T-lymphocyte that hinders enthusiasm for long-term cimetidine, which in other respects so far seems to be harmless. From a clinical standpoint, the suppression of gastric acid secretion in patients with duodenal ulcer given cimetidine is exhilarating indeed, but as I have already pointed out in the individual patient, the statistical benefit of cimetidine remains under study. The natural healing rate of duodenal ulcer varies widely from patient to patient, and from physician to physician, and so it seems to me that cimetidine may be considered simply to abolish such variations. I consider cimetidine indicated for the intractable duodenal ulcer patient, certainly before operation is considered. The patient being considered for operation for intractable pain should be endoscoped to be sure that an ulcer is present and should receive a six to eight week course of cimetidine, preferably in the hospital. I believe that cimetidine is also indicated for the patient with persistent night pain, and I suspect that sooner or later we will wean our patients off cimetidine at the end of the six to eight week course by giving them a night dose of cimetidine to cut out nocturnal acid secretion for a considerably longer period of time. I also suspect the current use of cimetidine four times a day may be more than is necessary and it would not surprise me to learn that cimetidine once or twice a day proves as effective as four times daily. When do I use cimetidine in my patients? On the one hand, I've emphasized that patients with duodenal ulcer become asymptomatic and seem to heal once they come to the attention of a physician, regardless of therapy; but, on the other side, I have to say that short-term cimetidine is remarkably free of side effects. We have not had enough long-term experience with the drug for me to be certain of that, but at present I am much impressed by the lack of side effects on a six to eight week course. Therefore, at present, I recommend that the patient take standard antacids and a modified diet for a few days before giving them cimetidine. If they respond immediately to antacids and small regular feeings, I have done enough. If they do not respond in a few days, or if the inconvenience of carrying antacids around is so great, I think that clinical evidence is strong enough to suggest that they take cimetidine three or four times a day. I do not, so far, see the superiority of cimetidine over standard therapies except for its convenience and the clear benefit in the intractable patient. I believe the drug should be given short term only, at least in the United States, but I do not know whether repeating the course after stopping it for two or three days qualifies as "short term" or "long term." I confess that I have given cimetidine at bedtime for longer than the standard eight week course.

We have much to learn about the therapy and the natural history of duodenal ulcer, and it is to the credit of a commercial pharmaceutical company that not only have they supported the research responsible for this remarkable advance in the management of a common disorder, but that their continued support of medical research has given us so much information about the natural history of duodenal ulcer.

References

1. Binder, H.J., Cocco, A., Crossley, R.J. et al: Cimetidine in the treatment of duodenal ulcer. Gastroenterology 74:380, 1978.
2. Carmichael, H.A., Nelson, L.M. and Russell, R.I.: Cimetidine and prostaglandins — evidence for different modes of action in the rat gastric mucosa. Gastroenterology 74:1229-1232, 1978.
3. Barros D'Sa, A.A., Bloom, S.R. and Baron, J.H.: Inhibition by Somatostatin of gastric acid and pepsin and of cellular release of gastrin. Gut 19:315-320, 1978.
4. Spiro, H.M.: Moynihan's Disease — The diagnosis of duodenal ulcer. N. Engl. J. Med. 291:567-569, 1974.
5. Peterson, W.L., Sturdevant, R.A., Frankl, H.D. et al: Healing of duodenal ulcer with an antacid regimen. N. Engl. J. Med. 297:341, 1977.
6. Gudjonsson, B. and Spiro, H.M.: Placebo response in ulcer disease. Am. J. Med. 65:399-402, 1978.

Self-Evaluation Quiz

1. Cimetidine is probably:
   a) Harmless for short periods
   b) Harmless for as long as necessary to clear up duodenal ulcer
   c) The cause of many side effects in duodenal ulcer patients

d) Only a minimal suppressant of gastric acid secretion in duodenal ulcer patients

2. H_2-blockers:
   a) Are always preferred for preventing acute ulceration
   b) Are never preferred for preventing acute ulceration
   c) May or may not be preferred for preventing acute ulceration
3. The conscientious therapist should:
   a) Cater to his patient's concern about pain
   b) Insist on the patient realizing that he is indeed a patient
   c) Not insist on the eradication of ulcer pain
4. Prostaglandins:
   a) May be cytoprotective
   b) Certainly do not protect cellular membranes
   c) Occur in normal gastric mucosa
   d) Do not protect against anything we know of in duodenal ulcer patients
5. Somatostatin:
   a) Should not be used for duodenal ulcer patients
   b) May be used in some duodenal ulcer patients
   c) Should not be used in any ulcer patients
   d) Is being phased out by the pharmaceutical industry merely because they cannot make enough profit from it
6. Ulcer pain correlates:
   a) Well with craters and domestic stress
   b) Poorly with craters
   c) Well with psychosomatic headaches and craters
   d) Poorly with domestic strife but well with craters
7. Kothari suggests:
   a) Forgetting craters
   b) Using the concept of "dyspeptic ulcer"
   c) Using the concept "apeptic ulcer"
   d) Using the concept "disparate ulcer pain"
8. Most peptic ulcers occur:
   a) At the boundary of acid-secreting mucosa with non-acid-secreting mucosa
   b) To the acid side of the boundary
   c) To the nonacid side of the boundary
   d) Equally distributed on one or the other side of the boundary

9. We should not be surprised if:
   a) Most ulcers in the upper gut heal
   b) Most ulcers in the lower gut heal
   c) Most ulcers in the middle gut heal
   d) Upper gut ulcers do not heal

Answers on page 721.

Current Experience With Parietal Cell Vagotomy in the Treatment of Duodenal Ulcer

John C. Goligher, M.D.

Objectives

To consider proximal gastric and other forms of vagotomy in regard to safety, recurrence of the condition being treated, diarrhea, and the Visick classification for overall assessment of postsurgical results in duodenal ulcer surgery.

Five years ago when I was privileged to give the E. Starr Judd Lecture in Minneapolis, I discussed the subject of gastric surgery, specifically the newly introduced, variously designated operation of selective proximal vagotomy, highly selective vagotomy, parietal cell vagotomy or proximal gastric vagotomy in the treatment of duodenal ulcer. This paper reports how the operation has stood the test of time in the management of duodenal ulcer. We have just recently completed a survey of our experience in my department from 1969 to the end of 1976.

We made use of this operation not only for duodenal ulcer but also for other conditions. Sometimes we employed it in patients with dyspepsia of unknown origin, in whom an ulcer was strongly suspected but at laparotomy no organic lesion was found. What should one do in such cases? One might close the abdomen without doing anything. Alternatively one might elect to perform this most minimal form of acid reducing surgery.

John C. Goligher, M.D., Consultant in General and Colorectal Surgery, Leeds, England; Emeritus Professor of Surgery, University of Leeds; formerly Surgeon, The General Infirmary at Leeds; Consulting Surgeon, St. Mark's Hospital for Diseases of the Rectum and Colon, London, England.

Sometimes we have combined it with operations for esophageal reflux. We have also done it for gastric ulcer, or for combined gastric and duodenal ulcer. But we have used it mostly for duodenal ulcer. I want to concentrate on the 323 *male* patients in order to make comparisons with our own experience with various other operations for duodenal ulcer. So I am going to make the issue clear by confining my remarks to 323 male duodenal ulcer patients treated by proximal gastric vagotomy without drainage. Actually, seven of those had a concomitant cholecystectomy and we have taken them out of consideration because those additional gallbladder operations might have influenced the results.

When you are trying to assess clinically the value of an operation for peptic ulcer, it seems to me that four things are important: (1) How safe is the operation? (2) How successful is it in curing the ulcer and preventing recurrence? (3) What side effects does it produce? Obviously, to cripple the patient severely with major side effects discredits the operation. (4) What are the overall results in terms of the patient's capacity for work and recreation?

With regard to the safety of the operation, that is very easily dealt with, for we have had no deaths in the 316 male patients, not even in the 40 who had the operation done as an emergency procedure for hemorrhage or perforation. We had one death in the 100-odd female patients with duodenal ulcer, and one death in the 50 or so gastric ulcer patients treated by this operation, which amounts to only two deaths in approximately 500 patients. So the operation seems pretty safe. However, I would not want to underrate the great safety of truncal vagotomy with drainage procedures. I am sure it is possible to perform several hundreds of these operations with perhaps only one death. In fact, we have done 450 elective truncal vagotomies and drainage procedures and have had only one death. Nonetheless, I consider that proximal gastric vagotomy is at least as safe as truncal vagotomy and drainage or perhaps safer, and that is the impression of most people who have used it. There is just one cloud on the horizon with regard to the safety of the operation — the complication known as "lesser curve necrosis." There have been quite a number of cases now recorded with this complication and, presumably, quite a number of cases not recorded. It is a serious occurrence because it seems to be associated with about a 50% mortality. I do not know the cause. It presumably has some technical explanation, injury to the lesser curve region of the stomach by forceps or diathermy during the dissection. I am happy to say that in our cases to date we have not had any instances of lesser curve necrosis and hope it will remain that way. Are there additional precautions that should be taken against leakage from the lesser curve due to necrosis? I now make it my practice to invaginate the lesser curve, to turn it in by a series of sutures between the anterior and the posterior gastric wall. I do what is the same as a fundoplication but at a lower level, on the lesser curve, a maneuver which I call a "corpoplication" rather than "fundoplication."

As regards the ability to protect against recurrent ulceration, initially our results from that point of view were exceedingly good. Where other surgeons were encountering quite a few recurrences we had none. But more recently that has changed. We now have had a number of recurrences. Actually in this series of 316 cases there have been 12 proven recurrences.

Here are some details regarding those 12 recurrent cases. Three of the recurrent ulcers were in the stomach, the rest were in the duodenum. Of course, all of the initial operations to which we are referring now were for duodenal ulcer. A point I would like to make is that in most of the recurrent cases good proximal gastric vagotomies had been performed with denervation to quite a low level on the antrum — mostly at 5.0 to 7.5 cm from the pyloroduodenal junction. The time of diagnosis of the recurrences varied from a few months to several years. As to treatment, four of the patients have had further operation. The rest have been treated medically, mostly by cimetidine, and maybe will come to operation eventually. So these are all proven ulcers, proven either at reoperation or by endoscopy.

In addition, there were five cases which were thought to be recurrences. All had the clinical manifestations of recurrence, but we could not demonstrate an ulcer at reoperation. Most of these patients came to further operation before the modern era of endoscopy. Several of those patients might not have been reoperated on, but with negative endoscopy would probably have been treated conservatively. But, back in 1970 to 1971, we felt that they needed an operation. At operation, no ulcer was found. As this was a reoperation, one felt obliged to do something, and most had another anti-ulcer operation.

There were another 21 patients with recurrent ulcer symptoms, but in whom we have been unable to prove the existence of a recurrence on endoscopy. In many of these cases, the symptoms have been transient, lasting only for a few weeks or months. In others they have caused a good deal of trouble, so much so that the patients regard the operation as unsatisfactory, even though we cannot demonstrate recurrences. As a consequence, some have been put into low Visick grades, 6 or 7 into the bottom grade (IV) because of recurrent pain.

Of course, it is very difficult to assess the true incidence of recurrence in a continuing series like this, where some of the patients have had operation only a year ago. A proper assessment really depends upon at least a five year follow-up. So we should really look at the patients who have had operations at least five years ago.

We have follow-up data on 120 patients traced for five to eight years since operation. Three of those patients were among the seven who had cholecystectomies and should be left out. Thus, we are left with 117 patients. I can compare the five-year results with the results we had after other operations. It obviously is not a controlled comparison and can be criticized on that score. All I can say is that the cases were done more or less in the same environment and for the same indications by approximately the same surgeons. The assessments were all done by the same group, by me and by various colleagues. Indeed, every patient to whom I refer has been seen and assessed by me on many occasions over the years.

We compared the results of proximal gastric vagotomy, in terms of recurrence, with the results of other operations, some of which were in a controlled Leeds-York trial, others not. We concentrate on the rates of proven recurrent ulceration and the incidence of recurrent symptoms. There were 4.3% proven recurrences after PGV, 6.7% after truncal vagotomy and pyloroplasty, 2.5% after truncal vagotomy and gastroenterostomy, none after truncal vagotomy and antrectomy and 0.9% after subtotal gastrectomy. In other words, the resection procedures are distinctly better in protecting against recurrent ulceration than are operations that involve vagotomy alone with or without drainage. As for vagotomy procedures, this new form of vagotomy without drainage seems to take its place alongside truncal vagotomy with gastroenterostomy or pyloroplasty. It is rather better than one and rather worse than the other, but the differences are not statistically significant. The incidence of recurrent symptoms is quite high after proximal gastric vagotomy, slightly less after truncal vagotomy and drainage, and a good deal less after truncal vagotomy and antrectomy or subtotal gastrectomy — the difference as against the resection procedures being statistically significant.

Other writers have reported recurrent ulceration rates following proximal gastric vagotomy to be higher than we found in our series, usually on the basis of shorter follow-ups and smaller series. One wonders what they will find when the follow-up lengthens. Some of these high recurrence rates may be due to technical inadequacies in the operation. Some surgeons have commented on the fact that when they have altered their techniques, they seemed to have fewer recurrences.

The side effects have been gone into endlessly over the last five or six years in our department and many other departments. Proximal gastric vagotomy does better than the other operations in regard to dumping and indeed almost completely eliminates this complaint. It also considerably reduces the incidence of diarrhea. There is just about the same incidence of diarrhea after this operation as there is after a subtotal gastrectomy without vagotomy. Diarrhea is distinctly less frequent than after truncal vagotomy with drainage or with antrectomy. With regard to other side effects with proximal gastric vagotomy, various claims have been made by us and by others. In fact, we have not been able to demonstrate a statistically significant advantage in this particular analysis. For example, bile vomiting is only slightly less frequent after PGV. We have to accept that only dumping and diarrhea are significantly reduced.

Diarrhea is such an important thing that we should analyze it further. Of course, much of the posttruncal vagotomy diarrhea is very mild. It gives the patient very little trouble. We should consider mainly severe diarrhea. In fact, some people say cynically that the best part of a truncal vagotomy operation is that it corrects a tendency to constipation and that a little looseness is often welcome. If you consider only the more severe forms of diarrhea, you can see this operation does quite well. We had two patients who had severe diarrhea. There seems to be a definite advantage with regard to avoidance of diarrhea. When you see bad postvagotomy diarrhea, even if it occurs only in a few patients in every 100 cases, you wish you had never done that operation, for we have virtually nothing to offer in the treatment of this form of diarrhea.

Now let us address the overall assessment. In Leeds, we use a system of grading of the overall results after gastric operations originally employed by a York surgeon, Hedley Visick. It is now referred to as the Visick classification.

The categories of that classification are as follows: Category I means literally perfect. Category II seems almost as good when you first start talking to the patient. But when you interrogate him a bit, you find that he does have a little trouble. In analyzing the results we generally bracket categories I and II together. Category III means that the patient really does have a fair amount of trouble, but in the final analysis, he says, "I think I am better off than I was before the operation." Category IV is where the patient has so much trouble from side effects he reckons that he is worse off than he was before the operation, or he has continued or recurrent ulceration.

Taking the top two categories together, 75% of the patients treated by proximal gastric vagotomy were I or II, compared with 70% after truncal vagotomy and gastroenterostomy, 68% after truncal vagotomy and pyloroplasty, and 78% or 77% for the two resection procedures. In category IV or failed cases, no less than 12% were in this group after proximal gastric vagotomy, mostly those patients who were having pain suggestive of recurrence but could not be demonstrated to have a definite recurrence. If it had not been for these cases, the Visick gradings would have been rather better for this operation.

Let us look in detail at the failures after PGV. There were 14 cases in category IV. Most of the failures were due to proven or suspected recurrent ulcer or to severe recurrent pain without being able to establish the presence of a further ulcer. Only one patient had gastric retention, which emphasizes the point that you do not need to do a drainage procedure with this operation, contrary to the continued recommendation of Fritz Holle of Munich, who was the originator of this operation, which he called selective proximal vagotomy, but which he has always accompanied by a drainage procedure. Our data show that whether or not this form of vagotomy is the best operation for duodenal ulcer, it can be done without drainage. It seems to me that drainage throws away the main advantage of the operation by causing many side effects that can be avoided. Some of the 14 category IV patients came to further operations which improved the Visick grading in some but not all.

In summary, now that I have reviewed these results, am I satisfied or dissatisfied? In one sense the results are as anticipated, insofar as you could not expect a proximal gastric vagotomy to do any better than a complete or truncal vagotomy plus drainage in preventing recurrence—although at one stage we almost convinced ourselves that it might turn out better in this respect! The operation certainly causes less dumping and diarrhea. I personally still do this operation instead of a truncal vagotomy and drainage because I have mastered the technique. The important question is whether I would recommend it to those who are doing truncal vagotomy and drainage at the present time. That is difficult to answer. Certainly if you are going to do the operation, you need to become thoroughly familiar with the technique. That means doing it in several nice thin female patients electively to start. If not many elective ulcer operations come your way — and they seem to be rather rare in the United States now due to the diminishing incidence of peptic ulcer — this experience may be difficult to get. There are some surgeons who feel that either of these operations — vagotomy and drainage, or proximal gastric vagotomy without drainage — does not give enough protection against recurrence and that avoidance of recurrence is most important. Therefore, they feel that the only satisfactory procedures are vagotomy and antrectomy or subtotal gastrectomy even though they carry greater risks to life. In England, that is not a popular view. British surgeons prefer to do a lesser operation in the first instance and accept a certain number of recurrences for which reoperation can be undertaken when necessary. After all, it takes many recurrences to equal one postoperative death. I personally accept the philosophy of an initial lesser operation, but whether it is to be a truncal vagotomy and drainage or a proximal gastric vagotomy without drainage is at present debatable. Provided the incidence of recurrence with the latter procedure does not escalate further, I would continue to opt for it.

Self-Evaluation Quiz

1. Proximal gastric vagotomy is also called:
   a) Selective proximal vagotomy
   b) Highly selective vagotomy
   c) Parietal cell vagotomy
   d) Sykes' duodenal vagotonic maneuver
2. The author believes that to inconvenience the patient with minor side effects discredits the operation.
   a) True
   b) False
3. How safe is truncal vagotomy with drainage procedures?
   a) Not at all
   b) Somewhat
   c) Very much so
   d) 100%
4. Among 450 elective truncal vagotomies with drainage procedure, the author reports:
   a) No deaths
   b) One death
   c) Four deaths
   d) Seven deaths
5. The cause of "lesser curve necrosis":
   a) Is definitely viral infection
   b) Is perhaps associated with iatrogenic factors
   c) Is definitely overuse of antibiotics
6. "Lesser curve necrosis" is associated with a mortality of:
   a) 25%
   b) 30%
   c) 40%
   d) 50%
7. Precautions taken to avoid leakage from the lesser curve due to necrosis include:
   a) Fundoplication

b) Pyloroplication
c) Corpoplication
d) Cardioplication

8. The author reported proven recurrent ulceration in:
   a) 10 of 250 cases
   b) 12 of 316 cases
   c) 14 of 400 cases
   d) No cases
9. What patient series is the author describing from his experience?
   a) 323 males
   b) 345 females
   c) 339 males and females
   d) None of the above

Answers on page 721.

Surgical Treatment of Duodenal Ulcer by Vagotomy and Drainage Procedure

E. R. Woodward, M.D., F.A.C.S.

Objectives

1. To establish the role of the vagus nerve in the pathogenesis of duodenal ulcer.
2. To review the clinical and laboratory results of truncal vagotomy and a drainage procedure in duodenal ulcer patients.

The late Lester Dragstedt revolutionized the surgical treatment of duodenal ulcer when on January 18, 1943, at the University of Chicago Clinics he performed a transthoracic truncal vagotomy in a patient with duodenal ulcer. Three cases were published later that year by Dragstedt and Owens [1]. Today all operations for duodenal ulcer include vagotomy as the single common denominator of the operative procedure. Three variations are currently in wide clinical use. I have been assigned one of these, vagotomy plus drainage procedure, since this was the first of the three to be widely used and well utilized in well over a thousand patients by Dragstedt during his career as a clinical surgeon.

Dragstedt began his career as a basic scientist with a career in physiology encompassing more than six decades. Much of his thought and endeavor during this long period had to do with

---

E. R. Woodward, M.D., F.A.C.S., Professor and Chairman, Department of Surgery, College of Medicine, University of Florida; Chief of Surgery, Shands Teaching Hospital and Clinics, Gainesville, Fla.

This work was performed at the University of Florida, Gainesville, and was supported by NIH grant AM-04178.

peptic ulcer — its pathogenesis, its pathophysiology and its treatment. His first paper on experimental peptic ulcer was published in 1917 [2]. He was well aware that this disorder occurred in man exclusively and did not afflict other mammals. Claude Bernard had shown that the gastric juice was capable of digesting living tissue under laboratory conditions [3]. The powerful proteolytic enzyme pepsin has the unique property of requiring an extremely low pH for its optimal function, ie, pH 3.5 and lower. This simple observation explains why all the activities of the physician and the surgeon are directed toward reducing hydrogen ion to alter gastric pH upward. Hay, Varco, Code and Wangensteen showed that prolonged overproduction of gastric juice would produce experimental peptic ulcer in the dog [4]. That this was not simple histamine toxicity was clearly demonstrated by Dragstedt and co-workers utilizing the dog prepared with the stomach entirely isolated from the gastrointestinal tract with its vagal innervation preserved [5]. Due to disturbances in feedback mechanisms inhibiting gastric secretion, these animals secrete enormous volumes of strongly acid gastric juice. Typical chronic peptic ulcers developed in a majority of the animals, confirming the hypothesis that an overproduction of gastric juice can overwhelm normal defense mechanisms and produce the lesion. If the vagus nerves were cut, secretion from the total stomach pouch was meager and no ulcers developed.

In all mammals except man the gastric secretory apparatus becomes completely quiescent during the interdigestive period, and no hydrogen ion is produced until the next meal. In man, however, there is usually a continuous secretion of acid-containing gastric juice, even in prolonged fasting. It seems a reasonable conjecture that this is a result of the development of the human cerebrum and that in this process the Pavlovian nervous phase of gastric secretion does not completely terminate. It has been known for many years that the human subject with duodenal ulcer has a stomach which will respond to a gastric secretory stimulant to a greater degree than that seen in normal individuals. Dragstedt and co-workers studied fasting human subjects *without* stimulation over a 12-hour nocturnal period [6]. They discovered that 85% of normal subjects secreted less than 20 mEq during this period, averaging 15 mEq, or approximately 1 mEq/hr. Duodenal ulcer patients, on the other hand, secreted acid over a much wider range. Seventy patients were studied in this manner prior to vagotomy and found to average 60 mEq, or 5 mEq/hr. Following transthoracic vagotomy with no other operative procedure performed, these 70 patients demonstrated a profound fall in their fasting or basal gastric secretory rate. This averaged 75% and correlated well with immediate and persistent relief of ulcer symptoms. The patient with a lesser reduction in gastric secretion was subject to persistence or recurrence of ulcer distress.

Dragstedt did not consider applying vagotomy to the treatment of duodenal ulcer because of apprehension that the parasympathetic denervation of the remaining abdominal viscera would have adverse effects. This reservation was laid to rest when esophagogastrectomy was performed in 1938 by Adams and Phemister [7]. Since both vagi were unavoidably sacrificed in this wide resection for cancer and the patients continued to have adequate function of the upper gastrointestinal tract and its appendages, the stage was set. When five years later a patient refused the standard subtotal gastrectomy of the time for his duodenal ulcer, the curtain opened on modern surgical therapy for duodenal ulcer. The patient accepted vagotomy as a less drastic substitute and was rewarded by prompt healing of his ulcer.

Adverse effects of vagotomy on gastric motility were very soon apparent. If vagotomy is adequate, gastric peristalsis is abolished with varying degrees of resultant gastric retention. When this was severe, a secondary drainage operation was performed. It is important to note, however, that in 155 patients treated by vagotomy alone, only one third required the secondary operative procedure. Nonetheless, by 1946 the Dragstedt group was routinely using posterior gastroenterostomy as a drainage operation. Through work in the autopsy suite an abdominal approach to the vagus just above the esophagogastric junction was found feasible. The entire operation, therefore, could be accomplished by the abdominal approach. Weinberg modified the standard two-layered, infolded, Heinecke-Mikulicz pyloroplasty by utilizing only a single layer of non-infolding sutures [8]. It was apparent at once that this procedure permitted adequate emptying of the vagotomized stomach in nearly all patients. Pyloroplasty has the advantages that (1) alkaline duodenal reflux into the stomach is presumably less than with gastrojejunostomy, (2) direct access to an acutely bleeding ulcer permits suture ligature, (3) operating time is saved, (4) more immediate function with regard to gastric emptying is assured and (5) gastrointestinal continuity is maintained, permitting activation of the growing multitude of hormones produced by the duodenum. The latter consideration appears to be more theoretical than real since malnutrition has been an equally rare postoperative sequel with both procedures. However, the dumping syndrome is less common with pyloroplasty.

We reported in 1969 the experience with the use of vagotomy plus drainage procedure at the University of Florida Affiliated Hospitals [9]. This encompassed 455 patients operated upon during the ten-year period 1958 to 1968. The usual male predominance was noted and the average age was 49 years. Three hundred and eighty patients underwent gastric analysis preoperatively, representing 95% of those having elective surgery. This consisted of a one-hour basal collection and a one-hour collection after Histalog (now pentagastrin). These figures demonstrate graphically our conviction that gastric analysis is important in the elective surgical treatment of duodenal ulcer. The procedure has very little diagnostic value because of the large overlap with the normal population. In fact, only 81% of these patients secreted more than 2 mEq/hr in the basal state. However, the test has highly significant prognostic implications. The same gastric analysis performed three to six months after surgical intervention will indicate clearly the surgeon's success in his objective, ie, reduction in gastric acid secretion by 75% or more. In a latter follow-up (1975) there was a close correlation between recurrence of ulcer and gastric analyses [10]. Only two patients with more than a 75% reduction in basal gastric secretion developed recurrent marginal or duodenal ulcer. Conversely, however, many patients with less than a 75% reduction in gastric secretion remained symptom free. If this group is studied separately the likelihood of recurrent marginal or duodenal ulcer is approximately 20%. The implications concerning preventive measures are obvious.

There were 401 (88%) elective operations and 54 (12%) emergency procedures. The most common indication for elective operation was intractability which was the decisive factor in 265 patients (66%). Unavailability of medical therapy, intercurrent hemorrhage and obstruction account for the remaining one third. Acute hemorrhage accounted for 85% of the emergency operations whereas definitive surgery was performed in only eight patients (15%) who presented with acute perforation. Operative mortality in elective cases was 1% (4/401). Two of these were clearly avoidable. Mortality in the emergency group consisted of only one death in 54 patients or 1.8%. This was an 83-year-old female with massive hemorrhage and preexisting severe cardiopulmonary disease.

In the 1969 study 16 patients were found to have proven or suspected recurrent peptic ulcer for an incidence of 3.6%. The same group of patients reevaluated in 1975 had a minimum follow-up of seven years and an average follow-up of ten years. Twenty-six patients had proven or suspected peptic ulcer for an incidence of 5.8%. Eighty-five patients had died in the interim, only one related to peptic ulcer. This patient died following emergency operation for bleeding marginal ulcer. It is interesting that only four of the recurrent ulcers were gastric in location and in every instance had a latent period of five years or longer. On the other hand, all the recurrent marginal or duodenal ulcers appeared within the first five years.

The dumping syndrome was reported in the 1969 study to be present in 65 patients (14%). This was of the early postprandial type in 60 and the late or hypoglycemic type in five. In the 1975 study adequate information could be obtained from 348 patients. Only ten (3%) still complained of this disorder: eight of the early postprandial variety and two with the hypoglycemic type. This unpleasant consequence of ablating the pyloric sphincter is clearly not a significant long-term deterrent to the use of vagotomy and pyloroplasty for duodenal ulcer.

Diarrhea, on the other hand, while less common in the earlier study, tended to be more persistent. In 1969, 21 or approximately 5% of the patients had postvagotomy diarrhea. This is distinguished from the diarrhea associated with the early postprandial dumping syndrome by its episodic nature, its nonrelationship to food intake, its failure to respond to a low carbohydrate diet and its not infrequent nocturnal character. In the 1975 study the incidence was approximately the same, ie,

5%, but unfortunately the system of data collection did not permit us to match patients. In one patient the disturbance was severe enough that remedial surgery was required.

It was possible to assess the clinical result both from the patient and by physician evaluation in the 1969 study. Seventy-seven percent of the patients were totally asymptomatic, whereas an additional 19% had only minor gastrointestinal symptoms for an overall patient satisfaction rate of 96%. Three percent of the patients were dissatisfied with the operation and 1% felt that they were unimproved or worse. The physician evaluation correlated rather closely. Seventy-six percent were considered to have an excellent result and 16% a good result for an overall satisfactory outcome in 92%. Two percent were thought to have only a fair clinical result and 6% a poor result. The difference in the lowest category represented a few patients with recurrent ulcer who were well controlled on medical management and therefore not dissatisfied. The 1975 study relied mainly on a questionnaire with only partial physician evaluation by telephone or clinic visit. The subjective evaluation of the patients with this much longer follow-up indicated that 87% were satisfied with the result of their operative procedure, 7% were dissatisfied and 6% felt that the operation had failed or that they were worse. We feel that the difference in the two studies is only partly related to the time interval and is largely the result in the earlier study of the impact of direct physician contact. We feel the later figures are more representative of the true long-term results of vagotomy-drainage.

In summary, vagotomy and pyloroplasty has during the past three decades proven to be a useful definitive and occasionally emergency procedure for the treatment of chronic duodenal ulcer and its complications. The procedure can be accomplished quickly with the advantages of less anesthesia and less operative trauma. More important, the hazards associated with a callous, penetrating, posterior wall duodenal ulcer near the pyloric ring are entirely avoided. Therefore, one is not faced with blown duodenal stumps and the associated high morbidity and mortality. The net result is a low morbidity and mortality, a short stay in the hospital and a quick return to normal activity. The incidence of "dumping" is relatively low; probably as a result of this, adequate nutrition is maintained in most patients. Most postoperative diarrhea is a manifestation of "dumping." However, idiopathic postvagotomy diarrhea is indeed a troublesome, if uncommon, complication. The reflux alkaline syndromes involving stomach and/or esophagus seem to be less frequent than after resective procedures, but quantitive data are lacking. The operation has the disadvantage as compared to vagotomy and antrectomy of a significant, although still relatively low, recurrence rate and probably should not be used in patients where recurrence of peptic ulcer would be particularly hazardous or unusually likely. The operation has some disadvantages compared to parietal cell vagotomy in that division of the pyloric sphincter inevitably results in some complications of dumping, diarrhea and the reflux alkaline syndromes.

A brief remark is in order regarding so-called selective vagotomy. By all means, this must not be confused with parietal cell vagotomy which is sometimes referred to as "super-selective vagotomy." This operation was based on extremely tenuous evidence that the hepatic and celiac branches of the vagus are important. In particular, vagal innervation to the small intestine might reduce postvagotomy diarrhea. Vagal innervation to the gallbladder might reduce the incidence of biliary tract disease. Preservation of vagal innervation to the pancreas might improve absorption through a lesser reduction in pancreatic secretion. None of these have proven to be the case. This needlessly tedious operative procedure is outmoded and has no place in the surgical treatment of duodenal ulcer today. On the other hand, Dragstedtian truncal vagotomy plus Weinberg pyloroplasty has withstood the test of time and in the appropriate case can be done with safety and with favorable definitive long-term results.

References

1. Dragstedt, L.R. and Owens, F.M.: Supra-diaphragmatic section of the vagus nerves in treatment of duodenal ulcer. Proc. Soc. Exp. Biol. Med. 53:152-154, 1943.
2. Dragstedt, L.R.: Contributions to the physiology of the stomach. XXXVIII. Gastric juice in duodenal and gastric ulcers. JAMA 68:330-333, 1917.

3. Grande, F. and Visscher, M.D. (eds.): Claude Bernard and Experimental Medicine. Cambridge, Massachusetts:Schenkman Publishers, 1967.
4. Hay, L.J., Varco, R.L., Code, C.F. et al: Experimental production of gastric and duodenal ulcers in laboratory animals by intramuscular injection of histamine in beeswax. Surg. Gynecol. Obstet. 75:170-182, 1942.
5. Neal, W.B., Harper, P.V. and Storer, E.H.: Secretory studies on the isolated stomach. Arch. Surg. 60:1-20, 1950.
6. Dragstedt, L.R.: The etiology of gastric and duodenal ulcers. Postgrad. Med. 15:99-103, 1954.
7. Adams, W.E. and Phemister, D.B.: Carcinoma of the lower thoracic esophagus. Report of a successful resection and esophagogastrectomy. J. Thorac. Surg. 7:621-632, 1938.
8. Weinberg, J.A., Stempien, S.J., Movius, H.J. et al: Vagotomy and pyloroplasty in the treatment of duodenal ulcer. Am. J. Surg. 92:202-207, 1956.
9. Eisenberg, M.M., Woodward, E.R., Dragstedt, L.R. et al: Vagotomy and drainage procedure for duodenal ulcer: The results of ten years' experience. Ann. Surg. 170:317-328, 1969.
10. O'Leary, J.P., Woodward, E.R., Dragstedt, L.R. et al: Vagotomy and drainage procedure for duodenal ulcer: The results of seventeen years experience. Ann. Surg. 183:613-618, 1976.

Self-Evaluation Quiz

1. The basic essential in all operations for duodenal ulcer is adequate vagal denervation of the parietal cell mass of the stomach.
   a) True
   b) False
2. Duodenal ulcer patients exhibit hypersecretion of gastric juice in the following percent of cases:
   a) 100%
   b) 80%
   c) 60%
   d) 40%
   e) 20%
3. The gastric enzyme pepsin is unique in that:
   a) The presence of bile acid is necessary for its proteolytic activity
   b) The enzyme is quickly inactivated by ingested food
   c) A drastically low pH, ie, less than 3.5, is required for its proteolytic activity

   d) The enzyme attacks only a mucosa of the stomach and duodenum
   e) The enzyme depends upon reflux of pancreatic bicarbonate for its proteolytic function
4. The Pavlovian nervous phase of gastric secretion is continuously active in all mammals, but only man develops spontaneous peptic ulcer. The reason is unknown.
   a) True
   b) False
5. Vagotomy inhibits gastric motility by:
   a) Paralysis of the gastric smooth muscle
   b) Stimulation of feedback inhibitory mechanisms to gastric motility
   c) Loss of parasympathetic augmenter influence on gastric smooth muscle
   d) Promotion of duodeno-gastric reflux
   e) Excessive release of catecholamines
6. The modified Heinecke-Mikulicz pyloroplasty is preferred over gastrojejunostomy because:
   a) Alkaline reflux is less
   b) Direct access to an acutely bleeding ulcer is available
   c) Operating time is shorter
   d) Gastrointestinal continuity promotes activation of duodenal hormones
   e) All of the above
7. Truncal vagotomy plus a drainage operation results in a recurrence rate of:
   a) .5%
   b) 5%
   c) 15%
   d) 25%
   e) 35%
8. Truncal vagotomy reduces gastric secretion by:
   a) 95%
   b) 75%
   c) 55%
   d) 35%
   e) 25%
9. Vagotomy plus a drainage operation produces a satisfactory long-term clinical result in the following percent of cases:

a) 90%
b) 80%
c) 70%
d) 60%
e) 50%

10. The low mortality and morbidity of vagotomy and drainage operations is due to the absence of dissection and division of disease in proximal duodenum.
    a) True
    b) False

Answers on page 721.

Antrectomy and Vagotomy in the Treatment of Peptic Ulcer Disease

H. William Scott, Jr., M.D.

Objectives

To review the recent historical development of vagotomy and hemigastrectomy (antrectomy) and the establishment of vagotomy plus antrectomy as the standard procedure in most clinics. To review the statistical results obtained in large series of patients with perforation, obstruction, hemorrhage and intractability.

Dr. Lester Dragstedt carried out a superb group of investigations that established truncal vagotomy as a means of controlling the acid hypersecretion of duodenal ulcer disease and permitted ulcers to heal. Dragstedt found that truncal vagotomy required an emptying procedure.

Drs. Leonard Edwards, Reginald Smithwick and David Johnston began in the mid-1940s to use vagotomy as described by Dragstedt with a small gastric resection. Although this operation had originally been done back in 1922 by Laterjet and reported in the French literature, it had been ignored. It remained for these three surgeons to initiate the use of what Smithwick called vagotomy and hemigastrectomy and what Edwards referred to as vagotomy and antrectomy.

The concept involved was substantiated and expanded by the subsequent experiments of Dragstedt and his associates, among them Woodward, which demonstrated that the antrum could be contributory to recurrence of ulcer after vagotomy with a drainage procedure. The combination of vagotomy,

---

H. William Scott, Jr., M.D., Chairman, Department of Surgery, Vanderbilt University, Nashville, Tennessee; Former President, American College of Surgeons.

eliminating the cephalic phase of gastric secretion, and antrectomy, eliminating the gastric phase, was found to be quite effective in controlling the duodenal ulcer diathesis and in preventing recurrence of duodenal ulcer. One could apply this operative procedure, as Edwards found early in his experience, to all of the complications of duodenal ulcer, including perforation, obstruction and bleeding, as well as intractability. If the duodenum permitted, one could resect the ulcer and do a primary anastomosis of the Billroth I type between the gastric stump and the duodenum or, as was originally done by Edwards, a Billroth II procedure, in preference.

The late Henry Harkins demonstrated that this combined operation, as he called it, of vagotomy and antral resection could be employed and the stomach anastomosed to the duodenum, thus avoiding bypass of the duodenum. He emphasized the value of this combination. In our early experience at Vanderbilt, we became enthusiastic about using a Billroth I anastomosis after vagotomy and antrectomy in the majority of patients, particularly in women.

By the mid-1950s we had adopted the operative procedure of vagotomy and antral resection for essentially routine use in treating patients with duodenal ulcer who required operation. In a series of almost 1,200 patients that was reported in the early 1960s, the indications for operation were tabulated. The categories, of course, have many overlappings. About 53% of the patients came to operation because of their own intractability or that of their ulcer. The average was about 12 years of medical management of ulcer before vagotomy-antrectomy was carried out. Hemorrhage, either massive or recurrent, was the principal indication in some 30% of patients; obstruction in 13%; and only a small group (4%) in this study came to definitive operation because of perforation.

Vagotomy-antrectomy has a profound effect in reduction of the hypersecretory state in patients with duodenal ulcer disease. Both as registered during daytime collections and night-time collections, volumes of gastric secretion were impressively reduced. The same is true of the reduction in acidity. Prior to operation 74.5 mEq acid was the mean value per day and postoperatively this value fell to a negligible figure of 1.24. The night-time secretion, as demonstrated by Dragstedt, represents the pure vagal secretory effect and was even more impressively reduced by vagotomy and antrectomy.

By the mid-1960s, we had accumulated in the four hospitals affiliated with Vanderbilt University an experience with some 1,750 patients with duodenal ulcer treated by vagotomy and antrectomy. In following these patients, our grading criteria were identical to those that have been alluded to by Goligher and Woodward, of the Visik one, two, three, or four. We found on follow-up that 94% of patients had a satisfactory result after this operative procedure. The mortality of 2.3% in this series of 1,750 patients, however, was a good deal higher than we had wanted. This occurred largely because of deaths after operation for massive bleeding in elderly patients. There were a few deaths which occurred as a result of technical errors. Therefore, we changed our policy of applying vagotomy-antrectomy to patients with all complications of duodenal ulcer disease, but restricted it to those patients who did *not* have massive bleeding and who represented good surgical risks. As a result of this change in policy, our mortality rate with vagotomy and pyloroplasty during this period rose to the level of 5%. The reason for this high mortality was the fact that we adopted the plan of using vagotomy-pyloroplasty and suture of the bleeder in virtually all patients who presented with massive bleeding from duodenal ulcer. This included all elderly patients. Through the years, this selective policy resulted in a reduction in mortality rates for vagotomy-antrectomy. By 1972, in the series of 3,584 patients with vagotomy-antrectomy that had accumulated, the mortality had dropped to the low figure of 1.6%. This figure is still higher than is desirable in treatment of benign disease.

Experience with this large group of patients was generally quite good. Gastric outlet obstruction was the most common source of morbidity in the postoperative period, whether the patient had a Billroth I or a Billroth II anastomosis. Duodenal stump leakage occurred in 18 patients, or 0.5% of this series. We learned to avoid resection or attempted resection of a large penetrating posterior duodenal ulcer but rather to exclude the ulcer from alimentary continuity and do a Billroth I anastomosis. This technique reduced the complication of postoperative stomal obstruction considerably.

In following up the results in this larger group of patients, they were essentially identical to those in the previous ten-year period, with only 6% representing unsatisfactory results. Most showed maintenance of the stable weight. Only 10% had a significant weight loss. Vagotomy and antrectomy resulted in an impressive drop in the basal acid output and the maximal acid output, as well as a fall in circulating serum gastrin concentration to extremely low levels.

These reductions in acid secretion account for the most impressive feature of vagotomy-antrectomy when applied to duodenal ulcer, namely, the achievement of the very low incidence of ulcer recurrence. In our large series recurrences have been documented in only 0.6%. A majority of these were due to proven incomplete vagotomy. Four missed Zollinger-Ellison tumors were responsible for another group. Several incomplete vagotomies were suspected in another group. The overall incidence of incomplete vagotomy in this group of patients when tested by the use of Hollander insulin testing has been approximately 20%. Despite this, the combination of vagotomy-antrectomy has been very effective in controlling duodenal ulcer diathesis. Proven recurrences took place in only three patients with a Billroth II anastomosis and in ten patients with a Billroth I anastomosis.

The experience in other clinics around the country and abroad with vagotomy-antrectomy has validated and confirmed the high incidence of satisfactory results, which approximate 90%, and the very low incidence of recurrence, usually less than 1%.

After reporting this large series of patients with vagotomy-antrectomy by retrospective review, in the last 15 years we have been interested in carrying out prospective randomized studies which attempt to compare the role of truncal vagotomy and antrectomy with the newer procedures that have been developed. During these last 15 years, we have compared by prospective randomized study in 143 patients truncal vagotomy and selective gastric vagotomy. In another group of 120 patients, selective gastric vagotomy was done in all and we compared antrectomy with pyloroplasty. More recently, Sawyers and Herrington, my colleagues, have compared proximal gastric vagotomy without drainage with truncal vagotomy and antrectomy, on the one hand, and with selective gastric vagotomy and pyloroplasty on the other. There were 174 men in one of their studies and 90 women in another. The results have emphasized the absolute importance of anatomic accuracy and completeness in carrying out vagotomy, irrespective of the type of vagotomy that is used. Further, they have shown antral resection to be a superb drainage procedure. When combined with accurate vagotomy in good risk patients, vagotomy-antrectomy controls duodenal ulcer disease with long-range satisfaction and with low mortality and morbidity. The low rate of ulcer recurrence after vagotomy and antrectomy has established the procedure in most clinics as the standard against which newer treatment modalities are measured. Our experience has confirmed the wisdom of Dragstedt whose concise summary of his many years of clinical experience and laboratory investigation was simply this: "If vagotomy is complete and drainage or emptying of the stomach satisfactory, duodenal ulcers will heal and will not recur."

Self-Evaluation Quiz

1. Dragstedt found that truncal vagotomy needs:
   a) Extensive chemistry work-up
   b) An emptying procedure
   c) Hemigastrectomy instead of antrectomy
   d) At least five years conservative medical treatment before it is justified
2. Smithwick's work with Edwards:
   a) Would have surprised Laterjet
   b) Had already been reported in the Danish literature
   c) Included the efforts of Johnston
   d) Began in the mid-1930s
3. The antrum can be:
   a) Contributory to ulcer recurrence after vagotomy with drainage
   b) Counted upon not to contribute to recurrence of ulcer after vagotomy with drainage
   c) Resected to eliminate the cephalic phase of gastric secretion
4. If the duodenum permits, you can resect the ulcer and do primary anastomosis of the Billroth I type between gastric

stump and duodenum, but Edwards found a Billroth II procedure unsatisfactory for this.
   a) True
   b) False
5. Henry Harkins showed how to bypass the duodenum and combined vagotomy and antral resection.
   a) True
   b) False
6. In a series of 1,200 patients hemorrhage was the principal indication in:
   a) 30%
   b) 35%
   c) 42%
   d) 48%
7. In the above series, obstruction was the principal indication in:
   a) 9%
   b) 13%
   c) 15%
   d) 19%
8. In the above series, perforation was the principal indication in:
   a) 4%
   b) 5%
   c) 7%
   d) None

Answers on page 721.

Whither Vagotomy

John Alexander-Williams, M.D.

Objectives

1. To determine how vagotomy has been refined in recent decades with an assessment of the relative advantages of selective and highly selective vagotomy over truncal vagotomy.
2. To consider whether it is possible for surgery to become more physiologically selective by attacking vagal nuclei, selective efferent secretory fibers or denervating specific end organs such as secretory cells.

Since the clinical application of vagotomy by Dragstedt in 1943, there have been gradual developments and refinements. The changing fashions have seen truncal vagotomy superseded by selective vagotomy and later by super selective, highly selective or proximal gastric vagotomy. The change from truncal to selective vagotomy brought about a reduction in the incidence of post vagotomy diarrhea; the change from selective to proximal gastric vagotomy meant that an innervated antrum could be retained and obviated the need for a drainage procedure. With this latest development, proximal gastric vagotomy, some surgeons consider that perfection has been achieved in the surgical treatment of duodenal ulcer. However, surgery never stands still and it is appropriate to consider the options open for vagotomy development in the future.

The aim of proximal gastric vagotomy is to denervate the acid-secreting part of the stomach, and failure to do so completely results in the only significant defect of the operation, recurrent ulceration. Can we become more accurate in our selection of the area to be denervated and more certain in our total denervation of that area? During the course of an

---

John Alexander-Williams, M.D., Chairman of Gastroenterology Group, University of Birmingham, Birmingham, England.

operation it is possible to map out with considerable accuracy the acid-secreting part of the stomach by means of pH testing of acid secretion in response to parenterally administered secretagogue [1]. This test is also used for an indication of the completeness of the vagotomy during operation, as is the test of vagally dependent motor function of the stomach [2]. Following an assessment of the value of these two tests in both delineating the acid-secreting area and in assisting surgeons to make a complete vagotomy, it was reported that the use of the intraoperative tests reduced the incidence of incomplete vagotomy from approximately 20% without testing to 0.6% using the test [3]. What will be the future of these tests? Although intraoperative testing undoubtedly improves the efficiency of the vagal denervation of the parietal cell area of the stomach, I think it is unlikely that the tests will become universally applied. Considerable persistence and expertise are necessary before the tests work reliably. The surgeon who treats duodenal ulcer only occasionally will not develop sufficient expertise to justify the investment of time or money. Most experienced surgeons throughout the world do not use or no longer use these tests in assisting them in performing proximal gastric vagotomy. Once they have perfected a technique of denervation that gives good clinical results, the cumbersome time-consuming intraoperative tests are usually abandoned. The tests have taught us that there are certain areas of the stomach that are particularly likely to be left innervated. The future will lead us to better anatomical selection in vagotomy.

Anatomical Selection

The areas of the stomach requiring particular attention during proximal gastric vagotomy are the following:

1. *The cardioesophageal junction.* It is essential to dissect carefully and thoroughly the distal 5 cm of the esophagus to insure that no fine vagal fibers are left embedded in the muscle. It is important also to insure that no fibers reach the lower esophagus and the stomach from the posterior vagal trunk as it crosses from behind to the right of the esophagus (criminal nerve). Failure to denervate adequately the cardioesophageal junction appears to be one of the principal causes of incomplete parietal cell denervation.

2. *The lesser curve.* It can be shown that the parietal cell area of the stomach extends to a variable extent toward the pylorus, in some patients reaching within 1 or 2 cm of the pyloric ring. Some surgeons insist that the whole of the acid-secreting area must be denervated; others state that as much as 10 cm of the lesser curve may be left with intact vagal innervation. In Britain and Scandinavia experienced surgeons, who enjoy a low recurrence rate after proximal gastric vagotomy, advise us to leave only 5 cm innervated. Although this may produce some temporary postoperative delay in gastric emptying, the experience in our unit suggests that it produces no significant disorder of gastric function in patients studied more than three months postoperatively.

3. *The greater curve.* Intraoperative pH testing following vagotomy shows that occasionally a small area of parietal cells is left innervated and functioning just proximal to the junction of the body and the antrum of the stomach along the greater curve. For this reason I consider that it is advisable to divide the gastroepiploic neurovascular bundle at the greater curve of the stomach, opposite the incisura angularis ventriculi.

4. *Do not overdo it.* Other suggested refinements of denervation of the parietal cell area of the stomach are unlikely to receive widespread acclaim in the future. These include splenectomy, division of the vasa brevia and division of the whole of the posterior trunk of the vagus, relying merely on the anterior nerve of Latarjet to leave sufficient of the motor innervation to the antrum. I do not think that they will "catch on."

Physiological Selection

If we have now reached the limits of anatomical selection of denervation, can we achieve anything by being more physiologically selective?

The vagal nerves connected to the stomach contain some fibers that stimulate secretion, some fibers that stimulate motor activity and many afferent fibers that transmit impulses from the stomach to the central nervous system. The secretory fibers represent only a relatively small proportion of the total bulk of the nerve. When we totally denervate the fundus or acid-secreting part of the stomach, we not only decrease acid secretion but decrease motility and deprive the central nervous system of stimuli via the afferent fibers. Total nerve division, even if anatomically selective, produces the results that we desire by reducing acid secretion. However, it also produces undesirable sequelae such as the loss of receptive relaxation of the body of the stomach and loss of normal coordination of intragastric movement. These unsought sequelae result in the early rapid gastric emptying of liquid meals and are responsible for the occasional dumping and diarrhea that occur even after proximal gastric vagotomy [4]. It is unlikely that selective secretory denervation with preservation of motor and afferent fibers will be achieved by physical dissection, even if vital staining allowed a visual differentiation between the different components of the fine vagal nerves. Also it seems unlikely that any specific chemical agent will be found that can selectively demonstrate, or destroy, the secretory fibers.

Therefore, it seems logical to consider attacking the secretory stimulating mechanism in an area where it is anatomically distinct from the motor or the afferent components of the nerve, that is, in the mid brain. Although accurate in vivo demonstration of the site of the secretory vagal nuclei can be achieved in experimental animals and, in theory, it might be possible to locate and destroy these areas by stereotactic neurosurgery, I think it is unlikely that this approach will supersede simple peripheral vagotomy in the foreseeable future.

Finally, the selective physiological attack could be directed toward the other end of the nerve system, that is, at the point of innervation of the parietal cell. The secretory fibers could be disconnected from the parietal cells they supply. Clearly with our present knowledge and techniques, this is outside the realm of the surgeon but now appears to be achieved by the pharmacologists who have produced safe histamine 2 receptor blocking agents. In my opinion these agents or their successors provide the ultimate in selective effective vagal denervation of the parietal cells and are likely to supersede surgical vagotomy for the majority of patients with duodenal ulcer. Therefore, I summarize the future of vagotomy as selection, ultra selection and extinction.

References

1. Grassi, G. and Orecchiac: A comparison of intra-operative tests of the completeness of vagal section. Surgery 75:155, 1974.
2. Burge, H. and Vane, J.R.: Method of testing for complete nerve section during vagotomy. Br. Med. J. 1:615, 1958.
3. Coupland, G.: Communication to the 6th World Congress of Gastroenterology, Madrid, 1978.
4. Donovan, I.A.: Different components of gastric emptying after gastric surgery. Ann. R. Coll. Surg. 58:368-373, 1976.

Self-Evaluation Quiz

1. The advantages of selective vagotomy over truncal vagotomy are:
   a) It is easier
   b) The recurrence rate is less
   c) There is less postvagotomy diarrhea
   d) It is reversible if complications ensue
2. The principal advantage of proximal gastric vagotomy over other vagotomies is:
   a) There is less postoperative diarrhea
   b) A drainage procedure is not needed
   c) There is a lower incidence of dysphagia
   d) It is technically easier
3. The most significant long-term complication of proximal gastric vagotomy is:
   a) Gastric retention
   b) Gastroesophageal reflux
   c) An increased tendency to gallstone formation
   d) Recurrent ulceration due to inadequate denervation
4. What test makes it possible to map out the acid-secreting part of the stomach during operation:
   a) pH testing of the mucosa of the stomach
   b) Muscular contraction in response to electrical stimulation of the vagus
   c) Fall in blood sugar in response to a glucose load
   d) Vital staining of nerve fibers
5. All but one of the following areas may be left innervated by surgeons performing proximal gastric vagotomy inexpertly:
   a) Mid portion of the lesser curve of the stomach
   b) The greater curve just proximal to the junction of body and antrum

   c) The lesser curve just proximal to the junction of body and antrum
   d) Near the cardioesophageal junction
6. The long-term effect of leaving only 5 cm of the distal antrum vagally innervated is persistent gastric stasis.
   a) True
   b) False
7. To ensure complete vagal denervation of the acid-secreting area of the greater curve of the stomach it is advisable to:
   a) Divide the vasa brevia
   b) Divide the gastroepiploic neurovascular bundle
   c) Divide the whole of the posterior trunk of the vagus
   d) Remove the spleen
8. In a vagal trunk the efferent fibers supplying the parietal cells represent only a small proportion of the total fibers of the nerve.
   a) True
   b) False
9. In what area of the body are the secretory nerves anatomically distinct from the motor nerve in the vagal system:
   a) Below the diaphragm
   b) In the chest
   c) In the neck
   d) In the mid brain

Answers on page 721.

Surgical Management of Gastric Ulcer

M. Michael Eisenberg, M.D.

Objectives

Benign gastric ulcer is a complicated disorder, the pathogenesis of which is only partially understood. Surgery in the past has been more aggressive and less precise than is currently available. The current theories on the cause of gastric ulcer allow tailoring the procedure to the disorder in ways which were not previously available. The following information is directed at an understanding of these concepts.

The evolution of attitudes toward the surgery of gastric ulcer remains incomplete. Just how important gastric malignancy is in the judgment of whether to operate or not remains open. Precise data on the incidence of gastric carcinoma in gastric ulcerating lesions are lacking, but it seems reasonable to conclude that a figure of 3% to 7% is appropriate. It does not seem plausible to recommend surgery for *all* gastric ulcers solely because of the often repeated exhortation that only operation conclusively rules out carcinoma, although this is true. Also, there is no real evidence that the overall longevity of patients with carcinoma, delayed in therapy, is significantly altered.

While the individual techniques for establishing or ruling out the diagnosis of gastric carcinoma are not in and of themselves sufficiently accurate for the surgeon to rely upon (perhaps 70% to 90% correct), the combination of techniques of cytology and x-ray, gastroscopy and x-ray, or x-ray, cytology, gastroscopy, and gastric analysis are most impressive (almost 100% accurate).

M. Michael Eisenberg, M.D., Head, Gastrointestinal Surgery, Department of Surgery, University of Minnesota Medical School, Minneapolis.

We feel confident therefore that the preoperative distinction between benign and malignant lesions, using currently available techniques, is quite precise. The surgeon, therefore, should and will know in a vast majority of cases whether or not he is dealing with cancer, allowing a more precise design of operation.

Pathogenesis of the Benign Gastric Ulcer

Du Plessis has stated that "gastric ulceration is not a single disease, but the result of a variety of conditions which lower gastric mucosal resistance, allowing peptic ulceration to occur." While there have been serious attempts recently to differentiate gastric ulcer from duodenal ulcer and, further, to categorize separate types of gastric ulcer, the area remains confused. For example, about 75% benign chronic gastric ulcers may exist as a single entity, but up to 40% may be associated with healed or active duodenal ulcer disease. Other gastric ulcers, although isolated, appear to be related to the chronic ingestion of anti-inflammatory drugs. Although some gastric ulcers are associated with stress, for the most part these tend to be acute and superficial. Finally, some distinction has been made between corpus gastric ulcer, that is, lying on the junction between the antrum and the parietal cell border, and those which have been termed prepyloric ulcer, within 1 to 2 cm of the antral-duodenal junction, and which appear to act both pathophysiologically and clinically much as do duodenal ulcers.

Although from a theoretical point of view distinction between the causes of these various lesions is interesting and perhaps even important, from a practical point of view surgical management tends to overlap. Still, it is desirable to delineate, when possible, identifiable elements in the pathogenesis of individual lesions and, if possible, to tailor the surgical approach in a way such that the underlying cause is rectified. A review of three hypotheses in the pathogenesis of gastric ulcer is appropriate.

The Dragstedt Hypothesis

Dragstedt advocated that antral stasis, with hyperrelease of gastrin secondary to food ingestion, causes gastric ulcer. He believed that while duodenal ulcer may be based on a hypersecretion of acid gastric juice due to overactivity of the central nervous system, gastric ulcer is related to hypergastrinemia during the digestive phase of gastric secretion. This hypothesis deserves attention and may have validity in that group of patients with evidence of some outlet obstruction such as may be seen in old duodenal ulcer disease. However, at most it can account for somewhat less than half of gastric ulcers and may account for no more than 25%.

The Davenport-Du Plessis Hypothesis

A second concept is based on relationships between the gastric mucosal barrier, back diffusion of acid, bile reflux, gastritis and pyloric sphincter dysfunction. It has been suggested that the reflux of bile and pancreatic juice may be related to the development of chronic gastritis and subsequently gastric ulcer. Du Plessis noted that of 75 stomachs resected for gastric ulceration, 65 displayed chronic gastritis extending from the pylorus for a variable distance proximally. The concentration of bile-acid conjugates in the fasting aspirates of patients with gastric ulcer was also noted to be abnormally high. He concluded that the refluxing probably acts by interfering with the protective layer of mucus and by allowing acid and pepsin free access to the mucus membrane.

The Dragstedt hypothesis has been somewhat difficult to justify, since most patients with unobstructed benign gastric ulcer tend to secrete normal or less than normal amounts of acid. Davenport, however, has suggested that the *apparent* hyposecretion may be related to excessive loss of hydrogen ion as a result of "back-diffusion" into gastric mucosa, the integrity of which is diminished or destroyed by a defective permeability barrier. In investigations designed to study the effect of a variety of agents (aspirin, alcohol, bile and pancreatic juice) he suggested that the lipoprotein layer of cell walls was damaged by these agents and permitted increased permeability of the stomach to acid. Clinical evidence corroborates this concept and lends further support to the idea that an abnormal gastric mucosal barrier may be at least one important factor in the pathogenesis of gastric ulcer.

The Oi Hypothesis

Oi in a series of three carefully executed and extremely important studies reported in 1959 examined the location of

170 gastric ulcers localized to the stomach alone and an additional 50 gastric ulcers associated with duodenal ulcer. He emphasized that the fundic and pyloric gland tissues form at their interface a junctional zone which constitutes what he called a *locus resistentiae minoris* (area of decreased resistance). He suggested that the cause of gastric ulcer is closely related to this local, congenital factor. He showed that all of the 170 gastric ulcers occurred at the most 1.5 cm from this junctional zone. In addition, in an examination of 114 surgical specimens with duodenal ulcer, he observed that they occurred in the region of the duodenal glands in 99.3% of the cases, at most 2 cm distant to the border of the pyloric antrum and the duodenal mucosa.

It is apparent that all three of these hypotheses have some merit. At the very least they emphasize that gastric ulcer is much more complex than previously appreciated. For purposes of the present discussion it is convenient to start with an assumption that in patients with pyloric stenosis due to old or active duodenal ulcer disease, Dragstedt's theory may apply. It is also reasonable to assume that for some — though not all — other gastric ulcers, the bile reflux theory may have merit. Adding the information available to us from Oi's studies, we now have a working hypothesis for the pathogenesis of most gastric ulcers and can proceed with surgical management accordingly.

Surgery for Gastric Ulcer

The ideal operation for the management of gastric ulcer should include (1) zero mortality, (2) zero recurrence rate, (3) zero morbidity and (4) perfect differentiation between benign and malignant diseases. While no operation meets all of these criteria, their achievement nonetheless represents a worthy goal.

A variety of operative approaches to the surgical management of gastric ulcer has been used in clinics throughout the world for the past 80 or 90 years. The majority, however, have fallen into disuse based primarily on changes in surgical "fashion," disappointment with morbidity, mortality and recurrence rates, or the introduction of improved techniques. In general, only two or three operations remain in widespread use today; one or two additional procedures, recently introduced, fall into the realm of experimental clinical trials.

Vagotomy (Truncal or Selective) With Drainage

Vagotomy with drainage for duodenal ulcer is a very effective operation. However, this operation is much less useful for the isolated gastric ulcer. Recurrence rates from 14.3% to 35.7% in seven years or less have been reported.

Subtotal Gastrectomy or Antrectomy

Total or extensive subtotal gastrectomy is curative, but it is excessive for benign lesions. Dumping and/or difficulty in maintaining body weight is closely related to the extent of gastric resection. Limited gastric resection is much better tolerated. Antrectomy, to include the ulcer, offers a very safe, very reliable and attractive form of therapy.

Vagotomy and Resection

The addition of vagotomy to limited gastric resection is used under specific circumstances. While the addition of vagotomy does not seem to decrease the quality of results, alterations in bowel habits and changes in biliary and pancreatic function may be a price which one pays, without significant improvement in cure rate. Nevertheless, in the presence of a combined benign gastric ulcer and duodenal ulcer, vagotomy is added to the resection. When it has been shown that the patient hypersecretes acid gastric juice, vagotomy is also added.

Highly Selective (Parietal Cell) Vagotomy With and Without Drainage

Highly selective vagotomy is currently being used in the form of randomized clinical trials. The reported data are thus far inconsistent, but it may well be that after further experience this operation may turn out to be the most effective yet devised.

The Current Approach to Surgery for Gastric Ulcer

The Decision To Operate

1. All of our patients are evaluated prior to recommendation for surgery by x-ray, endoscopy with biopsy, gastric

analysis and, sometimes, cytology. Unless all four of these modalities establish the benignancy of the lesion immediate operation is recommended.

2. If there is no evidence of malignancy, but the patient has failed a single test of healing (usually a 50% decrease in the size of the crater by endoscopy and x-ray within six weeks and complete or virtually complete healing within 12 weeks with standard medical therapy), operation is recommended.

3. If the patient has sustained a single episode of hemorrhage requiring transfusion, a prolonged test of healing is not advocated and early operation is advised.

4. If a patient has satisfactorily completed a test of healing but has developed a recurrence (in over 50% of patients who satisfactorily heal, the ulcer will recur within two years, up to 80% in five years), operation is recommended immediately. These criteria for immediate surgery, in our judgment, include the vast majority of patients with chronic benign gastric ulcer.

The Operation

We use one of two operative procedures: (1) limited subtotal gastrectomy (approximately 50%) to include the ulcer and most or all of the antrum and (2) truncal vagotomy plus the same type of limited subtotal gastrectomy.

1. *Limited subtotal gastrectomy.* If the patient has a benign gastric ulcer, satisfactorily established by the preoperative evaluation, has low acid secretion, does not have associated duodenal ulcer, is not dependent upon ulcerogenic drugs for other systemic disease (chronic arthritis, ulcerative colitis, regional enteritis, gout, etc.) and is not a chronic alcoholic, we prefer limited subtotal gastrectomy to include the ulcer and the antrum. This provides a total biopsy of the lesion, conclusively establishing the benignancy of the ulcer. This operative approach also eliminates Oi's *locus resistentiae minoris* and furthermore removes the area of decreased resistance due to the presence of the lesion or scar of the lesion. Although the operation cannot be claimed to reduce bile and pancreatic reflux, it does remove the areas most susceptible to injury. Finally, this operation eliminates the target organ hypothesized by Dragstedt's theory of antral stasis and, furthermore, improves gastric emptying in the presence of outlet obstruction.

Based on extensively reported data, as well as our own experience, this approach can be expected to bring about a virtually perfect cure rate with an extremely low mortality. Recurrence rate under these circumstances is small (0-4.4%), and morbidity in terms of dumping and weight loss is minimal.

2. *Limited subtotal gastrectomy with vagotomy.* If the patient has an associated duodenal ulcer, a prepyloric (1 to 2 cm proximal) ulcer, high normal or hypersecretory acid pattern, is a chronic alcoholic, is dependent upon ulcerogenic drugs or is a juvenile, we routinely add truncal vagotomy to limited (including the ulcer) gastric resection. This approach encompasses all of the beneficial aspects of limited gastric resection alone and affords added protection in terms of control of acid by parasympathetically denervating the residual stomach. Unfortunately, there are not yet hard data available to conclusively endorse this approach. We feel, however, that this attitude is warranted on the basis of theoretical physiologic grounds; subsequent appearance of data, which either support or contradict this rationale, will color future management.

Summary

Benign gastric ulcer is a complex disease, the pathogenesis of which is only partially understood. Differentiation between benignancy and malignancy in the lesion is important but with currently available techniques is virtually assured preoperatively. We recommend surgery for the vast majority of patients with proven benign chronic gastric ulcer, and we attempt to tailor the operation to the pathogenesis as we currently understand it. For most patients with chronic benign gastric ulcer, limited (50%) subtotal gastrectomy to include resection of the ulcer is the procedure of choice. Truncal vagotomy is added in a group of patients under certain specific criteria, which have been outlined.

Self-Evaluation Quiz

1. Preoperative distinction between benign and malignant lesions of the stomach is currently very accurate.
   a) True
   b) False

2. A combination of techniques for proving the presence of malignancy in a gastric ulcer, including cytology, x-ray, gastroscopy and gastric analysis approaches 100% accuracy.
   a) True
   b) False
3. The Dragstedt hypothesis suggests that the vagus nerves are primarily involved in the pathogenesis of benign gastric ulcer.
   a) True
   b) False
4. The Davenport-Du Plessis hypothesis of the pathogenesis of gastric ulcer is based on:
   a) An abnormally functioning antrum
   b) Reflux of duodenal contents
   c) Congenital weakness in the mucosa
   d) All of these
5. The Oi hypothesis is based on the concept that benign gastric ulcer is related to:
   a) Abnormally functioning antrum
   b) Reflux of duodenal contents
   c) Congenital weakness in the mucosa
   d) All of these

Answers on page 721.

Discussion

Moderator: William Silen, M.D.

Moderator: While we are waiting for the panel members to assemble, let me ask the members of the audience a question: How many of you have done proximal gastric vagotomy for duodenal ulcer? So there are a reasonable number, maybe 10% of those of the audience who have. One of the questions that keeps coming up about proximal gastric vagotomies has to do with this: Should you test the patient preoperatively for acid secretion? Dr. Spiro, do you want to answer that?

Dr. Spiro: I do not see any place in clinical medicine today and probably in the future for gastric acid secretory studies. I was surprised that Dr. Eisenberg suggested that it helped him in distinguishing gastric ulcer from gastric carcinoma. In the Veterans Administration statistics I saw that there was a 3.9% incidence of gastric cancer. Well, diagnostic accuracy depends upon prevalence. If Dr. Marshak had sat in front of his x-ray machine and had not turned the x-ray machine on, and had said that all of those patients had benign ulcers, he would be thought a better radiologist than he is today because he would have had only a 3.9% error rate.

Moderator: Dr. Goligher showed the BAO and the MAO and so does Dr. Scott. Dr. Woodward still uses a 30-year-old test called the overnight secretion. At any rate, Dr. Goligher, why do you measure acid? Dr. Spiro says it is not any good.

Dr. Goligher: I am inclined to agree with him that in actual practice it does not help very much. We have done a lot of gastric analysis on our patients, more for academic interest and so on, but it has not really influenced our decision about operations. Maybe those with very high acids should have been treated by more radical operations than proximal gastric vagotomy. We have not. I think many of the gastric analyses we did were really of academic interest alone.

Moderator: Dr. Goligher, I think I have asked you this before, but as I looked at your recurrent ulcers, almost all of them had MAOs preoperatively that were over 40 mEq. As you know, Professor Louw in South Africa has found that there is a level of approximately 25 mEq of maximal acid output above which truncal vagotomy and drainage does not seem to work very well. If you look at Terrence Kennedy's recent figures, almost all of his recurrences were in patients who had over 40 mEq per hour of maximal acid output. Should we not pay attention to that?

Dr. Goligher: I admit it is possible we should. In the past, we were anxious to explore this operation to the full, using it in all sorts of cases. Maybe we should be more selective, now that we know that there is a fair recurrence rate. Perhaps we should try to select the cases for parietal cell vagotomy and reserve it for people with lower acid levels on pentagastrin stimulation. But my experience is that if you accept that patients with acid levels above, say, 25 mEq/hr on pentagastrin stimulation should have vagotomy and antrectomy (or hemigastrectomy), you end up by treating most of your cases by this more radical operation.

Moderator: Dr. Eisenberg, did you want to comment on this?

Dr. Eisenberg: I think there are many reasons for using gastric secretory studies preoperatively. It is true that there is no single test yet developed that will help predict how one should tailor an operation either for duodenal or gastric ulcer. But the one that comes closest to it is the secretory test. First of all, it does give an indication of the virulence of the ulcer, which you just alluded to. Second, it gives a baseline, which helps evaluate postoperative therapy, if the patient should have recurrent symptoms. It helps to evaluate the possibility of the rare endocrine tumors. In general, it gives some measure of what the likelihood of successful medical management is going to be.

Moderator: I do not agree about telling you how virulent the ulcer is. After all, there are patients with gastrinomas who do not even have ulcers but who put out 100 mEq per hour. We have many questions that relate to this problem: How do you tell whether or not you have done a complete vagotomy? Dr. Alexander-Williams, would you like to comment? The questioner wants to know whether there is a test to tell whether or not you have done a complete vagotomy postoperatively. Let us forget the Grassi test and the Burge test and the methylene blue test. But how about deciding afterwards? What about insulin?

Dr. Alexander-Williams: No, the only test that will tell you whether or not you have done an adequate vagotomy is if the ulcer does not recur, and you need to follow the patient for a long time to know that that test is negative. But if you are monitoring your own efficacy as a vagotomist, I think there is much to be said for doing secretory tests postoperatively and probably the insulin test is of most value. It is a poor predictor of whether or not the patient will have a recurrence but at least it tells you whether you are as good as your colleagues or whether you are consistently leaving the patients Hollander positive while they are still in the hospital. If your patient's tests are often positive, you are probably doing a rather bad vagotomy and it is time you went back to gastrectomy.

Moderator: We are afraid to use the insulin test in this country because of some deaths that have been reported from myocardial infarction and cerebrovascular accident. So we tend to use other things. Dr. Scott, would you like to tell us what you use to decide whether or not you have done a complete vagotomy?

Dr. Scott: We have used the insulin test rather extensively in the past, despite the very sophisticated critiques of Dr. Eisenberg, who has written many papers about it. We have not used 2-deoxyglucose. I do not know if anyone here has had any experience with this, perhaps you have, Dr. Silen?

Moderator: No, I have not. We have tended to use the maximal acid output and the reduction in maximal acid output in assessing what we have achieved with the vagotomy. I am not saying that the MAO tells you whether you have done a complete vagotomy. I agree with Dr. Alexander-Williams. I do not know that there is any test that tells you, really. I think, as Dr. Eisenberg and others have pointed out, there are problems with knowing exactly what the response to an insulin test means. It is a very complex response. There are inhibitory reactions, as well as stimulatory ones. Dr. Woodward, please comment about the question of testing after vagotomy.

Dr. Woodward: I think it is easy to expect too much from a gastric analysis. If one is using a vagotomy pyloroplasty, the comparison between the preoperative and the postoperative basal and stimulated results correlates well with the recurrence of peptic ulcer. Almost none of the recurrences develop in patients who have had as much as a 75% reduction in both studies. It is true that only about 20% of those patients with an inadequate reduction in secretion will get a recurrent ulcer, but some will. We think it is useful for this purpose. But it is easy to expect too much of it. It does not have great diagnostic value. In fact it has very little. Dr. Oberhelman and I carefully studied the first 1,000 vagotomies done at the University of Chicago. There was absolutely no correlation whatever between the preoperative secretory rate and the incidence of recurrent peptic ulcer.

Moderator: Dr. Goligher wrote a very interesting paper in which he assessed the surgeons, as I recall, in terms of their insulin positivity or negativity after selective gastric vagotomy and truncal vagotomy. Do you want to comment about that study, Dr. Goligher?

Dr. Goligher: The gist of it was that, contrary to what we expected, the best results in terms of achieving complete vagotomy are not always obtained by the experienced surgeon. Sometimes their juniors do just as well or better.

Moderator: If I read that paper correctly, a surgeon nearly always seemed to do the same thing over and over. He was either good with the selective or he was good with the truncal. Did I read that correctly?

Dr. Goligher: There are such things as good vagotomists and bad vagotomists of whatever type.

Moderator: Dr. Woodward, one of the questions that has been asked by many members of the audience is the drainage operation that you use, the kind of pyloroplasty you use. Do you want to comment about that, as well as the use of the gastrostomy tube?

Dr. Woodward: To answer the last question first, we do not use gastrostomy nearly as extensively today because we do not decompress the stomach for nearly as long. We found that we were overdoing it. We treat them pretty much like any major abdominal operation. As soon as intestinal activity develops, we pull the nasogastric tubes.

Moderator: Dr. Scott, one group reported not using tubes at all with gastrectomies, and I can tell from personal experience I think that is perfectly feasible. Either with gastrectomy or with vagotomy, I think it is perfectly feasible in most instances not to use a tube at all. I see Dr. Alexander-Williams shaking his head. Do you agree with that?

Dr. Alexander-Williams: Yes, I do.

Moderator: The sacred tube may go.

Dr. Woodward: In the type of pyloroplasty, I think the Weinberg one layer noninfolding pyloroplasty is feasible, quick, safe and empties the vagotomized stomach very well. We seldom use a more complex procedure, unless the inflammatory mass is such that a Weinberg is not feasible, and then we tend to do a Jaboulay type of gastroduodenostomy.

Moderator: Dr. Goligher did a randomized trial, comparing pyloroplasty with gastroenterostomy. What were your results?

Dr. Goligher: No, we did not do that, but Terrence Kennedy of Belfast and a group in Glasgow carried out such trials.

Kennedy did not find any real advantage to pyloroplasty, just a little less bile vomiting but rather more recurrent ulcers after pyloroplasty. They found the same in Glasgow, except there was a significant advantage in lessening of bile vomiting with pyloroplasty.

Dr. Alexander-Williams, do you have a feeling about that?

Dr. Alexander-Williams: I cannot see why anybody does a drainage procedure anyway. I think that gastrojejunostomy is not an operation, it is a disease. Pyloroplasty is an incurable disease.

Moderator: Dr. Alexander-Williams, there are some people who think that pyloroplasty is a curable disease, because they are trying to put the pylorus back together again. Is that not going on in Leeds now? I think Terrence Kennedy is doing that. Dr. Eisenberg, do you have a comment?

Dr. Eisenberg: We put back a number of pyloruses, beginning in 1968. It is a very easy operation, done primarily for dumping. The problem is that if we could predict ahead of time, Dr. Alexander-Williams, we would not need a drainage procedure, and that would be fine. I think of Dr. Dragstedt's first 150 cases of vagotomy without drainage. Only about one third of them really got into trouble. Another third had some troubles but did not require any further operation, and the last third did not have any trouble at all. The question is: In which one would you not do drainage procedure with a truncal vagotomy? I know of no way of predicting.

Moderator: The sacred role of the drainage procedure is being assailed from all directions because there are small controlled trials on proximal gastric resections with and without drainage operations. It turns out that the patients without a drainage procedure do just as well and maybe better after a proximal gastrectomy. So maybe it is not quite as important as we formerly thought. We had better move along to some other questions about the diagnosis of the afferent loop syndrome versus the question of reflux gastritis. We have received several very good questions in relation to this: Is the afferent loop syndrome or what we formerly called the afferent loop syndrome something that is really and truly reflux gastritis, Dr. Woodward?

Dr. Woodward: Yes. Before we had the beautiful end-viewing panendoscope, we tended to call all bile vomiters afferent loop syndrome. I think that probably 90% of them were reflux gastritis and not the mechanical type of afferent loop syndrome. But the latter does, indeed, occur occasionally. I think that the differential can be made by history and then confirmed by endoscopic findings.

Moderator: I certainly agree with what you are saying. I think many of the patients we formerly called afferent loop syndrome really were reflux gastritis. Can you help us on that point, Dr. Marshak? Can you tell when we have an obstructed afferent loop, that is, one that is not acutely obstructed, but chronically low grade obstructed?

Dr. Marshak: No, I cannot help you too much with that. I can just tell you whether or not it is obstructed and nothing else.

Moderator: How about the diagnosis, Dr. Spiro, of bile gastritis, that Dr. Delaney told us about? How do you make that diagnosis? What about biopsy?

Dr. Spiro: I am a little bothered by the diagnosis. Gastroenterologists rarely recognized the afferent loop syndrome in the past. I have seen possibly three or four patients with bona fide findings in about 20 years. Most of the people who vomit after a drainage procedure vomit bile because the bile is there. I am bothered by the lack of controlled studies in this whole field. We usually find gastritis on biopsy in postgastrectomy stomachs. So I have some anxieties about the concept of bile gastritis, although I recognize that people who have Roux-Y procedures do get better.

Moderator: I think the big question is this: How do you select the patient who is going to get a Roux-Y operation? It was implied earlier in this course that there are many patients who have strange symptoms after gastrectomy. How are you going to select the patient who is going to get the operation? They all have a little peristomal gastritis that you can see. Can you help us on this point, Dr. Delaney?

Dr. Delaney: Not really, Dr. Silen.

Moderator: Do you want to biopsy those?

Dr. Delaney: I do not think biopsy helps. I think they all have some gastritis on biopsy. I do not think looking helps very much because most of them will have some visible gastritis. If you take the people who are having the trouble, that is, weight loss, pain that follows the right pattern and bile vomiting, they will be cured by the Roux-Y operation. There is probably a gray area where it is very difficult to select. That is the problem and I have no answer for it.

Moderator: Dr. Alexander-Williams has some studies on this question. Dr. Alexander-Williams, do you want to tell us about those studies?

Dr. Alexander-Williams: You cannot really make the diagnosis endoscopically or histologically, because if you look into a stomach that has had any gastric operation, even highly selective vagotomy, it is abnormal. We looked at 42 patients with quite severe symptoms and 42 control subjects, matched for operation, age and sex. Endoscopically and histologically, we could not differentiate between the symptomatic and the asymptomatic. The only clear-cut differentiation seemed to be the quantity of bile salt that was in the resting gastric juice. Everybody after a gastric operation has some reflux. It seems to be the absolute quantity of bile salt is in the resting gastric juice that is important. We produced an index, called "fasting bile reflux," which was a measure of bile salts in one half hour resting collection. It gave the best differentiation between symptomatic and asymptomatic.

Dr. Delaney: Dr. Alexander-Williams, you had the very interesting clinical experiment I recounted earlier of putting bile in through a duodenal tube. Have you ever extended that and put bile down a nasogastric tube in an attempt to ferret out those people who were sensitive to bile?

Dr. Alexander-Williams: Yes, we have done this. However, it is difficult to make the test very objective. Certainly, you take patients with the bile reflux syndrome and inject bile, usually somebody else's bile, into their stomach, they object to it strongly. It has proved rather difficult to do a properly controlled study of this test. We have only anecdotal evidence about the value of this test. It has not proved to be of great value to us. I know, Dr. Silen, you have tried that as well. What do you think about it?

Moderator: I tried it on one patient. I made up a solution of 4 mM sodium taurocholate and put it down after running some saline in. The lady said, "Wow, that is my pain," and she began vomiting bile. I think she would have been in the group that Dr. Delaney indicated had all the classical symptoms, namely, profound weight loss, severe epigastric pain, bile vomiting. She was indeed cured by the Roux-Y procedure. It is something to keep in mind as a sort of pseudo-Bernstein test, if you will.

Dr. Tom Gadacz at Johns Hopkins has looked at the question of the type of bile salt. He has found that there are high concentrations of deoxycholate, higher in symptomatic patients. As I pointed out, it is a more toxic bile salt, mole for mole.

One of the questions that many people have asked is about the Roux-Y technique. Dr. Scott, why not just do an enteroenterostomy, side-to-side below this Billroth II anastomosis?

Dr. Scott: For the simple reason that it does not work. We went into this experimentally some years ago, being interested predominantly in the alkaline esophagitis, so-called, that followed total gastrectomy, and trying to develop methods to prevent it. For instance, one can construct in the laboratory in dogs a simple high jejunal fistula, using a loop of jejunum as a control, and set up a model in which the animal will die of loss of fluid and electrolytes in the course of, let us say, five or six days without any supplementation. If you put an enteroenterostomy at the base of that loop, 1 foot, 2 feet, to as much as 4 feet from the exteriorized loop of jejunum, it has no effect in the rate of death of the dog. If you do a Roux-Y fistula which is what we are talking about here, with an isoperistaltic segment of jejunum representing the exteriorized limb, at least 12 to 18 inches in length, there will be no leakage at all and the animal will survive indefinitely.

Moderator: I think that has been learned clinically, too. You really do need an isoperistaltic loop that is going to be defunctionated, and by defunctionation I think most people would agree that you need about 18 inches, which is approximately 50 cm. I think regurgitation really does occur upward at least 1 foot probably. The other question about the technique is: Where do you divide the bowel? I will take the moderator's prerogative and say just a comfortable distance below the ligament of Treitz.

The other question about these loops is: Exactly how do you do it? If the patient has a Billroth II anastomosis I simply cut off the afferent loop and implant it below, a very simple thing to do. Are there any other comments about technique?

Dr. Woodward: The GI stapler makes this about a 20-minute operation.

Dr. Delaney: I was going to make the same comment. The side-to-side works very well, if you put a row of staples above the anastomosis on the afferent limb. I have used it quite a few times, but recently the first patient came back in whom the row of staples had broken through. So I am not so sure that it is a good method.

Moderator: Dr. Scott, how in the world can you exclude an ulcer and still leave it down there when you do the Billroth I operation in the bleeding patient?

Dr. Scott: The proximal stomach is a mobile organ and it will come over to the duodenum and one can leave the ulcer behind.

Moderator: You simply are covering that big bad posterior ulcer with the posterior wall of the stomach, is that correct?

Dr. Scott: Yes, in the same way that, for instance, if one had a marginal ulcer that has bedded down with an anterior gastrojejunostomy on the transverse colon, rather than resect the colon, one can leave the ulcer bed on the wall of the colon and do a definitive gastric procedure. It is the same basic principle.

Moderator: How are you sure that you have removed the antrum? There have been many questions about retained distal antrum. There are several questions about retained proximal antrum on the gastric side. What about that, Dr. Scott? What landmarks do you use to make sure that you do an antrectomy?

Dr. Scott: We now use the crow's foot as an anatomic boundary that Dr. Goligher has defined for us so clearly for the lesser curvature. We usually go a little higher on the greater curvature. We are not really worried about leaving antral tissue, as long as it is in the acid stream. When one leaves distal antral tissue excluded from the acid stream, then chronic gastrin stimulation occurs. To be sure that you have all of the distal antrum removed requires help from the pathologist. It is no great trick to transect the duodenum below the pylorus and have the pathologist look for a complete rim of duodenum on the specimen.

Moderator: Dr. Scott, would you not agree that the proximal margin of the antrum on the lesser curvature really is variable? It is my understanding that you cannot relate it to the crow's foot all the time. Patients with benign gastric ulcers have variable antrofundic junctions, do they not?

Dr. Scott: They seem to have. I was thinking specifically about duodenal ulcer, where I think antrectomy really is a superior drainage procedure more than anything else.

Moderator: Dr. Eisenberg, do you think a precise antrectomy is important? After all, I think you have pointed out that if you take the antrum out you can get a negative insulin test after operation even if you do not touch the vagus.

Dr. Eisenberg: We did report that. I not only think it is unimportant, as long as it is in the acid stream, I do not really know how, unless you are prepared to map the open stomach at the time of surgery, you can tell where the antral-duodenal border is. We conveniently think of it as a straight line, but it wanders all over the place. It has fingers and valleys and peaks. So I do not think you can tell where the antrum is, except in the case of gastric ulcer. If you believe Oi's hypothesis, and there is no reason to doubt it, the ulcer marks the antral-corpus junction.

Dr. Scott: May I remind you of Dr. Palumbo's experience in doing what he has called the small antrectomy and leaving the proximal antrum when doing a vagotomy and antrectomy. He has had remarkably fine results in a large series of well over 600 cases with a very small recurrence rate in patients treated for duodenal ulcer.

Dr. Eisenberg: That should not surprise anybody because he could take no antrum out at all and get a very low recurrence rate with a good vagotomy and a drainage procedure.

Moderator: Dr. Spiro, how do you treat postvagotomy diarrhea?

Dr. Spiro: One thing that has turned out to be very good is bismuth. In a controlled study in Europe codeine or Lomotil proved as good as anything else in patients in whom the physician excluded bacterial overgrowth and lactose intolerance.

Moderator: I think there is a controlled trial in England also showing quite clearly that cholestyramine was quite effective in treating postvagotomy diarrhea. I personally have had an experience with that and it is quite effective. To go along with that, there are changes in the bile salt concentrations in jejunal aspirates of vagotomized patients.

Dr. Spiro: Yes, but if you use cholestyramine, you must give fat-soluble vitamins. You are giving a product which is sequestering all kinds of substances that we are not really certain about. I think patients are better off with a little Lomotil or codeine than taking cholestyramine continuously.

Moderator: What about aluminum hydroxide, which has been shown to bind bile salts? Is that all right?

Dr. Spiro: A stand-off.

Moderator: Dr. Alexander-Williams, did you wish to comment?

Dr. Alexander-Williams: I was about to say that aluminum salts are as effective as is cholestyramine and considerably more palatable. I think the only people who can take cholestyramine are those who are addicted to eating fish manure.

Moderator: I should point out that one thing we really just learned is that patients who have cholecystectomies plus truncal vagotomy seem to have a much greater propensity for the development of postvagotomy diarrhea. This is something I do not understand, but perhaps the use of the proximal gastric vagotomy would avoid that.

Dr. Eisenberg: Dr. Silen, do you not think that much postvagotomy diarrhea is dumping? The first thing I do to treat postvagotomy diarrhea is to put the patient on a dry diet. I do not fool with cholestyramine or Lomotil or anything else.

Moderator: I think some are. I am talking about the real difficult diarrhea. Clearly there is such a group that should be distinguished from the dumping patients. They are really quite different.

Another question that many members of the audience asked is: What do you do about a patient with a perforated ulcer? Do you want to close the ulcer, or are you going to do one of the definitive operations? We might take the surgeons on the panel and ask them this question. Dr. Woodward, what do you do?

Dr. Woodward: We worry about the perforation first.

Moderator: Perforated duodenal ulcer.

Dr. Woodward: And about definitive therapy second. If this is a patient with chronic duodenal ulcer early after perforation and the tissues are not friable, we will do a vagotomy and pyloroplasty. We have done, as I recall, 36 such patients without one mortality. So it is very safe to do definitive surgery in the selected case. In the patient where this is a perforation out of the blue, with no preceding history, we are reluctant to do definitive surgery.

Moderator: How about the others? Does the length of time of the perforation at the time you are operating on the patient make a difference as to whether you will do the definitive operation or not on that patient?

Dr. Woodward: I do not pay any attention to the time. I pay attention to the character of the tissues.

Moderator: Let us say that the patient has been sick for 36 hours and there are peas, beans, garbage and pus in the peritoneal cavity and the patient has had symptoms for several years. Do you want to do a truncal vagotomy? I am not making that up. There are patients like that.

Dr. Woodward: Certainly. They are usually on the medical service.

Moderator: They have been there for a while. What do you do about those? Does that length of time and that degree of peritonitis bother you in doing a truncal vagotomy and a pyloroplasty?

Dr. Woodward: No, not particularly. We have found that there is very little correlation between the history of when the perforation occurred and the extent of the injury to the tissues. If the tissues are not friable and hold sutures well, we do not hesitate at all to clean up and do a definitive operation.

Moderator: Would you do a proximal gastric vagotomy, Dr. Goligher, on a patient like that?

Dr. Goligher: We have certainly done many proximal gastric vagotomies in the presence of perforation. If the patient comes in within a few hours of the perforation and has a good chronic ulcer, we would certainly do an elective operation at that time. With regard to your specific example, the patient with peas and vegetables in his peritoneal cavity with a perforation for 36 hours, well, I am not sure. I probably would just close that perforation. But we certainly do many proximal gastric vagotomies with perforations.

Moderator: Dr. Spiro, I have received many questions from the members of the audience about cimetidine. Would you treat with cimetidine a patient who just walks into your office off the street, and this is the first time he has had a duodenal ulcer?

Dr. Spiro: No, I do not want to do that, but everybody does. The patients have all read about it. It is an astonishingly harmless drug, as near as one can see. I prefer to treat the patient for a few days with small feedings and antacids. If he does not get better in two or three days, I give him cimetidine.

Moderator: Is it really completely innocuous? There is a question here about prolactin levels. You have pointed to the fact that you get gynecomastia.

Dr. Spiro: It is really impressive how little real data there are. *Lancet* always has an article or a letter on acute pancreatitis or mental confusion or various other kinds of things after cimetidine to make everybody worry.

Moderator: They have a letter in there every week about new and different complications like fever, neutropenia and rejection of renal homografts and God knows what else.

Dr. Spiro: In the ideal world, I would not use cimetidine unless it were needed. But in the world in which we live, everybody is getting it and everybody is giving it at the present time and I suspect that will continue.

Moderator: A member of the audience wants to know if you would treat reflux esophagitis with cimetidine?

Dr. Spiro: As I said earlier in this course, even in the absence of controlled studies I do tend and most gastroenterologists tend to treat reflux esophagitis at least at bedtime with one cimetidine tablet for six or eight weeks. Do I think that is proven? By no means is it proven.

Moderator: If you could get a patient to take antacids the way you wanted him to, would you choose cimetidine?

Dr. Spiro: Because I am conservative, I would choose regular medium dose liquid antacids on a regular basis until we know more about cimetidine. I am bothered by the duodenal ulcer recurrence rate, which runs from approximately 25% to 50%, depending upon whether you look at it endoscopically or symptomatically after cimetidine is stopped. I do not completely understand that. In a number of English studies, they suggest that as many as 75% of the patients will have a recurrence after cimetidine is stopped. There is something fishy because back before cimetidine, 75% of patients did not have a recurrence when they stopped taking whatever they were taking. So I do not understand all of the apparent changes in the natural history of duodenal ulcer. As I said to Dr. Goligher earlier today, I do not know that we are ever going to get a good controlled study of duodenal ulcers. Thanks to the US Food & Drug Administration, we enter the patient into the study, they get an endoscopy, and the minute they get an endoscopy, the observer affects the results. If you study patients who are willing to be endoscoped, the placebo rate is certainly going to be different from that of other people. So I do not know the answer to these questions.

Moderator: Dr. Spiro, I have several questions for you about diet therapy for duodenal and gastric ulcer.

Dr. Spiro: I live in an existential world. I do not think that there are any data to suggest that diet makes any difference. Nevertheless, in the society in which we live, people like small, regular feedings. They expect them to be rather bland; such a program cannot hurt and therefore I advise small, regular feedings and small amounts of antacids.

Moderator: Dr. Spiro, you must have something to fall back upon because patients always go off their diets. If a patient gets sick again, then Dr. Spiro says, "Well, you went off your diet, did you not?"

Dr. Spiro: No, I never do that, as a matter of fact. I tell patients that diet is simply for symptomatic relief and that there is no evidence other than for gluten-free diet and lactose-free diet, that diets affect the course of gastrointestinal diseases very significantly or specifically. So I have never punished patients by telling them, "You did that bad thing."

Moderator: You are a very different internist in that regard. Should patients on aspirin take buffering agents?

Dr. Spiro: Yes, I think probably such a patient with a duodenal ulcer will take either cimetidine or prostaglandins in a few years. At the moment, the average person without ulcer should take the cheapest aspirin that money can buy with a glass of water.

Moderator: In doing vagotomies, does anyone ever see postoperative achalasia? What is the phenomenon of dysphagia following vagotomy?

Dr. Goligher: It is quite common after proximal gastric vagotomy. It was not shown in my tables because they referred to the results after five years. But during the early postoperative weeks, there was quite an incidence of achalasia. I cannot give the precise figure. But certainly we have had two or three cases, and there have been one or two papers written on this subject. But it seems to rectify itself with time.

Moderator: Some people have suggested that it is the result of an intramural hematoma in the wall of the esophagus. These patients who appear to have achalasia do not have manometric changes. So it may be some sort of hematoma or fibrosis.

Zollinger-Ellison Syndrome

James C. Thompson, M.D.

Objectives

1. To understand the roles of gastrin and secretin in the Zollinger-Ellison syndrome.
2. To consider gastrectomy for Zollinger-Ellison syndrome.
3. To review the results of several representative cases, only some of which involved gastrectomy.

Drs. Robert Zollinger and Edward Ellison took care of two patients at Ohio State University who had a particularly virulent form of peptic ulcer disease. Upon operation, they were both found to have a pancreatic non-beta cell islet adenoma. Zollinger and Ellison reasoned that the tumor must produce a secretagogue which stimulated massive acid hypersecretion and that the only safe operative procedure was to totally excise the end-organ of that secretagogue, that is, to do a total gastrectomy. They reported their findings at the 1955 American Surgical Association meeting in Philadelphia.

The criteria that were proposed in 1955 have become familiar: massive gastric hypersecretion, a fulminant ulcer diathesis that usually gives rise to multiple peptic ulcers and a non-beta islet cell tumor of the pancreas. Gregory in Liverpool showed that the tumor secretagogue is gastrin. We now know that the invariable hallmark of the Zollinger-Ellison (Z-E) syndrome is a gastrin-producing tumor or a gastrinoma.

The normal value for serum gastrin in our laboratory is less than 200 pg/ml and in many laboratories, it is less than 150. All of the Z-E patients in our early experience had levels of gastrin of greater than 1,000 pg/ml and, for a while, we used that level

---

James C. Thompson, M.D., Professor and Chairman, Department of Surgery, The University of Texas Medical Branch, Galveston.

as the criterion for diagnosis. But as we gained experience, it became clear that there were patients with the Z-E syndrome who had levels not nearly that high. We also learned that gastrin levels fluctuate a great deal from time to time and that it is important to obtain multiple samples.

I would like to summarize our current knowledge of the Z-E syndrome and some of the developments that occurred in the last 23 years. It is difficult to be sure, but the incidence of this syndrome probably lies between 1:200 and 1:1,000 of all patients with duodenal ulcer. There is a slight preponderance of males. There are an estimated 200 to 400 new cases per year in this country and Canada. The diagnosis still depends upon a demonstration of acid hypersecretion and hypergastrinemia preoperatively. Radiography shows the ulcer and the changes that are incident to hypersecretion, edema and hypertrophy in the mucosa. At times it demonstrates the tumor by angiography. If gastrin levels are borderline, challenges with calcium and secretin determine the diagnosis.

At the University of Texas Medical Branch I have been involved in the treatment of 19 patients with the Z-E syndrome. Two had elevated gastrin levels with elevated calcium. After parathyroidectomy, the gastrins returned to normal and they have been asymptomatic. I am really not sure whether they really had the Z-E syndrome. We are still following them. We have a total of seven patients who have the multiple endocrine adenoma (MEA) syndrome, type I. All have had a parathyroidectomy. The two patients just mentioned had a return of gastrin levels to normal. One patient whom I shall discuss later had an elevated gastrin after parathyroidectomy, but had no ulcer symptoms. Four had a return of ulcer symptoms after a parathyroidectomy and underwent a later total gastrectomy. One patient refused operation. One patient with the MEA I syndrome had a parathyroidectomy and became asymptomatic, but had a persistently elevated gastrin. We were concerned that she had a functioning tumor which might be malignant. After demonstrating a pancreatic adenoma by angiography, we operated and did a distal pancreatectomy to remove a large gastrin-producing tumor. We did not do a total gastrectomy because she was asymptomatic.

Fifteen of the patients did have total gastrectomy without mortality. Six are now dead, all with metastatic tumor. Four of them died as a direct result of their tumor. Only one of the 19 currently has a normal gastrin level now for four years.

Of the 15 patients who underwent total gastrectomy, we found a primary tumor in ten, six of which were in the pancreas, two in the mesentery and two in the duodenum. Three of these patients had hepatic metastases at operation. Six are now dead. Nine are alive, eight with high levels of gastrin, which is indicative of functioning gastrinomas.

I will discuss several of these patients and suggest some generalizations for diagnosis and treatment. The first of these is a 41-year-old woman who died in our hospital recently. She had a total gastrectomy for the Z-E syndrome in 1969, at which time she was found to have numerous hepatic metastases. She was asymptomatic, nonetheless, until she noticed the gradual onset of symptoms caused by pressure from an enlarging liver.

Hepatic artery angiogram demonstrated a massive hepatic tumor. Her serum gastrin levels had been as high as 10,000 pg. We treated her in February, May and July 1974, with ten-day courses of selective hepatic artery infusion with 5-fluorouracil. During the second infusion she had an abrupt rise of gastrin to about 20,000, after which levels fell precipitously to 2,000. Her subsequent serum gastrins were all greater than 20,000. The hepatic artery thrombosed, so we were unable to continue the infusions. She had severe pain and a short time ago was brought into the hospital and died. At autopsy, her liver weighed 22 lb.

The next patient is a 74-year-old woman who never had a peptic ulcer. She was well until October 1969, when she had the onset of severe diarrhea, which caused a 50 lb weight loss, from 153 to 103 lb, in eight months. An upper gastrointestinal x-ray series showed no ulcer, but did show hypertrophic edematous folds of gastric and small bowel mucosa. These findings are suggestive of the Z-E syndrome. Gastric analysis revealed, to our surprise, a basal acid secretion of 50 mEq/hr, although she never had peptic ulcer symptoms — no heartburn, no pain. The upper limit of normal is 5 mEq/hr and anything above 15 is highly suggestive of the Z-E syndrome. Gastrin determinations revealed fasting levels of over 1,000 pg/ml. We resected a large tumor in the distal half of the pancreas. Unfortunately, she also had a large metastasis in the left lobe of the liver. We performed a total gastrectomy and reconstituted the GI tract with a

Roux-en-y esophagojejunostomy, end-to-end, our standard operation.

The histologic appearance of the pancreatic tumor showed well-differentiated cells arranged in cords and rosettes, separated by a highly vascular fibrous stroma. There are no histologic criteria to differentiate between benign and malignant tumors. In fact, there are no criteria to differentiate gastrinomas from carcinoid tumors, except that one produces gastrin and the other produces serotonin.

We operated on her more than seven years ago. For four years, she was completely asymptomatic, without any diarrhea, eating anything and everything she desired including enchiladas, which is our standard challenge.

About four years ago, she began to complain of pressure symptoms in the upper abdomen and her liver had obviously enlarged. Radiographic scans showed the growth of hepatic metastases, which began in September 1970.

Selective hepatic angiography revealed a large hepatic artery with multiple tumor nodules involving nearly the entire left lobe and the medial portion of the right lobe. One study was done in October 1973 and another in October 1974. The first study showed enlargement of the tumor and the growth of a large round satellite nodule at the bottom. We treated this metastatic tumor on four separate occasions with intrahepatic artery infusions of 5-fluorouracil, lasting from 8 to 14 days. Her gastrin levels fell after each infusion, but slowly went up again within two to three months. Even though gastrin levels were around 40,000, her only symptoms were directly attributable to pressure from the growth of the tumor itself. She never had any diarrhea postoperatively. The fact that patients with the Z-E syndrome *after* a total gastrectomy are able to tolerate extremely high levels of gastrin without any trouble indicates that diarrhea, as well as *all other* symptoms of the syndrome, is due to the massive secretion of water, acid and electrolytes by the stomach. It is not due to any intrinsic action of the hormone gastrin itself. Two years ago, this patient went into a coma at home and died within two weeks.

The next patient comes from a large family with multiple endocrine adenomatosis. He had been troubled with epigastric pain for 22 years and had had two previous gastric operations for ulcer disease. He had had a parathyroid adenoma excised one year before he came to us with massive GI bleeding. Figure 1 shows the family pedigree. The members involved in either the MEA I or the Z-E syndromes are shown in solid black. Our patient is number 11 on this diagram. Several members of his family had been found to have endocrine adenomas and a cousin had a total gastrectomy for the Z-E syndrome. His brother, number 13 (Fig. 1), also has the Z-E syndrome, but has refused operation. His nephew, number 41 (Fig. 1), is also one of our patients.

Measurement of basal gastrin revealed concentrations of only about 100 to 300 pg in this patient, even though we felt certain that he must have the Z-E syndrome. We infused calcium gluconate, which caused a rise in gastrin from a base of about 200 up to about 600 pg. On the basis of his family

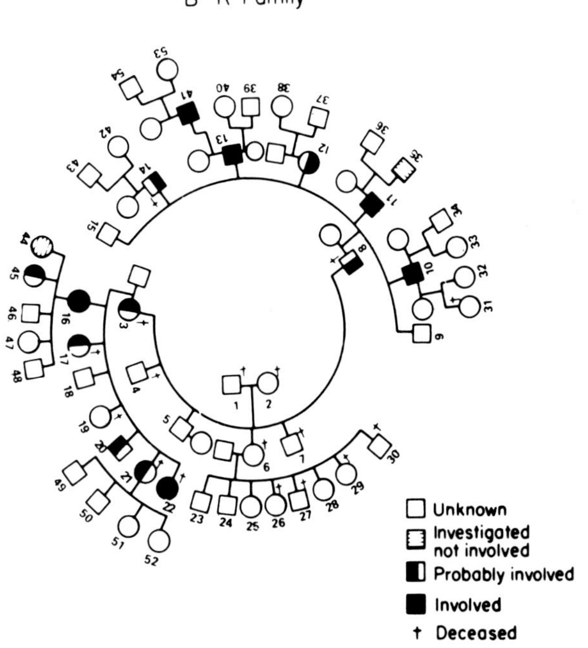

FIG. 1. Family pedigree showing members with MEA I syndrome. (Courtesy of Dr. M. Scurry.)

history, his acid hypersecretion and his gastrin studies, we made the preoperative diagnosis of the Z-E syndrome.

At operation, we explored the pancreas thoroughly and could find no tumor. After a lengthy search in which we sent 11 different nodules out for frozen section without success, we finally split the capsule of the pancreas in the region of the head over an area of questionably increased firmness and a nodule popped out. On histologic examination, it was found to be an islet cell adenoma and we performed a total gastrectomy. It had a gastrin concentration of more than 100,000,000 pg/gm.

Initially, he did well. Serial serum gastrin measurements after operation rose, indicating that he had either multiple primary tumors or metastases. He continued to do well. He worked full time as a cook on an offshore oil drilling platform until two years ago, when he was brought in by helicopter in coma with a blood sugar of 8 mg%. His glucose and insulin levels were strongly indicative of an insulinoma.

Initially he refused operation. However, as symptoms of confusion, sweating and blackouts became frequent and he had several automobile accidents, he finally decided to have an operation. In January 1977, we found a 2 cm adenoma in the uncinate process of the pancreas. Histologically, it was a beta-cell tumor which on assay was found to have 30,000 μU/gm of insulin. No gastrin activity was detected in the tumor. He is now asymptomatic with gastrin levels greater than 3,000. He is the only patient in our series with both gastrin- and insulin-producing tumors.

The next patient is a 37-year-old deaf mute woman with the multiple endocrine adenoma syndrome who came to us with ulcer symptoms and hypercalcemia. After parathyroidectomy, her gastrin levels fell precipitously. However, since they *never* fell to normal, we decided that we should look for a Z-E tumor. We obtained selective angiograms which beautifully demonstrated a small tumor in the body of the pancreas.

At operation, we found small tumor nodules. Both of the nodules were typical Z-E tumors. Because she was completely asymptomatic, we did not do a total gastrectomy. The gastrin levels remained low for about two months and we thought we might have cured her, but gradually the levels rose to around 500. She failed to keep her following appointments and we lost track of her. She recently died, but the cause of death is unknown.

The next patient is a 36-year-old man who came to us in 1972 as part of a routine kindred survey, since many members of his family were known to have the MEA I syndrome. Although he was completely asymptomatic, he had a basal acid output of 20 mEq/hr and borderline serum gastrin levels, which rose to 1,700 pg on calcium infusion. He was reluctant to undergo operation since he was asymptomatic. After six months, he developed severe epigastric pain, perhaps from worrying, and he returned. By that time, basal gastrin had risen to 1,200. Celiac arteriography demonstrated a tumor in the tail of the pancreas. He had developed a deep duodenal ulcer. At operation, we found a nodule and performed a two-thirds distal pancreatectomy, total gastrectomy and removal of a cortical adenoma from the left adrenal. The pathologist found an additional five separate islet cell adenomas of the pancreas, all of which were compatible with the Z-E syndrome. Of the 16 patients on whom we have operated, Z-E tumors have been found in ten. Of those ten, seven had multiple tumors.

The next patient had a perforated duodenal ulcer when he was 16 years old. He came to us five years later with hematochezia. Gastrin levels ranged as high as 2,200. Selective arteriograms failed to reveal any tumor.

At operation, we found no tumor in the pancreas. After an extensive search, we did find two small nodules in the gastrohepatic omentum. These were found to have no attachments to the pancreas or to any other organ. After excision of these nodules, the patient's gastrin levels fell to 72 pg/ml and have remained within normal limits to the present time, four years later, even though the tumors appeared to have been metastatic.

The next patient is a 41-year-old man who had symptoms of peptic ulcer for 11 years. Secretory studies and gastrin levels were compatible with the diagnosis. Arteriography showed no evidence of hepatic metastases. At operation, a nodule was palpated in the wall of the duodenum. It was excised and identified as an islet cell adenoma, consistent with gastrinoma. The acid secretion, which we were measuring intraoperatively, did not fall after removal of the duodenal adenomas, so we kept looking. Two Z-E tumors were also excised from the tail of the pancreas. Although his serum gastrin levels remain around 1,300, he is asymptomatic and is gainfully employed. The interesting thing about this patient and one other is that there has been a suggestion that Z-E tumors in the duodenum may not metastasize and that it may be wise to simply remove them and not do a total gastrectomy. This would not have worked in either patient because their postoperative gastrin levels were quite high.

The last patient I want to present is a 51-year-old woman who had abdominal pain and melena. She was treated for three months with cimetidine and did well until she developed symptoms of gastric outlet obstruction. Preoperative arteriography revealed an area that was suspicious for tumor in the head of the pancreas.

At operation, the mass was palpated in the second portion of the duodenum. This was excised and was found to be a gastrinoma. That excision did not cure her syndrome. Her gastrin levels rose to 2,800 postoperatively and we did a total gastrectomy. She is now asymptomatic and has returned to work. Her weight is stable at 113 lb. People with the Z-E syndrome tolerate total gastrectomy extremely well. We have one patient who weighs 210 lb and works full time as a stevedore. We have three other patients who consider themselves to be overweight.

To summarize the preoperative gastric acid secretory data in 12 Z-E patients: the normal upper limits are about 5 mEq/hr for basal and 40 mEq/hr for maximal; a basal acid output of greater than 15 mEq/hr is strongly suggestive of the Z-E syndrome; since endogenous gastrin from the Z-E tumor often drives the parietal cells to near maximal rates, many Z-E patients show little difference between basal and maximal stimulated acid output. Because basal serum gastrin levels fluctuate greatly, it is important to obtain multiple samples.

Since gastrin is usually circulating in massive excess in patients with the Z-E syndrome, the relatively small amounts of gastrin liberated from the antrum by a meal cause no significant change in gastrin levels. After total gastrectomy, however, there is a brisk serum gastrin response to food. This response is an enigma. We wonder what is the mechanism for this release of gastrin. How is the signal transmitted by food passing an esophagojejunostomy and proceeding down the small intestine? The gastrin obviously comes from tumor tissue, but the mechanism for its release is unknown. We suggest that the signal may be secretin because secretin does release gastrin from tumor tissue.

In caring for these patients, we have evolved a series of management protocols. This is the plan for diagnostic studies. After first carefully taking a history, performing a physical examination and getting routine laboratory studies, we obtain a basal gastrin level. Anything above 150 pg/ml is suspicious. We get an upper GI series, gastroscopy, gastric analysis and serum calcium determinations. An elevated calcium is often the best and sometimes the only clue to the MEA syndrome. If the patient provides good evidence of having the Z-E syndrome, we then proceed to challenge the gastrin level. Calcium is a strong stimulant of gastrin release in all patients, particularly Z-E patients. Secretin causes a fall in gastrin in normal and duodenal ulcer patients, but it causes a *rise* in Z-E syndrome patients; that it is an important discriminatory test. We then look for the tumor itself with arteriography and hepatic scans. We find it in about one out of three patients.

We must be alert for people who have the MEA I syndrome. Seven of our 19 patients, nearly one third, had the multiple endocrine adenoma syndrome. If the patient has hyperparathyroidism, we always operate on the parathyroids first to see what happens to the symptoms and to the serum gastrin levels.

The rise in gastrin after a calcium infusion is slow in some Z-E patients, but at four hours, most gastrin levels rise to 400% of basal.

The important thing to note about the effect of a secretin infusion in Z-E patients is rapid, nearly immediate, rise of gastrin within two minutes after the infusion of secretin. The important thing is that, as far as we know, secretin releases gastrin *only* from Z-E tumor tissues.

A recent study in postoperative patients showed that magnesium also has the capacity to release gastrin from tumor tissue, as does calcium. This may prove to be worthwhile.

We have certain criteria for diagnosis. The history and GI series and endoscopic findings should confirm an ulcer and the patient should have acid hypersecretion. Gastrin levels should be high and they should rise with calcium and secretin. High gastrin values are important only if the patient hypersecretes acid. It is particularly helpful if one can demonstrate the tumor by angiography.

We also have a protocol for the operative procedure itself. It is mandatory to make the diagnosis securely prior to operation. At operation, the surgeon should search for the tumor in the pancreas, omentum, peripancreatic and celiac nodes and in the duodenum and the liver. He should excise and get frozen section biopsies of all suspected tissue. All possible metastatic tumor tissue should be excised. The more tumor one takes out, the longer the patient will live. If you are sure of the diagnosis we think it is important to go ahead with total gastrectomy, even if tumor is not found.

A final word about the treatment of Z-E patients with the $histamine_2$ receptor blocking agent, cimetidine. Cimetidine will certainly block acid hypersecretion, temporarily at least, in nearly all Z-E patients. Gastroenterologists with experience vary in their assessment of the safety of cimetidine treatment. There is no question that cimetidine given at twice the standard dose, that is, at 600 mg tid and hs, for a total daily dose of 2.4 gm/day, will halt, at least temporarily, the massive acid hypersecretion. It is the suggestion that this may be used as a permanent treatment, in lieu of operation, that causes concern. Bonfils, a gastroenterologist in Paris, and Creutzfeldt, working in Goettingen, Germany, have each treated more than ten Z-E patients with cimetidine and both have found that in patients who initially had severe symptoms the patient escapes from cimetidine therapy and symptoms recur eventually. I am familiar with four patients treated on a long-term basis, all of whom have required or will require an operation. If control of the acid secretory symptoms is secured, and if the patient decides against total gastrectomy, I believe we should still make a strong argument for operation to excise the potentially malignant tumor. Even though the cure rate is low, it is at least as good as it is for, say, carcinoma of the stomach. No one would suggest that we not operate on gastric cancer. Although patients may live in symbiosis with the tumor for a long time, the tumor will eventually kill most. If we can excise the tumor early, we may provide a cure. In thinking of these tumors, it is worthwhile to use the carcinoid syndrome as a biologic model. We know that carcinoid patients will tolerate hepatic metastases for a long time. But when the metastases begin to grow, they may grow fiercely and kill their owners.

Cimetidine does afford an excellent means of preparing the patient for operation. It can totally defuse a potentially explosive secretory crisis and allow the surgeon to time the operation for when the patient is in optimal condition.

Self-Evaluation Quiz

1. Z-E syndrome is associated with:
   a) Gastrin hyposecretion
   b) Fulminating ulcer diathesis but never gastrinoma
   c) Gastric hyposecretion plus gastrinoma
   d) Gastric hypersecretion plus gastrinoma
2. A normal serum gastrin value would be about:
   a) 210 to 230 pg/ml
   b) 230 to 250 pg/ml
   c) 300 to 350 pg/ml
   d) Less than 200 or even 150, depending upon the laboratory
3. The number of new Z-E syndrome cases yearly is estimated at:
   a) 100 to 200
   b) 200 to 400
   c) 400 to 600
   d) 650 to 700
4. If gastrin levels are borderline:
   a) The patient may be lost before surgery is possible
   b) Dosage with magnesium and secretin may be sufficient therapy
   c) Challenge with calcium and secretin may help diagnosis
   d) Challenge with secretin and ferric sulfate may help diagnosis
5. The author's standard challenge for assessing postoperative success is:
   a) Calcium and secretin
   b) Enchiladas

   c) Strong tea
   d) Pablum
6. Diarrhea in patients with Z-E syndrome is:
   a) Caused intrinsically by gastrin
   b) Not caused intrinsically by gastrin
   c) Caused by too much challenging with calcium and synthetic gastrin
   d) Not caused by massive secretion of water, acid and electrolytes by the stools
7. Gastrin:
   a) Definitely does not come from tumor tissues
   b) Is released by secretin only in Z-E tumor tissues
   c) Is not elicited by calcium
   d) Is only weakly elicited by calcium
8. Cimetidine:
   a) Definitely does not block acid hypersecretion in Z-E patients
   b) Definitely does permanently block acid hypersecretion in Z-E patients
   c) Does block acid hypersecretion, at least temporarily, in about all Z-E patients
   d) Should not be considered a histamine-2 receptor blocker.

Answers on page 721.

Total Gastrectomy for Carcinoma of the Stomach

John Alexander-Williams, M.D.

Objectives

1. To consider the merits of total versus subtotal gastrectomy.
2. To review the criteria of decision for performing total gastrectomy.
3. To gain familiarity with a successful technique for total gastrectomy.

Master surgeons who deal with patients with carcinoma of the stomach usually develop such technique and expertise in the performance of gastric surgery that, in their hands, total gastrectomy for resectable carcinoma becomes a simple and safe procedure. Therefore, it is not surprising that they advocate total rather than subtotal gastrectomy for all potentially curable carcinomata of the stomach on the presumption that the more of the organ that is removed the greater the possibility of cure [1]. However, when reports of follow-up of large series of carcinoma of the stomach appear in the literature, invariably the results are better for subtotal than total gastrectomy in terms of the mean length of survival and the percentage of patients surviving five years [2]. Furthermore, studies of postoperative symptomatology and nutrition usually favor a lesser resection; total gastrectomy has a reputation of giving severe symptoms and being associated with gross malnutrition. Therefore, surgical teaching usually advocates that wherever possible a partial gastric resection is preferred to a total gastric resection for carcinoma.

John Alexander-Williams, M.D., Chairman of Gastroenterology Group, University of Birmingham, Birmingham, England.

This concept can be challenged on two grounds: (1) almost all reported series of survivals after total or partial gastrectomy for carcinoma of the stomach are retrospective analyses. In the reported series the selection of patients for total gastrectomy is inevitably biased toward those patients with extensive tumors or with proximal tumors and (2) the symptomatic and nutritional status of patients is good after a properly performed total gastrectomy.

It is well known that carcinoma of the stomach spreads in the submucosa, often for several centimeters beyond the apparent mucosal spread. Inevitably some patients having a partial gastric resection will have malignant cells left behind that might have been removed by total gastric resection. Furthermore, a gastric mucosa that develops one carcinoma is the type of mucosa that is particularly prone to develop another. I have known two patients who have developed a second, apparent primary carcinoma of the fundus of the stomach, having survived five years after partial gastrectomy for a proximal gastric carcinoma. The logic of performing total gastrectomy even for the earliest mucosal lesion is akin to the argument for performing a pan proctocolectomy for every patient with even the smallest colonic carcinoma; I would not wish to push the argument to absurd limits. However, a planned prospective randomized stratified survey is needed.

Another important argument of those who advocate partial gastric resection is that anastomoses of the bowel to the esophagus are prone to leak and that even if they do not, bad symptoms and malabsorption inevitably follow. There are important considerations of the technique of total gastrectomy that mitigate toward safety and symptomatic success. The technique to be described has been used for the past four years in a small consecutive series of 25 patients without anastomotic leakage and with good symptomatic results.

Total gastrectomy is designed to be employed as a curative operation. Where there is extension of tumor submucosally into the esophagus or to the adjacent organs or regional lymph nodes, total gastrectomy, although still technically possible in some cases, will give no better results than a limited palliative resection. For this reason I advocate early determination of the proximal spread of the disease by means of excision/biopsy of a strip of submucosal tissue at the cardioesophageal junction. Immediate frozen section histological examination will determine whether malignant cells are present. If they are, then other forms of palliation are preferred to total gastrectomy. If the biopsy is clear, then a total gastrectomy, splenectomy and removal of the omentum are performed. A bridge retractor elevating the costal margin enables the lower esophagus to be mobilized sufficiently for 1 to 2 cm to be removed and still gives good access to some of the intra-abdominal esophagus.

A loop of proximal mobile jejunum is selected as near as possible to the duodenal-jejunal junction. One vascular arcade is divided. The end of the distal limb of the jejunum is then crushed, ligated and buried with a purse-string suture, similar to the burial of an appendix stump. Through a hole in the meso-colon the closed end of the jejunum is brought up to the esophagus. A small hole, no more than 2 cm long, is made on the antimesenteric border of the apex of the loop, hemostasis being secured with diathermy. A two-layer anastomosis is made between the loop and the lower esophagus. For the outer layer I use interrupted mattress sutures of silk or Dexon and find that, despite the notorious difficulty of suturing the esophagus, it is always possible to make a useful posterior outer layer. A careful mucosa-to-mucosa suture is performed between the esophagus and jejunum. I prefer a continuous running catgut suture, although many surgeons feel safer using interrupted sutures through all layers. After completing the continuous suture, the anterior row of outer sutures is placed. Here it is possible to obtain good apposition between the serosa of the jejunum and the peritoneum over the hiatus that has been reflected when the esophagus was mobilized.

The duodenal end of the jejunum is then anastomosed to the side of the efferent loop, at least 50 cm distal to the esophago-jejunal anastomosis in the Roux-en-Y manner. I have found that a loop of less than 35 cm permits bile to reflux into the esophagus, whereas there is no detectable nutritional disadvantage in leaving a long loop. The long loop undergoes hypertrophy that can be demonstrated radiologically or at subsequent laparotomy to be sufficiently capacious to obviate the need to perform any type of jejunal pouch. Patients with such a Roux loop do not suffer from "small stomach syndrome." I find that they are much less susceptible to dumping than are most patients with a Billroth I hemigastrectomy. The duodenal stump is closed with two layers of continuous catgut.

The duodenum is mobilized sufficiently for a small balloon catheter to be inserted into its lateral border, usually 1 to 2 cm distal to the closed end. A catheter is inserted through a very small diathermy incision and is surrounded by a double purse-string suture of absorbable material. The balloon catheter is inflated with no more than 3 ml of fluid and the catheter is brought out laterally through the abdominal wall. This duodenostomy tube permits early decompression of the upper gastrointestinal tract. It also permits early administration of fluid.

I do not use a nasogastric tube, but the patients are permitted no more than sips of water until the seventh postoperative day. Then a water soluble contrast radiological study is performed to confirm the integrity of the esophagojejunal anastomosis. It is usually possible to give all the fluid and electrolyte requirements through the duodenostomy tube from the second postoperative day and, once bowel function is resumed, a blended normal diet can be given via the duodenostomy to maintain nutrition.

Most of the bad symptomatic results attributed to total gastrectomy in the past have resulted from the reflux of bile and pancreatic secretions into the esophagus. The creation of a Roux-en-Y anastomosis prevents any bile reflux. All my patients so treated have gained some weight following operation. I find there is no need for any vitamin or mineral supplements apart from vitamin B12 that is given parenterally at two monthly intervals.

A stomach that contains a carcinoma is usually hypo- or achlorhydria. It contains high concentrations of pathogenic microorganisms. In our institution five years ago the incidence of wound infection following elective operation for gastric cancer unprotected by antimicrobial prophylaxis was 60%. We now make a culture of the gastric content at the initial diagnostic endoscopy and so have an individual pattern of the gastric microflora and their sensitivity to apply appropriate prophylaxis. This policy has abolished all endogenous wound or intra-abdominal infections.

References

1. Lahey, S.H. and Marshall, S.F.: Should total gastrectomy be employed in early carcinoma of the stomach? Ann. Surg. 132:540, 1950.
2. Marshall, S.F. and Uram, H.: Total gastrectomy for gastric cancer: The effect upon mortality, morbidity and curability. Surg. Gynecol. Obstet. 99:657, 1954.

Self-Evaluation Quiz

1. The following are not considered to be good reasons for advocating total gastrectomy as opposed to partial gastrectomy:
   a) Gastric carcinoma spreads in the submucosa for several centimeters beyond the apparent mucosal spread
   b) Gastric mucosa that develops one carcinoma is predisposed to develop others
   c) Is more difficult to anastomose duodenum to the esophagus than to the distal end of the stomach
   d) Nutritional state of the patient is as good after total as after partial gastrectomy
2. Patients with a total gastrectomy and a Roux-en-y anastomosis usually experience a normal appetite.
   a) True
   b) False
3. The following are not considered to be important steps in the performance of a total gastrectomy for carcinoma:
   a) Frozen section at the proximal limit of dissection
   b) Splenectomy
   c) Removal of the greater omentum
   d) Ante-colic anastomosis
4. In the technique described it is recommended to join the cut end of the esophagus to the jejunal loop end to end rather than end to side.
   a) True
   b) False
5. The optimal length for the efferent loop in a Roux-en-y anastomosis is:
   a) 10 cm
   b) 20 cm
   c) 30 cm
   d) 50 cm

6. Those who advocate a long efferent loop do so because:
   a) It is easier to make the entero-enterostomy below the colon
   b) A long loop prevents bile refluxing into the esophagus
   c) There is less tension on the esophago-jejunal anastomosis
   d) It promotes digestion of carbohydrates
7. Patients after total gastrectomy require constant medication with:
   a) Antacids
   b) Bile salts binding agents
   c) Antibiotics
   d) Vitamin B12
8. The stomach containing a carcinoma usually contains a high concentration of bacteria because:
   a) There is hypochlorhydria
   b) Breaking down tumor is a good culture medium
   c) Patients have bad dental hygiene
   d) There is often a gastro-colic fistula

Answers on page 721.

Antacids in the Prophylaxis of Stress Ulceration

William Silen, M.D.

Objectives

To develop an awareness of the value of buffered luminal contents in the prevention of stress ulceration and acute gastrointestinal hemorrhage in critically ill patients.

Introduction

This report presents the results of a prospective randomized trial that was conducted in our institution and published in a recent issue of the *New England Journal of Medicine*. I am indebted to Drs. Paul Hastings, John Skillman, and Leonard Bushnell, my collaborators, who were largely responsible for the conduct of this investigation [1].

On the basis of our experimental work, it is clear that some acid must be present for stress-related ulceration to occur and that buffering of luminal content will protect against the development of ulceration induced by hemorrhagic shock [2]. We found that if luminal content was buffered to a pH of 3.5 or greater, protection would occur. A pH of 3.5 represents only about 1 mEq per liter of hydrogen ion concentration and when this pH is achieved experimentally, no ulcerations will occur in rabbits subjected to hemorrhagic shock [2]. These studies suggested that antacids might be used for prophylaxis against development of stress ulceration. It appeared to us that prophylaxis was far preferable to therapy since the development of overt gastrointestinal hemorrhage is associated with an extraordinarily high mortality, reaching 80% in some series.

William Silen, M.D., Johnson & Johnson Professor of Surgery, Harvard Medical School; Surgeon-in-Chief, Beth Israel Hospital, Boston, Mass.

Materials and Methods

One hundred patients were randomized into this study between March 1972 and March 1977. All patients were treated in the Surgical Intensive Care Unit of the Beth Israel Hospital during the study. Patients with one or more of the following problems were included: multiple trauma, major operative procedures, respiratory failure, hypotension to a systolic pressure of less than 100 mm Hg for more than two hours prior to randomization, sepsis, jaundice and renal failure.

Patients were excluded from randomization if they were receiving fluids or food by mouth, if they had undergone cardiac, gastric or esophageal operations, if their primary disease was a burn or a neurological problem, or if there was any evidence of gross gastrointestinal hemorrhage prior to the study. The definition of acute upper gastrointestinal bleeding in this study was the passage of bright red blood via the nasogastric tube or the presence of a 4+ positive guaiac test on nasogastric aspirate for three consecutive determinations within a 12-hour period.

Before the study began, the gastric contents were aspirated completely, the pH was tested by pH sensitive paper, and the results of the guaiac test were recorded. If the aspirate did not contain blood, the patients were randomized by a table of random numbers. The initial volume of antacid (Mylanta-II) was 30 ml. At the end of each hour the contents of the stomach were aspirated and the pH and volume of the aspirate were recorded. Thirty ml of antacid was instilled at the beginning of each subsequent hour provided the pH of the gastric content was 3.5 or greater. If the pH was less than 3.5, 60 ml of antacid was instilled. The nasogastric tube was flushed with 10 ml of tap water after each instillation of antacid. The tube was then clamped for 60 minutes and the sequence was repeated hourly. A guaiac test was performed on the aspirate every four hours and on the stool at least once daily. If regurgitation around the nasogastric tube occurred or if the total volume of antacid plus gastric content exceeded 150 ml at the end of one hour, the tube was clamped for 30 minutes and placed on intermittent suction for 30 minutes out of each hour until the aspirated volume was less than 150 ml.

In patients who were randomized not to receive antacid, the nasogastric tube was connected to intermittent low suction. The pH was determined and guaiac tests were performed on samples of gastric juice every four hours and stool guaiac tested as for the patients receiving antacid.

The two patients receiving antacid prophylaxis in whom evidence of bleeding developed continued to receive antacid medication to maintain the gastric aspirate above pH 3.5. Those in whom bleeding developed who were receiving no antacids were started on antacid therapy as described above. The study was terminated when a patient was discharged from the intensive care unit or was started on food either by tube or by mouth. Aluminum hydroxide was substituted for Mylanta-II in five patients whose renal failure was complicated by the development of noteworthy hypermagnesemia.

Results

Fifty-one of the 100 patients were randomized to receive antacids while forty-nine received no antacids initially. These two groups were similar with respect to age and the duration of the study. Figure 1 demonstrates that in consideration of the six major risk factors which have been shown to be associated with stress ulceration, the two groups of patients were quite similar. There were 110 risk factors in 51 patients in the antacid group, a mean of 2.2 risk factors per patient, while in the patients not receiving antacid prophylaxis, there were 150 risk factors in 49 patients, or a mean of 2.4 risk factors per patient. The degree of respiratory failure, renal failure and jaundice was not statistically different in the two groups. There were 11 deaths in the patients receiving antacids and 7 deaths in those not receiving antacid prophylaxis while they were in the intensive care unit. Gastrointestinal hemorrhage or complications relating to antacids were not thought to have contributed to the death of any patient in the study.

Figure 2 demonstrates that only 2 of 51 patients (4%) in the group receiving antacid bled, whereas 12 of 49 patients not receiving antacids (25%) bled. The difference between these two groups was highly significant ($P < 0.005$). Figure 2 also demonstrates the fact that there was an increasing incidence of

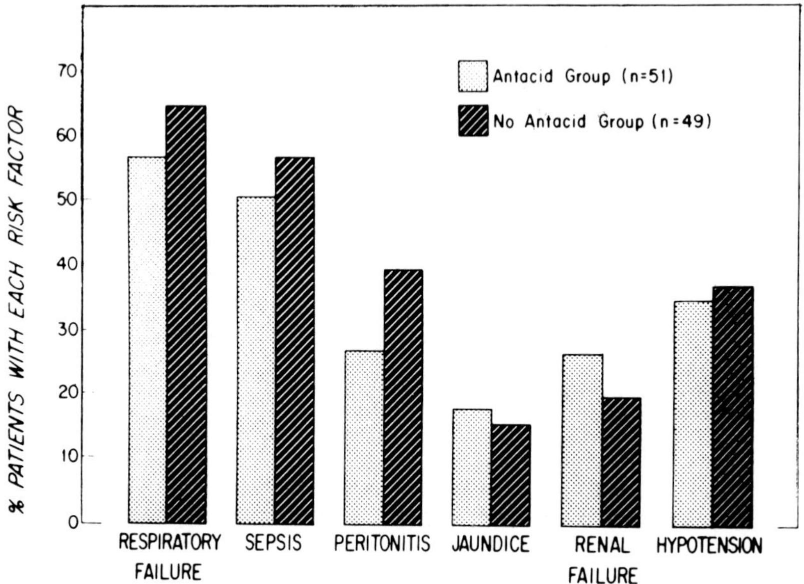

FIG. 1. Risk factors in patients receiving and those not receiving antacid prophylaxis. The similarity of the two groups is indicated by the almost equal rate of each risk factor. (From Hastings et al [1].)

gastrointestinal bleeding when the number of risk factors increased.

The pH of the gastric aspirate in patients receiving antacid medication was below 5 in only two cases in the entire study and usually ranged between 7 and 8. Consequently, a double dose (60 ml) of antacid was rarely necessary to achieve satisfactory buffering. The pH of the gastric content for patients not receiving antacids was variable in the same patient and between patients, the range being from 1 to 8.

Patients Who Develop Bleeding on Antacid Prophylaxis

Two patients in this group bled. One was a 58-year-old woman with respiratory failure, sepsis and peritonitis due to a perforated diverticulum of the colon. Her gastric aspirate became 4+ seven hours after she was placed on antacid therapy. Continued therapy maintaining the gastric pH above 5 resulted in conversion to guaiac negative after four hours. The second

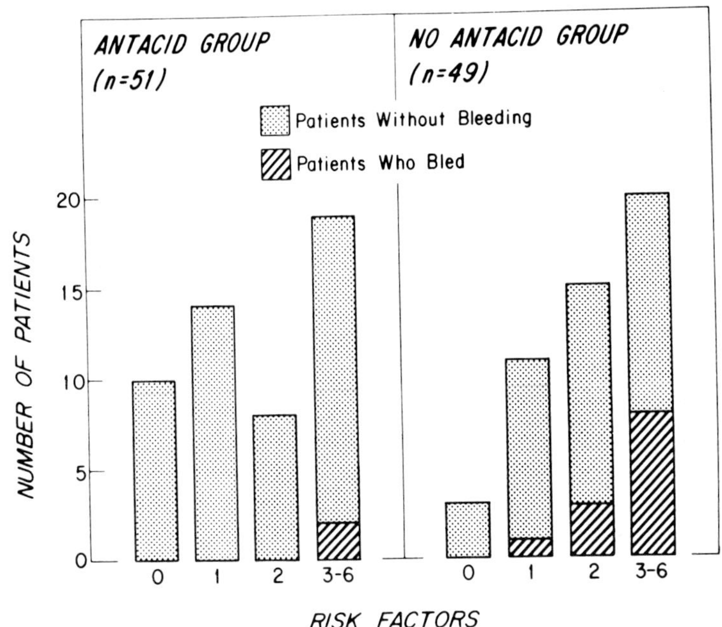

FIG. 2. Distribution of patients according to number of risk factors and number of patients who bled in each group. In the group given antacid prophylaxis only patients with the greatest number of risk factors (three to six) had evidence of bleeding. With one, two or three to six risk factors, the frequency of bleeding rose progressively in patients who did not receive antacid and was significantly different from that in the antacid group in each of these subgroups ($P < 0.05$ to $P < 0.005$). (From Hastings et al [1].)

patient who bled was an 87-year-old woman who had all six risk factors after cholecystectomy, common duct exploration and sphincteroplasty for ascending cholangitis. On the eighth postoperative day, she developed upper gastrointestinal hemorrhage which was shown to be the result of bleeding from the duodenotomy suture line. Superficial erosions were present in the fundus of the stomach but were not bleeding.

Patients Who Developed Bleeding While Receiving No Antacids

Twelve patients in this group developed gastrointestinal hemorrhage. None developed an exsanguinating hemorrhage and none required operation. Seven of the 12 who bled were treated with antacid titration and all subsequently converted to negative.

Complications of Antacid Use

Fifteen minor complications of antacid prophylaxis occurred, including diarrhea in ten, gross regurgitation in two and elevated serum magnesium in three. Diarrhea was treated variously by discontinuation of antacid treatment in one patient, change to a different antacid in two, continuation of the same antacid in four and feeding in three. The two patients with regurgitation were treated by stopping the antacid in one and by withholding the antacid for a few hours in the other. The three patients with slightly elevated magnesium levels were all asymptomatic and two of these were continued on the same antacid while the other one was changed to a preparation that did not contain magnesium.

Discussion

This study shows clearly that prophylactic antacid therapy decreases the risk of acute gastrointestinal bleeding in critically ill patients. Our data suggest that critically ill patients with renal failure, especially when associated with jaundice and hypotension, are at great risk for development of upper gastrointestinal bleeding since half of the patients with renal failure who did not receive the antacid had gastrointestinal bleeding, as defined by our study. Not only does this study show that antacids are effective in the prevention of bleeding. It is also of considerable importance that patients who were given antacids when they developed bleeding after having received none all responded to the antacid therapy with cessation of bleeding.

The conclusion that antacid prophylaxis prevents acute gastrointestinal bleeding in critically ill patients is in agreement with the results of a controlled randomized trial of antacid medication in selected patients with major burns [3]. Two other nonrandomized trials in critically ill patients came to the same conclusion [4, 5]. However, antacids have been reported to be ineffective in preventing bleeding in a randomized trial involving only 25 patients in hepatic failure [6]. The antacids in this study were given at four-hour intervals and only 35% of the aspirated samples taken at two-hour intervals were about pH 5. It is possible, therefore, that the lack of protective effect of antacids in that particular trial may be related to inadequate buffering of gastric acid. In that same trial it was shown that the H_2 antagonists were effective in protection against bleeding. This is the only trial in which the H_2 blocking agents have been prospectively and randomly assessed. We are currently involved in a trial which is comparing the use of cimetidine with antacids.

The incidence of acute gastrointestinal hemorrhage in seriously ill patients appears to be decreasing. The reason for this decline is uncertain, but may be related to the wider application of prophylactic antacid medication as well as other improvements in the metabolic care of critically ill patients.

Summary

One hundred critically ill patients at risk of developing acute gastrointestinal ulceration and bleeding have been randomized into two groups: one (51 patients) received antacid prophylaxis and the other (49 patients) received no specific form of prophylaxis. Hourly antacid titration kept the pH of the gastric contents above 3.5.

Two of the 51 patients who received antacid prophylaxis had gastrointestinal bleeding. Twelve of the 49 controlled patients bled ($P < 0.005$). Of the 12 patients in the control group who bled, seven were placed on antacid medication and all seven stopped bleeding. Analysis of all of the patients showed that an increasing prevalence of respiratory failure, sepsis, peritonitis, jaundice, renal failure and hypotension was correlated with a greater frequency of bleeding. No patients required operative treatment to control bleeding. These data indicate that the occurrence of acute gastrointestinal hemorrhage in critically ill patients can be reduced by antacid titration.

References

1. Hastings, P.R., Skillman, J.J., Bushnell, L.S. and Silen, W.: Antacid titration in the prevention of acute gastrointestinal bleeding. N. Engl. J. Med. 298:1041-1045, 1978.

2. Skillman, J.J., Gould, S.A., Chung, R.S.K. et al: The gastric mucosal barrier: Clinical and experimental studies in critically ill and normal man, and in the rabbit. Ann. Surg. 172:564-584, 1970.
3. McAlhany, F.C., Jr., Czafa, A.J. and Pruitt, B.A., Jr.: Antacid control of complications from acute gastroduodenal disease after burns. J. Trauma 16:645-649, 1976.
4. Curtis, L.E., Simonian, S., Buerk, C.A. et al: Evaluation of the effectiveness of controlled pH in the management of massive upper gastrointestinal bleeding. Am. J. Surg. 125:474-476, 1973.
5. Simonian, S.J. and Curtis, L.E.: Treatment of hemorrhagic gastritis by antacid. Ann. Surg. 184:429-434, 1976.
6. MacDougall, B.R.D., Bailey, R.J. and Williams, R.: H_2-receptor antagonists and antacids in the prevention of acute gastrointestinal hemorrhage in fulminant hepatic failure: Two controlled trials. Lancet 1:617-619, 1977.

Self-Evaluation Quiz

1. The luminal wall is protected against stress-related ulceration induced by hemorrhagic shock if the luminal content is buffered at:
   a) pH 2.5 or less
   b) pH 3.0
   c) pH 3.4
   d) pH 3.5 or greater
2. In some series of patients, overt gastrointestinal hemorrhage was associated with a mortality of:
   a) 50%
   b) 75%
   c) 80%
   d) 90%
3. Prophylactic antacids:
   a) Decrease the risk of acute GI bleeding in mildly ill patients
   b) Do not decrease the risk of GI bleeding in mildly ill patients
   c) Do not decrease the risk of GI bleeding in critically ill patients
   d) Decrease the risk of GI bleeding in critically ill patients
4. In patients given antacids when they developed bleeding after having received none:
   a) 50% ceased bleeding following antacid therapy
   b) 75% ceased bleeding following antacid therapy

c) All ceased bleeding following antacid therapy
d) None ceased bleeding following antacid therapy

5. Minor complications of antacid prophylaxis in this study were:
a) Diarrhea, cramping and elevated urinary Mg
b) Diarrhea and gross regurgitation
c) Elevated serum Mg and muscle cramping
d) Diarrhea, gross regurgitation and increased urinary Mg
e) Diarrhea, gross regurgitation and increased serum Mg

6. What patient was not included in the study?
a) One with a neurological problem
b) One with multiple trauma
c) One with respiratory failure
d) One with renal failure

7. Of the 11 deaths among the patients receiving antacids, how many were considered due to GI bleeding or complications related to antacids?
a) Five deaths
b) Ten deaths
c) None
d) All

8. Antacids in this study were given:
a) At four-hour intervals
b) At two-hour intervals
c) At one-hour intervals
d) *Pro re nata*

Answers on page 721.

Operation for the Prophylaxis of Stress Ulceration in Transplant Patients

George K. Kyriakides, M.D. and John S. Najarian, M.D.

Objectives

1. To consider indications for surgical prophylaxis and for medical treatment of peptic ulcer before transplant in renal patients.
2. To consider the statistical results obtained in a large series of transplant patients with ulceration.

Introduction

Peptic ulcer disease and its complications are associated with a high morbidity and mortality in transplant patients (Table 1). With increasing experience, emphasis has been placed on the prevention of peptic ulceration by establishing firm guidelines for prophylactic operations in uremic patients before transplantation.

The incidence of peptic ulceration in uremic patients is higher than in the general population [1, 2] because uremia is associated with hypergastrinemia and gastric acid hypersecretion [1, 3]. Furthermore, uremic patients have coagulopathy and platelet dysfunction which are made worse by the intermittent anticoagulation of hemodialysis [4, 5].

After transplantation the uremic state may recur during episodes of rejection; combined with the large doses of steroids used in the treatment of rejection, these posttransplant patients

---

George K. Kyriakides, M.D., Transplant Fellow, and John S. Najarian, M.D., Professor and Chairman, Department of Surgery, University of Minnesota Hospitals, Minneapolis.

Table 1. Incidence and Mortality of Gastroduodenal Ulceration

Author	*Year*	*Incidence (%)*	*Mortality (%)*
Penn et al	1968	5.0	55.0
Moore & Hume	1969	10.0	71.0
Hodjiyannakis et al	1971	11.5	50.0
Lewicki et al	1972	21.5	
Spanos et al	1974	2.1	62.0
Aldrete et al	1975	3.0	25.0
Berg et al	1975	8.0	58.0
Blohme	1975	10.0	37.0
Rasmussen et al	1975	6.1	
Owens et al	1976	19.4	25.0
Maxwell	1976	25.0	
Uhlschmid et al	1975	16.1	30.0
Najarian, Kyriakides	1978	2.9	81.0
Overall		11.6% (2.1-25.0%)	49.4% (25-81%)

are in a high-risk category for ulceration and bleeding. In addition, there is some evidence that stress-induced epinephrine release during rejection episodes may increase gastrin output [6] — increased histamine levels that result from rejection may increase the acid output even more [7].

Clinical Data

From 1968 to 1977, 1,050 renal transplants were done in 912 patients at the University of Minnesota. For the purpose of comparison this period is divided into phase I (from 1968 to 1973) and phase II (from 1973 to 1977). We chose this comparison because the indications for prophylactic operation were more carefully adhered to during the second period.

The indications for surgical prophylaxis for peptic ulcer disease before transplantation are (a) previous history of peptic ulcer disease, (b) present symptoms of peptic ulcer disease and (c) demonstration of ulcer by routine pretransplant upper gastrointestinal series.

Using these criteria, the diagnosis of peptic ulceration was made in 30 of 377 patients in phase I and 31 of 535 patients in phase II (Table 2). In phase I only three of 19 patients (15%)

Table 2. Patients With Ulcer History Before Transplantation

	Phase I	*Phase II*
Number of patients	30/377	31/535
Prophylactic surgery	19/30*	29/31†
posttransplant ulcer	3/19 (15%)	2/29 (7%)
No prophylactic surgery	11/30	2/31
posttransplant ulcer	9/11 (81%)	1/2 (50%)

*Vagotomy and pyloroplasty in 17, vagotomy and antrectomy in 2.

†Vagotomy and pyloroplasty in 28, vagotomy and antrectomy in 1.

who underwent prophylactic operation pretransplant developed posttransplant ulceration, whereas nine of the 11 patients (81%) who did not undergo prophylactic procedures developed ulcers posttransplant [8]. In phase II, 29 of the 31 ulcer patients underwent prophylaxis with only two recurrences of ulcers (7%) after transplant. Two of the 31 patients failed to undergo operation and one of them bled after transplantation. Despite prophylactic operations, five patients bled after transplantation, but four of them were in a high-risk category because of the presence of graft rejection or sepsis (Table 3).

There is, however, a small but definite group of patients with no previous evidence of ulcers who develop ulceration after transplantation, and who cannot be recognized before transplantation. Their ulcers, usually manifested by bleeding, are always secondary to predisposing conditions that follow transplantation.

We had 15 of these patients, three in phase I and 12 in phase II, an overall incidence of 1.8%. Only one of them did not have any recognizable predisposing factor. The other 14 patients had either rejection or sepsis, or both (Table 4).

The other four patients who developed posttransplant bleeding had a history of ulcer, but had no pretransplant prophylaxis. They also had recognizable factors predisposing to ulceration (Table 5). The predisposing conditions in posttransplant gastrointestinal bleeding were rejection-uremia (15 cases), infection (19 cases), heparinization (2 cases), and unknown causes (3 cases).

Table 3. Posttransplant Bleeding Pretransplant History of Ulcer With Prophylactic Operation Pretransplant

Patient	*Age*	*Donor*	*Source of Bleeding*	*Associated Conditions*	*Pretransplant Prophylactic Operation*	*Treatment*	*Outcome of Bleeding*	*Fate of Patient*
1	19	Cadaver	Gastric ulcer	Rejection	V&P	Antacids	Controlled	Survived
2	22	Living Related	Gastritis	Bladder leak, sepsis	V&P	Antacids	Rebled	Died of sepsis, bleeding
3	23	Cadaver	Gastric ulcer	–	V&P	Antacids	Controlled	Survived
4	29	Cadaver	Esophagitis	Posttransplant nephrectomy, wound sepsis	V&P	Antacids, tamponade	Controlled	Died of sepsis
5	46	Cadaver	Duodenal ulcer	Rejection	V&P	Antacids, gastrectomy	Rebled	Died of bleeding

Characteristics of Posttransplant Ulceration

Manifestation of ulcer disease in transplant patients usually occurs the first six months after transplantation (Fig. 1). The incidence is higher in males than in females (2:1) and significantly higher in cadaveric kidney recipients (3.5%) than in living related kidney recipients (1.5%).

Gastritis was the most common form of ulcer disease (12/25) followed by duodenal ulcer (7), gastric ulcer (5) and esophagitis (1). Before transplantation, most of the ulcers were duodenal. The most common manifestation of posttransplantation ulcers was bleeding (96%). In addition, there was one case of gastric outlet obstruction and one of gastric perforation. Most of the patients were already in critical condition when the bleeding started.

Treatment and Results

Initially, all patients were treated medically with ice-saline gastric lavage and hourly administration of antacids. Cimetidine was also used in three patients. Medical therapy successfully controlled bleeding in 12 of 24 patients. Of the 12 patients in whom medical treatment failed, eight underwent operation — vagotomy and pyloroplasty in five and gastrectomy in three. Bleeding was controlled in five patients. Six of the 16 patients who had only medical therapy survived, whereas of the eight patients who underwent surgery, one survived and seven died. The overall mortality was 71% (Table 6). Causes of death were sepsis in 11, continued gastrointestinal bleeding in two, and hyperkalemia, acute myocardial infarct, liver failure and respiratory failure in one case each.

The seven patients who survived were in relatively good general condition, ie, none had multisystem failure, six had discrete ulcer. The bleeding was mild and easily controlled medically in six patients.

Conclusion

Gastrointestinal ulceration with bleeding is frequently fatal in transplant patients. Surgical prophylaxis before transplantation in patients with known ulcer disease successfully prevents recurrence after transplantation. There is a group of patients,

Table 4. Posttransplant Bleeding No Pretransplant History of Ulcer

Patient	*Age*	*Donor*	*Source of Bleeding*	*Associated Conditions*	*Treatment*	*Outcome of Bleeding*	*Fate of Patient*
1	52	LR	Gastritis, esophagitis	Rejection	Vasopressin, antacids	Controlled	Died of sepsis
2	58	Cad	Duodenal ulcer	ATN	Antacids	Controlled	Survived
3	29	Cad	Gastritis	–	Antacids	Controlled	Survived
4	33	Cad	Duodenal ulcer	Bladder leak, thrombo-phlebitis	Cimetidine	Controlled	Survived
5	53	LR	Gastritis	Rejection, CMV	Antacids	Controlled	Died of CMV, sepsis
6	44	LR	Gastritis	Sepsis	Antacids	Controlled	Died of acute MI
7	49	Cad	Gastric ulcer	Rejection, CMV, liver failure	Antacids	Controlled	Died of liver failure
8	45	Cad	Gastritis	Rejection, sepsis	Antacids	Not Controlled	Died of sepsis

9	48	LR	Gastritis, esophagitis	Sepsis	Cimetidine, antacids, balloon tamponade	Controlled	Died of sepsis
10	45	Cad	(a) Duodenal ulcer	(a) ATN	(a) Antacids	(a) Controlled	
			(b) Gastritis (one month later)		(b) Vagotomy – gastrectomy	(b) Controlled	Survived
11	25	LR	Duodenal ulcer	Rejection, CMV cand.	Antacids – V & P	Rebled	Died of sepsis and bleeding
12	58	Cad	Duodenal ulcer	Thrombo-phlebitis	Pitressin, antacids V & P	Controlled	Died of CMV, sepsis
13	29	Cad	Gastritis	Rejection, CMV	Antacids V & P	Controlled	Died of hyperkalemia
14	30	LR	Gastritis	Rejection	Pitressin, antacids – total gastrectomy	Controlled	Died of sepsis
15	52	LR	Gastric ulcer	Sepsis, pancreatitis	Antacids V & P	Rebled	Died of sepsis and bleeding

Table 5. Posttransplant Bleeding Pretransplant History of Ulcer Without Prophylactic Operation Pretransplant

Patient	*Age*	*Donor*	*Source of Bleeding*	*Associated Conditions*	*Treatment*	*Outcome of Bleeding*	*Fate of Patients*
1	43	LR	Gastric ulcer	Posttransplant nephrectomy	Antacids	Controlled	Survived
2	39	Cad	Gastritis	Posttransplant nephrectomy	Antacids	Rebled	Died of bleeding
3	47	Cad	Gastritis	Rejection	Cimetidine, Antacids – V&P	Controlled	Died of respiratory arrest
4	51	Cad	Duodenal ulcer	Rejection	Antacids	Controlled	Died of sepsis

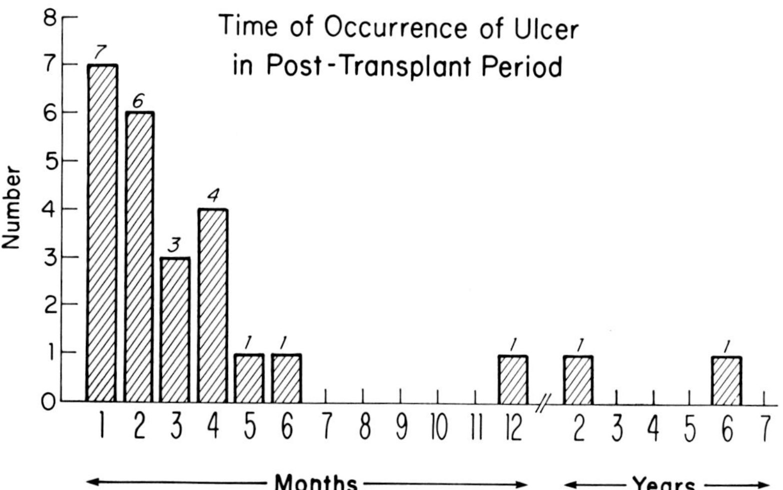

FIG. 1. The majority of ulcers occur in the early posttransplant period.

Table 6. Results of Treatment for Posttransplant Ulcer Bleeding

	Medical	*Surgical*	*Total*
No. of patients	16	8	24
Bleeding controlled	12	5	17 (71%)
Survived	6	1	7 (29%)
Died	10	7	17 (71%)

however, who develop bleeding as a result of predisposing conditions (rejection-infection) and not as a result of pre-existing ulcer disease. Unfortunately, there is no way to predict which patients will develop this sequence of complications; therefore, no prophylaxis can be instituted. An active program of prophylaxis, however, must be started as soon as the stress situation is recognized. Intensive antacid therapy will prevent bleeding in the majority of patients who receive treatment for rejection. Routine addition of cimetidine prophylaxis may further reduce the incidence of bleeding. Even when the bleeding was controlled by either medical or surgical means, the mortality was high because of sepsis or multisystem failure, of which bleeding was a manifestation and not a cause.

The high mortality of operative treatment reflects the grave condition of these patients when treatment is instituted. Graft nephrectomy should be considered early when bleeding is unresponsive to medical therapy. The deadly sequence of rejection, high dose immunosuppression, sepsis and bleeding must be interrupted.

References

1. Koman, M.G. and Laver, M.C.: Hypergastrinemia in chronic renal failure. Br. Med. J. 1:209, 1972.
2. Goldstein, H. et al: Gastric acid secretion in patients undergoing chronic dialysis. Arch. Intern. Med. 120:645, 1967.
3. Shepherd, A.M.M., Stewart, W.K. and Wormoly, K.G.: Peptic ulceration in chronic renal failure. Lancet 1:1357, 1973.
4. Horowitz, I.H.: Uremic toxins and platelet function. Arch. Intern. Med. 126:823, 1970.
5. von Kaulla, K.N., von Kaulla, E., Wasantupruck, S. et al: Blood coagulation in uremic patients before and after hemodialysis and transplantation of the kidney. Arch. Surg. 92184, 1966.
6. Stadil, F. and Rehfeld, J.F.: Release of gastrin by epinephrine in man. Gastroenterology 65:210, 1973.
7. Moore, T.C., Thompson, D.P. and Glassock, R.J.: Elevation in urinary and blood histamine following clinical renal transplantation. Ann. Surg. 173:381, 1971.
8. Spanos, P.K., Simmons, R.L., Rattazzi, L.C. et al: Peptic ulcer disease in the transplant recipient. Arch. Surg. 109:193, 1974.

Self-Evaluation Quiz

1. Uremic patients have coagulopathy and platelet dysfunction which are made worse by the intermittent anticoagulation of hemodialysis.

a) True
b) False

2. There is some evidence that stress-induced gastrin release during rejection episodes may increase epinephrine output.
   a) True
   b) False
3. Increased histamine levels resulting from rejection may increase acid output.
   a) True
   b) False
4. Indications for surgical prophylaxis for peptic ulcer disease before transplant are previous history of duodenal ulcer disease, present symptoms of duodenal ulcer disease, and demonstration of ulcer by routine pretransplant upper GI series.
   a) True
   b) False
5. The authors had what percentage of patients with no previous evidence of ulcers who develop ulceration after transplant, and who cannot be recognized before transplantation?
   a) 1.8%
   b) 2.3%
   c) 3.2%
   d) None
6. Initially, all patients were treated medically with:
   a) Ice-glucose lavage
   b) Saline at room temperature
   c) Antacids hourly
   d) Cimetidine
7. Manifestation of ulcer disease in transplant patients usually occurs ________ after transplantation.
   a) First month
   b) First six months
   c) First year
   d) Anytime
8. Gastrointestinal ulceration with bleeding is frequently fatal in transplant patients.
   a) True
   b) False

9. The most common form of ulcer disease was:
   a) Duodenal ulcer
   b) Gastritis
   c) Peptic ulcer
   d) None of the above

Answers on page 721.

The Management of Stress Ulceration

Ronald P. Fischer, M.D.

Objectives

The objectives of this paper are:

1. To describe the clinical spectrum of stress ulceration.
2. To offer an approach to the nonoperative management of stress ulceration.
3. To recommend appropriate operative procedures for the various forms of stress ulceration and to delineate the indications for operative control of stress ulceration.

Introduction

Clinically evident stress ulceration as manifested by gross upper gastrointestinal bleeding or perforation is a dreaded complication among severely traumatized or ill patients. The mortality of clinically evident stress ulceration has ranged from 40% to 95%. The high mortality relates principally to gram negative sepsis which precedes the development of clinically evident stress ulceration in at least three fourths of patients.

The spectrum of classic posttraumatic stress ulceration, as documented endoscopically [1-3], includes an early erosive phase which is uniformly observed within two days of injury (Fig. 1). With the rare exception of clinically evident bleeding from erosive fundic gastritis, this early erosive phase is clinically

Ronald P. Fischer, M.D., Department of Surgery, Saint Paul-Ramsey Hospital, Saint Paul, Minn., and the Department of Surgery, University of Minnesota Health Sciences Center, Minneapolis.

This study was supported by the Saint Paul-Ramsey Hospital Medical Education and Research Foundation.

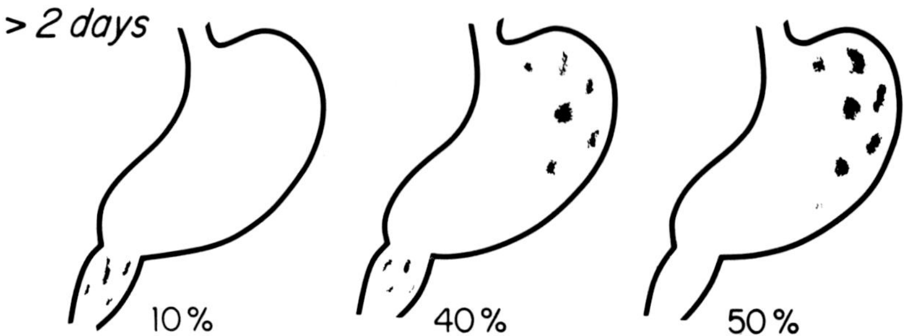

FIG. 1. Early erosive phase of stress ulceration.

covert. Approximately one half of severely traumatized patients subsequently develop ulcerations of the stomach and/or duodenum (Fig. 2). Some of the factors which have been implicated in the pathogenesis of this ulcerative phase are listed in Figure 2. Clinically evident bleeding or perforation occurs in approximately one third of the patients who develop gastric and/or duodenal ulceration, whereas, in another one third, clinically covert bleeding is evident by guaiac positive stools and nasogastric aspirates. In the overwhelming majority of patients, clinically evident stress ulceration arises from fundic ulcerative gastritis rather than from ulcerative duodenitis. Much of the confusion concerning stress ulceration arises because isolated

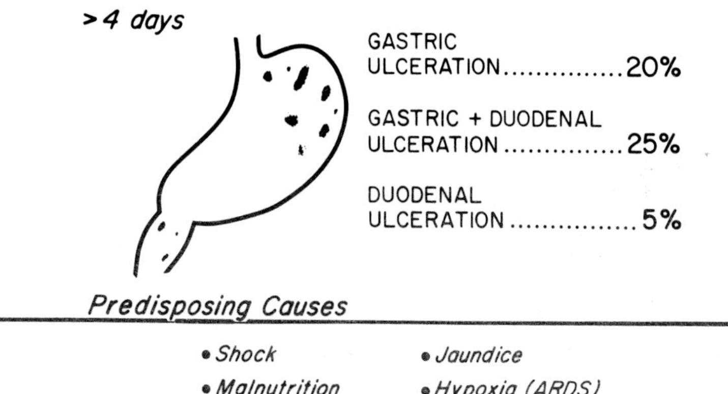

FIG. 2. Late ulcerative phase of stress ulceration.

duodenal ulcers and isolated gastric ulcers occurring in critically injured patients and also pre-existing gastritis in these patients have been termed stress ulcers. It is unlikely that isolated gastric or duodenal ulcers pathogenically relate to classic stress ulceration. More likely they predate the trauma or represent reactivation of dormant peptic ulcer disease, or are an expression of a predisposition toward peptic ulcer disease. Approximately 15% to 30% of patients with clinically evident stress ulceration have pre-existing peptic ulcer disease. Probably an equal percentage have ingested ulcerogenic drugs and/or alcohol prior to injury and/or have subsequently received ulcerogenic drugs.

The frequency of clinically evident stress ulceration and the distribution of the lesions among patients who have not received antacid prophylaxis are listed in Table 1. Fundic ulcerative gastritis has been the dominant lesion and the incidence of clinically evident stress ulceration has been high (15% to 35%). In contrast, among patients receiving acid-reducing regimens isolated gastric or duodenal ulcers have been the dominant stress lesions and the incidence of clinically evident stress ulceration has been low (2.8% to 41.%) [4-7] (Table 2). These data suggest that acid-reducing regimens effectively prevent fundic ulcerative gastritis, but less effectively prevent isolated duodenal or gastric ulcerations.

It should be noted that the majority of the reported series on stress ulceration are retrospective analyses which include patients with alcohol or aspirin gastritis, patients receiving ulcerogenic drugs and patients with pre-existing peptic ulcer disease and that the sites of stress ulceration are poorly

Table 1. Clinically Evident Stress Ulceration Among High-Risk Patients Not Receiving Acid-Reducing Regimens

	Incidence 15%–33%		
Distribution		*Presentation*	
Fundic ulcerative gastritis	40%–60%	Bleeding	90%–95%
Duodenal ulcer	30%–40%	Perforation	5%–10%
Fundic ulcerative gastritis + duodenal ulcer	10%–20%		
Other	1%– 2%		

Table 2. Clinically Evident Stress Ulceration Among High-Risk Patients Receiving Acid-Reducing Regimens [4-7]

Incidence 2.8%–4.1%			
Distribution [4-5]		*Presentation*	
Isolated gastric ulcer	50%	Bleeding	85%
Duodenal ulcer	40%	Perforation	15%
Fundic ulcerative gastritis	10%		

documented. Because these clinical data are imprecise, there exist conflicting management recommendations for clinically evident stress ulceration. High concentrations of gastric acid are necessary for the development of stress ulceration. Thus, both prophylaxis and management must include acid-reducing regimens. With the exception of gastric devascularization (to be discussed later), the operative procedures for stress ulceration include vagotomy to eliminate the dominant cephalic phase of gastric secretion. Vagotomy, when used in the treatment of fundic ulcerations, has the additional benefit of acutely reducing gastric mucosal blood flow.

Nonoperative Management of Bleeding Stress Ulceration

Three measures should be promptly and concurrently initiated: (1) Icewater gastric lavage, which reduces gastroduodenal blood flow by gastric hypothermia, stops or substantially reduces the rate of bleeding in approximately two thirds of all patients with upper gastrointestinal bleeding [8]. (2) Intravenous vasopressin should be administered continuously (40 units per hour) to decrease gastroduodenal blood flow [9]. Intermittent intravenous vasopressin is commonly used but affords only intermittent reduction of gastroduodenal blood flow. Thus, at least initially, continuous intravenous vasopressin should be employed. (3) Existing coagulopathies must be corrected.

Emergent gastroduodenoscopy should be performed as soon as the stomach has been emptied of blood clots. Endoscopy is 90% to 95% accurate in determining the site of bleeding in stress ulceration. Upper gastrointestinal x-rays are at best only 50% accurate because the bleeding often arises from erosions or superficial ulcerations which cannot be identified by contrast studies and because the bleeding may be mistakenly attributed to other identifiable upper gastrointestinal lesions. The site of bleeding will temper the timing of operative intervention, determine the site of selective intra-arterial catheter placement (if needed) and will provide a basis for predicting the probability of response to nonoperative treatment. If the site of bleeding has been established, operative intervention is expedited by eliminating unnecessary exploratory enterotomies.

The best method to control stress bleeding is gastric alkalinization. Experiments by Green and co-workers suggest that gastric pH should be maintained at neutrality [10]. Gastric alkalinization can be accomplished with antacids or with Tagamet (cimetidine), the commercially available H_2-histamine receptor antagonist. Because Tagamet is not approved by the Federal Drug Administration for this purpose or for stress ulcer prophylaxis, patients should provide informed consent. As summarized in Table 3, the success rate in stopping bleeding from fundic stress ulceration for the H_2-histamine receptor antagonists has been superior to that of antacids. Tagamet has the additional advantage that it can be administered parenterally or orally (300 mg q8h), whereas antacid regimens are tiresome and time consuming. For example, in Simonian's experience as much as 4300 ml of Riopan daily was required to maintain gastric neutrality in one patient [11]. Isolated duodenal ulcers or isolated gastric ulcers among stress patients, as presented in Table 3, are more resistant to management by gastric neutralization than are fundic ulcerations. Other modali-

Table 3. Gastric Neutralization for Bleeding Stress Ulceration

	Stopped Bleeding	*Operation*
Antacids – ulcerative gastritis* [11]	85%	10%
H_2-Histamine receptor antagonists – ulcerative gastritis† [17-19]	87%–100%	0%–15%
Duodenal ulcer† [18]	72%	22%
Gastric ulcer* [18]	62%	22%

*Primary treatment regimen
†Initiated after failure of other nonoperative treatment regimens

ties are of value in the management of bleeding stress ulceration: One is selective intra-arterial administration of vasopressin [12] or other vasoconstrictors, and selective arterial embolization. The site of selective arterial catheter placement depends upon the site of hemorrhage. Unfortunately, catheter placement is unsuccessful in approximately 20% to 25% of patients, the threat of catheter dislodgement is constantly present and both selective intra-arterial vasoconstrictor administration and embolization have potentially lethal complications. Thus, selective intra-arterial vasoconstrictor administration and/or embolization are usually reserved for critically ill patients who have failed to respond to other nonoperative treatment regimens. A second modality is gastric lavage with levarterenol. Because levarterenol gastric lavage has been accompanied by a high rebleeding rate (40%) [13], its use should also be reserved for similar patients. Other nonoperative regimens, such as gastric cooling, vitamin A therapy, endoscopic cauterization, fresh blood administration, etc., have been advocated to control bleeding stress ulceration, but insufficient data exist to quantitate their value.

Table 4 lists the indications for operative intervention for bleeding stress ulceration. Because so little is understood about isolated duodenal or gastric ulceration in stressed patients and

Table 4. Indications for Operative Intervention in Salvageable Patients With Bleeding Stress Ulceration

Exsanguinating bleeding
Hypotension
Continuing bleeding*†
1-2 units/day
or
>6 units – total
Rebleeding*†

*Not absolute indications for fundic ulcerative gastritis (see text).

†Continuing bleeding and rebleeding are indications for operative intervention in salvageable patients with isolated duodenal or isolated gastric ulcers, especially if they have preexisting peptic ulcer disease, are septic and/or are over the age of 60 years.

because no critical data are available for review, it seems reasonable to follow the proven indications for operative intervention for duodenal or gastric ulcers in nonstressed patients. Similarly, with two exceptions, it is reasonable to apply these criteria to patients bleeding from fundic ulcerative gastritis. A longer trial of nonoperative management seems justified for the rare patient with fundic ulcerative gastritis who is not critically ill and not septic. Such patients do not suffer the severe gastric mucosal reparative impairment of critically ill, malnourished, septic patients and thus are more likely to spontaneously heal mucosal ulcerations. The other patients with fundic ulcerative gastritis in whom early operative intervention is inappropriate are those in whom bleeding is but agonal manifestation of multi-organ failure secondary to uncontrolled gram negative sepsis. The decision to operate upon such patients is essentially a moral judgment, for they are unsalvageable unless sepsis can be controlled. On occasion this is possible by amputation of a septic extremity, by excision of a septic burn, by radical surgical debridement or by drainage of an intra-abdominal abscess. Many investigators have observed that bleeding from stress ulceration has stopped only when sepsis has been successfully eliminated.

Operative Procedures for Stress Ulceration

The mortality of clinically evident stress ulceration relates chiefly to the severity of patients' underlying injuries, illnesses or sepsis. Because no control series have been reported, and because many surgeons have subjectively preselected the operation used for bleeding stress ulceration, comparison of the reported mortalities for the various operations which have been used for stress ulceration is invalid.

There is general agreement that the preferred treatment for bleeding duodenal ulceration is oversewing of the ulcer with nonabsorbable sutures, ligation of the gastroduodenal artery combined with vagotomy and pyloroplasty [14]. The rebleeding rate for this procedure approximates 20%.

If the bleeding arises from an isolated gastric ulcer in the distal stomach, treatment consists of vagotomy and distal gastric resection to include the ulcer. Isolated ulcers in the proximal stomach are treated with oversewing with non-absorbable sutures combined with vagotomy and distal gastrectomy. In all probability, for both proximal and distal isolated gastric ulcers, vagotomy and pyloroplasty with oversewing of the ulcer or excision of the ulcer is an inferior operative procedure.

Three operative procedures are currently acceptable for the control of bleeding from fundic gastric ulceration. They are (1) vagotomy and distal gastric resection; (2) vagotomy and pyloroplasty; and (3) gastric devascularization. Included in all three operations is gastrotomy with oversewing of the bleeding sites. Because of its lower rebleeding rate (15% to 30%), the majority of authorities recommend oversewing of the ulcers combined with vagotomy and distal gastrectomy for fundic ulcerative gastritis. Several reports suggest that vagotomy and pyloroplasty plus oversewing of the fundic ulcers is as effective for ulcerative gastritis; however, excluding these conflicting reports, the rebleeding rates for vagotomy and pyloroplasty have been significantly greater than that reported for vagotomy and distal gastrectomy. Richardson and Aust reported gastric devascularization to be highly successful in controlling bleeding from fundic ulcerative gastritis [15]. Their rebleeding rate was only 10%. Gastric devascularization includes ligation of the right and left gastric arteries, ligation of the right and left gastroepiploic arteries combined with oversewing of the fundic bleeding sites. Surprisingly, these authors have performed gastric devascularization on patients who have undergone splenectomy without incurring postoperative gastric necrosis. Since gastric devascularization has only recently been reported and its effectiveness has not been confirmed from other institutions, it has not yet been widely accepted. Various other operative procedures — including total or near total gastrectomy, various forms of vagotomy with resectional and/or drainage procedures and proximal gastric vagotomy without drainage — have been employed for bleeding fundic stress ulceration. With the sole exception of Menguy's excellent results using total gastrectomy [16], insufficient clinical data presently exist to support the merit of these procedures. Distal gastrectomy without vagotomy has a rebleeding rate of at least 50% and is therefore an unacceptable procedure, as is oversewing of gastric ulcers when not combined with an acid-reducing operation, which has a rebleeding rate approximating 90%.

Immediate operative intervention is indicated for perforated stress ulcerations. The operative procedure indicated depends upon the site of perforation, the duration of perforation, the degree of peritoneal contamination and whether or not the patient has pre-existing peptic ulcer disease. Simple closure with an omental patch has been advocated for both duodenal and gastric perforations. The results of this approach are, however, poorly documented and simple closure probably is an inadequate operation at least for patients with pre-existing peptic ulcer disease and for critically ill patients with established gram negative sepsis. In these individuals the predisposing factors of stress ulceration remain unaltered postoperatively. It seems wiser, therefore, to provide such patients with an acid-reducing operation.

Vagotomy and pyloroplasty or drainage, vagotomy and distal gastrectomy, or proximal gastric vagotomy with omental closure are acceptable operative procedures for stress-induced duodenal perforation. Of these procedures, vagotomy and pyloroplasty is preferred if it is technically feasible to incorporate the perforation into the pyloroplasty incision. There is little to recommend proximal gastric vagotomy plus closure because few surgeons have documented expertise with this operation and it is tedious and time consuming.

Perforations of isolated ulcers of the distal stomach are managed by distal gastrectomy, to include the ulcer, plus vagotomy. Proximal isolated gastric ulcer perforations which cannot be included in the gastric resection are treated with oversewing combined with vagotomy and distal gastric resection. Such treatment has the theoretical advantage of being the most effective acid-reducing operative procedure and thus, in addition to effectively treating the offending ulcer, provides prophylaxis against the subsequent development of fundic ulcerative gastritis, which is a continuing threat in these critically ill patients.

The operative approach to perforated fundic ulceration includes an initial fundic gastrotomy and examination of the extent and severity of the concomitant nonperforating ulcers. If the perforation is solitary and the remaining ulcers do not appear to be in imminent danger of perforation, oversewing of the perforation and distal gastrectomy plus vagotomy is recommended. On rare occasions, the perforations are multiple, the remaining fundus is extensively and deeply ulcerated, or gastric malacia is present. These circumstances necessitate a total or near total gastrectomy.

Ancillary Management

Stress-induced perforated ulcer is easily corrected and stress-induced bleeding successfully responds to nonoperative management or operative management in approximately 95% of patients. Thus, the factors which predispose the critically injured patient to stress ulceration (Fig. 2) determine survival. These factors must be successfully corrected to prevent stress ulceration, to optimize the treatment response of stress ulceration and to insure against recurrent stress ulceration. Vigorous measures should be taken to avert or to correct cardiopulmonary instability or failure. Every effort should be taken to avert or to treat gram negative sepsis and its sequelae: jaundice, adult respiratory distress syndrome (ARDS) and renal failure. In many patients these predisposing factors cannot be prevented. Thus, the mortality among patients with clinically evident stress ulceration exceeds 50%. Malnutrition, however, can be averted. Elemental diets combined with a high-caloric, high-protein diet are an essential part of the treatment regimen of patients with a functionally intact gastrointestinal tract. Total parenteral nutrition is essential for patients unable to tolerate oral intake. Similarly, patients with renal failure should undergo "early" or prophylactic dialysis to keep the BUN below 100 mEq/L, plus receiving vigorous nutritional support. It should be assumed that all critically injured or ill patients have stress ulceration. All such patients should be maintained on vigorous prophylactic acid-reducing regimens. Similarly, all patients with clinically evident stress ulceration should be maintained on vigorous acid-reducing regimens. Because the optimal duration of such prophylaxis or treatment is unknown, these measures should be continued until the patient is ready for discharge.

References

1. Czaja, A.J., McAlhany, J.C. and Pruitt, B.A.: Acute gastroduodenal disease after thermal injury. N. Engl. J. Med. 291:925, 1974.
2. Lucas, C.E., Sugawa, C., Riggle, J. et al: Natural history and surgical dilemma of "stress" gastric bleeding. Arch. Surg. 102:266, 1971.
3. Czaja, A.J., McAlhany, J.C. and Pruitt, B.A.: Gastric acid secretion and acute duodenal disease after burns. Arch. Surg. 111:243, 1976.
4. Solem, L.D., Strate, R.G. and Fischer, R.P.: Antacid prophylaxis and nutritional supplementation in the prevention of Curling's ulcers. Surg. Gynecol. Obstet. 1978. In Press.
5. Watson, L.C. and Abston, S.: Prevention of upper gastrointestinal hemorrhage in 582 burned children. Am. J. Surg. 132:790, 1976.
6. Hastings, P.R., Skillman, J.J., Bushness, L.S. and Silen, W.: Antacid titration in the prevention of acute gastrointestinal bleeding. N. Engl. J. Med. 298:1041, 1978.
7. McAlhany, J.C., Czaja, A.J. and Pruitt, B.A.: Antacid control of complications from acute gastroduodenal disease after burns. J Trauma 16:645, 1976.
8. Palmer, E.D.: The vigorous diagnostic approach to upper gastrointestinal tract hemorrhage. JAMA 207:1477, 1969.
9. Thomford, N.R. and Sirnek, K.R.: Intravenous vasopressin in patients with portal hypertension: Advantages of continuous infusion. J. Surg. Res. 18:113, 1975.
10. Green, F.W., Kaplan, M.M., Curtis, L.E. and Levine, P.H.: Effect of acid and pepsin on blood coagulation and platelet aggregation. Gastroenterology 74:38, 1978.
11. Simonian, S.J. and Curtis, L.E.: Treatment of hemorrhagic gastritis by antacid. Ann. Surg. 184:429, 1976.
12. Athanasoulis, C.A., Brown, B. and Shapiro, J.H.: Angiography in the diagnosis and management of bleeding stress ulcers and gastritis. Am. J. Surg. 125:468, 1973.
13. Douglass, H.O.: Levarenterol irrigation. JAMA 230:1653, 1974.
14. Eisenberg, M.M.: Physiologic approach to the surgical management of duodenal ulcer. Current Problems in Surgery Vol. 14, No. 1, Jan. 1977
15. Richardson, J.D. and Aust, J.B.: Gastric devascularization. Ann. Surg. 185:649, 1977.
16. Menguy, R., Gadaez, T. and Zajtchuk, R.: The surgical management of acute gastric mucosal bleeding. Arch. Surg. 99:198. 1969.
17. MacDonald, A.S., Steele, B.J. and Bottombley, M.G.: Treatment of stress-induced upper gastrointestinal hemorrhage with metiamide. Lancet 1:68, 1976.
18. Dunn, D.H., Fischer, R.P., Silvis, S. et al: The treatment of hemorrhagic gastritis with cimetidine. Surg. Gynecol. Obstet. 147:737, 1978.
19. Burland, W.L. and Simkus, M.A. (eds.): Proceedings of the Second International Symposium on Histamine H_2-Receptor Antagonists. Amsterdam-Oxford:Excerpta Medica, 1977.

Self-Evaluation Quiz

1. Upper gastrointestinal bleeding is the most frequent presentation of clinically evident stress ulceration.
   a) True
   b) False
2. Icewater gastric lavage is an effective nonoperative mode of therapy for bleeding stress ulceration.
   a) True
   b) False
3. Continuous IV vasopressin is an effective nonoperative mode of therapy for bleeding stress ulceration.
   a) True
   b) False
4. Endoscopy is unnecessary in patients with clinically evident stress ulceration, because fundic stress ulceration is the most frequent cause of bleeding.
   a) True
   b) False
5. Gastric neutralization with antacids and/or with the H_2-histamine receptor antagonist Tagamet (cimetidine) effectively stops bleeding from stress ulceration.
   a) True
   b) False
6. Under all conditions, nonoperative management is preferred for bleeding stress ulceration.
   a) True
   b) False
7. Which of the following are accepted operations for bleeding fundic stress ulceration.
   a) Oversewing of the ulcers
   b) Gastric devascularization plus oversewing of the ulcers
   c) Distal gastrectomy plus oversewing of the ulcers
   d) Distal gastrectomy plus vagotomy plus oversewing of the ulcers
   e) Vagotomy and drainage plus oversewing of the ulcers
8. Which of the following are essential for either the prevention of or for the management of clinically evident stress ulceration?
   a) Gastric neutralization
   b) Prophylactic antibiotics

c) Nasogastric suction
d) Nutritional supplementation
e) Cardiopulmonary stability

Answers on page 721.

Discussion

Moderator: James C. Thompson, M.D.

Moderator: Dr. Beahrs, in what percentage of the people upon whom you do ileostomies do you do a Kock's ileostomy primarily? What percentage would you do secondarily?

Dr. Beahrs: For patients with a satisfactory body build (they cannot be obese) and chronic ulcerative colitis or familial polyposis, I do the procedure on all. Regarding the selection of the patients: there are four of us at our institution who are doing the procedure. There are other gastrointestinal surgeons who are not doing it. The internists' referral pattern acts as a selection of whether or not the patient gets the procedure. Roughly, overall, about one half of the patients are getting the pouch; the other half are not.

Moderator: Will the patients raise the question themselves? Or, if they do not mention it, will you talk to them about it?

Dr. Beahrs: I would say that most of the patients whom I see now have knowledge of the procedure, either through their referring physician or through an ileostomy club or some other associates. Most of the patients are somewhat knowledgeable regarding the Kock's pouch.

Moderator: How many of you have done this kind of continent ileostomy? I think Dr. Alexander-Williams has done three. Dr. Alexander-Williams, how did they do?

Dr. Alexander-Williams: They did badly!

Moderator: We did one at our institution 2½ years ago. He was a preacher. He did so splendidly that we just bring him back in every now and then and stroke him and admire him.

Dr. Silen, I have several questions related to the incidence of stress ulcer in 1978. I must say I am also interested in that because it seems as though this is a disappearing disease. In fact, I think many people have attempted to put together a prospective study and have not been able to find any patients.

If you do transplants, Dr. Najarian, I think you are going to find all kinds of problems. But if we put those aside, what about the incidence of this disease? If you do think that it has diminished in incidence, why?

Dr. Silen: I think stress ulcer has diminished in incidence. Everybody who has been an observer in this area has noticed this phenomenon. Clearly, it has decreased in our own unit, even in the patients who do not receive prophylactic antacids. I do not know why. It may be that we are managing these patients better from the standpoint of treating shock, acidosis, respiratory insufficiency and renal failure.

Moderator: Dr. Menguy, two or three years ago, proposed that one of the factors was a diminution in high energy phosphate stores in the mucosa. If that were true, do you think that perhaps the provision of greatly improved nutrition might be associated with fewer cases of stress ulcer?

Dr. Silen: In an experimental situation, if you give glucose orally to rats that are subjected to stress, you can decrease the incidence of stress ulcerations. It may be that with better nutrition and hyperalimentation, that is possible. I have my own doubts about it, but I think it is possible.

Moderator: How many people in the audience have done an operation for bleeding stress ulcer recently?

Dr. Alexander-Williams, what were the circumstances in which you operated?

Dr. Alexander-Williams: A young victim of an automobile accident who had been anticoagulated bled from erosive gastritis, had a vagotomy and antrectomy and rebled, had a Roux-en-Y bile diversion and rebled and came to total gastrectomy after which, of course, he did very well.

Moderator: Dr. Friesen, there are several questions about the syndrome of antral G-cell hyperplasia. How can we differentiate this from the ordinary duodenal ulcer? How can we suspect it?

Dr. Friesen: I am glad this question has arisen because we are getting more serum gastrin levels on patients who have severe ulcer disease and we are finding certain patients who have elevated serum gastrin levels, as contrasted to the normal or low level that you expect to find in an ordinary duodenal ulcer patient. So I think the first step in recognizing the possibility that a particular patient may have the Zollinger-Ellison syndrome at an intermediary stage is an intermediary level of serum gastrin. If it is, say, 400 or 500 picograms per milliliter, I would think that is the tip-off that this patient either has antral G-cell hyperplasia or the classic Zollinger-Ellison syndrome due to a tumor in the duodenum or pancreas. Then you have to do the tests I discussed, secretin and calcium stimulation. If these stimulate serum gastrin to elevated levels, then that patient probably has a tumor in the duodenum or pancreas rather than G-cell hyperplasia.

Moderator: There was an article not long ago raising the question of whether or not it is possible to reliably make the diagnosis of antral G-cell hyperplasia by endoscopic biopsy. The authors had strong evidence that it was not possible to do so. Would you comment, because there have been several communications which suggested that it is possible to do so.

Dr. Friesen: I have made those statements myself. I realize that it is difficult to confirm a relative increase in number of G cells in the antral mucosa. We do it by endoscopic biopsy, but we also do it at the time of operation when we take out a strip of mucosa and put it in glutaraldehyde so that it can be looked at properly by histologic methods. But this takes time. So I rarely depend upon a microscopic means to make the diagnosis preoperatively, even though it is absolutely diagnostic when present. The stimulation tests are better. I am confident that it occurs. You must have a pathologist who is accustomed to looking at G cells with special stains or you must have someone who has spent a lot of time looking at them over the years.

Moderator: Dr. Alexander-Williams, why in the world do you use a lateral duodenostomy? If you want to feed the patient, why not put a tube in the jejunum?

Dr. Alexander-Williams: Because the most dangerous complication of that procedure is a blowout of the duodenal stump. Everybody knows this. Dr. Thompson, I am surprised you asked this question.

Moderator: Are you really having trouble with blown stumps in patients with total gastrectomy?

Dr. Alexander-Williams: Formerly we did.

Moderator: Well, I would say then, that is probably a good thing for you to do. If you are interested in feeding, is that the main reason for your doing it? Or is this a decompression duodenostomy? That is really the basis of the question. Do you place that tube in order to protect the stump, or in order to feed the patient? What I am getting at is this: In what percentage of the patients do you use this for feeding?

Dr. Alexander-Williams: I do not feed my patients per os for seven days. It is much cheaper to give food through the duodenostomy than it is by parenteral nutrition. We have had some trouble with central line parenteral nutrition, and we are quite pleased to be able to avoid it. We have had fewer complications by feeding via the duodenostomy than we have with central feeding.

Moderator: I was just trying to sharpen up your thinking. You are trying to protect it from leaking, but you are then putting fluid in. I am a little surprised.

Dr. Alexander-Williams: Yes, I hope that you now grasp that concept.

Moderator: Dr. Alexander-Williams, what are the other bad operations? Several people say you have constructed straw men to destroy. When do you use a Hunt-Lawrence pouch or some other form of reservoir in patients with total gastrectomy? What do you consider to be the indications for the construction of a reservoir in patients with total gastrectomy?

Dr. Alexander-Williams: None. The jejunal loop hypertrophies to an amazing extent, and you can demonstrate this radiologically. The interesting thing is that patients do not experience the so-called small stomach syndrome after total gastrectomy with a Roux-en-Y. I find that the small stomach syndrome is much more common after a Billroth II gastrectomy for carcinoma of the stomach than after a total gastrectomy. I think that the so-called small stomach syndrome is due to bile reflux. In my opinion, a pouch is never required.

Dr. Silen: Dr. Alexander-Williams, would you do a total gastrectomy in a patient with a distal antral cancer?

Dr. Alexander-Williams: If the nature of the tumor was such that you were operating for cure, if it were node negative, then the answer is Yes. Recently, I have had two five-year survivors after partial gastrectomy for carcinoma of the stomach, both of whom have developed a second primary fundic carcinoma. I am speaking about small numbers of patients but I have to stick my neck out and say Yes, I would do a total gastrectomy for potentially curable antral carcinoma.

Moderator: And an obstructing pyloric tumor?

Dr. Alexander-Williams: Yes, I would.

Moderator: For an obstructing pyloric tumor, you would do a total gastrectomy?

Dr. Alexander-Williams: Yes, I would.

Moderator: How many would agree with Dr. Alexander-Williams' statement about the lack of need for a gastric reservoir after total gastrectomy for patients with carcinoma? Do you agree that the patients do not need a gastric reservoir?

Dr. Najarian: You do not agree?

Moderator: Yes, I agree entirely. I have never made one in my whole life.

Dr. Najarian: You should try it.

Moderator: Dr. Silen, would it be advantageous to use a continuous drip of antacid, rather than instillation? Do you routinely measure the pH after each instillation?

Dr. Silen: Yes, we do measure it at the end of a one-hour period. If the pH is running 6, we do not instill any antacid. We have not tried continuous drip, but its potential disadvantage is that a sudden increase in the volume of delivery could flood the stomach and cause vomiting and aspiration.

Moderator: Dr. Fischer, in your burn unit, what is your current regimen for prophylaxis against bleeding?

Dr. Fischer: Until very recently, namely, when Tagamet became available, we were using antacids for the first three or four days until the ileus was resolved and then feeding them up to 3 liters of Vivonex between meals without antacids. Under those circumstances, clinical stress ulceration occurred in 2.8% of patients over a five-year period. Those were high-risk patients who were burned over 40% of their bodies. Currently, the residents are using Tagamet for prophylaxis.

Moderator: That is what I really wanted to get at. How are you giving it?

Dr. Fischer: Not by design, we simply happened to find out that the residents have been using Tagamet for the last several months.

Dr. Silen: Dr. Thompson, it is as I have always said: The residents on the service always can set the policy a lot better than the professor can.

Moderator: I found out that we were using it routinely also. I wandered in one day to the ICU and I saw all of these IV cimetidine bottles sitting around. I had trouble getting it, but the residents talked to the detail man and had it flown in. That is a very important point. I think whenever any investigator sets about to write up his own experience, he had better go back and find out what his experience really was.

Dr. Najarian, you said something about your choice between a resection and vagotomy and an emptying procedure and vagotomy. There are several individuals who would like you to elaborate upon how you make that choice.

Dr. Najarian: If we have patients who are young, if they are hypersecretors, if they have an active ulcer at the time when they are evaluated pretransplant, then I believe that an antrectomy and vagotomy should be done. Otherwise, if there is just an ulcer history or perhaps a healed ulcer, then we do a vagotomy and pyloroplasty. We have performed an antrectomy and vagotomy in only four out of 60 patients.

Moderator: Does it trouble you that many people who study this problem have decided that perhaps resection may be too radical as therapy, and you are advocating it for prophylaxis? I am sure it does not bother you at all, but should it bother you?

Dr. Najarian: No.

Moderator: If you had an open mind, would it bother you?

Dr. Najarian: I was more concerned that Rod Carew was going to be traded than that. We have all kinds of strange people in medicine and there are all kinds of strange comments. I do not think that should affect your practice. But I will say that this is a virulent situation. David Hume first reported in the transplant population that bleeding peptic ulcers in his first series had an 85% mortality. As you saw in my presentation, the mortality of ulcer posttransplant is in excess of 50%. So we are not treating a situation that can be treated mildly. Under these circumstances, we have to give them the maximum operation when indicated. With an active duodenal ulcer, it is indicated.

Dr. Silen: Dr. Najarian, if I understand you correctly, these are all patients who had pre-existing ulcer, is that correct?

Dr. Najarian: Yes, these people all had a pre-existing ulcer or a history of pre-existing ulcer or had one demonstrated at the time. They all get a routine GI series and if there is any suspicion, they get an ulcer operation.

Dr. Silen: I would like to emphasize that that is a very special group and I am not sure that we would even call them stress ulcerations in the ordinary sense of the word. There is nothing that says that a patient with a pre-existing duodenal or gastric ulcer cannot have an exacerbation in the course of some other illness. It is important to emphasize that you are really treating pre-existing ulcer disease in your group of patients. This group has superimposed steroids, stress or whatever, and they are a particularly virulent group. I think that is a very different kind of situation than the kind of fundic erosions that we talked about that occur in nontransplant patients.

Dr. Najarian: Dr. Silen, you will recall from my presentation that of those without a previous history of ulcers — even under these stressful situations of rejection, high steroids, etc. — only 2% developed posttransplant ulcers. In fact, it is a very special group, and that is a way of protecting that special group.

Dr. Friesen: I think there is a similar situation, apart from the transplant patient, who probably does need an aggressive type of operation, that is, the patient with renal failure, with sepsis and massive bleeding. That patient probably cannot be handled with a V & P. That patient probably needs a total gastrectomy.

Dr. Najarian: I am talking about prophylaxis. You are talking about treatment. I agree with you 100% about treatment.

Dr. Alexander-Williams: May I comment? I wanted to mention the experience in Britain of using prophylactic highly selective vagotomy before transplantation in patients with a past history of peptic ulcer. They had absolutely disastrous results because of the high incidence of lesser curve necrosis. The series was abandoned. I just wondered whether Dr. Najarian has any experience with this.

Dr. Najarian: We have had no experience with highly selective vagotomies in these patients. However, the transplant patient, even in the pretransplant period, is a very difficult patient to get to heal gastrointestinal anastomoses. For instance, when we do a total gastrectomy to treat posttransplantation bleeding, we advocate stapling the lower end of the esophagus and bringing out a cervical esophagostomy, closing off the duodenum and not making any anastomosis until they are over the stress situation. We are dealing with a special group of patients. With a highly selective vagotomy, if anyone is going to have trouble with the lesser curvature, they are the patients who will do so. They do not heal well. You cannot make too many mistakes. Highly selective vagotomy could theoretically be the best prophylactic operation for these patients.

Moderator: Dr. Beahrs, I have two questions calling attention to the fact that a famous Cleveland surgeon has suggested that the Kock operation might be contraindicated ultimately because of troubles people get into catheterizing the stoma. I wonder if you would comment, because there is a lot of information going around about difficulties in catheterizing stomas.

Dr. Beahrs: The difficulty is really mechanical. When the nipple valve is not in proper position, that is the primary problem. There is an emotional problem in some patients, and these patients really should be selected out. Knowing what we know today, the problems are infrequent. Again, I refer back to the 10% figure. I really personally feel that the difficulty of intubation of the pouch is not a contraindication. However, I am not sure that the nipple valve is the final answer to the continence of the pouch.

Moderator: Would you elaborate on that? You said that there are some other things coming down the pike that looked as though they might be promising.

Dr. Beahrs: Many of you have heard of the magnetic ring, which they are using in Germany for colostomies. Something in the range of 20% to 50% of these have to be removed for a variety of reasons: infection, displacement, malposition, increase in body weight — all are factors that lead to extrusion of the magnetic ring. So that probably is not the answer. A group in California is experimenting with a carbon cone through which the bowel passes and, hopefully, the mucosa will heal to the skin edge, and this cone then can be plugged or capped. This method has been successful in the experimental animal. Whether or not it will be successful in man is uncertain. Another approach to the problem is to create the pouch with a straight conduit from the pouch to the surface and have an internal appliance that one can change periodically or clean periodically. It would require a one-way valve through which the catheter could be inserted for decompression of the pouch. With the catheter out, the valve closes and would prevent the outflow. With an appliance of this type inside the lumen, one does not have to be concerned about the infection problem. One concern, however, is whether or not pressure necrosis might occur that would lead to fistula formation. In several of our cases who have elected not to have a revision of the nipple valve because of leakage, we inserted a tracheal tube into the pouch, blew up the cuff, pulled it back and anchored it to the skin; that acts as a nice internal plug. They merely clamp the catheter and periodically open it. These are the devices that are being considered, which in the future might prove to be more successful than the anatomic nipple valve.

Dr. Silen: Dr. Beahrs, I noticed that you did not mention one of the things which I think Kock and others recently reported. We have seen at least one instance of ulceration in the pouch. Nystrom had a 20% to 25% incidence of ulceration in the pouch. Kock said it happens. These people have episodes of cramps, diarrhea, fever and he puts them on azulfadine and sometimes steroids, and he says they get better. What is that entity? Have you seen it? One of the reasons we have been very reluctant to do the operation in our patients with inflammatory bowel disease is the fear of such a complication. Would you comment?

Dr. Beahrs: There is a gradual change of the bacterial content of the pouch to that of the colonic flora. I am sure this leads to some complications with stagnation of the intestinal content in the intestine. There is dilatation of the pouch, which leads to a thinning out of the mucosa of the pouch. There is trauma of the tube periodically being inserted too far. We have had pressure necrosis in one or two, which led to perforation. To my knowledge, only one patient has perforated the pouch by inserting the tube. We have had several problems of increased outflow. One patient comes to mind, a young girl, which brings up the selection problem. She had a conversion from a Brooke ileostomy to a pouch and came back extremely sick with high output, 2,000 to 3,000 ml/day from the pouch. She had a monilial overgrowth within the pouch that led to erosion of the mucosa. In discussing this girl's problem with her and with her parents, we found that she had run away from home and had been eating potato chips for six months. It merely emphasizes the fact that nutrition is important. Selection of patients for the procedure is very important. There have really been no long-term ill effects nutritionally or as far as motility is concerned or ulceration, except for those patients with Crohn's disease. So our experience has not paralleled that of others in this respect.

Intestine

Role of Intestinal Gas in Functional Abdominal Complaints

Michael D. Levitt, M.D. and John H. Bond, M.D.

Objectives

1. To provide data on the composition, volume and source of intestinal gas.
2. To provide guidelines for therapy of intestinal gas problems.

Introduction

Complaints allegedly due to excessive intestinal gas usually take one of three forms: (1) excessive eructation; (2) abdominal pain and bloating and (3) passage of excessive gas per rectum. The goal of this communication is to briefly review available data with regard to the true role of gas in the genesis of each of these complaints.

Excessive Eructation

The composition of the gastric gas bubble is similar to that of the atmosphere (ie, about 79% N_2 and 21% O_2) with some additional CO_2 [1]. Thus, this air bubble appears to be almost entirely derived from "swallowed air" with minimal contribution from gases produced in the gut. Some cases of exploding belches, if true, presumably represent the combustion of H_2 or CH_4 (methane) produced by bacteria in the stomach due to severe gastric statis or reaching the stomach via a gastro-colic fistula.

Exactly how gas is "swallowed" is not clear. Apparently, air is carried along with a swallowed bolus of food, water or saliva.

Michael D. Levitt, M.D. and John H. Bond, M.D., Veterans Administration Hospital, Minneapolis, Minn.

Fluoroscopic observation of the gulping of liquids or solids suggests that some subjects may swallow several times as much air as liquids or solids. In some cases, the gas may actually be contained in the food, eg, an apple is said to contain 20% air by volume [1]. Last, air can be aspirated into the esophagus by inducing a negative pressure in the chest and relaxing the upper esophageal sphincter.

The occasional "healthy" belch following a meal can be shown to be derived from the gastric air bubble. On the other hand, the patient who complains of repeated eructation precedes each belch with an aspiration or swallowing maneuver and most of the gas entering the esophagus or pharynx never reaches the stomach but rather is immediately regurgitated. Thus, repeated eructation is a noisy nervous habit and rarely, if ever, truly represents an intestinal gas problem.

The patient who complains of repeated belching always precedes each belch with an elevation of the larynx as he aspirates air into the hypopharynx and esophagus. Given the origin of the problem, it is totally irrational to treat the patient with diet or medications such as anticholinergics or antacids. First of all, treatment consists of convincing the patient that his belching does not result from the presence of serious organic disease. Second, the physician must clearly demonstrate to the patient that his problem is a nervous habit related to air gulping. This can be done by showing the patient that each belch is preceded by a gulping maneuver. If the physician is able to belch at will, it is also highly effective therapy to belch at the patient several times. While such educational therapy does not always cure the patient, it usually breaks up the anxiety — air swallowing — anxiety cycle and some patients have improved markedly.

Functional Abdominal Pain and Bloating

There is a pervasive idea — held by both laymen and physicians — that functional abdominal pain associated with the feeling of distention is caused by excessive gas in the intestinal tract. The inability to measure this gas volume has made it difficult to test this concept objectively. Recently, the volume of gas present in the intestinal tract has been measured by a gas washout technique in which argon is rapidly infused in the upper small bowel [2]. The argon rapidly passes through the gut, washing out all the "native" intestinal gases, and all gas passed per rectum is collected and analyzed. Using this technique, normal subjects (either pre- or postprandial) have an average of about 150 ml of intestinal gas (range: 30 to 300 ml). As shown in Figure 1, entirely similar volumes of intestinal gas were observed in subjects complaining of abdominal pain and bloating which they attributed to excessive gas [3]. Similar results have been obtained in radiographic studies which have failed to demonstrate increased volumes of gas in subjects complaining of symptoms of "gaseousness." It seems highly unlikely that washout or radiographic studies could be "missing" the volume of gas required to produce the types of distention complained of by the typical patient with functional complaints. Figure 2 shows the volume required to produce a 2-inch increase in the circumference of a 12-inch-high cylinder representing the abdominal cavity. The volume required would be almost 1800 ml! It is not possible that such massive

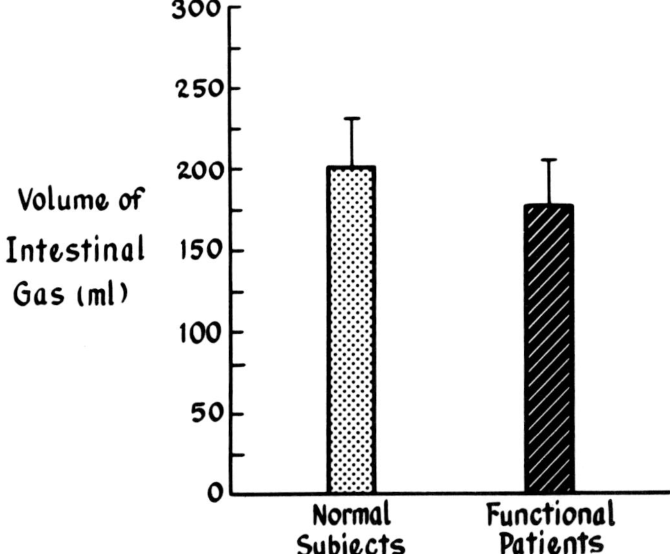

FIG. 1. Volume of intestinal gas measured by the washout technique in normal subjects and patients with functional bloating and abdominal pain.

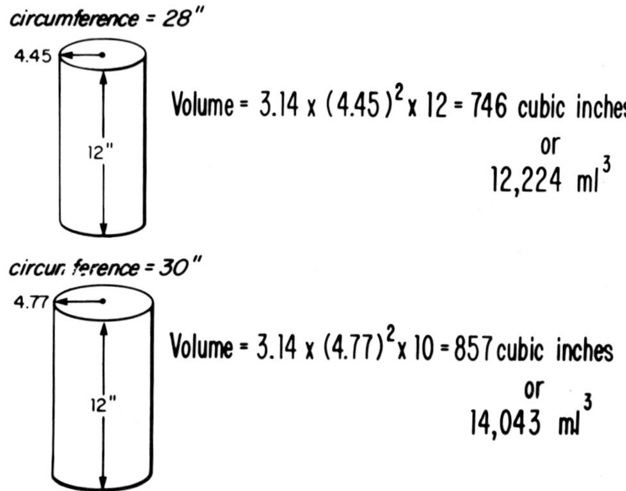

FIG. 2. Volume of gas required to increase the circumference of the abdomen schematically represented by a cylinder of 28″ circumference and 12″ height. An increase in circumference of 2′′ increases the volume by about 1800 ml.

quantities of gas would be overlooked on radiographic or washout studies.

However, patients with functional abdominal pain did differ from normal in that they complained of much more pain with the gas infusion than did controls (Fig. 3) and a larger fraction of the intestinally infused argon regurgitated back into the stomach of these patients. Thus, it seems likely that the primary abnormality of these subjects is some sort of motility disorder which disrupts the normally smooth transit of gas through the bowel and causes pain when the gut is distended by volumes of gas which are well tolerated by normal subjects.

What, then, is the explanation of the distended abdomen of these subjects? It appears that the patient is more comfortable with a protuberant abdomen and, therefore, lowers his diaphragm and relaxes his abdominal muscles — similar to the woman with pseudocyesis. The well-known observation that the

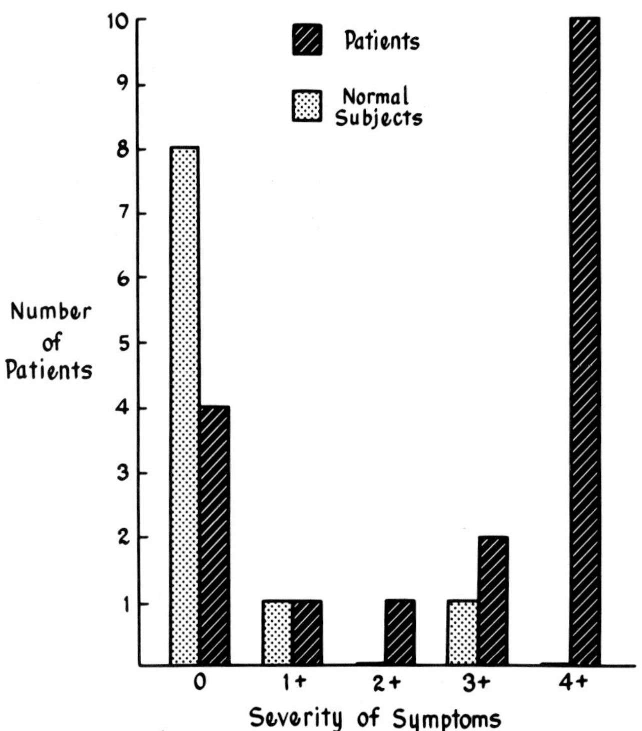

FIG. 3. Severity of symptoms during washout study in normals and patients with functional abdominal bloating and pain. "0" indicates no symptoms and "4+" such severe symptoms that gas infusion was discontinued.

distention of functionally bloated patient frequently disappears instantaneously when he reclines or exhales deeply supports this origin of the bloating.

The composition of the intestinal gas pool as measured by the washout technique [2] is variable, but N_2 is usually the predominant gas, there is very little O_2 (presumably due to metabolism by the mucosa and gut bacteria) and H_2, CH_4 and CO_2 are present in highly variable concentrations (Fig. 4).

The intestinal N_2 is derived from swallowed air. It is thought that at least several liters of N_2 are swallowed each day, yet only about 400 ml is passed per rectum and very little is absorbed from the gut. Thus, it appears that the bulk of swallowed N_2 is subsequently eructated with only a small

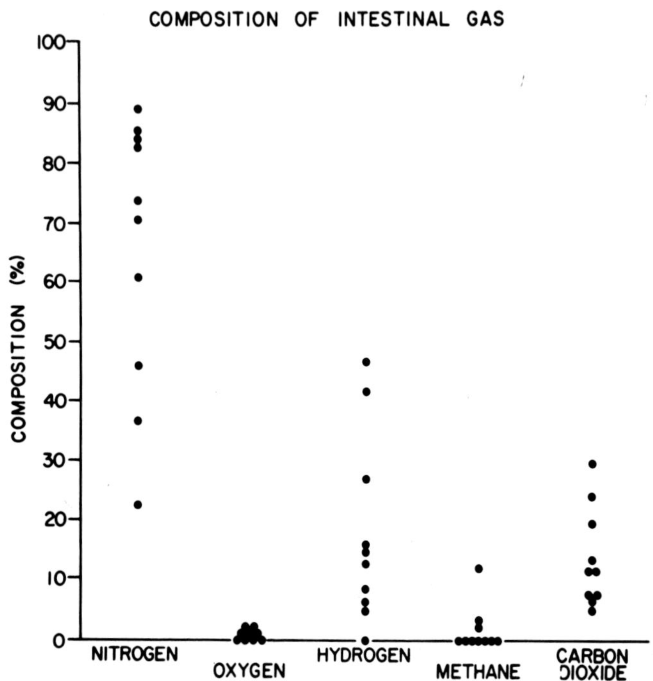

FIG. 4. Percentage composition of intestinal gas of normal subjects as measured by the washout technique.

fraction entering the intestine. Since the esophagus enters the posterior-superior aspect of the stomach, a fluid "trap" is formed at G-E junction when the patient assumes the supine position and this position should promote the passage of swallowed air into the duodenum.

H_2 and CH_4 are produced solely from the metabolism of the intestinal bacteria and, in normal subjects, the site of this production is limited to the colon. H_2 is only produced when a fermentable substrate (carbohydrate or protein) escapes absorption in the small bowel and is delivered to the colonic bacteria [4]. In gastrointestinal diseases, carbohydrates, which are totally absorbed by normal subjects, are malabsorbed yielding H_2 (and CO_2) production. Lactase deficiency is the most common example of this problem. In addition, a variety of vegetables (beans, cabbage) and grains contain oligosaccharides such as raffinose which are indigestible, even by normal subjects, and hence provide substrate for gas production [5].

CH_4 production appears to be a familial trait and is not influenced by diet [6]. CO_2 is produced both by bacterial metabolism of nonabsorbed carbohydrates and by the interaction of acid and bicarbonate (1 mEq HCO_3^- + 1 mEq $H^+ \rightarrow$ 22.4 ml CO_2).

If some sort of motor disorder underlies the problem of functional bloating and pain, the most rational form of therapy would be directed toward this problem. However there have been few double-blind studies that demonstrate benefit from pharmacologic therapy, including the anticholinergic drugs. The most convincing study to date showed that patients with functional abdominal pain were significantly improved during treatment with metoclopramide [7].

While these patients do not have excessive gas, they do appear to have pain from volumes of gas which are tolerated by normal subjects. Thus, efforts to minimize the volume of bowel gas may be helpful such as counseling regarding air swallowing and assuming a supine position after meals and avoidance of foods containing nonabsorbable carbohydrates. Lactose may not be completely absorbed, even by subjects with normal lactose tolerance curves, and a trial of a lactose-free diet may be useful even in the face of a normal lactose tolerance curve. Last, it seems possible that antacids might be helpful in that they reduce the H^+ and, hence, CO_2 production.

Excessive Passage of Gas per Rectum

Normal subjects pass an average of 700 ml of gas/24 hours (range: 300 to 2,000 ml) from the rectum and average about 13.6 ± 5 (1SD) gas passages per day [8]. The simplest way to determine the cause of excessive passage of gas is to analyze a rectal gas sample. If air swallowing is the cause, N_2 should be the predominant, whereas if H_2, CO_2 or CH_4 is predominate, it is apparent that the gas was produced in the bowel.

We recently studied a compulsive patient with a complaint of excessive flatulence who had recorded the exact time of each passage of rectal gas and each belch for a several year period [8]. The patient passed rectal gas about 34 ± 6 times per day, more than 3 SD above the normal mean. The patient's flatus consisted of largely CO_2 and H_2. When he drank nothing but 2 quarts of milk daily, he passed gas 141 times/day! The patient was lactose deficient and study with a rectal tube (Fig. 5) showed that he excreted excessive rectal gas when he ingested a test meal containing two glasses of milk or 50 gm of lactose.

We have also analyzed flatus of six additional patients with complaints of excessive flatus and, in each case, gases produced in the bowel (CO_2, H_2 and CH_4), rather than swallowed air, was the cause of the problem. In these patients, treatment should be directed toward determining what carbohydrate is being malabsorbed and presented to the colonic bacteria for gaseous fermentation reactions. Lactose malabsorption is by far the most common form of carbohydrate malabsorption in the United States and lactose restriction frequently alleviates the problem. Additional restriction of wheat products is usually helpful in the recalcitrant case. If N_2 is the major constituent of flatus, counseling concerning air swallowing is indicated.

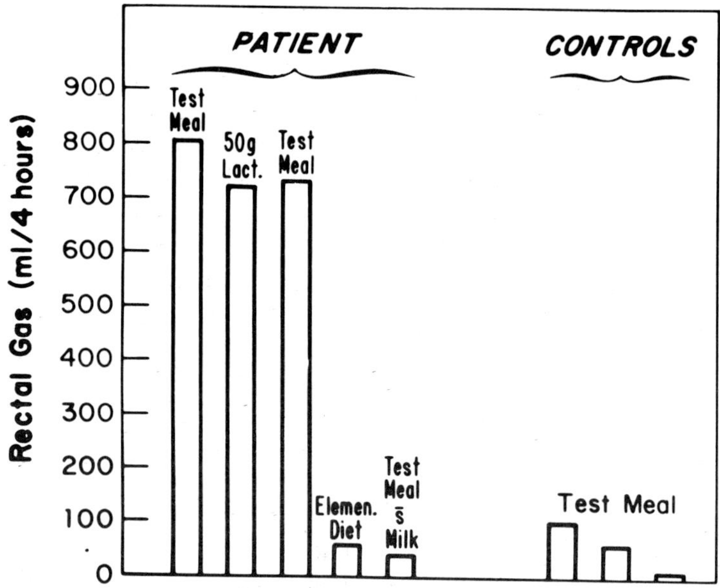

FIG. 5. Rectal gas passed by a lactose-deficient subject and controls after ingestion of a test meal (containing 2 cups of milk), 50 g of lactose and an elemental diet (Vivonex).

References

1. Calloway, D.H.: Gas in the alimentary canal. *In* Code, C.F.: Handbook of Physiology, Vol. V. Sect. 6, Alimentary Canal, pp. 2839-2859. Washington, D.C.:American Physiological Society, 1968.
2. Levitt, M.D.: Volume and composition of human intestinal gas determined by means of an intestinal washout technique. N. Engl. J. Med. 284:1394, 1971.
3. Lasser, R.B., Bond, J.H. and Levitt, M.D.: The role of intestinal gas in functional abdominal pain. N. Engl. J. Med. 293:524, 1975.
4. Levitt, M.D.: Production and excretion of hydrogen gas in man. N. Engl. J. Med. 281:122, 1969.
5. Steggerda, F.R: Gastrointestinal gas following food consumption. Ann. NY Acad. Sci. 150:57, 1968.
6. Bond, J.H., Engel, R.R. and Levitt, M.D.: Factors influencing pulmonary methane excretion in man. J. Exp. Med. 133:572, 1971.
7. Johnson, A.G.: Controlled trial of metoclopramide in the treatment of flatulent dyspepsia. Br. Med. J. 2:25-26, 1971.
8. Levitt, M.D., Lasser, R.B., Schwartz, J.S. and Bond, J.H.: Studies of a flatulent patient. N. Engl. J. Med. 295:260-262, 1976.

Self-Evaluation Quiz

1. Greater than 90% of intestinal gas is swallowed air.
   a) True
   b) False
2. The gas in a belch is usually produced in the bowel.
   a) True
   b) False
3. Most belching represents air which is swallowed or aspirated into the esophagus.
   a) True
   b) False
4. H_2 gas is produced by bacterial fermentation of carbohydrates.
   a) True
   b) False
5. Most H_2 gas in the bowel is produced in the stomach and small bowel.
   a) True
   b) False
6. Methane gas is produced by the digestion of fats by digestive enzymes secreted by the pancreas.

a) True
b) False

7. Only about one third of normal people produce methane in the bowel.
   a) True
   b) False
8. One source of CO_2 in the gut is swallowed air.
   a) True
   b) False
9. Bacteria may be important in the production of gut CO_2.
   a) True
   b) False
10. Excessive belching is best treated by anticholinergic medications.
   a) True
   b) False

Answers on page 721.

Recent Clinical and Pathological Aspects of Inflammatory Bowel Disease

Louis P. Dehner, M.D.

Objectives

1. To discuss recent or reemphasized aspects of neonatal necrotizing enterocolitis, pseudomembranous enterocolitis, ischemic enterocolitis, Crohn's disease and chronic ulcerative colitis.
2. To point out the morphological components of tissue reaction (inflammation, ulceration, necrosis, vascular changes, fibrosis and atrophy) in the above inflammatory bowel diseases.

Introduction

Inflammatory bowel disease is a general term to designate any number of clinicopathologic disorders in children and adults who present with similar clinical manifestations (fever, diarrhea with or without blood, distention) [1, 2]. Only through a meticulous diagnostic evaluation including a careful history and physical examination, laboratory and roentgenographic studies and endoscopic visualization usually with biopsies one can arrive at a reasonably specific interpretation. In addition to the well-known granulomatous enterocolitis (Crohn's disease), chronic ulcerative colitis and those infectious enterocolidites (tuberculosis, amebiasis, shigellosis, salmonellosis and yersiniosis), the diversified list has expanded with the inclusion of neonatal necrotizing enterocolitis, ischemic entero-

---

Louis P. Dehner, M.D., Professor, Department of Laboratory Medicine and Pathology (Division of Surgical Pathology), University of Minnesota Medical School, Minneapolis.

colitis and antibiotic-associated bowel disease. There are various clues such as age, extent of disease and anatomic localization that are important in differential diagnosis. From the perspective of the surgical pathologist, it is imperative that some clinical impressions are available at the time of the tissue examination.

This review will discuss some of the recent or reemphasized aspects of inflammatory disorders of the intestinal tract. Some points that should be stressed at the onset are that many gaps still exist in our understanding of etiology and pathogenesis of these diseases [1]. Inflammation alone is an inadequate characterization of the tissue reaction since ulceration, necrosis, vascular changes, fibrosis and atrophy are other important morphologic components regardless of the specific diagnostic terminology. These overlapping features are a constant source of potential confusion to the pathologist who examines these cases [2]. Some specific macro- and microscopic findings are important clues (microorganisms, granulomas, vasculitis, skip areas) when correlated with the appropriate clinical setting.

Neonatal Necrotizing Enterocolitis

One of the earliest forms of inflammatory bowel disease is represented by neonatal necrotizing enterocolitis (NEC) which has shown a progressive increase in frequency over the past five to six years [3-6]. It has emerged as a major problem in the newborn period, especially in premature or low-weight-for-dates infants. Approximately 30% of babies weighing 1200 gm or less can be anticipated to develop NEC [7]. At the University of Minnesota, nearly 5% of all neonatal admissions were for NEC [8]. Most series demonstrate an overwhelming predilection for premature babies (90%+) with the exception of Babies Hospital (Columbia University, New York) in which 20% of their cases were found in term infants [9, 10]. Some of these children had cardiac disorders or the delayed onset of symptoms. One proposed explanation for the apparent increase in the frequency of NEC is the improvement in resuscitative efforts of premature infants. The clinical and roentgenographic manifestations have been thoroughly reviewed in a number of other papers [11, 12]. It is sufficient to say that most children develop symptoms before ten days of age, and pneumatosis cystoides intestinalis is a pathognomonic roentgenographic sign which is present in 70% to 80% of cases (Fig. 1) [8, 11, 13]. There is debate whether the etiology(s) of NEC is ischemia, transmissible agents or hyperosmolar feedings [14, 15]. The transmissible agent hypothesis is suggested by the occurrence of cases in clusters even though a pathogen has not been identified as well as documented epidemics of "nonenteropathogenic" strain of *E. coli*, staphylococcus, *Clostridium butyricum* and coxsackie B [5, 16-19]. Ischemic or coagulative necrosis of the intestinal mucosa as the earliest lesion lends support to the vascular or hypoperfusion theory. Some cases have been associated with thrombosis of the abdominal aorta after catheterization of the umbilical artery or exchange transfusions through the umbilical veins. Those children who develop NEC after exchange transfusion have a delayed onset of disease, nearly exclusive colonic involvement and a mortality lower than the overall group. Disseminated intravascular coagulation with septicemia has likewise been implicated.

In the past, the pathologist encountered most cases of NEC as a postmortem finding but today, many centers are reporting survival rates of 70% or greater. Early diagnosis and clinical staging have reduced the need for surgical intervention. Most children requiring surgery have developed a grave complication such as multiple perforations. In those children who can be managed conservatively, the mortality is only 15% to 20% but increases to 40% or greater when surgery is required.

NEC is most frequently localized to the right side of the small and large intestine where the distal ileum and ascending colon are primarily affected [20]. Progressively more of the ileum, jejunum and colon is affected in a confluent fashion in the severe cases. Extension to the stomach has also been described. A dusky, hemorrhagic appearance as well as subserosal blebs of gas are encountered on the external surface (Fig. 2). Perforations are typically found in the distended ileocecal region but not exclusively. Adhesions and peritonitis are other operative or postmortem findings. The necrosis, hemorrhage and edema may be confined to the mucosa and submucosa with surprisingly minimal inflammation in the early lesion [9, 20] (Fig. 3). Transmural necrosis and inflammation occur somewhat later. Pneumatosis cystoides is represented by blebs or spaces in the submucosa, muscularis and serosa (Fig.

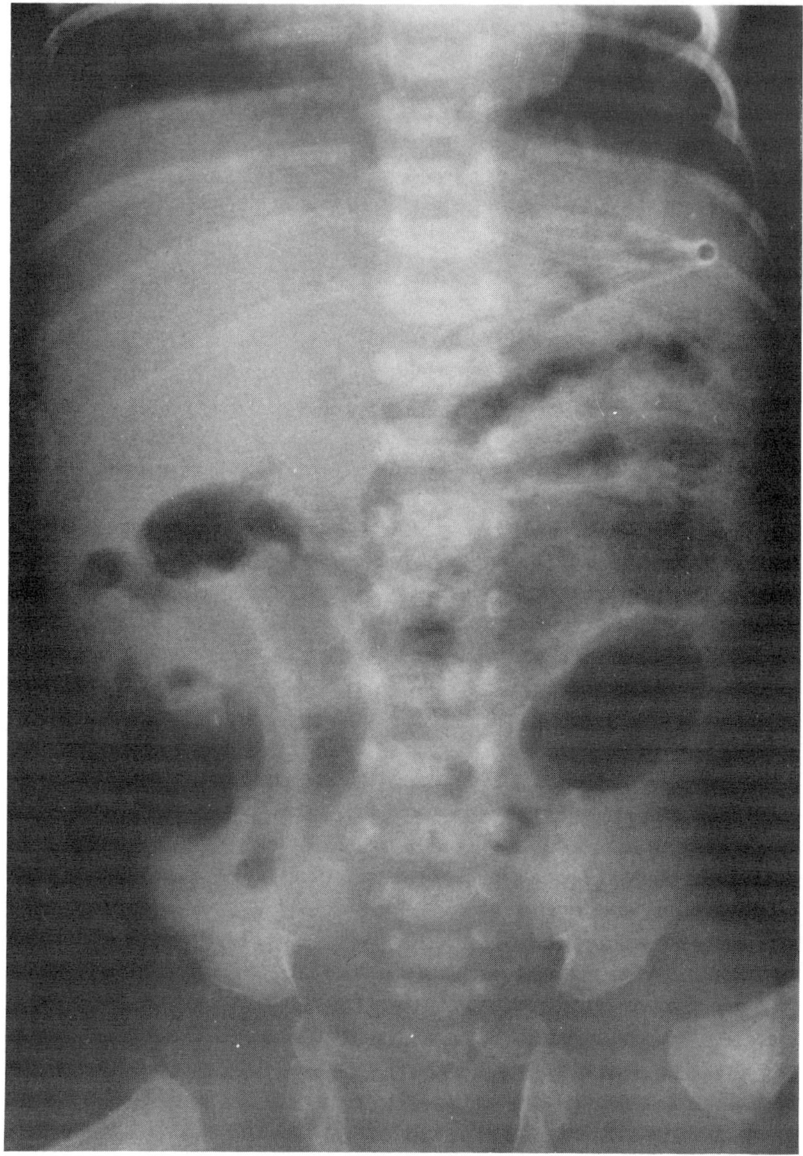

FIG. 1. Roentgenograph showing dilated loops of bowel and pneumatosis cystoides intestinalis primarily on the left side of the abdomen in an infant with NEC.

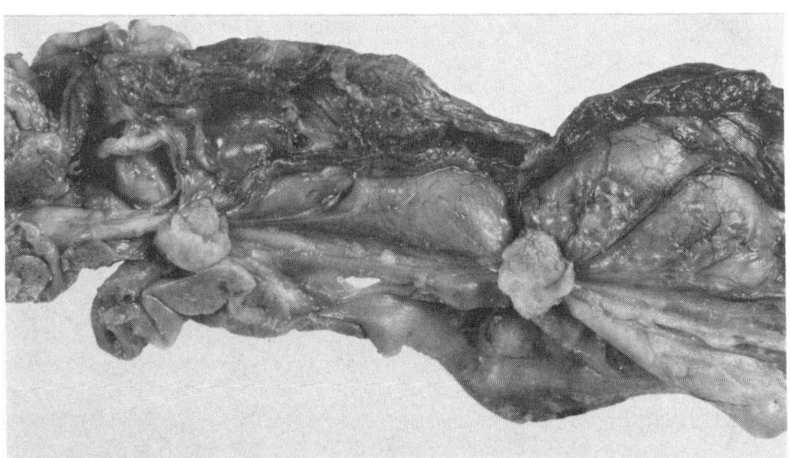

FIG. 2. Serosal aspect of a resected segment of bowel showing multiple blebs in a child with NEC.

3B). A giant cell reaction is usually lacking about these blebs. Platelet and fibrin thrombi are occasionally identified in the smaller submucosal and mural vessels, but their significance in the etiology of NEC is uncertain.

An important sequela of NEC is the development of one or more bowel strictures. Bell and associates reported this complication in eight of 56 babies (14%) [21]. There was an equal distribution of children between those treated medically and surgically. One difference was the presence of multiple strictures in the surgical group in addition to enterocyst formation. Some strictures were identified within a few days to months but not all were symptomatic. The histologic features are dependent upon the interval following the acute episode but reepithelialization, granulation tissue and fibrosis are the mucosal-submucosal findings. Eccentric hypertrophy of the muscularis interna and externa are late changes. The ganglion cells of the submucosal and myenteric plexi are normal appearing.

The differential diagnosis of NEC should include the necrotizing enterocolitis proximal to a congenitally stenotic segment of bowel, Hirschsprung's disease complicated by enterocolitis or thrombosis of the abdominal aorta after umbilical artery catheterization [22, 23]. Frozen section consultation may be sought to clarify the clinical problem. The

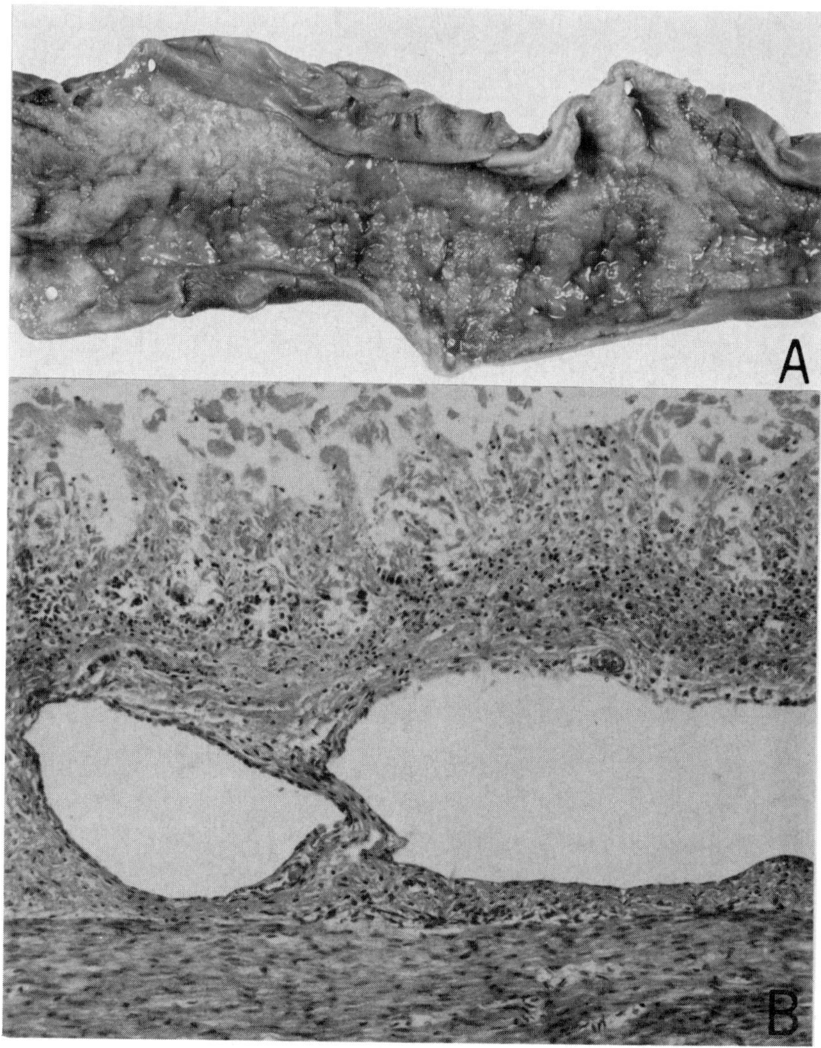

FIG. 3. (A) Mucosal surface of the small intestine showing ulceration and necrosis in NEC. (B) The mucosa is totally necrotic, yet there is a minimal inflammatory reaction. Pneumatosis cystoides is represented by the oval blebs in the submucosa (hematoxylin and eosin, × 145).

mortality for Hirschsprung's enterocolitis is as high as 25% to 30%. In some cases, the enterocolitis can persist in a chronic relapsing form in children who have had a pull-through procedure. The etiology remains obscure when re-biopsies of the colonic segment demonstrate apparently adequate numbers of ganglion cells.

Pseudomembranous Enterocolitis

This form of inflammatory bowel disease has received a great deal of recent attention because of its relationship to antibiotic therapy, particularly lincomycin and clindamycin (10% incidence) [24-27]. It had been recognized for some time earlier that pseudomembranous enterocolitis (PME) was a dread complication of broad spectrum antibiotics (ampicillin, tetracycline, chloramphenicol) other than clindamycin and lincomycin. Staphylococcus and Shigella both produce PME [28, 29]. A variety of debilitating diseases, colon proximal to an obstructing neoplasm and the postsurgical patient without other factors are conditions and situations complicated by PME [30-32] (Fig. 4). The majority of patients have been adults, but children are also affected [33]. In the past, the mortality has been impressively high but in the clindamycin-lincomycin cases, there have been very few deaths. Toxic megacolon has been reported in a rare case, and some patients have been explored with a simulated acute surgical abdomen [34, 35].

The pathogenesis of PME, except for those cases with a specific microbial etiology, remains speculative. Some investigators have considered PME part of the spectrum of ischemic enterocolitis or disseminated intravascular coagulopathy [36]. A hypersensitivity reaction is yet another theory and recently, toxin-producing clostridial organisms have been implicated in the antibiotic-associated PME [37, 38]. The argument about pathogenesis illustrates the problem of segregating the variables in the bowel when studying inflammatory diseases.

Multiple yellowish-white to yellowish-green plaques covering an edematous, erythematous mucosa are characteristic of the pseudomembranes (Fig. 4) [30, 39]. The early pseudomembranes measure 2 to 5 mm in diameter and with progres-

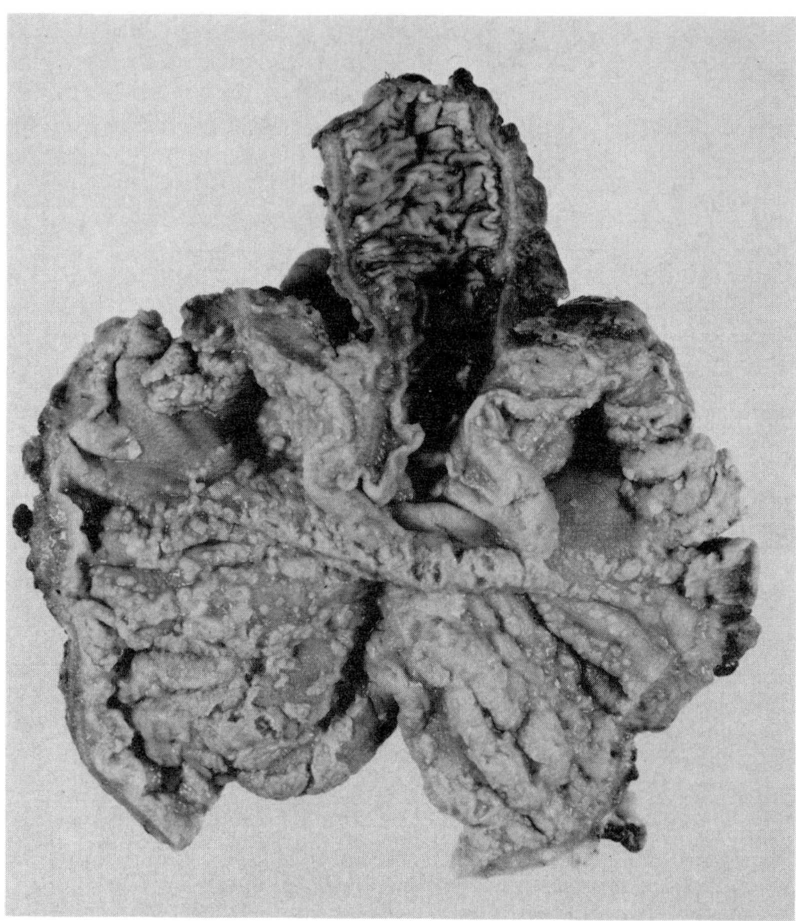

FIG. 4. Pseudomembranous enterocolitis with multiple yellowish-gray plaques which are coalescing in some areas.

sion, the mucosa becomes carpeted. A mixture of fibrin, neutrophils, mucin and degenerating epithelial cells is the composition of the pseudomembrane which is attached to the focally ulcerated surface [40, 41] (Fig. 5). The mushroom configuration of the pseudomembrane results from the narrow attachment and the layering effect over the surface. Mucosa between the pseudomembranes is intact. Acute and chronic inflammatory cells (lymphocytes and plasma cells) are present

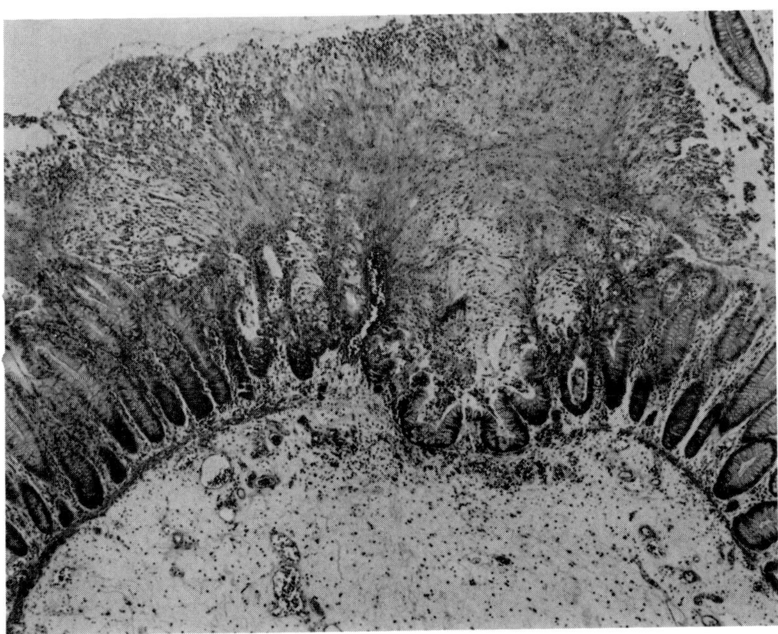

FIG. 5. Characteristic mushroom-shaped pseudomembrane composed of fibrin, mucin and neutrophils. The narrow point of attachment to the partially ulcerated and dilated glands is another typical feature of pseudomembranous enterocolitis (hematoxylin and eosin, ×60).

in varying numbers in the lamina propria. Crypt abscesses, deep ulceration and vascular thrombosis are atypical features. One difficulty with the rectal biopsy is that the plaque is visualized and presumably snared, but the microscopic section only demonstrates a nonspecific colitis. It must be realized that most of the pseudomembrane lacks an attachment and is, therefore, lost at the time of the biopsy or in tissue processing [40].

The gross extension of PME appears to differ between the postoperative cases and those associated with antibiotics as judged by postmortem and roentgenographic examinations [30, 42]. In a review of 107 postsurgical cases at the Mayo Clinic, the small intestine only (44 cases) or the small and large intestine together (24 cases) were the sites of predilection [30]. The large intestine is primarily and almost exclusively involved in the antibiotic-associated cases.

Ischemic Enterocolitis

It has been appreciated for many years that there existed a form of segmental, cicatrizing disease of the large and small intestines that was different from Crohn's disease. Ischemia of the intestinal tract was considered an acute process with infarction and the characteristic gross and microscopic changes of tissue necrosis. Marston and associates introduced the concept of "ischemic colitis" to include three general categories: (1) a gangrenous form (long, continuous segment involvement) due to large vessel occlusion or prolonged hypofusion; (2) nongangrenous ischemic stricture; and (3) transient ischemia [43]. The pathogenesis of ischemic enterocolitis would appear on the surface to be straightforward except for the relationship of pseudomembranous colitis. Alschibaja and Morson as noted previously include pseudomembranous colitis as part of the conceptual spectrum of ischemic colitis [36]. The umbrella of this latter disorder also includes the enteritis associated with enteric-coated potassium and neonatal necrotizing enterocolitis.

Thrombosis of an atherosclerotic superior mesenteric artery is the most common cause of intestinal infarction [44]. Ischemia is also a complication of aortic aneurysmectomy which infrequently is of clinical significance [45]. Occlusion of major and minor mesenteric vessels has been associated with various collagen vascular diseases (polyarteritis nodosa, rheumatoid arthritis, scleroderma), Degos' disease (malignant atrophic papulosis) and oral contraceptive agents [46, 47]. In the latter patients, the ischemic episodes may be transient or produce a major infarction [48]. Women who have taken an oral contraceptive for more than a year have a greater risk of thrombosis than those patients who have taken the hormones for a period of less than 12 months. The mortality is two times greater if the thrombosis is arterial rather than venous [48].

So-called nongangrenous ischemic enterocolitis, unlike the gangrenous form (shock), presents with colitic symptoms, ie, abdominal pain, bloody diarrhea and fever. Typically, a constricting process is present in the region of the descending, sigmoid colon or splenic flexure [43, 49, 50]. It is uncommon for ischemic colitis to occur in the right colon because of the rich vascular anastomoses. On the left side, there is a watershed effect between the superior and inferior mesenteric arteries.

Grossly, nongangrenous ischemic colitis is segmental and, therefore, may be confused with Crohn's disease, a constricting carcinoma or inflammatory diverticular disease. The mucosal appearance is dependent upon the age of the ischemic lesion. Ulceration, necrosis and hemorrhage are encountered mucosally and submucosally (Fig. 6). A biopsy at this stage shows ischemic glands with a ghostlike appearance near the ulcerated surface and viable ones nearer the submucosa (Fig. 7). Typically, the muscularis propria is preserved beneath the widened, edematous and hemorrhagic submucosa. It is during the stage of repair and fibrosis when difficulties are encountered in the macro- and microscopic interpretation. The mucosa may have a segmental cobblestone appearance reminiscent of Crohn's

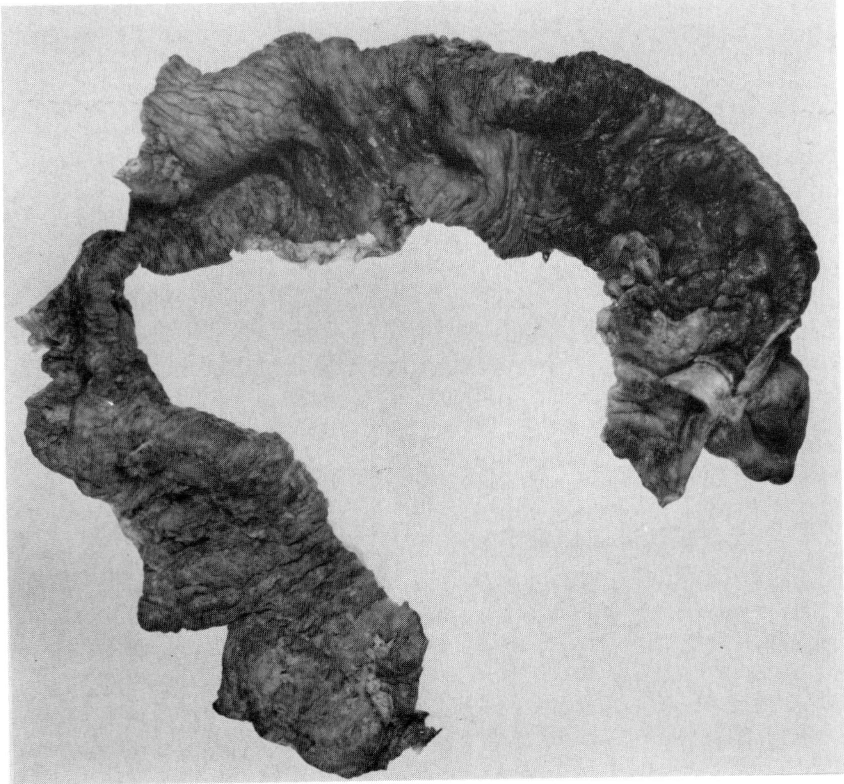

FIG. 6. Ischemic enteritis in a child who sustained a period of profound hypotension. The bowel subsequently became infected with *Candida albicans.*

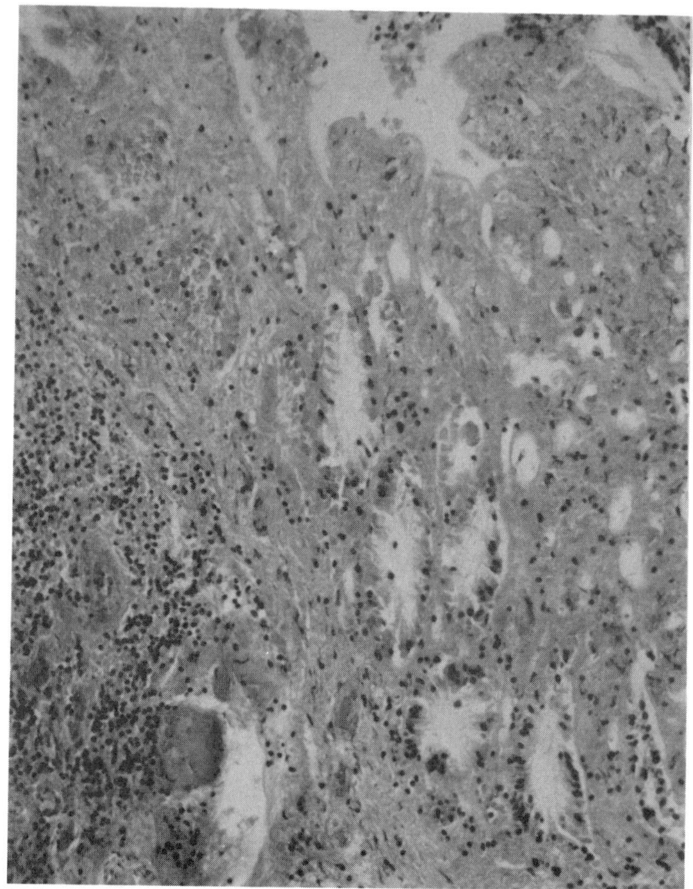

FIG. 7. Ischemic colitis showing necrotic "ghostlike" glands near the surface and better preserved glands near the muscularis mucosa (hematoxylin and eosin, ×160).

disease (Fig. 8). Histologically, the repair phase is characterized by residual focal ulceration, epithelial regeneration, granulation tissue, submucosal fibrosis and chronic inflammation. Metaplastic changes such as pseudopyloric mucosa in the small intestine and Paneth cells in the colon are relatively common. Repeated episodes of ischemia are evidenced by the presence of hemosiderin-containing macrophages in the submucosa. This finding among others is not encountered in Crohn's disease or

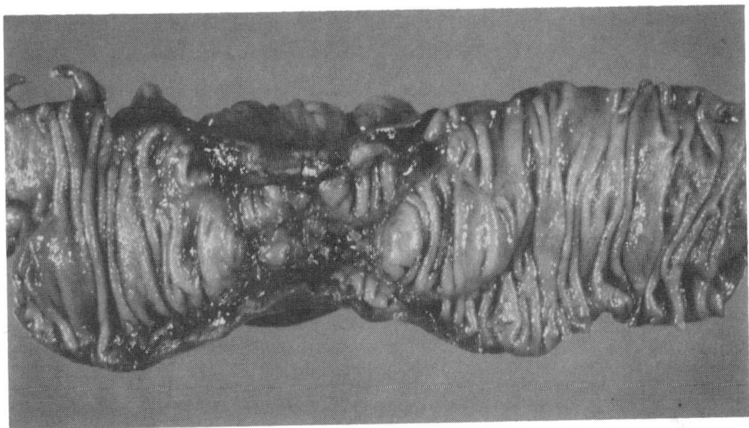

FIG. 8. Nongangrenous ischemic colitis showing focal constriction and mucosal irregularity resembling CD.

ulcerative colitis (Table 1). The stenotic or cicatricial stage is the one most frequently confused with Crohn's disease in our experience. An important differential feature in ischemic enterocolitis is the extension of fibrous tissue through the muscularis propria and into the circular smooth muscle. Transmural chronic inflammation and sarcoidal granulomas are absent in ischemic bowel disease.

Granulomatous Enterocolitis (Crohn's Disease) and Chronic Ulcerative Colitis

Every year literally dozens of papers are published on the numerous facets of these diseases known as Crohn's disease (CD) and chronic ulcerative colitis (CUC). The respective epidemiologies demonstrate that children and young adults are the usual victims but the age extremes are not spared [51, 52]. There is a seeming ethnic predilection with individuals of Jewish derivation especially prone to these diseases. Although the activity is centered upon the intestinal tract in CD and CUC, extra-intestinal manifestations are relatively common and may, in fact, become a predominant feature [53]. Arthropathies, cutaneous lesions (pyoderma gangrenosum, erythema nodosum) and chronic liver disease (chronic pericholangitis, chronic active hepatitis) are some of the more important extra-intestinal

Table 1. Morphologic Differential Diagnosis of Ischemic Enterocolitis From Idiopathic Inflammatory Bowel Disease

	Ischemic Enterocolitis	*Crohn's Disease*	*Ulcerative Colitis*
Typical distribution	Left colon (splenic flexure, sigmoid colon)	Ileum, colon	Colon (rectum)
Pattern of involvement	Segmental (sacculation)	Segmental (stenosing)	Continuous
"Toxic" dilatation	Occasional	Uncommon	Common
Transmural gangrene	Present	Absent	Absent
Mural thickening and serositis	Present	Present	Rare
Fistula formation	Absent	Present	Absent
Pseudopolyps	Uncommon	Common	Common
Cobblestone mucosa	Present	Present	Absent
Submucosal hemorrhage	Present	Absent	Absent
Pseudomembrane	Occasional	Absent	Absent
Fissuring ulcers	Micro-fissures to muscularis propria	Typical	Absent
Transmural inflammation	Absent	Typical	Absent
Hemosiderin-laden macrophages (mucosa-submucosa)	Present	Absent	Absent
Submucosal and muscular fibrosis	Present	Absent	Absent
Foreign body granulomas	Present	Present	Uncommon
Sarcoidal granulomas	Absent	Present (60%)	Absent
Goblet cell depletion and atypical mucosa	Absent	Absent	Present

disorders present in both diseases. The clinical courses of CD and CUC tend to be unpredictable with prolonged quiescent intervals in some patients and aggressive, unrelenting behavior in others. A chronic, relapsing course is the general rule [51]. As yet, the etiology remains elusive and essentially unknown for CD and CUC during a 40-year period of intensive research when infectious, toxic and immunologic factors have been considered, rejected and reconsidered [54, 55].

One heretical thought has occurred on the basis of recent clinical and pathologic observations that *possibly* we are *not* dealing with two separate diseases but rather one disease with slightly different tissue responses. The absolute distinctions which can be drawn between CD and CUC have dwindled to a few. If one can date the time when the sharp line began to fade, it occurred in the early 1960s with the recognition that CD could involve the colon exclusively or in conjunction with small intestinal disease [56]. There remain some differentiating morphologic features that have withstood the erosive phenomenon of time such as the restriction of CUC to the colon except for so-called backward ileitis and the invariable rectal involvement in CUC. CD has the ability to affect any segment of the enteric tract from the mouth to anus. Whereas CUC involves the colon in a continuous fashion, "skip" areas of normal mucosa between the areas of inflammation are characteristic of CD. Fissuring ulcers into the submucosa and muscularis, fistulae and sarcoidal granulomas in the bowel wall and lymph nodes are diagnostic findings in CD, but Price has even cast the specificity of the fissuring ulcer and transmural inflammation into doubt [57]. There is a small percentage of cases (10%) in which it is impossible to tell CD from CUC and represents "colitis indeterminate" [57, 60]. In the past, toxic megacolon, intestinal perforation and an increased cancer risk were thought to distinguish one from the other. That has been shown not to be the case in a number of recent reports [61-64].

Granulomatous Enterocolitis

CD suddenly appeared on the scene in 1932 in a report by Crohn and co-workers. Its clinical and pathologic similarity to tuberculous enteritis may have delayed its identification as a separate entity. The multifaceted aspects of this disease continue to emerge and thus dispel and modify concepts which were held to be valid in the preceding week, month or year. Because the tissue reactions of CD are so like those associated with infectious processes, this area of research continues to hold the attention of many investigators. Conflicting positive and negative reports claim the identification and isolation of viral-like agents and bacterial protoplasts whereas an adjacent paper denies the existence of transmissible agents [65-68]. Cave and co-workers have produced Crohn's-like lesions in the guts of rabbits who were fed filtered homogenates of human ileum and colon from patients with CD [69]. Immunologic studies have yielded interesting but difficult and sometimes contradictory data about CD [55]. Meuwissen and co-workers have examined the lymphoplasmacytic infiltrate and have found an abundant T-lymphocytic component in the deep inflammation of CD as compared to ulcerative colitis [70]. Janowitz and Sachar have reviewed other aspects of CD [71].

CD occurs as 2 to 4 cases per 100,000 population and there are epidemiologic data to suggest that the incidence is increasing especially in children [72]. Approximately 10% to 15% of patients (controls, 3% to 5%) have a positive family history for inflammatory bowel disease especially CD but also CUC [71, 73, 74]. The HL-A (W27) antigen is likewise present in the patients and their families. Most series show an average age at diagnosis between 28 and 32 years. Acute abdominal pain and diarrhea for a period of six months or less are the most common manifestations. Roentgenographic examination is a reliable method of diagnosis. Marshak has recently reviewed the roentgenographic aspects of CD [75].

The terminal ileum is the classic location for CD and thus the earliest designation of the disease as "regional ileitis" by Crohn. There is some variation from series to series about the percentage distribution of granulomatous enterocolitis but in general it is 60% ileum, 20% ileum-colon and colon only 15% to 20%. Marshak states, however, that 80% of patients with granulomatous colitis will have some small intestinal involvement [75]. CD may also involve the proximal small intestine (duodenum, jejunum), stomach, esophagus and even the oral cavity [76, 77]. Isolated appendiceal disease has also been described. A frustrating diagnostic problem is encountered in those patients with CD in an atypical location. Biopsies and even surgical resections show ulceration and transmural chronic inflammation but the sarcoidal granulomas are very difficult to identify. It is doubtful whether granulomas have ever been seen in Crohn's esophagitis. Even in ileal and colonic CD, the characteristic granulomas are found only in 60% to 70% of specimens.

Macroscopically, the features of CD have been often repeated and thus most observers have a reasonable concept of the changes. Linear ulcerations, cobblestone mucosa and pseudopolyps are the mucosal characteristics with contiguous areas of minimally altered or normal appearing mucosa [78] (Fig. 9). Through the thickened bowel wall, fistulous tracts can be identified in some cases. The serosa is congested and partially covered by fibrous adhesions. Mesenteric thickening and extension of the mesentery onto the serosa are other typical features. A surgical specimen can be extremely difficult to dissect because of the matted adhesions among loops of bowel and the interloop fistulae. Histopathologically, the intensely inflammed and partially ulcerated mucosa in the acute stages nearly always shows retention of goblet cells in contrast to CUC (Table 1). Fissure-like ulcers extending from the mucosa into the underlying bowel represent the nidus for the fistulae (Fig. 10). Large lymphoid aggregates are invariably present beneath the ulcerated mucosa which is the same relationship that the aphthoid ulcer, the earliest lesion of CD, has with the lymphoid follicles (Fig. 11) [79]. The sarcoidal granuloma is the only microscopic feature of CD which has not been denigrated by its presence in some other form of inflammatory bowel disease. Unfortunately, these granulomas are not present in all cases. In the mucosa and

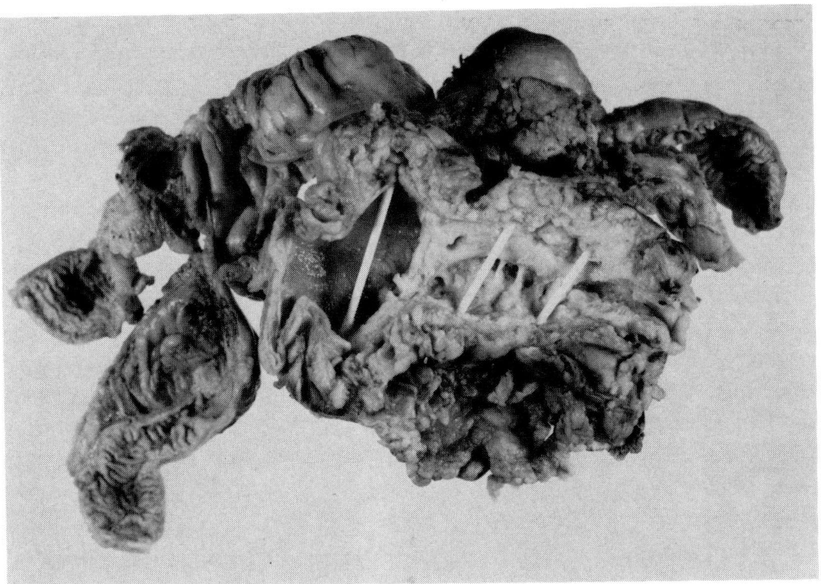

FIG. 9. CD showing narrowing of the lumen and marked thickening of the bowel wall. Multiple fistulae were present between intestinal loops.

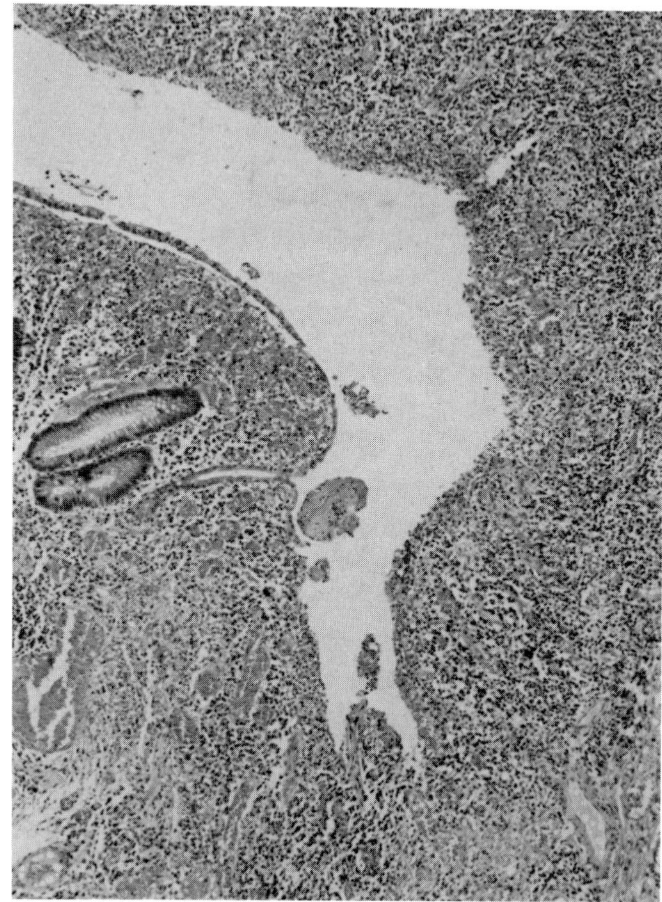

FIG. 10. A fissuring ulcer characteristic of Crohn's disease extending into the submucosa. Goblet cell retention is present in the adjacent glands (hematoxylin and eosin, ×60).

submucosa, the granuloma is composed mainly of epithelioid histiocytes with an occasional giant cell (Fig. 12A). The granulomas are better developed in the muscularis and lymph nodes (Fig. 12B). According to Glass and Baker, patients without granulomas in the bowel have a recurrence rate twice that of patients with granulomas [80]. This finding has not been corroborated by others as yet. When granulomas are found in mesenteric lymph nodes, the bowel likewise contains them. It

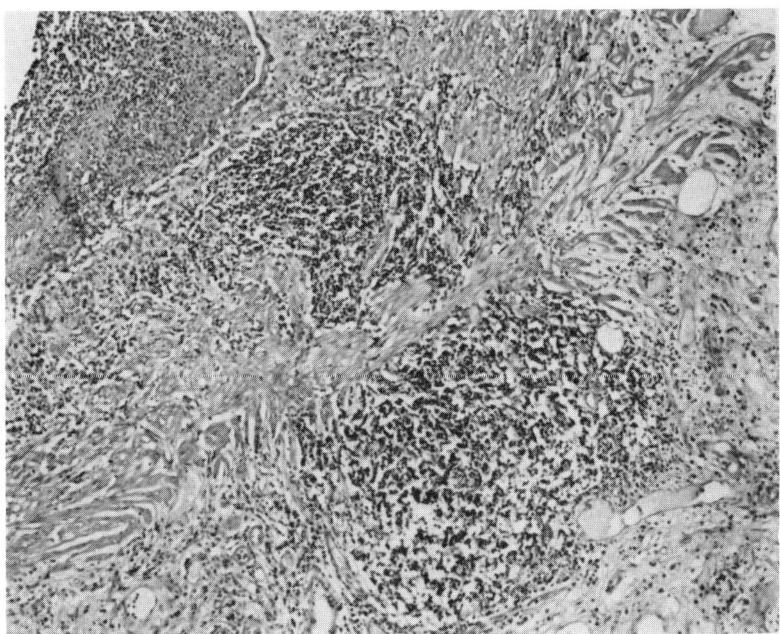

FIG. 11. Lymphoid follicles in the submucosa are typical features of CD. The overlying mucosa is ulcerated (hematoxylin and eosin, × 80).

is important in the differential diagnosis not to interpret a granulomatous reaction to vegetable or other foreign material which has penetrated the ulcerated mucosa in other types of inflammatory bowel disease as CD. Crypt abscesses and pseudopolyps, both thought to be characteristic of CUC, are not infrequent in CD (Fig. 13).

The role of frozen section examination during the course of a resection for CD is unsettled. Some surgeons consider the evaluation of margins for active disease as a guide to further segmental resections. There is no evidence to date that the recurrence rate which is substantial is less when inflammation is not present at the margins [81-83].

Rectal biopsy in the diagnosis of CD has been the subject of recent reviews [84, 85]. When granulomas are sought in rectal biopsies in patients with eventually proven CD, the yield is 8% to 20% overall but about 40% in granulomatous colitis. Approximately 10% of patients have rectal granulomas when

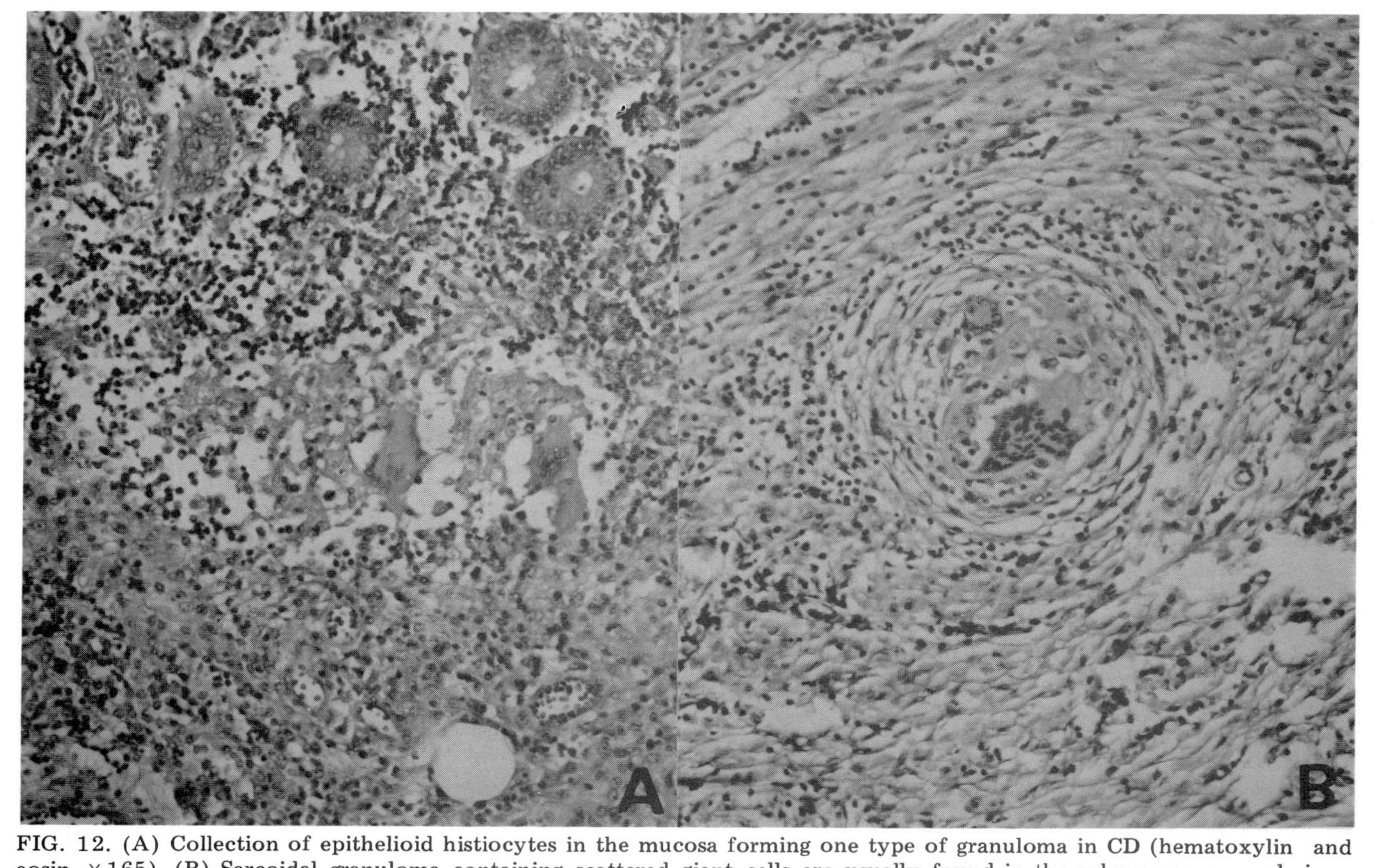

FIG. 12. (A) Collection of epithelioid histiocytes in the mucosa forming one type of granuloma in CD (hematoxylin and eosin, ×165). (B) Sarcoidal granuloma containing scattered giant cells are usually found in the submucosa, muscularis or regional lymph nodes (hematoxylin and eosin, ×170).

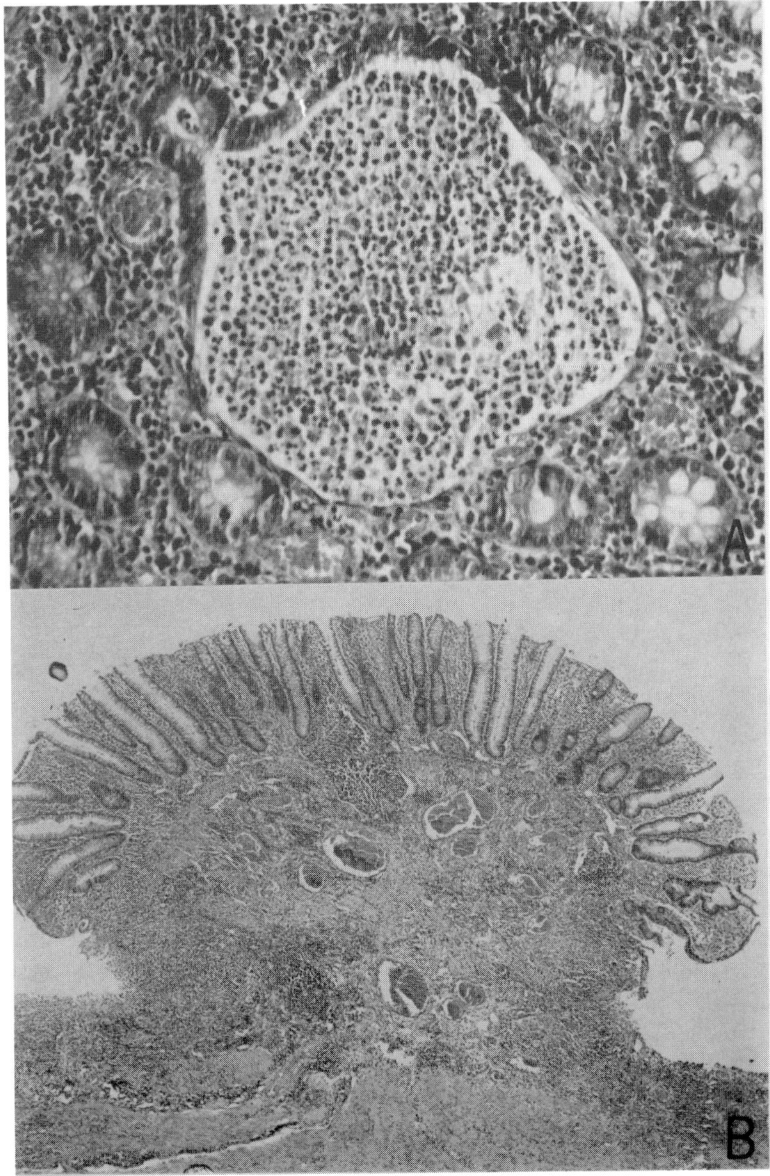

FIG. 13. (A) A crypt abscess in CD (hematoxylin and eosin, × 200). (B) The pseudopolyps in CD and CUC are indistinguishable microscopically (hematoxylin and eosin, × 30).

the disease is apparently localized to the ileum. Rotterdam and associates have emphasized the occurrence of microgranulomas in apparently normal mucosa in CD [86]. Fissures and ulcers in a rectal biopsy suggested a poorer outlook in patients with Crohn's colitis [87].

A disturbing feature of CD that has emerged in the last decade is the association with malignant tumors, primarily adenocarcinomas of the small intestine [88, 89]. It has been known for some time that CUC predisposed to carcinoma of the colon but it was thought that this risk did not exist in CD. In a follow-up study of 449 patients with CD at the Mayo Clinic, the incidence of colorectal cancer was 20 times greater than controls [64]. About 25% of carcinomas were diagnosed at the same time as CD. Approximately 30% of cancers occurred in bypassed loops of bowel [90]. Since the tumors tend to be constricting and infiltrating lesions, the ability to identify them grossly is reduced because of the similarity to active CD. This situation is analogous to that of CUC with a carcinoma. Most tumors are located in the ileum. The carcinomas are mainly well to moderately differentiated adenocarcinomas. Localized tumor-like masses simulating a polypoid or infiltrating carcinoma have been described in CUC and CD [91, 92]. Some of these lesions have been large pseudopolyps or exuberant granulation tissue.

One of the more serious extra-intestinal complications of CD is chronic inflammatory disease of the liver [53]. The incidence of significant liver disease is about 6% which is similar to that seen in CUC [93, 94]. On the basis of abnormalities in liver function studies, the incidence is about 50% [95]. Elevation of serum alkaline phosphatase is the most consistent finding. A chronic inflammatory reaction in the portal tracts consisting principally of lymphocytes surrounding bile ducts is the usual feature of the liver biopsy. There is variability in the degree of inflammation as well as the extent of periductular fibrosis. The entire response in the portal tract has been referred to as "pericholangitis." In some cases, the irregularity of the inflammatory infiltrate at the limiting plate with "piece-meal necrosis" and focal hepatocellular degeneration resemble chronic active hepatitis. This appearance is noted in a minority of cases. We have examined a liver biopsy from a patient with CD that had extensive sarcoidal granulomas in the portal triads. A consistent feature (20%) in biopsies is the presence of hepatocellular fat or steatosis [95]. In most cases, fat is contained in less than 50% of hepatocytes.

The differential diagnosis of CD in addition to the other forms of inflammatory bowel disease includes *tuberculosis*, *yersinosis* and *eosinophilic gastroenteritis*. *Tuberculous enteritis* has been reported in 2% of individuals with pulmonary tuberculosis [96]. The disease is characteristically localized to the ileocecal region like classic regional ileitis. There are many gross similarities that make the differentiation on the basis of macroscopic examination virtually impossible with cobblestoning and pseudopolyposis common to both. Tandon and Prakash have summarized the major morphologic differences [97]. Granulomas with caseation are present more often in tuberculosis. The mesenteric lymph nodes may contain granulomas where they are absent in the bowel wall which contrasts with CD. Fissuring ulcers, if present, are shallow but those in CD penetrate through the bowel. *Yersinia enteritis* likewise affects the terminal ileum with ulceration (aphthoid) and mucosal irregularity secondary to inflammation and edema [98-100]. The etiologic agent is *Yersinia enterocolitica*, a gram negative coccobacillus formly designated Pasturella pseudotuberculosis. Acute right lower quadrant pain simulating acute appendicitis is the presentation in 40% to 50% of patients. In children, it is a cause of mesenteric adenitis. Microscopically, the inflammatory reaction of acute and chronic inflammatory cells is confined to the mucosa and submucosa. Scattered microabscesses are present in the lymph nodes. *Eosinophilic gastroenteritis* is a rare disease characterized by recurrent abdominal pain, malabsorption, peripheral eosinophilia and a positive family history of allergy [101, 102]. Eosinophilic infiltration of the stomach, small intestine and regional lymph nodes is the microscopic appearance. Haberkern and associates reported a case in a 15-year-old female with eosinophilic ileocolitis which was very similar to CD [103]. Colonic involvement is very uncommon. When the eosinophils are confined to the mucosa, diarrhea, blood loss and malabsorption are the clinical features. Obstruction occurs with infiltration of the muscularis and ascites with serosal extension. The eosinophils are localized into polypoid lesions or diffuse infiltration of mucosa or muscularis.

Chronic Ulcerative Colitis

CUC is a disease older than CD in terms of its recognition as an entity. It may well date back into antiquity but it was Wilks over 100 years ago (1875) who provided a pathologic description of CUC that we could agree with today. Despite the time advantage of CUC for investigation, we know as much or little about it as we do about Crohn's disease.

It was alluded to previously that CUC and CD have many epidemiological, clinical and pathological similarities. CUC is more common than CD (4 to 7 cases per 100,000). The average age of onset also ranges from 28 to 32 years and 10% to 15% of patients develop their disease in childhood, even infancy [104-105]. It has been reasonably well documented that CUC in children is a more aggressive, virulent disease than the later onset form. According to Werlin and Grand, most children with severe colitis require surgery within two years of the initial attack [105]. One of the most serious early complications is the development of toxic dilatation or megacolon in 2% to 13% of cases [106]. The proper management of toxic megacolon (medical vs. surgical) is a subject of continued debate. Many of the extra-intestinal manifestations of CUC overlap with those of CD with differences mainly in frequency [53]. An area of intense interest and morphologic investigation has been the identification and significance of precancerous atypia and its relationship to adenocarcinoma of the colon [107-111].

In contrast to CD, CUC remains confined to the colon with some inflammation of the terminal ileum ("backward ileitis") in 5% to 10% of cases [59]. The rectum is universally involved with confluent disease in the adjacent sigmoid colon (protocolitis). Left-sided CUC is the general rule but pancolonic disease is usually present in surgical specimens which represent a skewed sampling. The rectum may appear remarkably normal in patients who have been treated with steroid enemas.

During the acute, active stage, a rectal biopsy may pose a diagnostic dilemma and it is not always possible to differentiate CUC from CD [2, 57, 58]. Price has emphasized the need to obtain a biopsy during a quiescent phase in order to identify the typical features of one or the other disease [57]. Acutely, the glandular epithelium may be totally denuded and the lamina propria replaced by ectatic blood vessels, acute and chronic (mononuclear) inflammatory cells and extravasated erythrocytes (Fig. 14). When this reaction is above the muscularis mucosa, a diagnosis of CUC is strongly suggested. If the inflammatory reaction has extended through the muscularis, it is well to recommend repeat biopsies during a less active phase. A biopsy which has adjacent, almost normal mucosa to an inflammed focus should suggest the diagnosis of CD. Depletion of globlet cells in an area of active or indolent inflammation is a highly reliable finding in CUC, but again Price's caveat should be kept in mind [57]. Goblet cell retention in similar circumstances supports an interpretation of CD. It has been our experience as well as others that crypt abscesses and pseudopolyps are not reliable differentiating histologic findings.

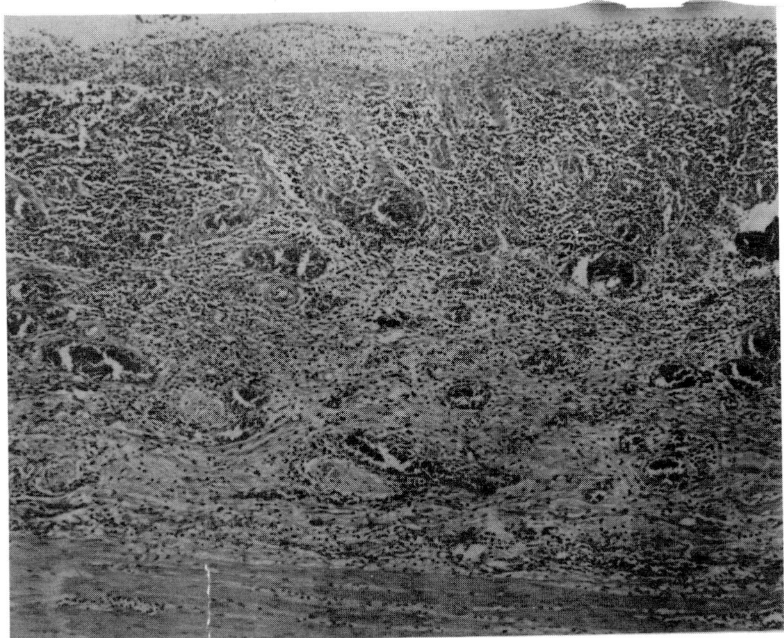

FIG. 14. Acute ulcerative colitis showing complete denudation of the mucosa and a mixture of acute and chronic inflammatory cells in the lamina propria. The muscularis is relatively uninvolved (hematoxylin and eosin, × 80).

Epithelial atypia and its implication have already been mentioned briefly. It is important not to overinterpret "regenerative atypia" that occurs as part of the repair phase of CUC with precancerous dysplasia (Fig. 15). Admittedly, this distinction is not always easy but to resolve any difficulties, we advise rebiopsy when the activity of the disease has diminished. The dysplastic epithelium remains whereas the "regenerative atypia" with its hyperchromatic, stratified nuclei and mitotic activity is no longer apparent. Isaacson has shown with the immunoperioxidase stain for carcinoembryonic antigen that the dysplastic and carcinomatous foci are positive and other areas are negative [112]. The colonic mucosa is atrophic in the inactive stage in those patients with chronic, intermittent disease (Fig. 16).

The risk of colonic carcinoma as a complication of CUC has been appreciated for the past 25 to 30 years [113]. There is an overall incidence of 3% to 5% which is some 20 times greater

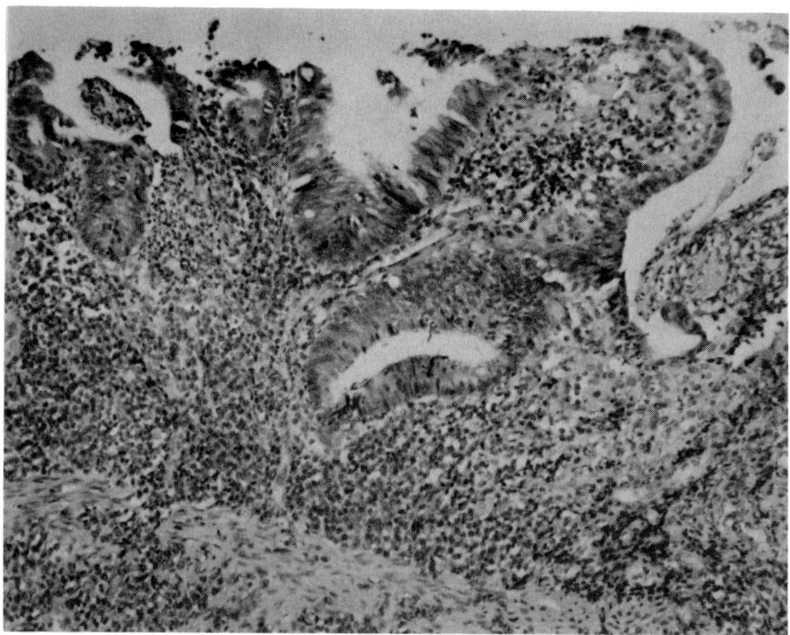

FIG. 15. "Regenerative atypia" in ulcerative colitis showing stratification of nuclei, hyperchromatism and abundant mitoses (hematoxylin and eosin, ×130).

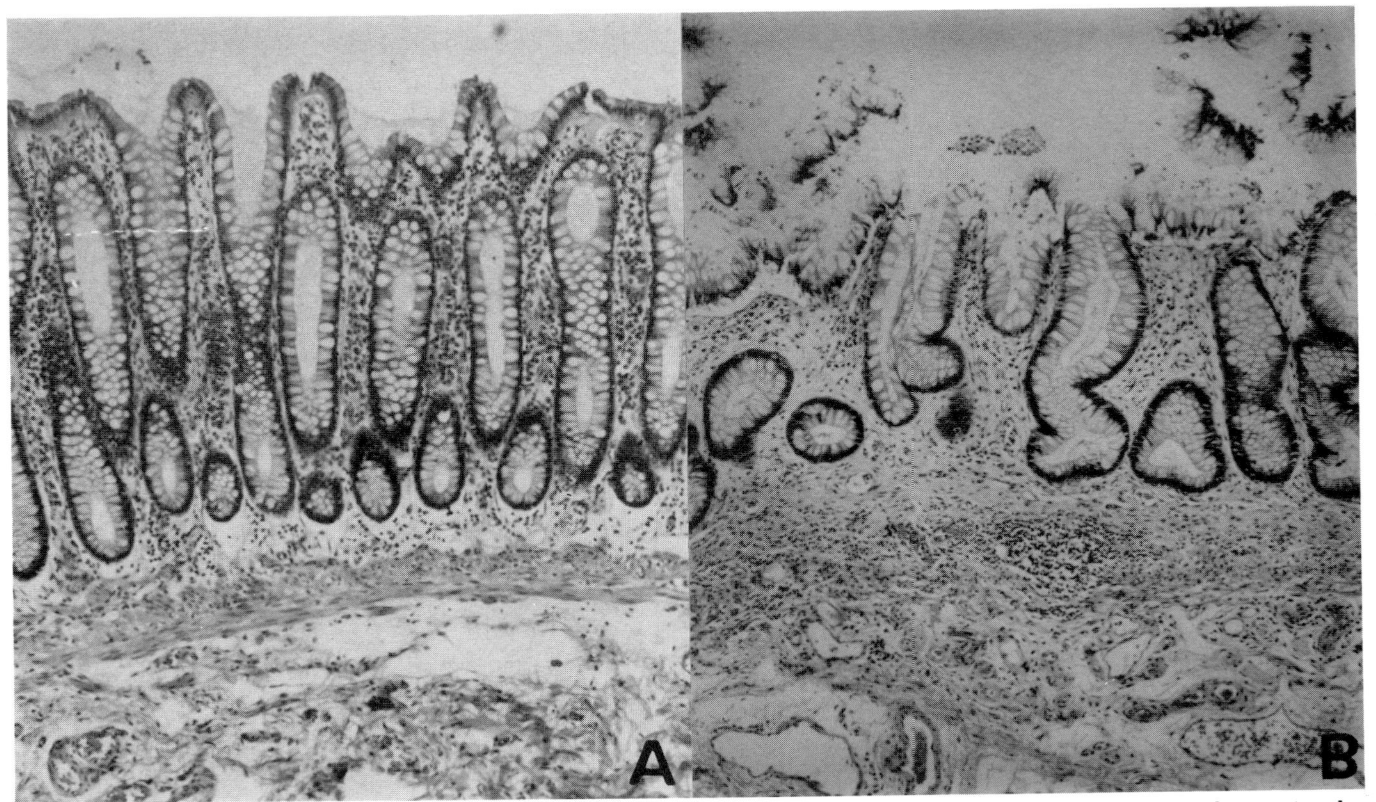

FIG. 16. (A) Normal colonic mucosa (hematoxylin and eosin, $\times 80$). (B) Inactive ulcerative colitis showing moderate atrophy of glands (hematoxylin and eosin, $\times 80$).

than the general population [110, 114]. It is also known that the risk of cancer is not the same for all patients with CUC, but the following factors enhance the probability of carcinoma: pancolonic involvement, onset of disease in childhood, a severe first attack and a continuous rather than intermittent course. After ten years of CUC in children, the risk of carcinoma is 20% per decade [115]. Unlike the sporadic carcinoma of the colon in the general population which occurs predominantly in the rectosigmoid colon, the CUC-related carcinomas arise in any segment of the colon and are multifocal in some cases. Because many of these carcinomas are flat, infiltrating lesions, it is extremely difficult for the endoscopist and radiologist to recognize them [116] (Fig. 17). Not all investigators agree that the prognosis is worse for the CUC-related carcinoma, a generally held view [117]. Recent reports indicate that some colonic neoplasms are nonepithelial and there is also an apparent increase in the frequency of carcinomas of the biliary tract [118, 119].

Morson and Pang were the first investigators to promote the role of the rectal biopsy as a means of identifying and monitoring the dysplastic epithelial changes in the colon [107]. Of their nine patients, five had one or more foci of invasive carcinoma. Dobbins and associates have recently reviewed a number of published series totaling 453 colectomies, 108 (24%) with carcinomas [111]. Precancerous dysplasia was present at some point in the colon in 95 (88%) specimens. When sections of the rectum were available for examination, dysplasia was noted in 15%. In another tabulation of 937 rectal biopsies with 53 (5.7%) precancerous dysplasias, the colectomies contained invasive carcinomas in 17 cases (32%). Over 80% of patients with dysplasia had CUC for greater than ten years. In addition to the review by Dobbins and associates [111], Riddell has also thoroughly evaluated this subject [108].

The presumption of a diagnosis of CUC is hazardous without a biopsy and for the pathologist, he must be mindful of *amebic colitis, shigellosis, salmonellosis, schistosomiasis*, various fungi (*Candida albicans, Histoplasma capsulatum, Aspergillus), cytomegalovirus colitis* and in children the *hemolytic-uremic syndrome* [2, 120]. Many of the clinical and pathologic features of amebic colitis are identical to CUC [121]. Despite

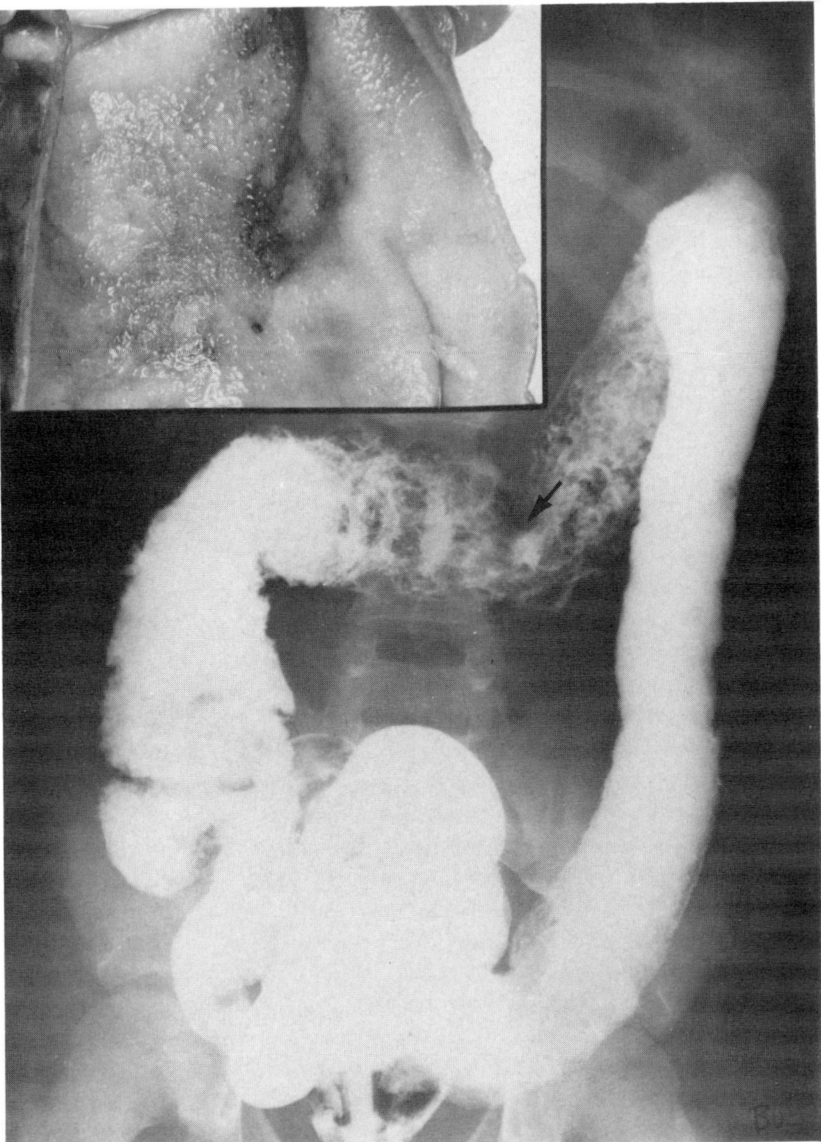

FIG. 17. Roentgenograph showing the appearance of total ulcerative colitis. A focus of depression and irregularity (*arrow*) later proved to represent a flat, infiltrating adenocarcinoma (*inset*).

repeated admonitions in the literature, the diagnosis continues to be overlooked in this country [122]. The trophozoites of *Entamoeba histolytica* are present in the exudate on the ulcerated surface. A periodic acid-Schiff stain (PAS) facilitates the identification of the organisms and it is not a bad policy to perform this stain routinely in all cases of acute colitis. Infectious colitis of bacterial etiology is characterized by a predominant neutrophilic reaction rather than the mixed inflammatory response of CUC [123]. Cytomegalovirus (CMV) *colitis* also produces changes very similar to CUC (Fig. 18). In

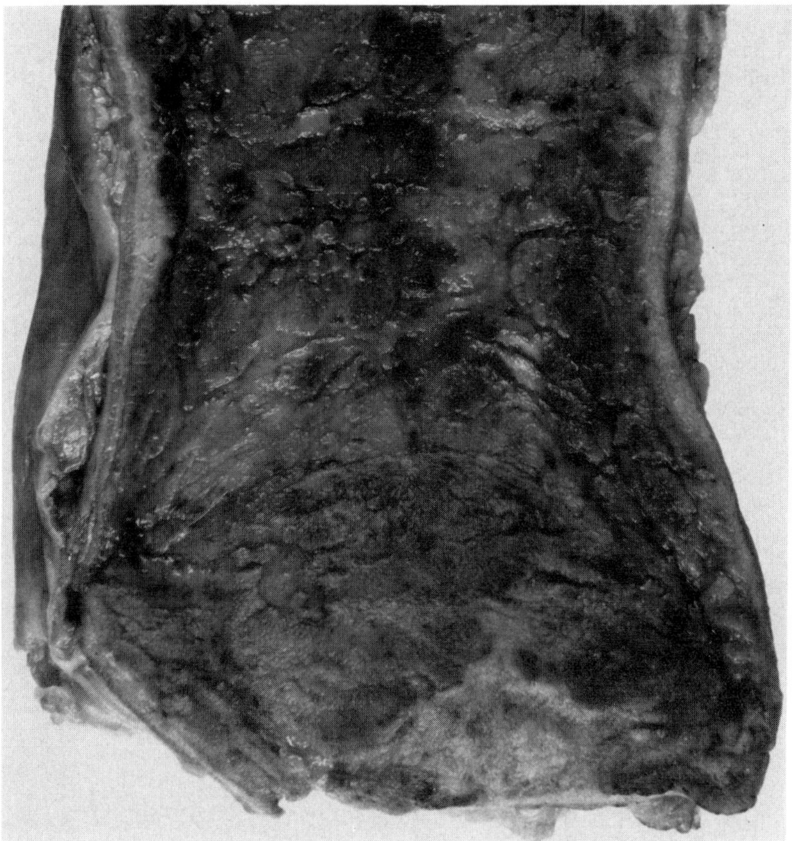

FIG. 18. Cytomegalovirus colitis in a renal transplant patient at autopsy. The lumen is dilated and the mucosa is diffusely ulcerated, an appearance identical to ulcerative colitis.

generalized cytomegalic inclusion disease in adults, the intestinal tract is infected in 66% of patients [124]. Most of these patients have predisposing debilitating illnesses and in our institution, the recipient of a renal transplant is especially vulnerable [125]. Cooper and co-workers made an interesting observation that six of their 46 patients (13%) requiring resection for ulcerative colitis had CMV inclusions in the colon [126]. These six patients were all males over 47 years old and five of the six presented with toxic megacolon. Histopathologically, the viruses are present in the nuclei of epithelial and endothelial cells as well as fibroblasts [127]. The CUC-like presentation of the *hemolytic-uremic syndrome* is most likely the result of intravascular coagulopathy [128]. Although there is a paucity of histologic material, it is suspected that mucosal ischemia and thrombi in the microvasculature are the principal findings [129].

References

1. Kirsner, J.B.: Inflammatory bowel disease. Considerations of etiology and pathogenesis. Am. J. Gastroenterol. 69:253-271, 1978.
2. Price, A.B. and Morson, B.C.: Inflammatory bowel disease. The surgical pathology of Crohn's disease and ulcerative colitis. Hum. Pathol. 6:7-29, 1975.
3. Touloukian, R.J.: Neonatal necrotizing enterocolitis: An update on etiology, diagnosis, and treatment. Surg. Clin. North Am. 56:281-298, 1976.
4. Bunton, G.L., Durbin, G.M., McIntosh, N. et al: Necrotizing enterocolitis. Controlled study of 3 years' experience in a neonatal intensive care unit. Arch. Dis. Child. 52:772-777, 1977.
5. Book, L.S., Overall, J.C., Jr., Herbst, J.J. et al: Clustering of neonatal necrotizing enterocolitis. Interruption by infection-control measures. N. Engl. J. Med. 297:984-986, 1977.
6. Bell, M.J., Ternberg, J.L., Feigin, R.E. et al: Neonatal necrotizing enterocolitis. Therapeutic decisions based upon clinical staging. Ann. Surg. 187:1-7, 1978.
7. Editorial: Necrotising enterocolitis. Lancet 1:459-460, 1977.
8. Frantz, I.D., III, L'Heureux, P., Engel, R.R. et al: Necrotizing enterocolitis. J. Pediatr. 86:259-263, 1975.
9. Santulli, T.V., Schullinger, J.N., Heird, W.C. et al: Acute necrotizing enterocolitis in infancy: A review of 64 cases. Pediatrics 55:376-387, 1975.
10. Polin, R.A., Pollack, P.F., Barlow, B. et al: Necrotizing enterocolitis in term infants. J. Pediatr. 89:460-462, 1976.

11. Bell, R.S., Graham, C.B. and Stevenson, J.K.: Roentgenologic and clinical manifestations of neonatal necrotizing enterocolitis. Experience with 43 cases. AJR 112:123-134, 1971.
12. Lister, J. and Rickham, P.P.: Necrotizing enterocolitis: Bacterial and meconium peritonitis. *In* Rickham, P.P., Lister, J. and Irving, I.M.: Neonatal Surgery, ed. 2. London:Butterworths, 1978, pp. 419-423.
13. Daneman, A., Woodward, S. and deSilva, M.: The radiology of neonatal necrotizing enterocolitis (NEC). A review of 47 cases and literature. Pediatr. Radiol. 7:70-77, 1978.
14. Gough, M.H.: The perinatal aspects of intestinal ischaemia. Clin. Gastroenterol. 1:675-687, 1972.
15. deSa, D.J.: The spectrum of ischemic bowel disease in the newborn. Perspect. Pediatr. Pathol. 3:273-309, 1976.
16. Gutman, L.T., Idriss, Z.H., Gehlbach, S. et al: Neonatal staphylococcal enterocolitis: Association with indwelling feeding catheters and S. aureus colonization. J. Pediatr. 88:836-839, 1976.
17. Speer, M.E., Taber, L.H., Yow, M.D. et al: Fulminant neonatal sepsis and necrotizing enterocolitis associated with "nonenteropathogenic" strain of Escherichia coli. J. Pediatr. 89:91-95, 1976.
18. Johnson, F.E., Crnic, P.M., Simmons, M.A. et al: Association of fatal Coxsackie B2 viral infection and necrotizing enterocolitis. Arch. Dis. Child. 52:802-804, 1977.
19. Howard, F.M., Flynn, D.M., Bradley, J.M. et al: Outbreak of necrotizing enterocolitis caused by Clostridium butyricum. Lancet 2:1099-1102, 1977.
20. Hopkins, G.B., Gould, V.E., Stevenson, J.K. et al: Necrotizing enterocolitis in premature infants. A clinical and pathologic evaluation of autopsy material. Am. J. Dis. Child. 120:229-232, 1970.
21. Bell, M.J., Ternberg, J.L., Askin, F.B. et al: Intestinal stricture in necrotizing enterocolitis. J. Pediatr. Surg. 11:319-327, 1976.
22. Bill, A.H., Jr. and Chapman, N.D.: The enterocolitis of Hirschsprung's disease. Its natural history and treatment. Am. J. Surg. 103:70-74, 1962.
23. Joshi, V.V., Draper, D.A. and Bates, R.D., III: Neonatal necrotizing enterocolitis. Occurrence secondary to thrombosis of abdominal aorta following umbilical arteral catheterization. Arch. Pathol. 99:540-543, 1975.
24. Bartlett, J.G. and Gorbach, S.L.: Pseudomembranous enterocolitis (antibiotic-related colitis). Adv. Int. Med. 22:455-476, 1977.
25. Tedesco, F.J., Barton, R.W. and Alpers, D.H.: Clindamycin-associated colitis. A prospective study. Ann. Intern. Med. 81:429-433, 1974.
26. Tedesco, F.J.: Clindamycin and colitis: A review. J. Infect. Dis. 135(Suppl.):S95-S98, 1977.
27. Editorial: Pseudomembranous enterocolitis. Lancet 1:839-840, 1977.
28. Gorbach, S.L. and Bartlett, J.G.: Pseudomembranous enterocolitis: A review of its diverse forms. J. Infect. Dis. 135(Suppl.):S89-S94, 1977.
29. Kelber, M. and Ament, M.E.: Shigella dysenteriae I: A forgotten cause of pseudomembranous colitis. J. Pediatr. 89:595-596, 1976.

30. Pettet, J.D., Baggenstoss, A.H., Dearing, W.H. et al: Postoperative pseudomembranous enterocolitis. Surg. Gynecol. Obstet. 98:546-5521 1954.
31. Tietjen, G.W. and Markowitz, A.M.: Colitis proximal to obstructing colonic carcinoma. Arch. Surg. 110:1133-1138, 1975.
32. Feldman, P.S.: Ulcerative disease of the colon proximal to partially obstructive lesions: Report of two cases and review of the literature. Dis. Colon Rectum 18:601-612, 1975.
33. Buts, J.-P., Weber, A.M., Roy, C.C. et al: Pseudomembranous enterocolitis in childhood. Gastroenterology 73:823-827, 1977.
34. Hoogland, T., Cooperman, A.M., Farmer, R.G. et al: Toxic megacolon-unusual complication of pseudomembranous colitis. Cleve. Clin. Q. 44:149-155, 1977 (Winter).
35. Tedesco, F.J., Anderson, C.B. and Ballinger, W.F.: Drug-induced colitis mimicking an acute surgical condition of the abdomen. Arch. Surg. 110:481-484, 1975.
36. Alschibaja, T. and Morson, B.C.: Ischaemic bowel disease. J. Clin. Pathol. 30(Suppl.): 68-77, 1977.
37. Rifkin, G.D., Fekety, F.R., Silva, J., Jr. et al: Antibiotic-induced colitis implication of a toxin neutralized by Clostridium sordellii antitoxin. Lancet 2:1103-1106, 1977.
38. Bartlett, J.G., Chang, T.W., Gurwith, M. et al: Antibiotic-associated pseudomembranous colitis due to toxin producing clostridia. N. Engl. J. Med. 298:531-534, 1978.
39. Price, A.B. and Davies, D.R.: Pseudomembranous colitis. J. Clin. Pathol. 30:1-12, 1977.
40. Sumner, H.W. and Tedesco, F.J.: Rectal biopsy in clindamycin associated colitis. An analysis of 23 cases. Arch. Pathol. 99:237-241, 1975.
41. Medline, A., Shin, D.H. and Medline, N.M.: Pseudomembranous colitis associated with antibiotics. Hum. Pathol. 7:693-703, 1976.
42. Stanley, R.J., Melson, G.L., Tedesco, F.J. et al: Plain-film findings in severe pseudomembranous colitis. Radiology 118:7-11, 1976.
43. Marston, A., Pheils, M.T., Lea Thomas, M. et al: Ischaemic colitis. Gut 7:1-15, 1966.
44. Mavor, G.E.: Acute occlusion of the superior mesenteric artery. Clin. Gastroenterol. 1:639-653, 1972.
45. Ernst, C.B., Hagihara, P.F., Daugherty, M.E. et al: Ischemic colitis incidence following abdominal aortic reconstruction: A prospective study. Surgery 80:417-421, 1976.
46. Kumar, P.J. and Dawson, A.M.: Vasculitis of the alimentary tract. Clin. Gastroenterol. 1:719-743, 1972.
47. Rodriquez, M.A.: Ischemic colitis and malignant atrophic papulosis. Am. J. Gastroenterol. 67:163-166, 1977.
48. Hoyle, M., Kennedy, A., Prior, A.L. et al: Small bowel ischaemia and infarction in young women taking oral contraceptives and progestational agents. Br. J. Surg. 64:533-537, 1977.
49. Marcuson, R.W.: Ischaemic colitis. Clin. Gastroenterol. 1:745-763, 1972.

50. McDonald, G.S.A. and O'B. Hourihane, D.: Ischaemic lesions of the alimentary tract. J. Clin. Pathol. 25:99-105, 1972.
51. Farmer, R.G., Hawk, W.A. and Turnbull, R.B.: Clinical patterns in Crohn's disease: A statistical study of 615 cases. Gastroenterology 68:627-635, 1975.
52. Ament, M.E.: Inflammatory disease of the colon: Ulcerative colitis and Crohn's colitis. J. Pediatr. 86:322-334, 1975.
53. Greenstein, A.J., Janowitz, H.D. and Sachar, D.B.: The extra-intestinal complications of Crohn's disease and ulcerative colitis: A study of 700 patients. Medicine (Baltimore) 55:401-412, 1976.
54. Ward, M.: The pathogenesis of Crohn's disease. Lancet 2:903-905, 1977.
55. Whorwell, P.J. and Wright, R.: Immunological aspects of inflammatory bowel disease. Clin. Gastroenterol. 5:303-321, 1976.
56. Lockhart-Mummery, H.E. and Morson, B.C.: Crohn's disease of the large intestine. Gut 5:493-509, 1964.
57. Price, A.B.: Overlap in the spectrum of non-specific inflammatory bowel disease — 'colitis indeterminate." J. Clin. Pathol. 31:567-577, 1978.
58. Price, A.B.: Difficulties in the differential diagnosis of ulcerative colitis and Crohn's disease. *In* Yardley, J.H., Morson, B.C. and Abell, M.R. (eds.): The Gastrointestinal Tract. Baltimore:The Williams and Wilkins Company, 1977, pp. 1-14.
59. Morson, B.C. and Dawson, I.M.P.: Gastrointestinal Pathology. Oxford:Blackwell Scientific Publications, 1972, pp. 448-486.
60. Margulis, A.R., Goldberg, H.I., Lawson, T.L. et al: The overlapping spectrum of ulcerative and granulomatous colitis: A roentgenographic-pathologic study. AJR 113:325-334, 1971.
61. Editorial: Toxic megacolon may complicate Crohn's disease. Br. Med. J. 3:723-724, 1975.
62. Homan, W.P., Tang, C-K. and Thorbjarnarson, B.: Acute massive hemorrhage from intestinal Crohn disease. Report of seven cases and review of the literature. Arch. Surg. 111:901-905, 1976.
63. Fisher, J., Mantz, F. and Calkins, W.G.: Colonic perforation in Crohn's disease. Gastroenterology 71:835-838, 1976.
64. Weedon, D.D., Shorter, R.G., Ilstrup, D.M. et al: Crohn's disease and cancer. N. Engl. J. Med. 289:1099-1103, 1973.
65. Bergstrand, O. and Holmstrom, B.: Recent studies on transmissible agents in Crohn's disease. Acta Chir. Scand. 482 (Suppl.):41-44, 1978.
66. Ahlberg, J., Bergstrand, O., Gillstrom, P. et al: Negative findings in search for a transmissible agent in Crohn's disease. Acta Chir. Scand. 482(Suppl.):45-47, 1978.
67. Beeken, W.L., Mitchell, D.N. and Cave, D.R.: Evidence for a transmissible agent in Crohn's disease. Clin. Gastroenterol. 5:289-302, 1976.
68. Parent, K. and Mitchell, P.: Cell wall-defective variants of Pseudomonas-like (group Va) bacteria in Crohn's disease. Gastroenterology 75:368-372, 1978.

69. Cave, D.R., Mitchell, D.N. and Brooke, B.N.: Experimental animal studies of the etiology and pathogenesis of Crohn's disease. Gastroenterology 68:618-624, 1975.
70. Meuwissen, S.G.M., Feltkamp-Vroom, T.M. and de la Riviere, A.B.: Analysis of the lympho-plasmacytic infiltrate in Crohn's disease with special reference to identification of lymphocyte-subpopulation. Gut 17:770-780, 1976.
71. Janowitz, H.D. and Sachar, D.B.: New observations in Crohn's disease. Annu. Rev. Med. 27:269-285, 1976.
72. Gryboski, J.D. and Spiro, H.M.: Prognosis in children with Crohn's disease. Gastroenterology 74:807-817, 1978.
73. Singer, H.C., Anderson, J.G.D., Frischer, H. et al: Familial aspects of inflammatory bowel disease. Gastroenterology 61:423-430, 1971.
74. Lewkonia, R.M. and McConnell, R.B.: Familial inflammatory bowel disease — heredity or environment? Gut 17:235-243, 1976.
75. Marshak, R.H.: Granulomatous disease of the intestinal tract (Crohn's disease). Radiology 114:3-22, 1974.
76. Haggitt, R.C. and Meissner, W.A.: Crohn's disease of the upper gastrointestinal tract. Am. J. Clin. Pathol. 59:613-622, 1973.
77. Cynn, W-S., Chon, H., Gureghian, P.A.: Crohn's disease of the esophagus. AJR 125:359-364, 1975.
78. Sommers, S.C.: Ulcerative and granulomatous colitis. AJR 130:817-823, 1978.
79. Laufer, I. and Costopoulos, L.: Early lesions of Crohn's disease. AJR 130:307-311, 1978.
80. Glass, R.E. and Baker, W.N.W.: Role of the granuloma in recurrent Crohn's disease. Gut 17:75-77, 1976.
81. Fawaz, K.A., Glotzer, D.J., Goldman, H. et al: Ulcerative colitis and Crohn's disease of the colon — a comparison of the long term postoperative courses. Gastroenterology 71:372-378, 1976.
82. Truelove, S.C. and Pena, A.S.: Course and prognosis of Crohn's disease. Gut 17:192-201, 1970.
83. Greenstein, A.J., Sachar, D.B., Pasternack, B.S. et al: Reoperation and recurrence in Crohn's colitis and ileocolitis. Crude and cumulative rates. N. Engl. J. Med. 293:685-690, 1975.
84. Goodman, M.J., Kirsner, J.B. and Riddell, R.H.: Usefulness of rectal biopsy in inflammatory bowel disease. Gastroenterology 72:952-956, 1977.
85. Korelitz, B.I. and Sommers, S.C.: Rectal biopsy in patients with Crohn's disease. Normal mucosa on sigmoidoscopic examination. JAMA 237:2742-2744, 1977.
86. Rotterdam, H., Korelitz, B.I. and Sommers, S.C.: Microgranulomas in grossly normal rectal mucosa in Crohn's disease. Am. J. Clin. Pathol. 67:550-554, 1977.
87. Ward, M. and Webb, J.N.: Rectal biopsy as a prognostic guide in Crohn's colitis. J. Clin. Pathol. 30:126-131, 1977.
88. Valdes-Dapena, A., Rudolph, I., Hidayat, A. et al: Adenocarcinoma of the small bowel in association with regional enteritis. Four new cases. Cancer 37:2938-294711976.

89. Nesbit, R.R., Jr., Elbadawi, N.A., Morton, J.H. et al: Carcinoma of the small bowel. A complication of regional enteritis. Cancer 37:2948-2959, 1976.
90. Greenstein, A.J., Sachar, D., Pucillo, A. et al: Cancer in Crohn's disease after diversion surgery. A report of seven carcinomas occurring in excluded bowel. Am. J. Surg. 135:86-90, 1978.
91. Fishman, R.S., Fleming, C.R. and Stephens, D.H.: Roentgenographic simulation of colonic cancer by benign masses in Crohn's colitis. Mayo Clin. Proc. 53:447-449, 1978.
92. Martinez, C.R., Siegelman, S.S., Saba, G.P. et al: Localized tumor-like lesions in ulcerative colitis and Crohn's disease of the colon. Johns Hopkins Med. J. 140:249-259, 1977.
93. Dordal, E., Glagov, S. and Kirsner, J.B.: Hepatic lesions in chronic inflammatory bowel disease. I. Clinical correlation with liver biopsy diagnoses in 103 patients. Gastroenterology 52:239-258, 1967.
94. Eade, M.N., Cooke, W.T., Brooke, B.N. et al: Liver disease in Crohn's colitis. A study of 21 consecutive patients having colectomy. Ann. Intern. Med. 74:518-528, 1971.
95. Kern, F., Jr.: Hepatobiliary disorders in inflammatory bowel disease. Prog. Liver Dis. 5:575-589, 1976.
96. Hill, G.S., Jr., Tabrisky, J. and Peter, M.E.: Tuberculous enteritis. West. J. Med. 124:440-445, 1976.
97. Tandon, H.D. and Prakash, A.: Pathology of intestinal tuberculosis and its distinction from Crohn's disease. Gut 13:260-269, 1972.
98. Kohl, S., Jacobson, J.A. and Nahmias, A.: Yersinia enterocolitica infections in children. J. Pediatr. 89:77-79, 1976.
99. Ekberg, Ol, Sjostrom, B. and Brahme, F.: Radiological findings in Yersinia ileitis. Radiology 123:15-19, 1977.
100. Vantrappen, G., Agg, H.O., Ponette, E. et al: Yersinia enteritis and enterocolitis: Gastroenterological aspects. Gastroenterology 72:220-227, 1977.
101. Klein, N.C., Hargrove, R.L., Sleisenger, M.H. et al: Eosinophilic gastroenteritis. Medicine (Baltimore) 49:299-319, 1970.
102. Robert, F., Omura, E. and Durant, J.R.: Mucosal eosinophilic gastroenteritis with systemic involvement. Am. J. Med. 77:139-143, 1977.
103. Haberkern, C.M., Christie, D.L. and Haas, J.E.: Eosinophilic gastroenteritis presenting as ileocolitis. Gastroenterology 74:896-899, 1978.
104. Foglia, R., Ament, M.E., Fleisher, D. et al: Surgical management of ulcerative colitis in childhood. Am. J. Surg. 134:58-63, 1977.
105. Werlin, S.L. and Grand, R.J.: Severe colitis in children and adolescents: Diagnosis, course, and treatment. Gastroenterology 73:828-832, 1977.
106. Strauss, R.J., Flint, G.W., Platt, N., et al.: The surgical management of toxic dilatation of the colon: A report of 28 cases and review of the literature. Ann. Surg. 184:682-688, 1976.
107. Morson, B.C. and Pang, L.S.C.: Rectal biopsy as an aid to cancer control in ulcerative colitis. Gut 8:423-434, 1967.

108. Riddell, R.H.: The precarcinomatous phase of ulcerative colitis. Curr. Top. Pathol. 63:179-220, 1976.
109. Gewertz, B.L., Dent, T.L. and Appelman, H.D.: Implications of precancerous rectal biopsy in patients with inflammatory bowel disease. Arch. Surg. 111:326-329, 1976.
110. Lennard-Jones, J.E., Morson, B.C., Ritchie, J.K. et al: Cancer in colitis: Assessment of the individual risk by clinical and histological criteria. Gastroenterology 73:1280-1289, 1977.
111. Dobbins, W.O., III, Stock, M. and Ginsberg, A.L.: Early detection and prevention of carcinoma of the colon in patients with ulcerative colitis. Cancer 40:2542-2548, 1977.
112. Isaacson, P.: Tissue demonstration of carcinoembryonic antigen (CEA) in ulcerative colitis. Gut 17:561-567, 1976.
113. Cavell, B., Hildebrand, H.: Meeuwisse, G.W. et al: Chronic inflammatory bowel disease. Clin. Gastroenterol. 6:481-486, 1977.
114. Morowitz, D.A. and Kirsner, J.B.: Mortality in ulcerative colitis: 1930 to 1966. Gastroenterology 57:481-490, 1969.
115. Devroede, G.J., Taylor, W.F., Sauer, W.G. et al: Cancer risk and life expectancy of children with ulcerative colitis. N. Engl. J. Med. 285:17-21, 1971.
116. James, E.M. and Carlson, H.C.: Chronic ulcerative colitis and colon cancer: Can radiographic appearance predict survival patterns? AJR 130:825-830, 1978.
117. Hughes, R.G., Hall, T.J., Block, G.E., et al.: The prognosis of carcinoma of the colon and rectum complicating ulcerative colitis. Surg. Gynecol. Obstet. 146:46-48, 1978.
118. Wagonfeld, J.B., Platz, C.E., Fishman, F.L. et al: Multicentric colonic lymphoma complicating ulcerative colitis. Am. J. Dig. Dis. 22:502-508, 1977.
119. Akwari, O.E., Van Heerden, J.A., Foulk, W.T. et al: Cancer of the bile ducts associated with ulcerative colitis. Ann. Surg. 181:303-309, 1975.
120. Yardley, J.H. and Donowitz, M.: Colo-rectal biopsy in inflammatory bowel disease. *In* Yardley, J.H., Morson, B.C. and Abell, M.R. (eds.): The Gastrointestinal Tract. Baltimore:The Williams and Wilkins Company, 1977, pp. 50-94.
121. Giacchino, J.L., Pickleman, J., Bartizal, J.R. et al: The therapeutic dilemma of acute amebic colitis and ulcerative colitis. Surg. Gynecol. Obstet. 146:599-603, 1978.
122. Tucker, P.C., Webster, P.D. and Kilpatrick, E.M.: Amebic colitis mistaken for inflammatory bowel disease. Arch. Intern. Med. 135:681-685, 1975.
123. Day, D.W., Mandal, B.K. and Morson, B.C.: The rectal biopsy appearance in Salmonella colitis. Histopathology 2:117-131, 1978.
124. Henson, D.: Cytomegalovirus inclusion bodies in the gastrointestinal tract. Am. J. Clin. Pathol. 93:477-482, 1972.
125. Simmons, R.L., Matas, A.J., Rattazzi, L.C. et al: Clinical characteristics of the lethal cytomegalovirus infection following renal transplantation. Surgery 82:537-546, 1977.

126. Cooper, H.S., Raffensperger, E.C., Jonas, L. et al: Cytomegalovirus inclusions in patients with ulcerative colitis and toxic dilatation requiring colonic resection. Gastroenterology 72:1253-1256, 1977.
127. Keren, O.F., Strandberg, J.D. and Yardley, J.H.: Intercurrent cytomegalovirus colitis in a patient with ulcerative colitis. Johns Hopkins Med. J. 136:178-182, 1975.
128. Peterson, R.B., Meseroll, W.P., Shrago, G.G. et al: Radiographic features of colitis associated with the hemolytic-uremic syndrome. Radiology 118:667-671, 1976.
129. Schwartz, D.L., Becker, J.M., So, H.B. et al: Segmental colonic gangrene: A surgical emergency in the hemolytic-uremic syndrome. Pediatrics 62:54-56, 1978.

Self-Evaluation Quiz

1. Surgical management of NEC in children is associated with a mortality of:
   a) 10%
   b) 30%
   c) 40%
   d) 60%
2. The differential diagnosis of NEC should include the necrotizing enterocolitis proximal to a congenitally stenotic segment of bowel, Hirschsprung's disease complicated by enterocolitis or thrombosis of the abdominal aorta after umbilical artery catheterization.
   a) True
   b) False
3. The mortality for Hirschsprung's colitis is as high as 25% to 30%.
   a) True
   b) False
4. Chronic inflammatory disease of the liver is one of the more serious complications of Crohn's disease.
   a) True
   b) False
5. Crypt abscesses, deep ulceration and vascular thrombosis are atypical features of pseudomembranous enterocolitis.
   a) True
   b) False
6. In a review of 107 postsurgical cases at Mayo Clinic, the small intestine only, or the small and large intestines together, were the sites of predilection for:

a) CUC
b) PME
c) Ischemic enterocolitis
d) CD

7. CD occurs to what extent in the population?
a) 6 to 8 cases/100,000
b) 8 to 14 cases/100,000
c) 2 to 4 cases/100,000
d) 2 to 4 cases/10,000

8. Neonatal necrotizing enterocolitis is most frequently localized to the left side of the small and large intestine.
a) True
b) False

Answers on page 721.

Medical Therapy in Inflammatory Bowel Disease: 1978

Howard M. Spiro, M.D.

Objectives

1. To recognize that ulcerative colitis is now seen as a result of differing host response rather than as the effect of a specific pathogen.
2. To recognize the disease's changing incidence and changing clinical expression, especially involving Crohn's disease.
3. To consider cancer prophylaxis in patients with ulcerative colitis.

Introduction

Inflammatory bowel disease seems to me to be a disorder which has changed considerably over the past 25 years, not only in the way it presents, but also in its frequency, its complications and even the people whom it affects. Five major problems are apparent.

No Clear Etiology

Bargen 25 years ago thought that bacilli, especially the Bargen bacillus, was the cause of ulcerative colitis. In 1978 viruses are thought to be the leading candidates for the cause of ulcerative colitis, or at least Crohn's colitis, but this is far from proven. Host factors, especially immune responses in the tissues, are popular items for consideration. Many gastroenterologists regard the spectrum of inflammatory bowel disease, which is now so wide, as simply the results of differing host responses to one or more infectious agents.

Howard M. Spiro, M.D., Yale University School of Medicine, New Haven, Conn.

One thing is certain — clinicians have returned to regarding "ulcerative colitis" as the end result of many different infectious disorders and that classical idiopathic ulcerative colitis is what is left over after specific infections have been excluded. Although it has long been known that shigellosis, tuberculosis and amebiasis can simulate ulcerative colitis sigmoidoscopically and even radiographically, it has not been so widely recognized that other infections can mimic ulcerative colitis. Over the past five years, in Connecticut at least, Salmonella has increasingly been associated with an acute fulminant bloody diarrhea and with a sigmoidoscopic and histologic picture difficult to tell from ulcerative colitis except for the rapid improvement without therapy and the recovery of Salmonella from the sigmoid culture. Presumably, some strains of Salmonella can now penetrate the mucosa just like Shigella. I now think first of Salmonella when I see a patient with acute bloody diarrhea without other symptoms.

One big conceptual advance in the physiology of diarrhea over the past ten years has been the demonstration of a general mechanism for watery diarrhea, the stimulation of intestinal secretion by a whole host of agents (cholera is the prototype) all of which seem to stimulate adenyl cyclase to bring about intestinal secretion. Our old friend *E. coli* has several injurious strains one of which produces a short-lived watery diarrhea, but another and probably equally important strain is not so well known because it can be detected only by sophisticated laboratory techniques requiring the eye of a rabbit. This strain is invasive and penetrates the mucosa to produce acute bloody diarrhea histologically and radiographically identical to ulcerative colitis. I believe that some of the acute short-lived bloody diarrheas which resemble ulcerative colitis and from which no specific agents have been recovered very probably are the result of an invasive *E. coli.* Such patients should not be deemed to have ulcerative colitis, as has been the case in the past, too often, especially when microabscesses have been found on biopsy because microabscesses are not as specific as believed 25 years ago. The microabscess has been found as a result of various toxins and even in ischemic colitis.

In these days of sexual freedom the wary clinician must keep in mind that rectal gonorrhea and venereally transmitted amebiasis are more common, as a cause of ulcerative proctitis, than ten years ago.

Changing Incidence [1]

Once a rare disease, which seemed to predominate among whites and particularly Jews, inflammatory bowel disease is now much more widespread. Where blacks constituted only six of 250 patients with inflammatory bowel disease admitted to the Yale-New Haven Hospital before 1970, they now seem much more frequently afflicted with Crohn's disease. In the Southwest ten years ago gastroenterologists did not recognize inflammatory bowel disease at all, but now they see it quite frequently. Whether this is a result of migration from the Northeast of susceptible patients, aggressive infectious agents, or simply gastroenterologists to make the diagnosis remains uncertain, but the phenomenon seems to be a real one. Inflammatory bowel disease is still rare among Asians, but patients are being reported from the West Coast.

It may seem paradoxical that the gastroenterologist suggests that ulcerative colitis, regional enteritis and Crohn's colitis which would sometimes seem so easy to separate often merge in a spectrum of inflammatory bowel disease. When the disorders are clearly separable, the prognosis is clearly different and the fact that we cannot separate 30% of our patients into clear categories should not make us conclude that when the categories are clear that the prognosis is the same. Children with terminal ileal disease alone do very much better than children with ileocolitis, and patients with Crohn's disease of the colon do very much worse than patients with ulcerative colitis. For that reason the clinician needs to have some kind of criteria, for prognostic reasons, if for no other even though currently therapy is about the same. Clinical "eyeball" criteria for Crohn's colitis include (a) normal rectal mucosa, (b) segmental colonic disease, (c) involvement of more than a foot of ileum or of the upper bowel or stomach, (d) anal and perianal disease and (e) confined perforations or fistulas. Clinically and histologically the fistula is the most important manifestation of the host response which we call Crohn's disease and is more important than the granuloma. Indeed, many of the clinical manifestations which the clinician thinks of as characteristic of Crohn's disease are simply the end result of fistulas and fissures.

Changing Clinical Manifestations [2]

A number of fascinating clinical observations remain for statistical confirmation. The apparent emergence of Crohn's colitis as a separate clinical disorder in the 1960s and its ever increasing predominance in hospitalized patients with inflammatory bowel disease in the 1970s is the most striking. Because fissures and fistulas are the hallmark of this disorder, it seems unlikely that the horrible anal disease, the fistulas which reach to almost all parts of the body, and the extensive recurrences after operation could have been overlooked by clinicians in the 1940s and 1950s. I am convinced that this is more than simply our awareness of the disorder.

Some changing manifestations are easy to pinpoint. Crohn's disease used to be a disease of the terminal ileum and is now much more often a disease of the colon. At Yale-New Haven Hospital in the decade 1955 to 1965 40% of patients under the age of 20 had only ileal disease but in 1965 to 1975 only 20% of patients had terminal ileal disease and 50% had ileocolitis. Part of this may be a change in referral patterns, but as most other centers are noting the same phenomenon, it seems to be a real one. This change in the major site of the disease is an important characteristic because in the 1970s the long-term prognosis of Crohn's disease seems to depend upon the site of the disease, that is, the small bowel is the easiest to treat and ileocolitis the most refractory.

Toxic megacolon seemed to be a very common problem in the 1960s, when it was first described as an entity, but many gastroenterologists now believe that it has become quite rare. Only one or two patients are seen a year at the Yale-New Haven Hospital now and very few seem to be present around the state in the hospitals of the Yale Affiliated Gastroenterology Program. Whether this is because of better therapy, an increasing number of gastroenterologists, or the result of some other influence I do not know.

What has happened to the familial incidence of the disorder is fascinating: Before 1955 the familial incidence of inflammatory bowel disease went unrecognized, but by the decade 1955 to 1965 the familial incidence rose to the 5% to 10% level, whereas in 1965 to 1975 the familial incidence at Yale-New Haven Hospital runs around 20%. These figures are echoed in different parts of the United States and go along with what appears to be a real increase in the disease.

Indeed the outlook after total colectomy depends upon whether the predominant response of the bowel is Crohn's colitis or ulcerative colitis. At Yale-New Haven Hospital 40% of patients whose colon was removed for Crohn's disease, followed for an average of nine years after colectomy, developed recurrent disease in the distal ileum and many have required a second operation. In contrast, no patient whose colon was removed for ulcerative colitis has had a recurrence in the distal ileum. Such experience suggests that the host response determines the outlook, and the way in which inflammatory bowel disease manifests itself is very important. Crohn's disease tends to be refractory to therapy.

Therapy of Crohn's Disease [1]

For a disorder as varied in presentation, and possibly in origin, as Crohn's disease, I despair of ever getting therapeutic answers for the individual patient from controlled studies. I note in part the great difficulty that such studies have in collecting comparable patients and the problems of (1) stratification, (2) observer bias and influence and (3) the general questions which controlled clinical studies, however popular, have raised. I note how inflammatory bowel disease generally and regional enteritis particularly have changed over the past 20 years and I believe that old studies are no longer pertinent. For such reasons I take a relatively empirical approach to the management of inflammatory bowel disease, keeping firmly in mind that (1) the physician should not make patients out of people from a misguided notion of what therapy can do and (2) the physician as placebo still has a large role in therapy, as studies of cimetidine in duodenal ulcer have taught. Therefore, I tell the person with regional enteritis discovered at an annual "health examination" who has neither diarrhea, weight loss nor abdominal pain to go about his business without thought to his x-rays.

In the patient with symptoms, however, I believe that dietary restriction is useful even if no very good controlled studies have proven the value of restricted fiber or low lactose programs. After all, vegetables and fruits have fiber now much vaunted to overcome constipation, contain such natural laxatives as oxyphenisatin and do hold much water in their fibrous interstices; moreover, fiber can obstruct the narrowed lumen. Therefore, it makes sense to me to restrict fiber in patients with cramps or diarrhea, but for symptomatic relief only; the patient should understand that fiber does not injure the bowel or worsen the disease, but its reduction simply makes life with an inflamed bowel more comfortable. In New Haven, where so many patients with regional enteritis are of Italian or Jewish background, I look for lactose intolerance, not because lactose has anything to do with the genesis of regional enteritis, but because the lesser fluid and osmotic load of a restricted lactose diet is easier for the secreting inflamed bowel to handle. If dietary restriction does not help, I abandon it.

Even after 30 years, sulfasalazine has a better press from the advertisers than from controlled studies. Some of the reservations already noted apply, but despite evidence of symptomatic improvement in some patients, the benefits of sulfasalazine in patients with regional enteritis remain far from obvious. Presumably, sulfasalazine helps some patients with Crohn's colitis or with regional enteritis and bacterial overgrowth in the small bowel because bacteria convert the parent drug into sulfapyridine and 5-amino salicylate and this latter compound inhibits prostaglandin synthesis and therefore decreases diarrhea [3]. Although I believe its possible benefits are somewhat greater in patients with colonic disease, I often try the effect of sulfasalazine in patients with symptoms from regional enteritis without any overwhelming expectations. I am convinced that sulfasalazine has no place in the prophylactic management of regional enteritis.

For the patient with diarrhea alone, I use a combination of dietary restriction, a hydrophylic colloid such as Metamucil, and drugs such as Lomotil, Imodium or codeine. It is sometimes hard to convince referring physicians that codeine 15 to 30 mg four times a day for diarrhea will not make drug addicts of their patients, but I prefer to use the small amount of codeine or Lomotil necessary for control of bowels rather than running the risks of continued administration of prednisone.

Although controlled studies are few, clinical experience convinces me that steroids have a place in the management of many patients with regional enteritis, even if they should be used more cautiously than is often the case. In the patient with anorexia, weight loss or malabsorption, 20 mg of prednisone twice daily often brings about rapid improvement of symptoms; after a week or so I usually suggest that the dose be cut by 5 mg every three or four days down to 20 mg per day. I advise that the 20 mg be taken as one dose in the morning to avoid upsetting the diurnal cycle [4]; after a week or two of continued clinical benefit, I ask the patient to continue to try to cut the steroid dosage by 2.5 mg over the next few weeks. Sometimes this is successful, but sometimes the steroid dosage needs to be maintained for several months; I keep trying to stop the steroids to avoid their long-term side effects. I find that many physicians do not rely on other measures to stop diarrhea and so increase the steroid dosage for its antidiarrheal effect, something I find unnecessary.

The patient ill enough to be in the hospital, I believe, benefits from intravenous steroids, if only to avoid the question of whether the oral dose is adequately absorbed. A controlled study could not detect any great difference between the effect of 40 mg of ACTH or 300 mg of hydrocortisone in an eight-hour drip, and so I use either one, preferring hydrocortisone for the patient who has taken steroids before entering the hospital. There has been no study of which I am aware measuring the effect of a 24-hour steroid drip, and so I do not give steroids for more than 8 hours, and I take its benefit to be pharmacological and not physiological. If IV steroids have not helped in the hospital after ten days, and in the patient with acute toxic megacolon in three, I advise colectomy; but over the past few years we have seen many fewer such patients, as the incidence of Crohn's colitis has increased and that of classical ulcerative colitis lessened.

None of the controlled studies of azathioprine in patients with Crohn's disease, including our own in patients with extensive regional enteritis, have convinced me that immunosuppression has much more to offer than a placebo. I have generally abandoned the use of azathioprine in patients with regional enteritis except in a very occasional patient to reduce steroid dosage or as a last ditch effort when neither operation nor other therapy has been helpful. A few reports suggest that fistulas may close under the benefit of immunosuppression, but I await the results of the national Crohn's disease study without great expectations.

Finally, there may be a place in therapy for metronidazole, but attempts to set up controlled studies have met with opposition from the FDA. I do not know whether levamisole, chromalyn or other drugs will be at all helpful.

Cancer Prophylaxis [5]

I am aware that carcinoma of the colon is apparently increased in frequency in patients with ulcerative colitis, that it is most likely to afflict patients who have had the disease since childhood and for more than ten years and who have total colonic involvement. I think that the incidence of cancer increases impressively somewhere between 10 and 20 years after the onset of colitis. I fear that studies at such large referral institutions as the Mayo Clinic may magnify the problem, however, simply because their superb clinical skills attract the most refractory patients who may have long resisted operation; statistics at such institutions often differ from others around the country. Since pathologists, radiologists and internists cannot always tell Crohn's colitis from ulcerative colitis, I find it easy to believe that there may be an increased occurrence of carcinoma in patients with Crohn's colitis equal to that in patients with ulcerative colitis, given the predilection of most chronic inflammatory processes to lead to an increased incidence of cancer. Yet in New Haven some years ago, only 0.2% of 250 patients who had been in the Yale-New Haven Hospital with ulcerative colitis had developed cancer of the colon, in part because total colectomy had already been carried out in two thirds of the patients with ulcerative colitis for intractability and one third of the patients with Crohn's colitis for anal and perianal disease. I therefore suspect that an aggressive surgical approach, in the past at least, has prevented the development of cancer in some patients. Total colectomy at Yale as an elective procedure still has a mortality rate of 3.1%, and the incidence of prestomal ileitis in patients after total colectomy for Crohn's colitis is 33%, so I do not advise an operation without firm reasons.

In the individual patient, therefore, I have adopted the concept that clinical criteria are useful but not absolute signposts to colon cancer susceptibility. Routinely for the past several years I have advised patients with ulcerative colitis, regardless of radiological extent, to undergo colonoscopy and multiple biopsies at about 10 cm intervals after they have had the disease for ten years. What the outcome of this study will be I do not know, but two patients have been instructive. The first had been asymptomatic for ten years after a single attack of toxic megacolon; since biopsies showed "dysplasia" without evidence of inflammation, he underwent "prophylactic" total colectomy, with the discovery of a grade B Dukes' colon carcinoma which had not been seen at colonoscopy. Another patient, with Crohn's colitis, had had colonoscopy in 1976 with normal findings at biopsy and returned in 1977 asking for a repeat colonoscopy which I was loathe to offer. Biopsies revealed considerable dysplasia, and he too underwent colectomy with a discovery of a grade B colon cancer not seen at colonoscopy.

Such anecdotal experiences, taken with the growing judgment in the literature, make me continue to believe that colonoscopy with multiple biopsies makes better sense than prophylactic colectomy, but I do not know how often colonoscopy should be carried out. At present I suggest a two- or three-year interval, but I advise patients who have had colitis for ten years to undergo sigmoidoscopy and rectal biopsy in the year in which they do not undergo colonoscopy.

References

1. Spiro, H.M.: Clinical Gastroenterology. Ulcerative Colitis. New York: Macmillan, 1977, pp. 739-752.
2. Gryboski, J.D. and Spiro, H.M.: Prognosis in children with Crohn's disease. Gastroenterology 74:807-817, 1978.
3. Khan, A.K., Piris, P. and Truelove, S.C.: An experiment to determine the active therapeutic moiety of sulfasalazine. Lancet 2:892-895, 1977.
4. Streeten, D.H.: Corticosteroids therapy. JAMA 232:944-947, 1975.
5. Dobbins, W.O.: Current status of the precancer lesion in ulcerative colitis. Gastroenterology 73:1431-33, 1977.

Self-Evaluation Quiz

1. Ulcerative colitis is more common now because of:
   a) *E. coli*
   b) Gonorrhea
   c) *Trichomonas vaginalis*
   d) Benzene derivatives in foodstuffs
2. Inflammatory bowel disease is rarer in Jews than in Asians.
   a) True
   b) False
3. Clinical "eyeball" criteria for Crohn's colitis include:
   a) Pathologic rectal mucosa
   b) Segmental colonic disease
   c) Involvement of less than 6 inches of ileum
   d) Absence of anal and perianal pathology
4. Clinically and histopathologically, the fistula is the most important evidence of host response, even more important than granuloma.
   a) True
   b) False
5. In patients with symptoms of Crohn's disease, dietary restriction is:
   a) Useful
   b) Useless
   c) Mandatory
   d) Good only if the patient suggests it
6. There is no place in the prophylactic management of regional enteritis for:
   a) Metamucil
   b) Sulfasalazine
   c) Codeine
   d) Lomotil
7. Mayo Clinic statistics should be used *cum grano salis* because:
   a) Undue numbers of refractory patients are attracted there
   b) Mayo statistics are unreliable at the $p = 0.05$ level
   c) All Mayo cases are terminal
   d) All Mayo cases are from only one demographic stratum
8. Total colectomy as an elective procedure at Yale has a mortality rate of:

a) 2.0%
b) 3.1%
c) 4.2%
d) 5.1%

9. Incidence of prestomal ileitis in patients after total colectomy for Crohn's colitis (at Yale) is:
   a) 16%
   b) 22%
   c) 33%
   d) 46%

Answers on page 721.

Surgical Aspects of Regional Enteritis

John C. Goligher, M.D.

Objectives

To differentiate large bowel Crohn's disease from the classical type and to become familiar with the pathognomy, diagnosis, treatment and frequency of ileal recurrence and other postsurgical problems.

Regional enteritis, or, as we prefer to call it in England, Crohn's disease [1], comes in many different forms and can occur anywhere in the alimentary tract from the mouth to the anus or entirely outside the gastrointestinal system, as in the skin of the submammary region. But in the vast majority of the cases the intestine is affected. From the practical surgical point of view it is convenient to recognize two forms. One is classical Crohn's disease, as described by Crohn and his collaborators in the early 1930s, where the condition affects mainly the small bowel, particularly the distal ileum, sometimes extending into the cecum or right colon.

In typical classical Crohn's ileitis, the bowel is thickened and congested. One cannot easily convey the heavy feel of the bowel, which resembles that of a piece of hosepipe. Actually, Crohn was preceded in his description of this disease by a surgeon in Glasgow, Sir Kennedy Dalziel [2], who described a number of cases 15 or 20 years earlier. He referred to the feel of the diseased segment as being like that of "an eel in a state of rigor mortis!" I have never felt an eel in a state of rigor mortis

John C. Goligher, M.D., Consultant in General and Colorectal Surgery, Leeds, England; Emeritus Professor of Surgery, University of Leeds; formerly Surgeon, The General Infirmary at Leeds; Consulting Surgeon, St. Mark's Hospital for Diseases of the Rectum and Colon, London, England.

but have handled a hosepipe quite frequently and can assure you that this is the characteristic feel of Crohn's enteritis.

Another feature of Crohn's disease of the small bowel is "skipping" which is present in 25% or 30% of the cases. I have operated on a number of patients who have had as many as 25 to 30 "skip" lesions throughout the small intestine.

Classical Crohn's disease, if it comes to operation, usually involves small bowel resection, often a terminal ileal segment with or without a partial right colectomy. By and large, the results of this treatment are not very satisfactory. In fact, there is a rather depressingly high incidence of recurrence. Most surgeons are very familiar with the manifestations and its treatment. Therefore, I will concentrate my discussion mainly on the other form of Crohn's disease — the form to which our attention was drawn in the late 1950s and early 1960s by a number of workers, such as Bryan Brooke [3] and Charles Wells [4] in England, Richard Marshak [5] in the United States and, above all, by Lockhart-Mummery and Morson [6], who really put this condition on the map. Large bowel Crohn's disease may affect perhaps a small segment of the colon or of the rectum, looking rather like a rectal carcinoma. But usually it is more extensive, involving the whole of the large intestine. In addition it may show "skipping" as in the small intestine. But perhaps the most typical appearance of large bowel Crohn's disease is when the condition affects the terminal ileum, the right colon, the transverse colon, the descending colon and then fades out in the sigmoid or upper rectum [6A].

My experience with Crohn's disease has been concerned much more with the large bowel type. About 70% of the 517 patients I personally have treated have had the large bowel type, which is a much higher proportion than seen in most other series. Why is that so? I think it is because I have had a special interest in ulcerative colitis and that has resulted in many referrals of patients labeled as suffering from colitis, who, when more carefully examined, are found to have, not colitis, but Crohn's disease of the large bowel. The distinction is actually quite easy, as a rule. It can be made on radiological, clinical and sigmoidoscopic findings. I am not going to mention the radiologic findings, as Marshak has explained with clarity and forcefulness the differences between Crohn's colitis and ordinary ulcerative colitis. But I shall say something about the clinical differentiation.

One of the things that often distinguishes these patients very quickly is the anal manifestations. The presence of broad anal fissures or fistulas is very suggestive that what you are dealing with is not ulcerative colitis but Crohn's colitis. Edema of the anal region is also strongly indicative of Crohn's colitis. Very severe ulceration of the anal and perianal region is absolutely pathognomonic of Crohn's disease. On sigmoidoscopy, if the rectum is normal in a patient with radiologic colitis, that makes the diagnosis pretty definitely one of Crohn's colitis. Or, if the rectum is involved in a patchy manner, that is highly diagnostic of Crohn's disease. Then you can proceed to biopsies. This would seem to be a potentially very helpful step, but I would like to emphasize that the biopsy is only as good as the pathologist. Many pathologists are not very interested in this differentiation and they return equivocal reports which are of little use to the clinician.

About treatment of Crohn's disease of the large bowel, I would like to make an important point, namely, that Crohn's disease of the large bowel often does very well on medical treatment of exactly the same kind used for ulcerative colitis. Contrary to what many people think, it pursues an up-and-down course rather like colitis. If you can get over a severe exacerbation with steroids and azulfadine the patient may be very well for a year or so without significant symptoms. There is much to be said for trying the full gamut of medical treatment, and that is my policy. Of the 352 patients with large bowel Crohn's disease I have treated [6A], no less than 70% have come to operation, whereas in most other published series the operation rate is more like 40% or 35%. I do not think I am more inclined to operate than others; the reason so many of my patients have come to operation is that they are referred to me so often specifically for operation after many courses of medical treatment have failed. Though I may stall on surgical treatment for a while, in many instances it becomes necessary.

If the lesion is localized, it may be possible to do a limited resection with anastomosis. But far more frequently the disease is extensive in the large bowel and it is necessary to do the same sort of wide excision that is employed in the treatment of ulcerative colitis — colectomy and ileostomy, proctocolectomy and ileostomy, colectomy and ileorectal anastomosis. I would like to mention that last operation first, because I am not a great enthusiast for colectomy and ileorectal anastomosis for ordinary ulcerative colitis insofar as it means keeping and using a diseased rectum. But in 25% to 30% of cases of Crohn's disease of the large bowel, the rectum is normal and there would seem to be a good indication here for colectomy and ileorectal anastomosis.

Forty-eight of my patients [6A] were treated by this operation, none suffering from acute phases of the disease. No less than three leaked in the immediate postoperative period, one of whom died, the other two being saved by a relaparotomy and dismantling of the anastomosis, bringing out the ileum as an ileostomy. One other patient was lost to follow-up. Forty-four patients were available for follow-up who had operations performed between 1960 and 1977. Nearly 60% have developed recurrences, which is very daunting. Other people have had similar experiences, for example, St. Mark's Hospital [7] and Birmingham, in England [8]. Turnbull [9] of Cleveland is a great advocate of this procedure for Crohn's disease, but if you study his results or talk to him, you find that he has quite a lot of recurrences also. It is true to say also that he uses this operation infrequently — I think in only about 4% of all the Crohn's cases at the Cleveland Clinic [10]. We have used it rather more frequently and that may be responsible for our particularly bad results. I imagine that surgeons will continue to employ this operation and, when people get recurrences, to reoperate and convert to a terminal ileostomy and rectal excision. There is a reasonable argument for doing a loop ileostomy just proximal to an ileorectal anastomosis as a safety precaution against anastomotic leakage or rather the serious consequences of such leakage. My own inclination when I have a patient with Crohn's disease which does not seem to involve the rectum, and there is doubt about whether it involves the sigmoid, is to do a subtotal colectomy and ileostomy leaving a rectal stump. Then, after 6 or 12 months, if on repeated sigmoidoscopic surveys the rectum remains normal, the patient regains normal health and is keen to be joined up again, I am willing to try a secondary ileorectal anastomosis provided that the patient fully understands that success cannot be guaranteed. By that stage many of the patients have become content with their ileostomies and prefer not to gamble on a further major operation.

Far more frequently the surgeon must advise an operation involving an ileostomy, with proctocolectomy or subtotal colectomy or, occasionally, in cases with very localized rectal lesions, an abdominoperineal excision with an iliac colostomy. When surgery for this form of Crohn's disease began in the early 1960s, the idea gained credence that people with large bowel Crohn's disease were going to do better than people with small bowel lesions treated surgically. I have been interested over the period that has elapsed since to see what has happened in actual practice. The series reported by Nugent et al [11] from the Lahey Clinic had almost no recurrences. The series from St. Mark's Hospital in London, Ritchie and Lockhart-Mummery [12], had also a low recurrence rate. But the series from Birmingham, England [13], showed frequent recurrences, as did the series from Mt. Sinai Hospital [14] with incidences of nearly 100% in patients followed for 15 years. A series of our own, reported nearly ten years ago [15], came somewhere in between these other groups with regard to recurrence, but rather closer to Nugent et al [11] and Lockhart-Mummery [6]. How does one explain these differences? I do not know. But when I am faced with such differences in evidence the best solution is to see what the results are in my own patients. That is obviously more relevant for my practice than what is being seen at Mt. Sinai or at Birmingham or at St. Mark's Hospital.

So recently I surveyed my results in the cases I treated from 1960 to 1977 by ileostomy and excision or colostomy and excision [6A]. No patients who had previous resections or bypass operations were included. There were 15 operative deaths, which may seem quite a high mortality, but as I explained, Crohn's disease of the large bowel is very like ulcerative colitis in its presentation. We get many patients presenting with acute manifestations of toxic megacolon who require the same sort of urgent surgical treatment as ulcerative colitis. Of the 15 deaths, ten were in the group of 35 patients who were operated on in acute stages. Allowing for that fact, the elective operative mortality is not so discreditable. A certain number of the patients were subsequently converted from ileostomy and subtotal colectomy to an ileorectal anastomosis and were deleted from this survey of the results of patients with stomas. A certain number died subsequently from related or unrelated causes and a few were lost to follow-up. So we were left with 144 patients who have been followed after operation, some of the operations being done as long ago as 1960, others as recently as one year ago.

The recurrence rate in that series is 13.2%. I am referring to ileal recurrence. With a subtotal colectomy and an ileostomy in a certain number of those patients, disease appears in the rectum, either as a continuation of the condition at the time of the operation or as a subsequent recurrence. Let us not confuse the issue by dealing with rectal manifestations, but consider only the ileal recurrences.

First, the recurrences take place usually just above the stoma. When you get recurrences after an anastomotic operation for Crohn's disease, it nearly always is proximal to the anastomosis. When it recurs after an operation giving the patient a stoma, the recurrence is usually just above the stoma. That generalization applies to most recurrences but not quite all; there are a very few who had recurrence higher up in the small intestine.

Second, you might think that the people more likely to get recurrence would be those who had involvement not only of the large bowel but also of the terminal ileum. But analysis of our cases shows that there is no significant difference in the incidence of ileal recurrence depending upon whether the lower ileum had been involved at the time of the original operation.

Third, people who have Crohn's disease when they are young tend to do rather badly. That certainly applies to my large bowel cases for there have been more recurrences in young patients.

Fourth, the most important thing is the length of follow-up. There are all sorts of sophisticated ways of expressing the cumulative incidence of recurrence with graphs which tend to conceal the fact that the longer you follow the cases, the smaller the series becomes and the less valid the conclusions to be drawn from it. The recurrence for the whole series followed for 1 to 18 years is 13%. When you consider only patients who have been followed for at least five years, it is approximately 18%. For those who have been followed for ten years and more it is 37%, and for those with at least a 15 year follow-up it is 43%. In other words, our experience confirms a trend revealed by other writers [13, 14], although the rate of accumulation of recurrences is not as rapid as in these other two series.

What are you to do about patients with ileal recurrence? They present a problem because they have usually had some ileum removed at the time of that original operation in addition to a proctocolectomy or subtotal colectomy. Further surgery means sacrifice of more small bowel. Yet, quite a number of my patients have come to further operation because they have had troublesome abscesses or fistulae in connection with ileal recurrent disease or have had other symptoms that have forced an operation. I have operated on these patients and on quite a number of others with recurrence who have been referred. I have operated on 75 patients for recurrence [6A]. Some of them after ileostomy and colectomy or proctocolectomy, others after colectomy and ileorectal anastomosis. They have all been treated by excision of the recurrence and a fresh ileostomy. There were three operative deaths, no patients were lost to follow-up and there were only two subsequent deaths, which left 70 patients for follow-up. How have they behaved?

Comparing the results of that follow-up for subsequent or second recurrence with the figures for recurrence after excision of primary large bowel Crohn's disease, we found that the incidence of recurrence was not very different in the two series: 13% vs. 17%, 18% vs. 26%, 37% vs. 33% and 43% vs. 37% for follow-ups of 1 to 18 years, 5 to 18 years, 10 to 18 years and 15 to 18 years, respectively. It is rather surprising that recurrence is not more frequent in the reoperation cases, because you might have expected that a patient who has had recurrent Crohn's disease and who has another operation would be more predisposed to further recurrence. But that does not seem to be true in our experience. There is some consolation in these figures because it could be that a patient might have an operation for primary Crohn's disease of the large bowel, do very well for 10 or 12 years, and then get a recurrence, have another operation and go on for another 10 or 12 years. But, nonetheless, this high recurrence rate is disappointing and I think one must admit that surgical treatment of Crohn's disease of the colon and rectum leaves a great deal to be desired in comparison with that for ordinary ulcerative colitis.

I have emphasized the frequency of recurrence, which is the main shortcoming of operation for Crohn's disease of the large bowel. However I must draw attention to two or three other weaknesses of large bowel Crohn's surgery. One is that after operation there is often considerable difficulty in securing healing of the perineal wound if the rectum is excised. Although some healed primarily or at least fairly quickly, others took a long while, some seemed to go on forever. A number have required further operations, some successful, others have permanent sinuses. It appears at first sight a very unsatisfactory state of affairs, but in fact sometimes the sinus is not much trouble to the patient, though it is obviously a blemish on the results of one's efforts. But I know of no way of avoiding sinuses in some patients after rectal excision.

Another snag to large bowel Crohn's surgery is that these operations are labeled proctocolectomy or subtotal colectomy or colectomy with ileorectal anastomosis, but that is not the whole story. Nearly always there is a bit of terminal ileum and sometimes a lot of terminal ileum removed. This may have considerable influence on the patient with an ileostomy, for the fecal discharge will tend to be a good deal more liquid than that of the average ulcerative colitis patient, which will make stoma care more difficult. Usually these patients must employ antidiarrheal drugs like codeine, Lomotil or, perhaps best of all, loperamide to try to make the motion firmer. They must be very careful about the skin, using agents such as Stomahesive to keep the appliance in position and avoid leakage.

I recently made a survey of some of our patients to see just how much trouble they were having with their ileostomies. A number had no trouble at all, a certain number had minor troubles but they did not find ileostomy much of an inconvenience. However, a certain number really had considerable trouble. As you would expect, the people who had had reresections and consequently more ileum removed were the ones who had less satisfactory results.

Yet another drawback to operations for Crohn's disease of the large bowel, relating also to the frequent necessity for sacrifice of some of the precious lower small bowel, is the interference with the enterohepatic circulation of bile acids and consequent predisposition to the formation of cholesterol gallstones, as a recent study of my cases has shown [16].

A general overall assessment of the patients, rather like the Visick grading which we apply to our patients who have had operations for peptic ulcer, indicates that 81% of my patients having operations for primary disease were really very pleased, 15% were somewhat dissatisfied and 4% had poor results. With operations for recurrent disease, obviously the results were not so good.

References

1. Crohn, B.B., Ginsburg, L. and Oppenheimer, G.D.: Regional enteritis. JAMA 99:1323, 1932.
2. Dalziel, T.K.: Chronic interstitial enteritis. Br. Med. J. 2:1068, 1913.
3. Brooke, B.N.: Granulomatous disease of the intestine. Lancet 2:745, 1959.
4. Wells, C.A.: Ulcerative colitis and Crohn's disease. Ann. R. Coll. Surg. Engl. 11:105, 1952.
5. Marshak, R.H., Wolf, B.S. and Eliasoph, J.: Segmental colitis. Radiology 73:707, 1959.
6. Lockhart-Mummery, H.E. and Morson, B.C.: Crohn's disease (regional enteritis) of the large intestine and its distinction from ulcerative colitis. Gut 1:87, 1960.

6A. Goligher, J.C.: The outcome of excision for Crohn's disease of the large bowel. Surg. Gynecol. Obstet. In press, 1979.

7. Baker, W.N.W.: Ileorectal anastomosis for Crohn's disease of the colon. Gut 12:427, 1971.
8. Burman, J.H., Cooke, W.T. and Williams, J.A.: The fate of ileorectal anastomosis in Crohn's disease. Gut 12:432, 1971.
9. Turnbull, R.B., Jr.: The surgical approach to the treatment of inflammatory bowel disease: A personal view of techniques and prognosis. *In* Kirsner, J.B. and Shortner, R.G. (eds.): Inflammatory Bowel Disease. Philadelphia:Lee and Febiger, 1975, p. 338.
10. Lefton, H.B., Farmer, R.G. and Fazid, V.: Ileorectal anastomosis for Crohn's disease of the colon. Gastroenterology 69:612, 1975.
11. Nugent, F.W., Veidenheimer, M.C., Meissner, W.A. and Haggitt, R.C.: Prognosis after colonic resection for Crohn's disease of the colon. Gastroenterology 65:398, 1973.
12. Ritchie, J.K. and Lockhart-Mummery, H.E.: Non-restorative surgery in the treatment of Crohn's disease of the large bowel. Gut 14:263, 1973.
13. Steinberg, D.M., Allan, R.N., Thompson, A. et al: Excisional surgery with ileostomy for Crohn's colitis with particular reference to factors affecting recurrence. Gut 15:845, 1974.

14. Korelitz, B.I., Present, D.H., Alpert, L.I. et al: Recurrent regional ileitis after ileostomy and colectomy for granulomatous colitis. N. Engl. J. Med. 287:110, 1972.
15. De Dombal, F.T., Burton, I. and Goligher, J.C.: Recurrence of Crohn's disease after primary excisional surgery. Gut 12:519, 1971.
16. Hill, G.L., Mair, W.S.T. and Goligher, J.C.: Gallstones after ileostomy and ileal resection. Gut 16:932, 1975.

Self-Evaluation Quiz

1. A drawback to surgery for Crohn's disease of the large bowel is the interference with the enterohepatic circulation of bile acids and consequent predisposition to:
   a) Phosphate renal stones
   b) Excess cholesterol in the blood
   c) Cholesterol gallstones
   d) Bile overflow
2. The study of Hill, Mair and Goligher deals with:
   a) Pituitary influence on gravel in Crohn's disease patients
   b) Bile acids and gallstones
   c) Hepatotoxic feedback
   d) Nothing to do with Crohn's disease
3. The rectum is normal in what percentage of Crohn's large bowel disease?
   a) 20%
   b) 25% to 30%
   c) 37% to 47%
   d) 80%
4. Recurrences take place usually just above the stoma.
   a) True
   b) False
5. Recurrences after an anastomotic operation for Crohn's disease are:
   a) Always proximal to the anastomosis
   b) Nearly always proximal to the anastomosis
   c) Nearly always distal to the anastomosis
   d) Always (ie, every case of the author's) distal to the anastomosis
6. What feature of Crohn's disease of the small bowel occurs in 25% or 30% of the patients?
   a) Edematous foci
   b) Stricture

   c) Skipping
   d) Masking
7. Surgically, Crohn's disease can be classified as:
   a) Classical, subclassical and large bowel
   b) Classical and large bowel
   c) Crohn's ileitis and classical
   d) Crohn's ileitis, subclassical and classical
8. Crohn's large bowel disease often does very well on medical treatment of exactly the same kind used for ulcerative colitis.
   a) True
   b) False

Answers on page 721.

The Operative Approach to Ulcerative Colitis

John Alexander-Williams, M.D.

Objectives

1. To review the indications for emergency surgery in ulcerative colitis.
2. To review the indications for elective surgery.
3. To consider details of the management of the posterior space.

Introduction

Before the achievements of Brooke, Crile and Turnbull in perfecting the eversion ileostomy, surgery was considered the last desperate resort in the treatment of ulcerative colitis. By 1952 Brooke had achieved such good technical results in ileostomy management that he stated that a proctocolectomy and a permanent ileostomy could be offered to all patients suffering chronic ill-health or socially devastating diarrhea.

Twenty-five years ago once the patient had a full knowledge of the significance of the operation for ulcerative colitis, the operative approach was to perform a panproctocolectomy, either in one or two stages. Our opinions have changed somewhat during the last 25 years. At present the indications for surgical intervention in ulcerative colitis in patients treated on our Unit in Birmingham are as follows:

1. Emergency Operations
    a. Unresponsive fulminant disease
    b. Toxic dilatation or perforation
    c. Hemorrhage

John Alexander-Williams, M.D., Chairman of Gastroenterology Group, University of Birmingham, Birmingham, England.

2. Elective Operations
   a. Incapacitating diarrhea
   b. Chronic ill-health
   c. Malignancy

Emergency Operations

Indications

1. If a patient with acute fulminant ulcerative colitis fails to respond adequately to 48 hours of intensive medical therapy. Such a definition allows room to maneuver around the definition of the terms adequate and intensive. If a patient is admitted ill and dehydrated with profuse diarrhea, electrolyte disturbance and usually anemia, we treat him or her with bed rest, intravenous fluid blood replacement and parenteral steroid therapy. Less ill patients who are taking well by mouth are given sulfasalazine. Seriously ill patients are treated with continuous nasogastric suction. Unless a local septic complication is evident, systemic antibiotics are not given. Failure of improvement of the vital signs or abdominal signs within 48 hours leads us to consider emergency surgical treatment. However, these rules are not adequate. Patients with some signs of improvement are reassessed repeatedly.

2. Some patients are admitted in a state of toxic dilatation. Fortunately rarely, some patients are admitted with free perforation and peritonitis. We consider that both complications are avoidable by prompt medical treatment of acute exacerbations of colitis. During the past ten years we have had to operate on a patient with toxic dilatation of the colon only rarely and in the past eight years no patient with perforation of the colon due to colitis has been seen in our Unit.

3. Continued hemorrhage from the large bowel requiring repeated transfusions is now a rare indication for surgical treatment in ulcerative colitis. In our experience it is much less common now than it was 20 years ago.

Colonic bleeding in ulcerative colitis almost always stops in response to adequate medical treatment. However, continued severe bleeding, particularly in the young person, is an indication for mesenteric angiography to demonstrate the bleeding site. In our experience sigmoidoscopy and colonoscopy are poor means of demonstrating the site of bleeding.

Management

1. Emergency operation for fulminant disease should be a total colectomy with preservation of the rectum and a small portion of the sigmoid, sufficient to allow it to reach the abdominal wall as a mucous fistula. The only exceptions to this policy are patients who are known to be bleeding actively from the rectum and patients who are known to have a rectum so severely damaged that they were considered for elective panproctocolectomy before the acute exacerbation that necessitated emergency surgery. My reasons for advocating retention of the rectum in emergency surgery are (1) not removing the rectum decreases the length and severity of the emergency operation and decreases the blood loss and (2) patients having to be operated upon because of an acute exacerbation, particularly if it is early in the course of the disease, may have a rectal mucosa capable of recovery sufficient to permit later ileorectal anastomosis.

Alternatives to the creation of a mucous fistula of the distal bowel are to close the rectal stump. Even with extraperitoneal isolation this is a dangerous maneuver and not to be recommended. There is significant risk of breakdown of the rectal closure, with disastrous results. A second alternative is primary ileorectal anastomosis. I have used this to good effect in patients with fulminant disease principally affecting the descending colon and transverse colon with relative rectal sparing. In this situation I perform a total colectomy with a primary ileorectal anastomosis at the level of the pelvic brim, protecting the anastomosis and bypassing the rectum by means of a temporary loop ileostomy. Once anastomotic integrity has been confirmed by contrast radiology and the patient's health returned to normal the loop ileostomy is closed.

2. Toxic dilatation perforation. If a surgeon finds himself in the potentially disastrous situation of operating on a patient with perforated necrotic bowel as a result of neglected fulminant ulcerative colitis, the recommended operation is still a total colectomy and, if the sigmoid is viable, a mucous fistula. In this situation I strongly advise against the ileostomy and multiple "blow-hole" colostomies. Even in the rare instance when there is a walled-off intraperitoneal abscess as a result of perforated fulminant colitis, I still do not advise "blow-hole"

colostomy management. The walling off and isolation of the perforation is rarely adequate to be trusted. I have shared with many others the disasters of employing this technique after it was first advocated. If the colon has not yet perforated, even though it is necrotic and friable, total colectomy can be achieved by very careful dissection. If perforation has occurred, or occurs during the operation, the patient is at risk of succumbing to overwhelming sepsis. I believe that such a situation can be transformed from potential disaster to success by careful physical debridement of all phlegmenous exudate from the peritoneal cavity and repeated lavage with 10 liters of normal saline. One liter is instilled into the peritoneal cavity, agitated and then aspirated as completely as possible. Even if as much as 100 ml remain after drainage of the peritoneal cavity, a tenfold dilution of the contaminant will have been achieved. Ten tenfold dilutions will reduce even the grossest contamination to insignificant levels. Appropriate chemotherapy against both aerobic and anaerobic organisms further decreases the risk.

Elective Operations

Indications

1. The most common indications for elective surgery in ulcerative colitis are persistent incapacitating symptoms such as urgency and frequency of stools. Patients whose social and working life is marred by the constant necessity to defecate will frequently choose an ileostomy life in preference to a colitis life.

2. Chronic ill-health as a result of loss of blood and protein from the ulcerated bowel will cause physicians to advise removal of the ulcerated bowel.

3. Elective operations for ulcerative colitis were once advised because of cancer risk. To operate when symptomatic cancer supervenes is far too late and, if the patient was known to be suffering from colitis, indicates inadequate supervision.

It is well known that patients with ulcerative colitis have an increased risk of developing colonic carcinoma. If the colitis is confined to the rectum and distal sigmoid, the risk does not appear to be significantly greater than that in the normal population. If more of the colon is involved, the risk becomes significant, particularly when the patient has had the disease for more than 10 years. Those particularly at risk are patients whose colitis began at an early age, involves the whole colon and runs a chronic continuous course.

Management

Patients suffering urgent diarrhea are rarely suitable candidates for a total colectomy and ileorectal anastomosis. Most require panproctocolectomy and permanent ileostomy.

Patients operated upon because of chronic blood and protein loss may have relative rectal sparing. In such situations many authorities have reported a 70% permanent success rate with total colectomy and ileorectal anastomosis. Our own series has begun too recently for a good long-term assessment to be made, but in the short term more than 50% of our patients having ileorectal anastomosis are symptomatically well controlled.

At one time patients were advised to have a prophylactic proctocolectomy after eight to ten years if they were considered to be at high risk. We should now be able to detect cancer at an early and curable stage. At one time it was felt that carcinoma complicating ulcerative colitis had a poorer prognosis than carcinoma of the colon in the rest of the population. Our experience does not support this view; with early detection by colonoscopy/biopsy, it should be possible to detect early lesions at a curable stage and spare the majority, who will not develop carcinoma, from having unnecessary ablative surgery.

The problem with the early detection of carcinoma in ulcerative colitis is that the malignant lesions are not like ordinary carcinoma of the colon and do not necessarily begin in polyps or produce proliferative lesions. They often begin as infiltrating flat malignant plaques that do not give the characteristic radiological signs of colonic carcinoma. Furthermore, their appearance on colonoscopy is not typical of carcinoma and so multiple biopsies are essential for adequate surveillance.

Before the advent of colonoscopy I advised subtotal colectomy with an ileorectal or ileo-distal-sigmoid anastomosis in patients at high cancer risk who had relatively quiescent colitis. I advised this operation in order to bring the remaining large bowel mucosa within the reach of regular sigmoidoscopic review. This has been a rewarding approach and so has saved many people who otherwise might have had a panproctectomy. I believe that such a policy is still justifiable, particularly if colonoscopic review presents difficulties. In a series of 18 patients so treated none have developed rectal carcinoma during a follow-up of seven years. One practical problem with this approach is that the soft feces that coat the residual rectum make mucosal inspection difficult. Furthermore, there is frequently some degree of mucosal inflammation in the rectum, and it is not easy to detect early carcinomata. I advise careful preparation of the rectum before sigmoidoscopy and in some patients perform annual sigmoidoscopy under general anesthesia to facilitate thorough inspection and biopsy.

Management of Posterior Space

The space in the pelvis left where the rectum has been excised for inflammatory bowel disease is a frequent site of complication. Since the space is bounded by the fixed bony pelvis it does not collapse and obliterate and is therefore particularly prone to collect blood and serum after the operation. The collection may become infected and the subsequent slow drainage of the abscess can cause a persistent perineal sinus.

In my experience the optimum method of posterior space management is primary closure of the pelvic peritoneum and primary closure of the perineal skin with vacuum drainage of the resultant space. If this is performed in the noncontaminated pelvis with adequate hemostasis, the vacuum suction pulls down the sutured peritoneum and pulls up the perineal skin so that, despite the fixed lateral bony walls, the space is obliterated. I prefer to bring the vacuum drainage tubes out through the abdomen since this is easier for nursing than routing the drainage tube through the perineum. If obliteration of the space can be achieved, there is a high chance of primary healing. However, if there is a contaminated pelvis, the chances of success fall from 80% to 40%.

A second method of management is to close the pelvic muscle floor and perianal skin and to leave the pelvic peritoneum wide open to allow blood or serum free access to the general peritoneal cavity from whence they can be absorbed. This method can be improved by the mobilization of a tongue of omentum that is brought down into the pelvis. One problem with this method of management is that in the female the uterus and adnexa often fall into and become adherent to the raw pelvic space. This may have a subsequent deleterious effect on fertility.

Intersphincteric dissection is not an easy technique to perform, but may be successful in ulcerative colitis. It is usually so difficult in Crohn's disease that I do not recommend it.

In some females having a proctectomy for carcinoma of the rectum, I excise the posterior vaginal wall, allowing the posterior space to drain freely into the vagina and then perform a primary suture of the posterior wound as far as the posterior vaginal fourchette. In ladies having proctectomy for ulcerative colitis in whom there has been pelvic contamination or difficult hemostasis I have employed this technique with great success. However, in some patients with perianal complications, particularly those in whom there is a possibility of Crohn's disease, I am cautious in using the technique because of the disastrous results that follow complete posterior wound breakdown.

Persistent Perineal Sinus

With a high success rate of primary healing, we now rarely encounter patients with persistent perineal sinuses. I have been referred one patient with persistent perineal sinus resulting from incomplete secondary perineal removal of a rectal stump so that a large area of functioning colonic mucosa was left behind at the top of the perineal wound. However, by far the most common cause of persistent perineal sinus is the slow healing of an infected and poorly drained posterior space when the superficial part of the wound heals more rapidly than the deep part. The deeper part is held apart by the rigid bony wall of the pelvis and the resultant flasklike cavity does not heal and constantly discharges purulent serum.

The key to successful management of a persistent sinus is to provide free drainage. The sound is therefore guttered. If the coccyx has not been removed this should be done. I also use bone nibblers to cut away any lower part of the sacrum that might be preventing free drainage. If the edges of the wound are very large but with clean granulating tissue, I occasionally apply skin grafts. These may shorten the time taken for complete epithelialization.

Self-Evaluation Quiz

1. The following is not an indication for emergency operation:
   a) Continued hemorrhage
   b) Toxic dilatation
   c) Unresponsive fulminant disease
   d) Premalignant changes on the mucosa
2. In a patient admitted ill with fulminant ulcerative colitis the treatment regime does not include:
   a) Frequent steroid enemas
   b) Fluid replacement
   c) Blood transfusion
   d) Parenteral steroid therapy
3. Toxic dilatation can usually be avoided by prompt medical treatment of acute exacerbations.
   a) True
   b) False
4. Acute hemorrhage in ulcerative colitis rarely responds to medical treatment alone and usually requires emergency surgery.
   a) True
   b) False
5. Mesenteric angiography is better at determining the site of acute bleeding in ulcerative colitis than is colonoscopy.
   a) True
   b) False
6. One of the following is not a reason for preserving the rectum when undertaking emergency total colectomy for colitis:
   a) It decreases the operating time in a sick patient
   b) The rectum may be reserved for a later ileorectal anastomosis
   c) There is a lower rate of malignancy
   d) There is less blood loss during the emergency operation

7. After removing the whole colon but leaving the rectum it is best to close the rectal stump and bury it extraperitoneally.
   a) True
   b) False
8. Important measures in reducing the morbidity and mortality of perforation in acute colitis do not include:
   a) Steroid therapy
   b) Physical debridement of all the phlegmonous peritoneal exudate
   c) Repeated peritoneal lavage with large volumes of normal saline
   d) Appropriate aerobic and anaerobic chemotherapy
9. Patients with colitis at greatest risk of developing cancer are:
   a) Those who develop colitis late in life
   b) When the colitis is confined to the rectum and distal sigmoid
   c) When the disease runs an intermittent course
   d) When the disease has been present for more than ten years

Answers on page 721.

Radiation Injury to the Intestine

Jerome J. DeCosse, M.D., Ph.D.

Objectives

Radiation injury of the intestine results from a vasculitis and can lead to ulceration, necrosis or perforation. The discussion will center on the diagnosis as well as the conservative and surgical management of this injury.

Introduction

Radiation injury to the intestine is probably being recognized more frequently. Although improved quality control has undoubtedly resulted in greater precision and safety of radiation therapy, indications for radiation therapy have also become more common. In the past, it was rare to see a man with radiation injury of the rectum but during recent years, radiation therapy for carcinoma of the prostate has resulted in rectal injury. An additional important factor in a possible increased prevalence of patients with radiation injury is more frequent use of chemotherapeutic drugs in conjunction with radiation therapy. Many of these drugs enhance the effect of radiation on tissues and are called radiomimetic. Actinomycin, bleomycin, adriamycin and cytoxan are among such agents. Efforts are under way to develop radioprotective drugs, agents that will protect adjacent normal tissues when administered during radiation therapy. In experimental studies, only prednisolone has actually provided radioprotection.

The true incidence of radiation injury of the intestine is difficult to assess. Physical costs of an operation are known within a few days whereas the consequences of radiation therapy may not be apparent for many years. Many, perhaps

---

Jerome J. DeCosse, M.D., Ph.D., Professor and Chairman, Department of Surgery, Medical College of Wisconsin, Milwaukee.

most, patients treated with radiation therapy for carcinoma of the cervix or endometrium will have transient diarrhea during therapy. The cause is impaired mucosal renewal from an alteration in cell kinetics of intestinal epithelium; at completion of treatment, recovery regularly occurs.

Chronic radiation injury is due primarily to progressive obliterative endarteritis and tissue fibrosis (Fig. 1). Vasculitis can result in tissue hypoxia which progresses to necrosis, ulceration and perforation. Low-flow cardiovascular states such as congestive failure or arteriolar narrowing from atherosclerosis or hypertension add to the effects of radiation-induced vasculitis until cellular oxygenation and nutrition fall below critical levels and necrosis develops. If collagen deposition predominates, fibrosis can lead to obstruction of the damaged hollow viscus.

Therefore, patients with systemic causes of vascular constriction such as atherosclerosis, diabetes and hypertension are at greater risk for injury. In addition, previous abdominal surgery and pelvic inflammatory disease may cause loops of

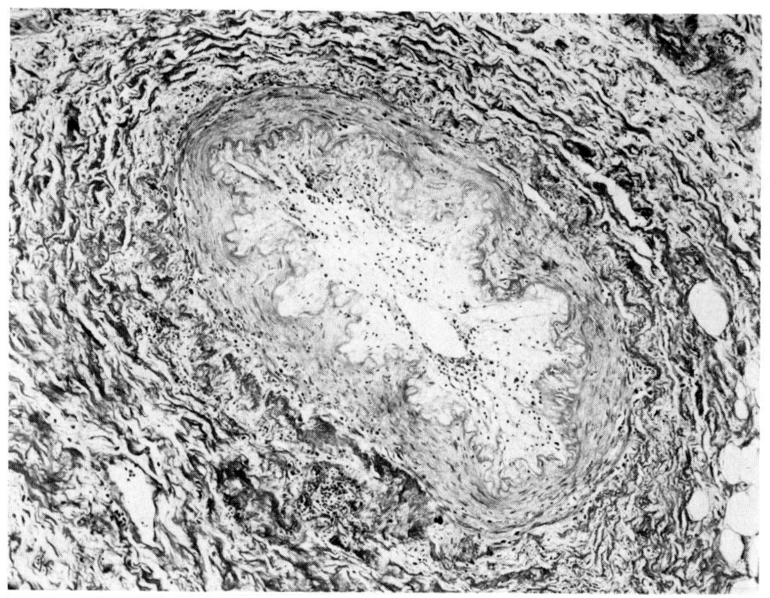

FIG. 1. Severe radiation vasculitis. (From Sabiston, D.C.: *Davis-Christopher Textbook of Surgery*. Philadelphia:W.B. Saunders Co., 1977.)

intestine to agglutinate to pelvic structures and, by limiting mobility of the intestine, enhance the likelihood of radiation injury. For this reason, patients who are going to have postoperative radiation should have the pelvic floor reconstructed whenever possible.

In many cases, radiation injury can be attributed to the physical factors of radiation treatment. Often, however, no apparent cause can be identified; it must be assumed that some patients have an unusual tissue sensitivity to radiation.

Most intestinal complications of radiation therapy appear within 24 months, but there may be a delay of many years before symptoms develop. In contrast, most recurrences of carcinoma of the cervix and endometrium will be evident within 12 to 18 months. The patient who appears well and maintains his or her body weight but continues to have crampy abdominal pain more often has radiation injury, not residual or recurrent cancer.

Diagnosis of Radiation Injury

Rectal Injury

As a consequence of radiation therapy of pelvic malignancies, such as carcinoma of the cervix, endometrium or prostate, persistent diarrhea, often bloody, with tenesmus may develop as the hallmarks of rectal injury. Rectal pain can be excruciating; a brief general anesthesia can be a kindly and helpful maneuver to adequately perform the necessary proctosigmoidoscopy. At the same time, pelvic examination and biopsies, if warranted, can be carried out. Ordinarily the rectal mucosa is reddened and hyperemic. Usually, a factitial ulcer is located anteriorly about 6 to 8 cm from the anal verge in apposition to the cervix; unlike tumors, a factitial ulcer has a flat edge and a grayish base.

Rectal stenosis may also be a late consequence of radiation therapy. An unusually proliferative fibrotic response causes marked narrowing of the rectum and may be confused with recurrent tumor. The clinical expression of a rectovaginal fistula is readily evident; however, a rectovaginal fistula may obscure an associated small intestinal fistula. These patients should have assessment by small bowel contrast studies and fistulograms for associated small bowel injury.

Frequently, rectal damage is associated with injury to the sigmoid colon. A barium enema x-ray examination and, possibly, colonoscopy may be necessary. Often, rectal injury is associated with small bowel damage and symptoms of partial small bowel obstruction may be obscured by rectal symptoms. At least one half of patients with rectal damage from radiation therapy will also have involvement of genitourinary structures. Radiation-induced nephritis may also be present. In some, a fibrotic response may cause ureteral narrowing, easily mistaken as due to recurrent pelvic tumor; cystoscopy and intravenous pyelography are warranted.

Small Intestinal Injury

As is also the case with regional enteritis, symptoms of chronic partial intestinal obstruction from radiation damage may be limited. Seemingly minor postprandial distention, cramps and nausea may herald the presence of substantial radiation damage to the intestine. Small bowel barium examinations, however, are not always reliable. In the presence of colonic and rectal damage, it may be difficult to detect small intestinal injury. In this circumstance, the presence of malabsorption with its consequences, namely, excessive fat in the stool, vitamin B_{12} deficiencies and hypocalcemia may be a clue to small intestinal damage. It has recently been recognized that patients may have steatorrhea from radiation therapy to the pancreas.

The symptoms and findings described above relate to chronic partial intestinal obstruction. Complete intestinal obstruction, abscess formation, fistulization and perforation with diffuse peritonitis may also result from radiation injury.

Management of Radiation Injury

In a patient with chronic partial intestinal obstruction or factitial proctitis without irreversible damage, the basic strategy of management is conservative. Entry into the peritoneal cavity should be avoided unless forced by complete obstruction, abscess formation, perforation or fistula formation. Symptoms of partial obstruction or factitial proctitis usually can be controlled with a combination of a low residue diet, stool softeners, antidiarrheal medications (Lomotil® or codeine phosphate), prednisone, Azulfidine® (salicylazosulfapyridine) and general supportive measures. In addition to drugs to reduce hypermotility, cholestyramine (Questran®) may be of value. The majority of patients with radiation injury do not require operative intervention; the consequences of inappropriate surgery can be devastating to the patient.

Irreversible Rectal Damage

Operative treatment is necessary for the patient with a rectovaginal fistula, an obstructing rectal stenosis or massive uncontrollable bleeding from proctitis. The first step is a proximal sigmoid or descending colon colostomy constructed outside of the radiation portal because a colostomy in radiated tissues has a substantial risk of stenosis and necrosis. If the rectovaginal fistula is small and high and there is normal distal rectal mucosa, subsequent excision and restoration of gastrointestinal continuity can be planned and occasionally achieved. A very distal rectal anastomosis may be accomplished with a transsacral or posterior approach. A low rectal anastomosis in a patient with radiation damage should always be protected by a temporary defunctionalizing transverse colostomy.

During the first few years after radiation therapy, concern for recurrent malignancy is often present. Dense pelvic fibrosis from radiation damage can be easily confused with recurrent cancer; a policy of always seeking biopsy proof of malignancy is important.

With a combination of severe bladder and rectal damage, the appropriate life-saving treatment may be an exenteration with construction of an ileal conduit and a permanent sigmoid colostomy.

Many of these patients are critically ill with severe malnutrition and sepsis. In this circumstance, one of the major advances of recent years is hyperalimentation and gut rest. One useful maneuver is an examination under anesthesia shortly after admission. At this time the exact extent of radiation damage can be more easily assessed and subclavian catheters introduced. In addition, adequate drainage can be provided for possible loculated abscesses in order to accelerate healing and prepare the patient for subsequent definitive operation.

Irreversible Small Bowel Injury

In the presence of vascular compromise or complete obstruction, operative intervention is necessary: in the former urgently and in the latter after nasogastric intubation for decompression, and fluid and electrolyte replacement. In the presence of necrosis or peritonitis, exteriorization of small bowel is necessary. When exploration is necessary for small bowel injury, inappropriate lysis of adhesions must be avoided. Damaged small bowel is thickened, has a grayish serositis and demonstrates impaired motility. Loops of bowel are often agglutinated by fibrinous or fibrous adhesions. The thick and stenotic bowel may suggest regional enteritis or even recurrent cancer.

In general, an extensive resection is preferable to limited resection or bypass. The consequences of a blind loop syndrome should be avoided. With pelvic radiation the cecum is often damaged; removal of the cecum and ascending colon should be included with distal small intestinal resection and the anastomosis established in unirradiated transverse colon. Occasionally, when loops of small bowel are densely adherent in the pelvis, a bypass is the appropriate procedure.

Above all, it is imperative that an anastomosis be performed in tissues that have not been subjected to radiation damage. We find that frozen section has limited value. The gross appearance of normal bowel and recognition that the bowel, such as transverse colon, is outside of pelvic radiation portals, have been more useful.

Bibliography

DeCosse, J.J.: Radiation injury to the intestine. *In* Sabiston, D.C. (ed.): Davis-Christopher Textbook of Surgery. 11th edition. Philadelphia: W.B. Saunders Co., 1977, pp. 1057-1062.

DeCosse, J.J., Rhodes, R.S., Wentz, W.B. et al: The natural history and management of radiation induced injury of the gastrointestinal tract. Ann. Surg. 170:369-384, 1969.

Deveney, C.W., Lewis, F.R., Jr. and Schrock, T.R.: Surgical management of radiation injury of the small and large intestine. Dis. Colon Rectum 19:25-29, 1976.

LoIudice, T., Baxter, D. and Balint, J.: Effects of abdominal surgery on the development of radiation enteropathy. Gastroenterology 73:1093-1097, 1977.

Palmer, J.A. and Bush, R.S.: Radiation injuries to the bowel associated with the treatment of carcinoma of the cervix. Surgery 80:458-464, 1976.

Phillips, T.L., Wharam, M.D. and Margolis, L.W.: Modification of radiation injury to normal tissues by chemotherapeutic agents. Cancer 35:1678-1684, 1975.

Van Nagell, J.R., Jr., Parker, J.C., Jr., Maruyama, Y. et al: The effect of pelvic inflammatory disease on enteric complications following radiation therapy for cervical cancer. Am. J. Obstet. Gynecol. 128:767-771, 1977.

Self-Evaluation Quiz

1. Which of the following drugs is *not* radiomimetic, that is, the effect of radiation on tissues is not enhanced by the agent?
   a) Actinomycin
   b) Bleomycin
   c) Adriamycin
   d) 5-Fluorouracil
   e) Cytoxan
2. Most recurrences of carcinoma of the cervix and endometrium will be evident within:
   a) 6 months
   b) 12 months
   c) 24 months
   d) 36 months
   e) 48 months
3. A factitial (radiation-induced) ulcer is ordinarily found:
   a) At the anal verge
   b) About 6 cm posteriorly from the anal verge
   c) About 6 to 8 cm anteriorly
   d) At the rectosigmoid junction
   e) In the mid-sigmoid colon
4. What proportion of patients with rectal damage from radiation injury will also have involvement of the genitourinary system?
   a) 10%
   b) 25%
   c) 50%
   d) 70%
   e) 90%

5. Which of the following is *not* associated with malabsorption from radiation injury?
   a) Excessive fat in the stool
   b) Vitamin B12 deficiency
   c) Hypocalcemia
   d) Weight loss
   e) Lactase deficiency

Answers on page 721.

Current Results in Treatment of Intestinal Fistulas

J. Englebert Dunphy, M.D., F.A.C.S., F.R.C.S.

Objectives

To delineate supportive and operative management of intestinal fistulas, especially the high-output type, by emphasizing fluid replacement without overloading, drainage of abscesses, total parenteral nutrition, sepsis control, closure of fistulas and major mistakes to avoid.

Introduction

My first acquaintance with this disease on a large scale came when I was in Oregon, when we encountered a number of very depleted patients — septic, emaciated, with very complicated problems. We soon found that if we were able to provide adequate nutrition, that is, optimal nutrition, we had a substantially improved result. At that time, as a result of these observations, we set down certain criteria for the management of intestinal fistulas, particularly of the high output type. The overall mortality in the Oregon series before we adhered to these principles is shown in Table 1.

The sequences in resuscitation, diagnosis and control of the fistula are outlined in Tables 2-5. The first priority is fluid replacement, but this takes time, as these patients are not only dehydrated, but "hypoproteinemic." An initial fluid overload will throw them into pulmonary edema. The second step is to drain obvious, easily accessible abscesses; then get control of the

J. Englebert Dunphy, M.D., F.A.C.S., F.R.C.S., Professor of Surgery Emeritus, University of California School of Medicine, San Francisco; Associate Chief of Staff for Education, Veterans Administration Hospital, San Francisco, Calif.

Table 1.

Method of Management	*Operations*	*Success*	*% Success*
Resection	16	7	56%
Closure	7	1	14%
Bypass	4	1	25%
Cecostomy closure	3	3	100%
Surgical total	30	12	40%
Supportive total	33	18	55%

Table 2. Treatment Priorities

Immediate Measures

1. Restore blood volume and begin correction of fluid and electrolyte imbalance.
2. Drain surgically accessible abscesses and control sepsis with appropriate antibiotics.
3. Control fistula drainage, protect skin, collect and measure volume and electrolyte losses.

Table 3. Treatment Priorities

Second Priority – Up to 2 days

1. Continued correction of electrolyte imbalances.
2. Replace ongoing fluid and electrolyte losses.
3. Intravenous hyperalimentation.

Table 4. Treatment Priorities

Third Priority – 5 to 10 days

1. Consider replacing TPN by feeding tube through the fistula or oral feeding if fistula is low jejunal or ileal.
2. Complete anatomic delineation of the fistula by GI series, small bowel series, barium enema and sinogram.

Table 5. Treatment Priorities

Fourth Priority – After 5 days

1. Maintain full nutritional support (3000 calories per day).
2. Operate to control sepsis.
3. Resect or totally bypass fistula if it fails to close.

fistula by protecting the skin and collecting and measuring the losses. Over the next day or two, continue to correct the electrolyte imbalance. Once the patient is stable, attention should be given to nutrition; in complicated situations, and most of these cases fit that category, total parenteral nutrition (TPN) should be started. However, it must be noted that TPN has not improved our results. At the University of California, the figures for closure of fistula, spontaneously or by operation, and the morbidity and mortality are the same. TPN may seem easier, but it should not be used to the exclusion of alimentation. Many fistulas can be handled very simply by feeding the patient through the fistula or above the fistula. There may be times, even today, when a feeding jejunostomy is useful.

Table 4 lists some of the maneuvers used before total parenteral nutrition was available, and often these are still applicable. Feeding tubes through the fistula, nasogastric feeding, often with a tube passed beyond the fistula; jejunostomy only if necessary, but also, hyperalimentation only if necessary. It is very important, once sepsis is controlled and the patient is in reasonable condition, to define the fistula by GI series, small bowel series, barium enema and a sinogram. The precise anatomy of the fistula will often predict whether or not it will close spontaneously.

The most critical issue is to control sepsis. Never attempt operative closure of a fistula in the face of severe sepsis. If the patient remains septic, and is not gaining ground, but no definite abscess cavity can be located by physical examination, scanning or ultrasound, exploratory laparotomy is essential. Never allow a patient to go steadily downhill because of unexplained sepsis without reoperating and opening the whole abdomen, if necessary, to find and drain sepsis. Spontaneous closure of a fistula will take place fairly promptly after sepsis is controlled and nutrition is adequate. Complicating factors include distal obstruction, large local cavities or a wide open fistula in direct contact with skin. In any of these situations it will soon become evident that spontaneous closure is not occurring and operation is necessary.

Results under these circumstances at the University of California, San Francisco, in comparison with other series are shown in Table 6. These are older figures, but the trend to a 10% to 12% mortality rate with good management is obvious. The results at the University of California before and after the use of TPN are shown in Table 7.

Operative Technique

There are several important points of technique in the operative closure of a fistula. First, enter through a clean area, not through the fistula. Sometimes an incision can be extended above or below the fistula. Sometimes it is better to make an

Table 6. Mortality of Small Bowel Fistulas (1933 - 1969)

	% Mortality	*Years*
University of California	14%	1963-69
Boston City Hospital	38%	1962-66
University of Chicago	38%	1959-68
University of Oregon	65%	1933-63
University of Utah	35%	1945-69
University of Mississippi	32%	1945-62
Lahey Clinic	25%	1933-66
Massachusetts General Hospital	45%	1946-59

Table 7. Enterocutaneous Fistula UCSF 1968 - 1977

Treatment	*1968-71*	*1972-77*
Nonoperative (Total)	25 (35%)	56 (49%)
Nonoperative (Successful)	19 (76%)	40 (71%)
Operative (Total)	47 (65%)	58 (51%)
Operative (Successful)	39 (83%)	49 (84%)
Fistula Deaths	9 (13%)	11 (10%)

entirely separate incision, or to use a transverse incision across a longitudinal one. Avoid cutting into the fistula until it has been completely "surrounded." These are some basic rules about how to divide adhesions: If you can see through it, cut it. If you cannot see through it, feel it. Squeeze it. Then cut it. If it bleeds, it is the wrong place. Leave it alone and work someplace else. In most cases, by the time operative closure is elected the adhesions should be well fibrosed. If one stays in the right plane, it is a relatively bloodless operation. It is critical not to make repeated "inadvertent" openings into the bowel. Sometimes it is not necessary to take down adhesions well away from the fistula, but in most cases, everything must be taken down. In our large personal experience, we have not used long tubes or plication of the bowel. Where there are very obvious raw surfaces, loops of bowel can be approximated with one or two sutures to hold them together until raw surfaces rapidly glue together.

If it is necessary to sacrifice large areas of the abdominal wall, no effort need be made to close it. Because of the obvious risk of infection, rotating flaps or undermining skin should be avoided. If the intestines are covered with fine Marlex mesh, granulations will form and the wound will close spontaneously by contraction of full thickness skin and subcutaneous tissue. Then at a later date reconstruction of the fascial defect can be undertaken.

Finally, never expose a suture line to an open wound. Every effort should be made to cover incisions in the bowel with omentum or another loop of bowel. I am convinced that peritoneal fluid plays an important role in the healing of bowel. A suture line in either small or large bowel is prone to break down if it is exposed to the air.

There are times when loops of bowel are so densely bound together that it is impossible to separate them. Usually this is the case close to the fistula. Under these circumstances, good judgment will indicate that it is better to resect several loops of bowel rather than persist in a *futile* dissection.

These are the major mistakes to be avoided: (1) Inadequate drainage of pus. (2) Attempts at direct closure of fistula by putting a stitch into it at the bottom of a widely open cavity. Ninety percent of the time it will break down with a larger hole.

(3) Premature attempts to close a fistula in the presence of uncontrolled sepsis. (4) Inadequate nutrition.

There is no hurry. Once a fistula is controlled, sepsis is eliminated and nutrition adequate, a wait and see policy is in order. Let the fistula tract mature, then if it fails to close spontaneously, operate.

Conclusion

The mortality should be about 10%. Failures are due primarily to the underlying disease, cancer, severe irradiation damage, or uncontrollable pulmonary or hepatic sepsis.

Bibliography

Chapman, R., Foran, R. and Dunphy, J.E.: Management of intestinal fistulas. Am. J. Surg. 108:157, 1964.

Reber, H.A., Roberts, C., Way, L.W. and Dunphy, J.E.: Management of external gastrointestinal fistulas. Ann Surg 188:460, 1978.

Sheldon, G.F., Gardiner, B.N., Way, L.W. and Dunphy, J.E.: Management of gastrointestinal fistulas. Surg. Gynecol. Obstet. 133:385, 1971.

Webster, M.W. and Carey, L.C.: Fistulae of the Intestinal Tract. *In* Current Problems in Surgery, Vol. XIII. Chicago:Year Book Medical Publishers, June 1976.

Self-Evaluation Quiz

1. The first principle in the management of intestinal fistulas is fluid replacement in patients who are:
   a) Not yet dehydrated
   b) Hyperproteinemic
   c) Already dehydrated
   d) Suffering from pulmonary edema
2. Severe sepsis:
   a) Should deter closure of a fistula
   b) Is always associated with a clearly manifested abscess
   c) Should always inspire scanning or ultrasound exploration, even when the sepsis is from a clearly manifested abscess
   d) Should delay closure until cleared up
3. Rotary flaps:
   a) Are useful to combat infection
   b) Should be avoided

c) Should be used to close up after sacrifice of large areas of abdominal wall

4. Expose a suture line to an open wound:
   a) Only in cases of infection
   b) Only in cases of perfect asepsis
   c) Never
   d) Usually
5. In operative closure of a fistula:
   a) Always enter through the fistula itself
   b) Never enter through the fistula itself
   c) Enter through the fistula if surgically convenient

Answers on page 721.

Discussion

Moderator: Mark M. Ravitch, M.D.

Moderator: I have a number of questions on regional enteritis which have to do with the patient who comes in, suspected of having acute appendicitis, and is found to have a few inches of red bowel with the fat creeping up from the mesentery. What do you do? Is it true that 50% of these people get well if you do nothing? Dr. Goligher, would you like to answer that question?

Dr. Goligher: You are forced into an operation because you think the patient has appendicitis. In most of these people it is our policy to do nothing other than perhaps remove the appendix. We would not remove the acute ileitis itself, for subsequently, a lot of these acute cases seem to do well. Indeed there is evidence that many are really suffering from Yersinia infection and not from an early stage of regional enteritis.

Moderator: Dr. Spiro, do we know that this is regional enteritis? We have not resected it.

Dr. Spiro: If they have regional enteritis in these circumstances, do I want it resected? No, I do not.

Moderator: The patient comes in with acute appendicitis but he turns out to have what looks like regional enteritis in a small segment.

Dr. Spiro: All I want the surgeon to do is to take out the appendix so that later on I will not be worried, when giving the patient steroids, that he has a confined perforation that is masked. My biggest problem is with the patient who is on 20 mg of prednisone, and someone increases the dose when the patient has an acute abdominal pain. I like to get the appendix out.

Moderator: Neither of you is worried about the alleged development of fecal fistulas from the appendiceal stump.

Dr. Spiro: As far as I know, studies suggest that it makes no difference whether or not the appendix is removed. We rarely see fistulas. In fact, I would ask some of the older clinicians whether the abdominal fistulas in regional enteritis of the small bowel exist the way they did 15 or 20 years ago.

Moderator: I am not one of the older clinicians! Dr. Dunphy, would you answer for one of the older clinicians, if he were here?

Dr. Spiro: Dr. Dunphy was one of my teachers.

Moderator: He still has a long way to go. Just keep trying. Dr. Dunphy, the question Dr. Spiro asked was whether or not 20 or 30 years ago spontaneous fistulas in regional enteritis occurred as often as they seem to occur now.

Dr. Dunphy: I think it is about the same. I really think that the Crohn's fistula is a unique problem. It should not be operated on immediately. We have seen fistulas from Crohn's disease heal spontaneously. If the patient is not suffering from it and does not have a high output fistula, one can be quite conservative. It is a different problem from the mechanical, postsurgical traumatic high output fistula.

Dr. Goligher: To go back to the question that you originally asked, about fistula following appendicectomy: I said that it was safe to remove the appendix in most of these cases. That is based on an experience of perhaps 50 appendicectomies in such cases without a fistula. It is safe, contrary to the teaching that says that one should not remove the appendix.

Moderator: I agree. I think when fistula comes, it probably comes from small bowel that was traumatized during the procedure.

Dr. Dunphy: I would like to respond to the question, too. I think that if the appendix and the tip of the cecum are involved, one should not do an appendectomy. But if the disease is in the small bowel, it is very important to remove the appendix because subsequent attacks of ileitis are easily confused with appendicitis.

Moderator: There are a number of questions related to the matter of the perianal fistulas. There is a question that deals with Crohn's statement, made many years ago, that if the disease in the bowel is resected when the rectum otherwise is not involved, these fistulas heal. There are other questions about whether the presence of anal fistulas in themselves constitutes an indication for operation. Dr. Goligher, would you like to respond to those questions?

Dr. Goligher: If a patient has a fistula in the anal region, not associated with immediate rectal disease, but with Crohn's of the ileum, the correct thing is to deal with the ileal lesion. You will find very frequently that fistula in the anal region either heals or eventually requires a very small operation. But today we see so many fistulas in the anal region that are part of the rectal disease. Then the problem is rather different because you may be faced with radical surgery, taking out the rectum and removing the fistula at the same time.

Dr. Spiro: The point that Dr. Goligher just made is very important. I was taught by Dr. Dunphy that when one sees an anal fistula, one thinks of Crohn's disease of the small bowel. Today, when I see anal fistulas, most of the time I expect to see Crohn's colitis. Dr. Marshak has been seeing these patients for years and he might have an opinion.

Dr. Marshak: Dr. Ravitch knows that I have seen 25,000 cases of Crohn's disease of the intestine. He knows that better than anyone else. Except for him, I always had to tell surgeons what to do. I never told him what to do, though.

Moderator: Dr. Marshak, please comment on the many questions about the apparent increased incidence of cancer in the colon in Crohn's disease and whether or not this constitutes an indication for removing any colon with this disease.

Dr. Marshak: I cannot agree with the published reports that there is an increased incidence of carcinoma in Crohn's disease of the colon. I think what happens that differentiates Crohn's disease of the colon and ulcerative colitis is that operation is done sooner in Crohn's. It is unusual that a patient with Crohn's disease of the colon goes any length of time without some sort of surgery. Therefore, I do not see an increased incidence of carcinoma of the colon in this disease. But I think it is due to surgery. However, I cannot disagree with those who perhaps watch Crohn's disease of the colon longer and find an increased incidence. It is just not in my statistics.

Dr. Spiro: I wish that Dr. Marshak would cross the Hudson River and East River a little more often because we have problems in Connecticut being sure that we can tell them apart. That being the case, we have followed the general trend over the past several years of recognizing that in inflammatory bowel disease generally there seems to be an increased incidence of cancer. We colonoscope our patients at the end of ten years following the Morson hypothesis about dysplasia in the colon. In patients without inflammation in the biopsy but with marked evidence of dysplasia of the epithelial cells, we have recommended total colectomy in two patients in the past 1½ years. We have found, as the literature suggests, that the colonoscopists — whom Dr. Marshak does not like, anyway — do not see the cancers. The cancers are just kind of flat mural lesions. The biopsies show dysplasia. Often the carcinoma is under the dysplasia. We have continued to recommend colonoscopy after ten years in people with inflammatory bowel disease of the colon, whether called ulcerative colitis or Crohn's colitis or granulomatous colitis. How often that should be done I do not know. But I am impressed with the fact that my colleagues in different parts of the country seem to be having the same kinds of experiences.

Dr. Marshak: I think it would be a mistake to equate ulcerative colitis with Crohn's disease of the colon. Although I have the greatest respect for Basil Morson, dysplasia in Crohn's disease of the colon means absolutely nothing to me. In ulcerative colitis, it means a great deal. I have never had any difficulty distinguishing a carcinoma in the colon from Crohn's disease. It is unusual in Crohn's disease of the colon to get a single small lesion without evidence of other lesions elsewhere. I think to equate the two diseases in terms of malignancy would be wrong.

Dr. Goligher: There is good evidence of carcinoma arising in ulcerative colitis. But there is not good evidence that carcinoma arises in Crohn's colitis. I have studied the literature very carefully. There seems to be some evidence that there is an increased predisposition to carcinoma in small bowel Crohn's disease, but not in Crohn's of the large bowel. So, in practical terms, we do not think of carcinoma when we are planning treatment of Crohn's disease of the large intestine and are prepared to leave diseased bowel, if necessary.

Dr. Marshak: Some patients who have total small bowel involvement and marked stenosis, but cannot have an operation, we have watched for 20 or 25 years. These are the patients who have carcinoma. Primary carcinoma of the small bowel is a rare lesion. Therefore, when you get 12 cases out of thousands of Crohn's disease examined, it is an increased incidence.

Moderator: While we are on the subject of carcinoma, can we agree that at some point along the line for garden variety ulcerative colitis, the bowel should be removed simply because it has been diseased for X number of years? Is that right, Dr. Marshak?

Dr. Marshak: I do not understand the question. Could you restate it?

Moderator: The statement is generally made that the longer you observe a group of patients with chronic ulcerative colitis, the greater is the incidence of carcinoma of the bowel. At some point along the line, 10 or 12 or 15 years, even if the patient is tolerating the retained bowel well, he should have a total colectomy. Is that correct?

Dr. Marshak: The problem is prophylactic colectomy in ulcerative colitis.

Dr. Marshak: I have noticed among my distinguished gastroenterological colleagues that no two agree. These patients come in with mild ulcerative colitis, some people call it by different names. I am not impressed with the dysplasia of Basil Morson. I am not convinced. Dr. Spiro is absolutely right. On x-ray, we cannot see an early carcinoma in ulcerative colitis. I think it takes the combined experience of the distinguished members of this panel to decide whether or not prophylactic colectomy should be done in any individual case. You cannot take a 36-year-old or 40-year-old female who started at the age of 20 in good health who has one bowel movement a day and who has minimal ulcerative colitis and take that colon out. Yet, that is what many people are doing in the United States. I know they are doing this at the Lahey Clinic. Janowitz varies. He tosses a coin. He does one and he does not do the next one. I see now everybody is being colonoscoped every year. It drives our pathologists crazy to study these tiny bits of tissue. They send them to Basil Morson in England, and he says the tissue was lost in the mail. I have no objection to anyone who does a prophylactic colectomy in ulcerative colitis that started in childhood. We all agree on that, if it starts in childhood. However, to do it later on, it takes a tremendous degree of sympathy and intelligence, not just a dysplastic cell.

Dr. Spiro: I would like to come back to the issue of ulcerative colitis and Crohn's colitis simply for one reason: Not everybody has Dr. Marshak or Basil Morson available at his own institution. In those circumstances, I think it would be a disservice to the people in the audience if we leave them with the impression that everybody can tell ulcerative colitis from Crohn's colitis. British studies have shown that when two pathologists get together and decide the criteria for ulcerative colitis and for Crohn's colitis, and then they go over a group of patients, their intra-observer variation is extraordinary. It varies from 10% for a microabscess or a granuloma all the way up to 30% for some of the less tangible lesions. If the pathologists cannot agree, when they have worked together, then it seems to me that very few, other than Dr. Marshak and Dr. Morson, can really tell those disorders apart. In the United States generally, the surgeons, gastroenterologists and radiologists ought to say, "Well, I am not sure what the disease is." I think we have to do colonoscopies even if I am not sure how often they should be done. Still, colonoscopy gets around the issue that Dr. Marshak has raised of prophylactic colectomy in someone who is well. At least if biopsies show nothing, or just a little inflammation, we can delay.

Dr. Goligher: For quite a while I advocated prophylactic proctocolectomy and I may have even influenced some people to adopt that philosophy. That was for patients who had had total colitis for ten or more years and particularly if they started with the disease in childhood, because we know there is quite a risk of their getting carcinoma. But I quite take Dr. Marshak's point that many of these people have remarkably little inconvenience from bowel symptoms. They have come to terms with their colitis. They have perhaps two or three motions a day, which they regard as normal. They are fit and well. When you talk about giving them an operation with a bag, they almost jump out the window. It is very difficult to sell this operation to such people. I can recall a number of patients in that situation to whom I have advised prophylactic proctocolectomy. They refused it and within three years were back with carcinoma. So I know there is a real risk. What has changed many people's attitude in Britain is Basil Morson's concept of epithelial dysplasia in rectal and colonoscopic biopsies. He postulates, and at the moment it is just a postulate, that if a patient is going to get a carcinoma anywhere in the colon in colitis, he will develop diffuse precancerous changes in colon and rectum beforehand. If you spot these on a rectal biopsy, you can select that patient for prophylactic proctocolectomy. In other words, you take the same indications that I had, but narrow the field still further by doing colonoscopic and rectal biopsies every year. That is what many people are doing in Britain. I myself am doing that. But you need a good pathologist.

Moderator: Dr. Dunphy, in my mind you are always associated with inflammatory bowel disease, back to an occasion at the American Surgical Association, when our banquet speaker was President Dwight Eisenhower, and when there were long papers presented from the Lahey Clinic and the Mayo Clinic on regional enteritis. When Dr. Ravdin was asked to speak, he discussed a patient who remained nameless. Obviously, he referred to President Eisenhower. When he finished, the presiding officer, Dr. Dunphy, said: "You know, every time we have a big meeting of a scientific society, people get up and discuss hundreds of cases. There is always a country practitioner with hay in his hair and cow dung on his shoes talking about one single case." Dr. Dunphy, would you tell us about your attitude toward the possibility of cancer in ulcerative colitis?

Dr. Dunphy: You would like to hear about my case, would you? I think this is a very controversial area. There is no doubt, from Dr. Goligher's studies, that there is a definite increased risk in a child with total colitis who is 10 years or 20 years down the road. However, I still find it very difficult to advise a prophylactic colectomy, under these circumstances, if the patient is really quite well. Our gastroenterologists at the University of California are very conservative about this. What we like is the patient who still is having difficulty after ten years and is not quite well. Then it is easy to push for total colectomy. But in the patient who is well, we are seeing a shift toward repeated observation, hoping to recognize cancer early. Our pathologists have not been as convinced as Basil Morson about his ability to detect early changes in the rectal biopsy. It is a controversial area. Faced with the problem, as a practicing surgeon, all you can do is to present the situation to the patient. Make him aware that he has an increased risk of carcinoma. If he elects to have the operation, that is fine. I think you should say this: "We do not know for sure what your particular chances are. Everyone does not get cancer, even though in this situation they are at higher risk." Suppose the risk is 30%. Well, there is a 70% chance that they will not get cancer. Or if it is 50%, then it is 50-50. Most of us, faced with the 50-50 choice of losing our colon, or dying of cancer, will probably choose to take the risk and then hope that the cancer, when it comes, will not be an advanced one. That is my position.

Dr. Spiro: As a nonpathologist I would like to make the point that if you are going to use the biopsies as Dr. Goligher has indicated, you had better be sure that there is no inflammation in the specimen itself. You cannot rely upon the epithelial changes, if there are many inflammatory changes in the bowel at that point. Therefore, histology is not terribly useful in a patient who is having continuing symptoms at the time of the colonoscopy.

Dr. Marshak: Dr. Ravitch, I have noticed that the incidence of carcinoma in ulcerative colitis in the last few years has dropped. Is this due to the fact that all the colons with ulcerative colitis have already been taken out in the United States?

Moderator: Dr. Marshak, I do not know. I have not taken out as many as I would have liked. I would predict, however, that the biopsy, whether by sigmoidoscopy or colonoscopy, will prove not to be worthwhile. First, there is such an enormous area to be examined. Second, due to the nature of the disease, it is frequently not possible to pass the colonoscope very far. Third, frequently when the specimen is opened, the pathologist does not recognize the cancer and finds it only by chance on microscopic section. Fourth, and this has already been alluded to earlier, frequently the tumor actually arises in the wall of the bowel where a crypt has been buried over by scar tissue and the regenerative cells have finally developed a carcinoma with perfectly innocent scar or granulation tissue or even regenerating mucosa on the surface. This is a guess and a prediction.

Dr. DeCosse, is colonoscopy helpful or dangerous in the assessment of colon irradiation injury? Is it good or bad?

Dr. DeCosse: Colonoscopy is useful in assessment of injury that is above the reach of the proctosigmoidoscope.

Moderator: You have no fear of tearing the rigid bowel?

Dr. DeCosse: It depends upon the patient's findings. Basically there ought not be fear, and one has the problem of differentiating recurrent cancer or even a new tumor from irradiation injury.

Moderator: Dr. DeCosse, and Dr. Marshak, would you please both respond to this question: Can you identify chronic radiation change in the small or large bowel by x-ray?

Dr. DeCosse: I think Dr. Marshak should respond.

Moderator: No, Dr. DeCosse, it is directed to you and Dr. Marshak will follow you.

Dr. DeCosse: May I ask Dr. Marshak a question first?

Moderator: Dr. Marshak, would you be good enough to respond?

Dr. DeCosse: In my own comments earlier, I made the statement that small bowel x-ray series are very hard to interpret. One may often have substantial pathology from radiation damage in the small bowel with minimal or no radiological findings. That is a comment that perhaps Dr. Marshak would like to challenge.

Dr. Marshak: I would agree with that. I make the diagnosis of radiation enteritis by exclusion. I rule out the different diseases. Then, of course, unlike many radiologists, I take a history. If a patient has had a seminoma of the testicle and extensive irradiation and I see changes in the small bowel, I shall blame it on the radiation first. It looks like regional enteritis, except less marked and these patients do not have a history of regional enteritis. I agree with you that it is a difficult diagnosis to make without a history.

Moderator: Dr. Simmons, a number of people in the audience have already ordered heparin to be ready the next time they do a laparotomy. They want to know how much heparin, whether it interferes with healing, whether it really prevents adhesions, whether you really believe what you said, whether with heparin you can really leave dead gut in the abdomen which then just serves as a protein supplement. Would you respond, Dr. Simmons?

Dr. Simmons: If you are a dog, it is good for you. But I do not know whether or not it is good in patients. There have not been any studies in patients. We have used it in patients with peritonitis in whom we felt that there was a poor prognosis due to the advanced state of the disease. We use the typical miniheparin dose that one might use for prevention of thromboembolic disease, ie, 5,000 units for a normal sized person every eight hours. It may be useful in lesser doses, namely, 3,000 units, because we cannot afford to have bleeding in the peritoneal cavity. So when you are choosing between an experimental hope like heparin and a known danger of bleeding I prefer to prevent the bleeding.

Moderator: So the message is to call the office and tell them to hold the heparin?

Dr. Simmons: I think there really is a place for doing the appropriate studies here.

Moderator: Dr. Dunphy, you have had a long interest in wound healing. What are the facts about the prevention of adhesions by heparin? If they can be prevented, is that good or bad or indifferent?

Dr. Dunphy: It is a very indeterminate situation. There is no question that the patient who is under heavy anticoagulation has a risk of hematoma formation with retardation of healing and the risk of sepsis. With low dose heparin, you can believe whatever you like. There are many groups who say they have no difficulty. There are others who say they have had a very significant increase in bleeding. I do not really have a solid answer. I am onthe fence. If it were me, I do not think I would take the heparin. But I might give it to Dr. Simmons.

Moderator: Dr. DeCosse, do you have any feeling about heparin in wound healing and adhesions?

Dr. DeCosse: No, sir, none whatsoever.

Moderator: Dr. Simmons just said that his work was in rats. Someone in the audience who is sharp eyed and who is good at filling out questions pointed out that in an experiment to demonstrate the diaphragmatic circulation within the peritoneum, a slide showed the injection of bacteria into the pelvis and showed where they went. That slide showed a little of the right lobe and left lobe, the gallbladder, a sigmoid, an ascending colon, a transverse colon, a descending colon and so forth. The interpretation was that the slide showed the needle going into the pelvis of a human. Where did you find the volunteer?

Dr. Simmons: That slide was from an animal, which generally has the same viscera that humans have. A similar study has been done in man, using dye, and showing that the dye migrates after a few minutes in the same direction in humans.

Moderator: The experiment was obviously not done in humans and that is the important thing. It was done in animals.

Dr. Levitt, here are three questions about the malodorous flatus which afflicts Dr. Scott's patients after he does a gastrojejunoileal shunt. Do you have a cure for that?

Dr. Levitt: I do not think I have a cure. Presumably, the cause is the malabsorption of something that the bacteria convert into a compound that is odoriferous. We have to consider both quality and quantity. The odoriferous factors represent a miniscule faction of the total intestinal but virtually no one has studied them. Presumably fats and proteins which are not absorbed get into the colon and the bacteria convert them into volatile odoriferous compounds.

Moderator: What about the quantity? Do these people actually have a large quantity of flatus?

Dr. Levitt: The quantity is different. Large volumes of gas generally result from carbohydrate which reaches the colon and is then fermented releasing large amounts of carbon dioxide and hydrogen. Neither of those gases have any odor. So one must postulate that bacteria work on something other than simple carbohydrates to produce the odoriferous gases. I should mention that the gases which have an odor are relatively rapidly absorbed from the bowel. I think when one is producing much hydrogen and carbon dioxide, there is not enough time for the odoriferous gases to be absorbed. There is a fairly close correlation between quantity and quality most of the time.

Moderator: Have you had an opportunity to study gas quantitatively in a large number of these patients?

Dr. Levitt: No, I have not.

Moderator: Dr. Dunphy likes to talk about gas.

Dr. Dunphy: I would like to ask Dr. Levitt a question. An old and great clinician at Harvard, John Homans, always maintained that flatus passed in the living room was small in quantity but high in odor, whereas flatus passed postoperatively was high in quantity but without odor. Is that correct?

Dr. Levitt: I think it is absolutely correct. You have to be eating protein or fat in order to feed the colonic bacteria something from which they can produce odoriferous gas.

Moderator: Dr. DeCosse, if small bowel obstruction due to radiation damage forces one to bypass bowel which is extremely adherent to the pelvic mass, would a side-to-side or an end-to-side ileocolostomy be preferred?

Dr. DeCosse: I argue for the principle that excision is better than bypass. But I also implied that there are times when the prudent maneuver is a bypass. There are occasions of greatly adherent bowel in the pelvis when simple side-to-side bypass of the bowel is best.

Moderator: Dr. Dunphy, what is your opinion of a simple bypass in an obstruction in the bowel?

Dr. Dunphy: I think it is to be avoided if possible. It produces a blind loop. It does not solve the problem. Ordinarily, depending upon what you are doing the bypass for, it is better to do a divided mucus fistula and then come back and resect the lesion. Bypasses have their place. We have that great case of Ravdin's, which was successful. But generally speaking I think a simple bypass is not a good operation.

Dr. Goligher: Is this question related to Crohn's disease?

Moderator: No, not specifically, irradiation colitis, intestinal obstruction, carcinoma or whatever.

Dr. Goligher: I would prefer to excise, if possible. But, as Dr. DeCosse recognized, there are cases when it is safer to do a bypass and I would not hesitate to do so.

Moderator: I have a question from the West Coast which asks about the new treatment for Crohn's disease.

Dr. Spiro: On the West Coast, it is claimed that ampicillin helps patients with colitis. In the East, at Columbia Presbyterian Hospital, they have a drug called coherin, which has had more publicity than it deserves. It comes from somewhere in the head and is supposed to regulate intestinal peristalsis. I do not know its value. I do not know what other drugs the questioner had in mind.

Moderator: Dr. Simmons, assuming that all of your patients do not escape an abscess, do you advise a transperitoneal or extraperitoneal approach for subdiaphragmatic abscesses?

Dr. Simmons: Retroperitoneal dissection, finding the abscess with a needle and then draining it works in a large percentage of the patients. However, we have been struck by the repeated observation that in a patient with a subphrenic abscess there is another intraperitoneal abscess or retroperitoneal abscess 20% to 30% of the time. You are going to miss these abscesses by the blind technique of subphrenic abscess drainage. In general, in the healthy but febrile patient with a subphrenic abscess, the retroperitoneal approach is a very nice clean one. In the patient who is septic and has a subphrenic abscess, I think abdominal exploration and transperitoneal drainage is safer.

Dr. Dunphy: I would agree with Dr. Simmons. You have to be selective and make your decision in the particular patient. But with the number of times when you have multiple problems, it is better to take a look at the whole show. In the patient who has had a subphrenic collection after a biliary operation, or something of that sort, you should be able to zero in directly on the lesion.

Moderator: I would like to put this thesis to Dr. Goligher: These are all sick patients and exploration may be difficult and dangerous. One in general does not *explore* for pus, but drains it when one has localized it. Is that an acceptable thesis, Dr. Goligher?

Dr. Goligher: I gather you are asking me the same question you asked Dr. Dunphy?

Moderator: The thesis I would like to put to you is this: The septic patient is not a patient who tolerates an abdominal exploration for pus very well. You are likely to get fistulas and bleeding or you might even miss the pus. In general one localizes the abscess by physical examination with a needle and then drains the abscess one has found. Is that an acceptable thesis, Dr. Goligher?

Dr. Goligher: No, I quite frequently explore. I find it easier to find abscesses in that way. It is sometimes quite difficult to find them by more limited means. So I have quite frequently gone back, opened them up and looked in extensively.

Moderator: I surely hope none of my house staff is here because I will be undone if they have heard that.

Dr. Dunphy: Dr. Ravitch, I think we have to clarify the situation. Here is a patient who has had an appendectomy for advanced appendicitis and has an obvious pelvic abscess. I think we would all drain it through the rectum or through the vagina and wait and see. But if we are talking about a patient who has had multiple problems with sepsis and we have difficulty finding and localizing it by ultrasound, or whatever, I think it is a mistake to just drain locally and allow the patient to remain profoundly septic. You must go in and take a total look.

Moderator: Dr. Simmons addressed himself to that earlier and said that in the patient who obviously has pus here, there and everywhere wide exploration is indicated. You will remember that Claude Welch 10 or 15 years ago presented perhaps half a dozen patients like that who were saved by this kind of a last ditch desperate and dangerous operation.

Dr. Simmons: I think the major problem is with a condition which can be called "surgical denial." If we have operated on the patient for the first time, then it is always a "last ditch exploration." If someone else has operated on the patient the first time, then it is "early re-exploration to rule out sepsis." It is important to recognize that all of the diagnostic tools that the radiologist and the nuclear medicine specialist have offered us have a high incidence of false negatives. Ultrasound is wonderful, but if you have left the wound open the first time around due to sepsis, the ultrasonographer will not go anywhere near you. CAT scans only localize purulent collections with firm abscess walls. Gallium scans are virtually worthless. We found that Indium scanning, in which you take tag white cells with Indium-111, and inject them, will frequently localize infection in 24 hours. But most of the time it seems to me the safest thing when you have a high suspicion of sepsis is to re-explore.

Moderator: To put it another way, the last man to see the necessity for the second operation is the man who did the first one. That is the time to get a consultant, when your patient is in trouble.

Reappraisal of the Bowel Obstruction Problem

Owen H. Wangensteen, M.D.

Objectives

To review historically the development of understanding and skills in managing intestinal obstruction. To recognize the need to concentrate on mastering more of the acute obstruction problem, particularly mesenteric vascular occlusions, venous and arterial and strangulating obstructions.

Early History

The 4th century B.C. Greek surgeon Praxagoras put on record an instance in which he saved the life of a patient with a strangulated inguinal hernia by incising the bowel in the groin, leaving the patient with an external fistula, a practice emulated with success by Pierre Franco in Bern in 1561 and by Pigray of Rouen in 1615. In the early decades of the 18th century at Hôtel-Dieu in Paris, a succession of bold surgeons duplicated the performance of Praxagoras and Franco on several occasions, not only on strangulations of external hernias, but also on internal strangulated bowel within the peritoneal cavity. In the early 19th century, the famous surgeons Dupuytren of Paris and Astley Cooper of London exhausted all measures of depletion, including phlebotomy, leeches and purging before resorting to operation for strangulated hernia.

For two centuries from the time of Sydenham (1676) to Hugh Owen Thomas (1879), better known as an orthopedic surgeon, conservatism remained the chief guide in the management of intestinal obstruction. Both Sydenham and Thomas

---

Owen H. Wangensteen, M.D., Regents' Professor Emeritus, Department of Surgery, University of Minnesota Medical School, Minneapolis.

were exponents of the liberal use of morphine, believing that most types of bowel obstruction were essentially functional and not mechanical in origin. Other frequently used agents were mobile metallic mercury, faradic electrical stimulation, gastric lavage, tobacco enemas and percutaneous intestinal puncture.

The Liverpool physician Greves (1884) called in his surgical colleague Mr. Pughe after strenuous efforts over several days with taxis, enemas and intestinal insufflation had proved futile in an obstructed patient. Operating under Listerian precautions, Pughe divided an obstructing band enveloping the terminal ileum with recovery of the patient, an experience that lent considerable impetus in Britain to the rationale of early operative management of acute intestinal obstruction.

However, safe techniques of operative management had to be developed. In the second edition (1899) of his monograph on Intestinal Obstructions, Treves said it was safer to jump from the Clifton suspension bridge 275 feet above the Avon River than to suffer intestinal obstruction and decline operation, a statement that accelerated acceptance of operative management of obstruction. As late as 1916 in his Textbook of Operative Surgery, Kocher illustrated and adopted the unacceptable enterostomy of Nélaton of 1842. Nor was the method of drainage of the obstructed bowel by that great surgeon Lord Moynihan (1926) a safe method by which to drain the distended obstructed bowel.

As the senior surgical resident in our University Hospitals in 1925, I had witnessed my surgical teachers perform either a Stamm-Kader or a Witzel type of enterostomy without isolating the distended bowel between clamps prior to inserting the decompression catheter. Moreover, a number 30 F rectal tube was conventionally used as the drainage tube. The result was inevitable leakage at every stitch site. The obvious remedy was utilization of the Witzel technique upon a deflated, isolated segment of bowel, employing a 14 F catheter. The difference in achievement was astounding. The recorded mortalities of C. Jeff Miller of the Charité Hospital in New Orleans of 65% and that of Allen Whipple and his associates at the Presbyterian Hospital in New York of 70% shrank, with refinement of the enterostomy technique, to 10% and over the years became progressively less because leakage at the needle sites was completely eliminated, constituting the first significant reduction in the operative management of acute bowel obstruction in this clinic in the 1925 to 1927 period.

Recognition of Acute Intestinal Obstruction

Jeff Miller complained that his operative mortality had rivaled that of the prior nonoperative era because it was not possible to diagnose acute obstruction early. Miller very obviously overlooked the circumstance that the only pathognomonic finding of bowel obstruction was *intestinal colic.* In acute cases, a high metallic tinkle is audible with the stethoscope at the very height of each intermittent colicky abdominal pain, a characteristic finding in all early instances of acute intestinal obstruction.

After 24 to 30 hours, because of delay in fluid absorption from the distended bowel, a gurgling sound is heard at the acme of the colic. The diagnosis of bowel obstruction is essentially clinical. Scout x-ray films of the abdomen help to locate the site of the obstruction, yet a well-taken history suffices to indicate whether the obstruction is in the small or large intestine. Well into the late 1930s, one read in textbooks of surgery that obstruction of the colon was heralded by feculent vomiting, a holdover from the pre-elective surgical era, when the ills of the body cavities fell under the supervision and aegis of the physician. For more than a century, in the writings of their books, with three or more honored compilations of the subject matter of an earlier period before them, not being able to distinguish fact from fiction, successions of physicians put a bit of each into their new compositions.

My first observation of an obstructed patient without vomiting and with huge distention delimited to the colon came in 1929. There was slight tenderness over the cecum. At operation, an obstructive carcinoma was observed in the sigmoid. Peritoneal tears, without leakage, sufficed to explain the tenderness. The operation was completed by performance of a loop colostomy in the transverse colon. By 1934, additional obstructed patients had been seen to justify this sequence of events as characteristic of colon obstruction, an occurrence attributable to the competency of the ileocecal valve precluding retrograde reflux into the terminal ileum. In 1944, my colleague Clarence Dennis reviewed our observed instances of acute colon obstruction, noting that the sequence just depicted occurred in 61% of instances. It had become patently clear by 1934 that feculent vomiting is consistently observed in obstruction of the small bowel, not the colon.

I have characterized that 16th century prince of military surgeons, Ambroise Paré, as a surgeon who believed what he observed rather than what he had been taught to believe. Every premise needs to be tested. Having once seen an orange, the surgeon who believes what he sees will recognize it for what it is in subsequent encounters.

Recognition of Strangulating Types of Intestinal Obstruction

Establishment of the presence of strangulating types of intestinal obstruction is not so readily made as is detection of simple obstruction, which has just been described. Venous mesenteric occlusions are far more readily identified than the arterial. In a series of papers in 1932, Horace Scott and I established the consistent presence of a greatly increased density of the bowel in the area of 60% when the veins to a segment of jejunoileum 4 to 5 feet in length were obstructed. In occlusions of arteries to similar lengths of bowel only a very slight increase in density of the bowel was observed. The 1932 observations were put to practical use by John Perry in the laboratory and in this clinic in 1956 when he observed that the introduction of 500 to 700 cc of air into the peritoneal cavity made short and long segments of mesenteric venous occlusion stand out as if the loops had been filled with barium, a reliable method by which to identify the presence of venous mesenteric occlusion. In 1970, Ghanem, Goodale and associates pointed out that when the arterial supply to short or long segments of the small bowel was occluded in mice, rats and dogs, high levels of peritoneal leukocytosis were observed regularly at eight to ten hours following occlusion, far in excess of that in the peripheral blood. The method, a variant of the methods used by Harlan Root and John Perry, in the recognition of injury attending abdominal trauma, deserve to be applied clinically in the recognition of arterial mesenteric occlusions. Of methods currently available, peritoneal lavage probably will prove to be the most reliable manner in which to establish the presence of mesenteric arterial occlusion in time to salvage the situation. Early placement of a dialysis catheter through a short mid-line suprapubic incision into the peritoneal cavity will permit periodic assessment of peritoneal leukocytosis.

Experiments and Observations with Practical Implications for Management of Obstruction

In the early 1930s, Charles Rea and this author divided the cervical esophagus followed by division and obstruction of the terminal ileum; only when the distal aperture of the divided esophagus was occluded were we able to exclude inhaled air from the GI tract, demonstrating that swallowed air is the chief source of intestinal distention in obstruction. As long as the distal end of the divided cervical esophagus is open, air is breathed into the stomach. Several dogs maintained on a glucose-saline solution survived as long as eight weeks; at autopsy, only minimal amounts of gas were observed in the obstructed bowel.

Clinical and experimental observations served to establish the fact that obstructions in the small intestine were accompanied usually by intraluminal pressures lower than capillary blood pressure, actually in the range of 14 cm of saline solution; the highest pressure observed in either dog or man under circumstances of complete obstruction was 19 cm of saline solution. On the contrary, in the "closed loop" obstruction in the colon, pressures as high as 52 cm of saline solution have been observed, accounting for the circumstance that perforation of the cecum not uncommonly follows neglected instances of acute colic obstruction.

Intestinal Decompression by Peroral Intubation

In observations in the 1929 to 1931 period upon fluid losses through an enterostomy catheter in three patients with acute obstruction of the small bowel at various levels, it was noted that in patients with incomplete intestinal obstruction after a few days, the fluid losses through the enterostomy catheter diminished markedly, indicating that the continuity of the bowel had been reestablished. When persistent losses of fluid and gas continued through the enterostomy catheter we knew that a complete obstruction was present, necessitating reentry to deal with the obstructive mechanism. These observations served to suggest that perhaps in some instances of intestinal obstruction, decompression could be established by an indwelling duodenal catheter. Three patients with incomplete obstruction of the small intestine were successfully decompressed in this manner by suction applied to an indwelling duodenal tube. The report was submitted first to an experimental journal and subsequently to a clinical journal but rejected by both. I then resorted to the device of submerging the report in a longer account titled Diagnosis and Treatment of Acute Intestinal Obstruction and it appeared in print in January 1932.

A monograph on the subject, which won the Samuel D. Gross Prize of the Philadelphia Academy of Surgery in 1935, failed to find a publisher. In fact, the manuscript was submitted to four publishers before the 1935 thesis appeared in print in 1937.

Considerable progress has been made in recent years in advancing peroral intestinal intubation, making it possible to decompress the bowel within the space of eight to ten hours, permitting the surgeon to deal with the obstructing mechanism at operation in the absence of distention with an almost totally decompressed bowel. The surgeon finds it necessary only to release the obstructing mechanism, finding no need to perform either enterotomy or enterostomy. Improved methods by my colleagues Arnold Leonard and Richard Edlich of intubating the duodenojejunum, hastening the descent of an inlying long intestinal tube, have proved to be a very significant factor in lowering the mortality of acute bowel obstruction.

Another very striking development in lowering the mortality of obstruction has occurred in congenital intestinal atresia and stenosis. Two decades ago its surgical relief commanded a formidable mortality. Today many pediatric surgeons have been able to deal with this serious challenge with surprisingly low mortalities of less than 3%.

Mastery of the distention factor in obstruction has been achieved. The remaining serious challenge is the strangulating obstruction. Methods of recognition are available to detect their presence. Their early application in all patients under suspicion of harboring a strangulating type of intestinal obstruction will yield impressive dividends. Detection and immediate recourse to surgical exploration, with excision of dead or dying bowel, will suffice to meet this remaining serious challenge of strangulating acute intestinal obstruction. Acceptance of the guidelines outlined above by current day surgeons will make an additional significant contribution to the lowering of mortality in acute intestinal obstruction.

Antibiotics Afford No Protection in Strangulating Obstructions

In the literature of the past two decades, there are to be found champions of the role of antibiotics in protecting against the lethal factor in strangulating obstruction. Whereas there is some suggestive evidence in experiments upon animals with strangulating obstructions that life can be prolonged in this manner, there is no convincing evidence that antibiotics have a useful role in protecting against the lethal factors of strangulating obstruction. The only reliable method is excision of the dead bowel at the earliest possible moment. No one doubts the validity of this thesis in dealing with dead tissue attending trauma to the extremities and elsewhere. All the antibiotics in all the pharmacies and hospitals of the Twin Cities cannot compete with early abdominal exploration and excision of dead bowel; any alternative procedure spells disaster.

The Autointoxication Theory

The Paris surgeon Amussat (1839) formulated the thesis of autointoxication as the responsible cause of death in bowel obstruction, a suggestion that lessened his sorrow on losing at operation Broussais, his friend and teacher. Amussat's thesis has since been a source of solace to generations of surgeons over the past 75 years under similar circumstances. The studies of George H. Whipple (1913-17), Nobel Laureate who isolated a toxic proteose from the filtrate in obstructed intestinal loops in canine experiments, appeared to justify the correctness of Amussat's views. Proof of its invalidity came in the experiments of Hartwell and Hoguet (1912) who observed that the administration of saline solution to dogs obstructed in the high jejunum enabled them to survive for as long as three weeks. Haden and Orr (1923 to 1924) subscribed to Amussat's thesis, confirming the observation of Hartwell and Hoguet but rationalized that the role of the saline was to detoxify the absorbed toxin. Clarification of the mystery came when Gamble and his associates (1925) demonstrated that saline solution served as an excellent substitute for the fluid and electrolytes lost by vomiting, confirming the earlier observations of O'Shaughnessy (1831 to 1932) and of Schmidt (1850) that the severe diarrhea of cholera and dysentery could, in many instances, be neutered by the liberal administration of fluid, and electrolytes in the quantities noted in diarrheal stools.

Current Achievement with Serious Common Abdominal Surgical Challenges

Over the years since 1930, the most striking improvement in serious surgical abdominal emergencies has been achieved with appendicitis. In 1930, there were 15.3 deaths per 100,000 population from acute appendicitis in the United States. For the year 1973, only 1066 deaths from appendicitis were recorded in the Vital Statistics of the United States, representing a reduction of approximately 99%. With acceptance of early excision, before perforation, we may anticipate nearing the challenge of C.N. McBurney of the Roosevelt Hospital in New York who envisioned in 1889 no mortality from the disorder with early operation. Appendicitis, despite its name, is not primarily an infection but an obstruction. The high intraluminal secretory pressure exceeding diastolic blood pressure, in the presence of an obstructing fecalith, is the responsible cause for the ensuant perforation or gangrene of the appendix.

There has been a decrease in the mortality of intestinal obstruction between the years 1930 and 1973 of approximately 68%, a nice achievement in the light of the serious nature of the challenge. It is surprising to learn from the recorded Vital Statistics for 1973 that 45% of the overall mortality of operations for hernia occurs in the absence of obstruction, a situation certainly susceptible of considerable improvement.

Over many years, the mortality from peptic ulcer and its complications of hemorrhage and perforation continued with little suggestion of improvement. In recent years, however, owing to introduction of more conservative surgical measures and effective medical measures in controlling gastric acidity with antacids and HCl blocking agents (cimetidine), there has been a discernible decrease in the number of deaths from massive gastric hemorrhage.

Special Areas of Concern in Acute Obstruction

The Vital Statistics for the year 1973, reported in 1977, record 37,745 deaths from colon cancer, exclusive of the rectum. Unfortunately, a figure for the number dying from obstruction is not available, probably, however, not in excess of 5%, but still a shocking number. The vigorous attack being launched by my colleague Victor Gilbertsen on early detection of colic cancer may evolve a method to reduce the mortality of cancer of the colon. As Sølve Welin (1955) of Malmö pointed out, barium air-contrast studies can detect colic lesions less than 1 cm in diameter. An ordinary barium enema is valueless in the detection of lesions of this size in the colon.

The Vital Statistics for the year 1973 records 3830 deaths from mesenteric venous and arterial occlusion. The guidelines sketched herein for early detection, if followed, could make a durable and favorable impression upon the mortality of these disorders. There have been a few recent reports attesting the importance of sharper attention to the clinical data of peritoneal tenderness, fever, tachycardia and peripheral leukocytosis in the recognition of strangulating varieties of obstruction (Nyhus and colleagues, *Annals of Surgery* 187:189-193, 1978). However, their employment over the past three decades delineates an uncomfortable record begging for improvement.

Adhesive obstructions accounted for 2368 deaths in 1973, a formidable figure, certainly susceptible of improvement by criteria well known to our profession.

Only 60 patients died from intussusception in 1973, a creditable achievement when compared with 145 deaths in 1930, but also susceptible of betterment. Paralytic ileus took 297 deaths in 1973 in which uncontrolled sepsis undoubtedly played a dominant role.

Conclusions

Great progress has been made in the management of acute intestinal obstruction over the past half century. Several surgical clinics with a special and sustained interest and concern for acute intestinal obstruction have achieved hospital mortalities in the area of 5%, an accomplishment too that can be bettered. Remaining areas of special concern are hernias, both obstructed and unobstructed. The large number of annual deaths from cancer of the colon is a reproach of defiance to the medical profession, a record certainly susceptible of considerable betterment; of that large number, probably 1500 or more die of acute obstruction.

Of the various types of intestinal obstruction, mesenteric vascular occlusions and strangulating obstruction probably constitute the most difficult and continuing challenge to our profession. Yet the tools to recognize and deal with these modalities of obstruction, before inundation of the peritoneal cavity with uncontrollable sepsis, are known to us. Earlier operative action is the only solution.

It comes as a shocking surprise, after the profession's strenuous wrestle with the bowel obstruction problem over half a century, that 2368 lives were lost from adhesive obstructive bands in 1973. A tight band behaves like a saw, dividing the bowel wall like a blade of steel in four to seven days, a situation demanding that the surgeon decompress completely the distended and fluid-containing segment of bowel before searching at operation for the point of occlusion.

Surgeons may take much encouragement over their current accomplishment in the difficult chapter of intestinal obstructions. It is the author's belief that in the next decade we may anticipate that surgeons addressing themselves to the special concerns of hernia, cancer of the colon, mesenteric venous and arterial occlusion and the threat of obstructive adhesive bands will reduce very materially the current mortality of acute intestinal obstruction. It is a challenge that the well-trained surgeons of today are capable of meeting.

Acknowledgments

The author acknowledges with gratitude the helpful support in these studies from the Ralph and Marian Falk Research Foundation, the Margaret W. Harmon and the Alice M. O'Brien Research Funds.

Bibliography

Wangensteen, O.H.: Intestinal Obstructions, 3rd edition. Springfield, Illinois:Charles C Thomas, 1955.

Wangensteen, O.H.: Historical aspects of the management of acute intestinal obstruction. Surgery 65(2):363-383, 1969.

Wangensteen, O.H.: Understanding the bowel obstruction problem. Am. J. Surg. 135(2):131-149, 1978.

Self-Evaluation Quiz

1. Moynihan's drainage was:
   a) Safe for distended obstructed bowel
   b) Unsafe for distended obstructed bowel
   c) A brilliant maneuver, but only for good surgeons
   d) Never used on distended bowel unless a metallic tinkle was audible
2. In acute obstruction, a metallic tinkle is heard:
   a) At the height of each colicky pain
   b) Just preceding each pain
   c) Just after each pain
   d) Only rarely in moribund patients
3. Venous mesenteric occlusions:
   a) Are less readily detected than are arterial ones
   b) Are just as readily detected as are arterial ones
   c) May be more or may be less easily detected than arterial ones
   d) Are more readily detected than are arterial ones
4. Observations established that obstructions in the small intestine were accompanied by intraluminal pressures:
   a) Lower than capillary blood pressure
   b) Higher than capillary blood pressure
   c) Sometimes lower and sometimes higher than 14 cm saline
   d) Always greater than 30 cm saline
5. Closed loop obstructions in the colon have been associated with pressures:
   a) As high as 74 cm saline
   b) As high as 52 cm saline
   c) Of any magnitude
   d) Far too low to account for a perforated cecum

6. Intubation of the duodenojejunum and hastening the descent of an inlying long intestinal tube helped lower mortality from acute bowel obstruction.
   a) True
   b) False
7. Congenital intestinal atresia and stenosis is now associated with a mortality of:
   a) Less than 1.5%
   b) Less than 3%
   c) Less than 5%
   d) Over 5%
8. As a problem, the strangulating obstruction has been overcome. The distention factor, too, has been mastered.
   a) Both statements are true
   b) Both statements are false
   c) Only the first statement is true
   d) Only the second statement is true

Answers on page 721.

Intussusception in Infants and Children

Mark M. Ravitch, M.D.

Objectives

To define the etiology, diagnosis and various modes of therapy for intussusception in children, especially the author's 8-step barium-enema procedure.

Intussusception, the inversion of one loop of intestine into the next, occurs classically in the 5- to 8-month-old, healthy male infant. It is announced by vomiting, severe abdominal pain and frequently collapse or lethargy. The child passes one normal stool and, thereafter, bloody mucus — the currant jelly stool. A palpable mass becomes apparent, usually sausage-shaped. This is the classic picture and the diagnosis can hardly be missed.

The causative factors are uncertain in the large majority of cases. In 6% of the cases or less, a predisposing lesion, such as a polyp, Meckel's diverticulum, or congenital malformation serves as a leading point for the intussusception. In a small number of cases, masses of submucosal lymphoid tissue in the terminal ileum are identified as causing the intussusception. In most cases, no obvious mechanical explanation is found. However, the now well-demonstrated incidence of antecedent respiratory infections, the Sheffield studies showing a higher incidence of positive stool cultures for several viral strains in children with intussusception than in a control group all suggest that lymphatic tissue enlargement in the terminal ileum may be responsible for many intussusceptions. Henoch's purpura, submucosal hemorrhage, leukemic infiltrations, the inverted appen-

---

Mark M. Ravitch, M.D., Professor and Head, Department of Surgery, Montefiore Hospital, Pittsburgh, Pa.

dix and a variety of even rarer lesions may initiate an intussusception. Intussusception is also common in children with cystic fibrosis.

Errors in the diagnosis of intussusception are made (a) because the intestine is not completely obstructed, (b) because the mass lies behind the liver and not palpated, (c) because the diagnosis of dysentery is made, particularly if some stool continues to be mixed with the blood and the child is febrile, as is common with intussusception, (d) if the intussusception occurs in the course of an established disease (an exanthem, pneumonia, etc.) and (e) because the diagnosis is not made even when all of the signs and symptoms point to it!

Spontaneous reduction occurs probably more frequently than is suspected. Prior to the end of the 19th century, if recovery occurred at all, it was when the intussusception became gangrenous and sloughed before the child died of intestinal obstruction. From 1890 to 1940, there was vigorous discussion as to whether the appropriate treatment was immediate operation or an attempt at hydrostatic (or pneumatic) reduction. In this country, there is now general agreement that a very large proportion of patients can have the intussusception safely and completely reduced by barium enema.

Our own position is that barium enema should be resorted to when the possibility of intussusception has been raised. The duration of the intussusception and the condition of the child do not affect this recommendation except in the unusual case when peritonitis is manifestly present and operation must be undertaken at once.

Our procedure involves the following regimen:

1. Placement of a nasogastric tube.
2. Initiation of antibiotic therapy as in any patient with a diagnosis of potential strangulating intestinal obstruction.
3. Institution of intravenous therapy with electrolytes, plasma, or blood as the child's condition indicates.
4. Calling the operating room and formally scheduling the child for operation.
5. Initiation of the barium enema: (a) cannister no higher than 3′ or 3′6″ above the table, (b) no anesthesia, (c) child's legs strapped together, (d) ungreased Foley balloon catheter in the rectum, balloon pulled back against the levators, and

buttocks taped, (e) continuous flow of the barium with intermittent fluoroscopy, (f) persistence so long as there is any change in the shape, location, or density of the head of the barium column, (g) avoidance of any palpation of the abdomen (the patient may be turned face down to separate the cecum and the sigmoid) and (h) upon *free-filling* of multiple loops of small bowel, the catheter is deflated and removed and a post-evacuation film taken to demonstrate multiple loops of small bowel framed by the now contracted, emptied colon.

6. If there is any doubt about complete reduction, immediate operation through a McBurney incision.

7. Admission to the hospital and continuation of systemic antibiotics and oral, poorly absorbed sulfonamides or neomycin.

8. Administration of charcoal by a nasogastric tube to be recovered by enema in six hours as proof of restoration of patency of the gastrointestinal tract.

This regimen will reduce upwards of 75% of the intussusceptions completely, depending upon the precision and persistence with which it is performed. Those intussusceptions which are not completely reduced by barium enema will, in almost every case, be reduced to the right colon, permitting a right lower quadrant laparotomy instead of a midline laparotomy with its attendant major intra-abdominal manipulation. Furthermore, of those children operated upon because the intussusception was thought not to have been reduced, one quarter will be found to have the intussusception, in fact, completely reduced. Recurrences in a range of 4% to 6% occur both with manual reduction and with hydrostatic pressure reduction. A significant incidence of intestinal obstruction due to adhesions occurs months or years later in all series of manual reductions, but has not been reported in patients who have had hydrostatic pressure reduction.

The incidence of resection is invariably higher in series in which all patients are operated upon. The mortality, formerly much higher for primary operation, now is the same for primary operative or primary hydrostatic pressure reduction. In major centers today, the only deaths from intussusception are in those children admitted moribund, or with fatal complicating diseases.

Self-Evaluation Quiz

1. Intussusception occurs classically in the healthy male aged:
   a) 2-4 months
   b) 5-8 months
   c) 9-12 months
   d) Any age
2. Lymphatic tissue enlargement in the terminal ileum may be responsible for many cases of intussusception.
   a) True
   b) False
3. If there is any doubt about complete reduction by barium enema, immediately operate through a McBurney incision.
   a) True
   b) False
4. Proof of restoration of GI tract patency is administration of charcoal by nasogastric tube and its recovery in ______ hours:
   a) 3
   b) 4
   c) 6
   d) 12
5. The author's regimen will reduce how much of the intussusception completely?
   a) Less than 60%
   b) Upwards of 75%
   c) Upwards of 85%
   d) Almost 100%
6. Intussusceptions not completely reduced by enema are usually reduced to the right colon, permitting a right lower quadrant aspiration.
   a) True
   b) False
7. There is general agreement in the United States that many cases of intussusception can be safely and completely reduced by:
   a) Magnesium sulfate bolus
   b) Barium enema
   c) Hydrostatic pressure
   d) Pneumatic pressure
8. Intussusception is announced by vomiting, severe abdominal pain and frequently hyperexcitation.

a) True
b) False

9. A significant incidence of intestinal obstruction due to adhesions occurs months or years later in some series of manual reductions, but has not been reported in patients who have had hydrostatic pressure reduction.
   a) True
   b) False

Answers on page 721.

Current Status of Jejunoileal Bypass for the Treatment of Morbid Obesity

Philip D. Schneider, M.D. and Henry Buchwald, M.D., Ph.D.

Objectives

1. To offer the background for and a short history of jejunoileal bypass surgery for obesity.
2. To discuss the indications and general technique of the operation.
3. To develop an understanding of the normal sequelae and potential complications of the procedure and the means of treating them.
4. To discuss follow-up care and responsibilities for the jejunoileal bypass patient.
5. To review the beneficial effects and the therapeutic role of the procedure.

Background

There is no debate regarding the lethality and morbidity of obesity. Morbidly obese patients — 100 pounds or more over ideal weight — have a host of health problems stemming from their disease state that lead to an increased mortality in comparison to an age-matched nonobese population [1]. In addition, there are psychosocial and economic factors related to obesity that prevent the patient from functioning effectively in society. Table 1 lists several of these problems resulting from morbid obesity.

Surgical therapy for obesity is receiving increasing attention and support in the medical community because of the dramatic

---

Philip D. Schneider, M.D. and Henry Buchwald, M.D., Ph.D., Department of Surgery, University of Minnesota Medical School, Minneapolis.

Table 1. Problems Associated With Morbid Obesity

A. *Medical Problems*
- Hypertension
- Diabetes mellitus
- Cerebral vascular accidents
- Myocardial infarctions
- Respiratory insufficiency – Pickwickian syndrome
- Cholelithiasis
- Cirrhosis – hepatic failure
- Traumatic arthritis
- Low back syndrome – herniated disc syndrome
- Venous insufficiency
- Thrombophlebitis – pulmonary embolism
- Genitourinary dysfunction
- Carcinoma of endometrium
- Carcinoma of breast

B. *Psychosocial*
- Impaired self-esteem
- Limited physical activity
- Social ostracism

C. *Economic*
- Limited capacity to work
- Unsightly image – job discrimination
- Insurance limitations

weight reduction achieved and, most importantly, the low rate of recidivism — the major limitation and cause of failure of all current diet, drug and behavior modification programs.

The greatest experience with the surgical treatment of morbidly obese patients is with jejunoileal bypass. Many major centers have each treated from 200 to 850 patients in the past ten years. Selection criteria have become fairly standardized. Basically, these criteria are as follows: (1) the patient must be massively obese, generally defined as 100 or more pounds overweight; (2) the patient must have been obese for five years duration; (3) the patient's overweight condition must have persisted despite attempts at weight reduction by diet and counseling efforts; (4) the patient must have no evidence of correctable endocrinopathy which may be a basis for his/her obesity; and (5) the patient must have the mental capacity and the emotional stability to tolerate the procedure and the postoperative sequelae. We also believe it is important that patients have no history of alcoholism, and we secure a commitment from the individual to avoid alcoholic beverages for a minimum of three years subsequent to surgery. Patients have to consent to a program of vigorous and intensive postoperative follow-up care, including percutaneous needle biopsy of the liver for three years and other hospitalization as indicated. Thus, all patients require a full discussion of the procedure and the postoperative course before therapy is initiated; anything short of this does not fall under the purview of true informed consent.

Intestinal bypass for obesity, since its initial employment in the 1950s, has taken several forms. Gradually, several technical factors have been shown to provide the most predictable and reliable results and maximum weight reduction with relative safety. These techniques employ jejunoileal bypass in which 36 to 40 cm of proximal jejunum are anastomosed end-to-end to a segment of distal ileum varying in length from 4 to 20 cm. Thus (1) the ileocecal valve is left intact and in continuity and (2) the bypassed bowel must be drained by a second anastomosis. The length of bowel is critical, since numerous authors have shown that the degree of malabsorption and the resulting weight loss are determined by the amount of bowel left in continuity [2-4]. Scott has demonstrated a difference in the percentage of patients achieving successful weight loss related to a difference of only 2 inches of bowel in the absorptive pathway [4]. In our experience at the University of Minnesota, an anastomosis of 40 cm of jejunum to the terminal 4 cm of ileum results in 90% of patients losing weight to within 50 pounds of ideal [2]. Series reporting procedures that leave 18 to 24 cm of terminal ileum document that 70% of patients attain near ideal weight [3,4]. The importance of not making the jejunoileal bypass anastomosis end-to-side stems from the experience of certain authors showing that some patients with such an operation will eventually regain excessive amounts of weight or not lose weight to near ideal, secondary to reflux into the bypassed loop [2-4].

Technique of Preparation for Surgery and Conduct of the Procedure

The importance of preoperative preparation and intraoperative technique cannot be overemphasized. These patients are at excess risk for morbid and mortal complications indirectly due to obesity alone and, additionally, because certain obesity-related complications, such as hypertension and diabetes, add an excess risk of their own. These individuals are unlikely to tolerate breaks in technique. Therefore, we stress (1) adequate bowel preparation, both mechanical and antibacterial; (2) prophylactic systemic antibiotics in the perioperative period; (3) preoperative, intraoperative and postoperative prophylaxis against thromboembolism, including lower extremity elastic support and early ambulation.

A transverse abdominal incision causes less compromise of ventilatory function in these obese patients following surgery than does a vertical incision. Strict observance of aseptic technique during the procedure — wound protection by a plastic drape; change of gloves, gowns, and instruments prior to closure; and subcutaneous wound suction drainage, which decreases the accumulation of liquid fat and serum in the wound — all contribute to the low wound complication rate seen in our patients (2%). We feel that omission of any one of these precautions exposes patients to an increased risk of operative complications.

Immediate Results

Despite the nature of the population being operated upon, the operative mortality of jejunoileal bypass has been surprisingly low. Reported operative mortality ranges from 0.5% to 2.9% [2,4,5]. By careful adherence to the previously mentioned preoperative and intraoperative techniques, one can expect a wound infection rate close to 2% despite the obesity of these patients. In addition, 4% to 11% of patients have prolonged drainage from the catheters left in the wound without evidence of infection. An incidence of thrombophlebitis of 4% with a 2% incidence of pulmonary embolization would seem to be acceptable results at this time [2,4]. Wound dehiscence and evisceration should not occur; we have had one in 850 patients.

Follow-up Care

Postoperative care, including prophylactic mineral supplements and medications, and careful follow-up care are as important in recognizing and preventing late complications as preoperative preparation and intraoperative wound precautions are to decreasing operative morbidity and mortality. The side effects and unique complications of jejunoileal bypass have been fairly well identified (Table 2).

Thus, an adequate and rational program of follow-up can be devised: (1) Immediately postoperatively, patients should be started on diphenoxylate hydrochloride and atropine sulfate to control diarrhea. (2) Patients must be placed on oral calcium and potassium supplements prior to discharge to compensate for the temporarily decreased absorption of these electrolytes. We have found it advisable to continue oral calcium indefinitely to prevent oxalate kidney stones [6]. (3) Patients should receive vitamin B_{12} therapy. It is our recommendation that patients receive 1,000 μg of vitamin B_{12} intramuscularly every six weeks. This may be unnecessary in instances where longer segments of ileum are left intact. Indeed, in certain patients with 4 cm of ileum, adequate B_{12} absorption can reappear by the end of the first postoperative year. However, this is not uniform and, until further information is available, we routinely give vitamin B_{12} injections to all jejunoileal bypass patients. (4) The patients should be discharged on low fat, low oxalate, low caffeine and high protein diets. Patients will discover that for them certain foods may increase diarrhea or induce nausea.

Table 2. Side Effects and Complications of Jejunoileal Bypass

Side Effects – 100% of Patients
Diarrhea
Electrolyte deficiency: potassium, calcium, possibly magnesium
Vitamin deficiencies, primarily vitamin B_{12}
Qualitative dietary restriction: low fat, low oxalate, low caffeine, high protein
Unique Complications – 8%-10% of Patients
Gas-bloat syndrome; flatulence
Arthritis/arthralgia
Nephrolithiasis
Liver failure
Unknown Potential Risks
Carcinoma of the colon – not demonstrated to date
Cholelithiasis – not demonstrated to date
Significant late weight gain – rare

Surprisingly, the caloric intake of the majority of patients does decrease. It has been demonstrated that a significant cause for the weight loss which occurs following jejunoileal bypass is related to unconscious calorie restriction by these patients [7].

We recommend that all post-jejunoileal bypass patients adhere to a careful follow-up program including as a minimum 3, 6, 9 and 12 month appointments for physical examination, electrolyte, hepatic and renal function studies; followed by similar studies at two, three, four, and five years. Liver biopsies are performed one, two, and three years postoperatively and as indicated clinically.

Long-term Beneficial Effects

The main aim of the surgery is, of course, weight loss. Ninety percent of patients lose to within 50 pounds of ideal weight; that is, patients generally achieve 70% to 90% of the targeted weight loss and this occurs without conscious limitation of oral intake. It is the rare patient who experiences anorexia or nausea. Weight loss occurs primarily during the first year (90.6 lb average), continues to maximum in the second year (106.7 lb average) and stabilizes by the third year (100 lb average) with a slight regaining of weight in the majority of patients [8].

In addition to weight loss, certain documented beneficial results can be expected [2]. Preexistent hypertension is decreased or absent; insulin requirements are markedly decreased or eliminated in diabetics; cardiac and ventilatory functions are improved, particularly in those with Pickwickian syndrome preoperatively. Definite benefit for orthopedic problems has been documented. Lower extremity venous circulation is improved and lower extremity thrombophlebitis decreases in incidence. Intertriginous skin problems are generally cured after weight loss occurs and hygiene improves as a result.

Additional benefits resulting from weight loss may include improvement and regression of atherosclerotic cardiovascular disease and decreased risk of developing certain cancers.

Views of the psychological nature of these obese patients are undergoing a radical change. Bypassed patients have been documented to have increased self-esteem, and social opportunity and participation have improved for many [9]. The view that the obese person is a psychologically damaged patient who eats and becomes obese because of a poor self-image is no longer tenable. Some psychiatrists have been unable to demonstrate any manifestations of psychological disorder in the post weight-loss individual, suggesting that in the morbidly obese, obesity may precede certain characteristic psychological aberrations [9-11].

Additionally and importantly, intestinal bypass surgery offers advantages not available with weight reductive therapy by gastric bypass or gastroplasty: lipid reduction is marked and obligatory, with a mean decrease in serum cholesterol of 40% and a mean decrease in serum triglyceride of 65% documented in several centers [2,4]. Secondary arrest of progression of atherosclerosis has yet to be adequately documented, but this is certainly a potential advantage of the procedure over the long term.

Long-term Side Effects and Complications

In discussing these undesirable consequences of intestinal bypass for obesity, it is important to differentiate the side effects, which are to be expected in 100% of the patients, and the complications which are unique and occur in only 8% to 10%.

Side effects should be expected from the short bowel syndrome alone and generally include diarrhea and electrolyte imbalances, as well as certain vitamin deficiencies, which have already been discussed. In the majority of patients these side effects are under control and tolerable by the end of the first postoperative year. In a small number, electrolyte imbalance is a persistent problem and may require increased supplementation, in some for a lifetime or, rarely, may necessitate additional operative intervention.

The unique complications ascribed to jejunoileal bypass include gas-bloat syndrome, arthralgias and arthritis, oxaluria and oxalic acid renal calculi, and hepatic fibrosis and hepatic failure. These complications are often discussed in the literature, but it now appears that only 2% to 5% of patients eventually require takedown or revision of their jejunoileal bypass for medical reasons.

The gas-bloat syndrome and excessive flatulence can be two of the most troublesome complaints of the post-jejunoileal bypass patient. We have employed a wide spectrum of remedies for these problems and have found that bismuth subgallate, a lactose-free diet and antibiotics (eg, tetracycline), singly or in combination, to be the most effective.

Arthralgias and arthritis have been uniquely associated with jejunoileal bypass. The precise basis for this problem is unknown. However, the rheumatoid-like, but serologically negative, arthritis/arthralgia is often relieved by a course of tetracycline or metronidazole, suggesting that the etiology of this syndrome may be anaerobic bacterial overgrowth in the bypassed segment.

Nephrolithiasis, secondary to oxaluria, is the major metabolic complication of jejunoileal bypass. The reported incidence of this occurrence ranges from 10% to 30% [6,12,13]. Despite the fact that this is the most troublesome and the most frequent of bypass complications, therapy for this problem is available and the etiology is well understood. Increased oxalate absorption occurs when ingested calcium, which normally binds oxalates, is not available because it is bound to the excess of unabsorbed fat. Excess absorption leads to increased oxalate in the urine and, on exceeding the coefficient of formation in the nephron, precipitation may occur. It was noted that patients taking calcium supplements on a regular basis for prevention of hypocalcemia were also those with the lowest incidence of nephrolithiasis. In a controlled study at the University of Minnesota, it has been shown that low oxalate diets coupled with calcium supplementation can lower the incidence of nephrolithiasis from 10% to 2% [6].

Liver failure is an infrequent (5%), but much discussed, complication of jejunoileal bypass. In fact, only 1% to 2% of patients will require reversal of jejunoileal bypass for the treatment of liver failure [2]. There are several theories regarding the possible etiology of liver failure. Currently the major focus is on a pseudo-blind-loop syndrome with toxic products from the bypassed loop affecting hepatic function and morphology, and a possible nutritional etiology based on the concept of relative protein malnutrition such as occurs in the disease Kwashiorkor. There is some evidence that antibacterial agents effective against anaerobes may ameliorate some cases of hepatic failure. This therapy is not always effective and present efforts must be directed at improving nutrition, primarily protein availability, until further research defines the problem in more detail.

In gastric bypass there is a theoretical potential for the development of cancer in the proximal or distal pouch. Likewise, with jejunoileal bypass there are potential complications which have not as yet had sufficient time to develop and may not develop, but nevertheless must be anticipated. For instance, carcinoma of the colon secondary to increased colonic mucosal contact with bile acids is a theoretical possibility. Potentially, a higher incidence of cholelithiasis exists, though in our ten-year experience this has not been borne out. The possible complications of gastric hypersecretion noted with the short bowel have not been proven to be present in patients undergoing jejunoileal bypass [14].

Summary

Jejunoileal bypass can be performed safely with a recorded mortality of less than 0.5% and with an expected immediate morbidity of 2% to 4%. Jejunoileal bypass may result in more significant weight loss than does gastric bypass, and jejunoileal bypass cannot be outeaten while gastric bypass can. Careful attention to preoperative, intraoperative and postoperative details will protect most of the jejunoileal bypass patients from the well-known side effects and unique complications of this procedure and allow the morbidly obese to achieve the maximum benefit from intestinal bypass with fewer adverse results. Finally, it must be admitted that all gastrointestinal surgery for morbid obesity is an approximation for a rational therapy for a disease of poorly understood etiology.

References

1. Proceedings of the National Institutes of Health Consensus Development Conference on Surgical Treatment of Morbid Obesity. Am. J. Clin. Nutr. To be published.
2. Buchwald, H., Varco, R.L., Moore, R.G. and Schwartz, M.Z.: Intestinal bypass procedures: Partial ileal bypass for hyperlipidemia and jejunoileal bypass for obesity. Curr. Prob. Surg., April 1975.

3. Salmon, P.A.: The results of small intestinal bypass operations for the treatment of obesity. Surg. Gynecol. Obstet. 132:965, 1971.
4. Scott, H.W., Jr.: Jejunoileal bypass in patients with morbid obesity. *In* Buchwald, H. (ed.): Metabolic Surgery. New York:Grune and Stratton, 1978, p. 59.
5. Payne, J.H. and DeWind, L.T.: Surgical treatment of obesity. Am. J. Surg. 118:141, 1969.
6. Clayman, R.G., Buchwald, H., Varco, R.L. and Williams, R.D.: Urolithiasis in jejunal-ileal bypass patients: The role of calcium carbonate. J. Surg. Res. (In press.)
7. Bray, G.A., Barry, R.E., Benfield, J.R. and Pasaro, E.: Intestinal bypass operation as a treatment for obesity. Ann. Intern. Med. 85:97-109, 1976.
8. Guzman, I.J., Varco, R.L. and Buchwald, H.: Factors determining weight loss following jejunoileal bypass for obesity. J. Surg. Res. 18:399, 1975.
9. Eckert, E.D., Leon, G.R., Teed, P. and Buchwald, H.: Physical, psychological, and eating changes after intestinal bypass surgery for massive obesity. Arch. Gen. Psych. (In press.)
10. Crisp, A.H.: Experiential aspects of obesity. Proceedings 2nd International Congress on Obesity, 1978. (In press.)
11. Solow, C., Silberfarb, P.M. and Swift, K.: Psycho-social effects of intestinal bypass surgery for severe obesity. N. Engl. J. Med. 290:300, 1974.
12. O'Leary, J.P., Thomas, W.C., Jr. and Woodward, E.R.: Urinary tract stones after small bowel bypass for morbid obesity. Am. J. Surg. 127:142, 1974.
13. Dickstein, S.S. and Frame, B.: Urinary tract calculi after intestinal shunt operations for the treatment of obesity. Surg. Gynecol. Obstet. 136:257, 1977.
14. Coyle, J.J., Varco, R.L. and Buchwald, H.: Gastric secretion and serum gastrin in human small bowel bypass. Arch. Surg. 110:1036, 1975.

Self-Evaluation Quiz

1. Support for surgical treatment of morbid obesity is increasing in the general medical community.
   a) True
   b) False
2. Diets, counseling and drug therapy for morbid obesity are not generally effective because most patients regain any weight lost through treatment.
   a) True
   b) False

3. Varying the bowel length in the absorptive pathway by only 5 cm does not affect the chances of successful weight loss in the morbidly obese.
   a) True
   b) False
4. All weight loss from small bowel bypass is due to malabsorption.
   a) True
   b) False
5. As expected, the operative mortality of jejunoileal bypass is high.
   a) True
   b) False
6. Weight loss in jejunoileal bypass patients is cosmetically beneficial but has no objective health benefit.
   a) True
   b) False
7. The major metabolic complication of jejunoileal bypass is oxaluria and oxalic acid nephrolithiasis.
   a) True
   b) False
8. Liver failure occurs in only 5% of jejunoileal bypass patients and only 1% to 2% of patients require takedown of the bypass to manage liver failure.
   a) True
   b) False

Answers on page 721.

Gastric Bypass for Morbid Obesity

Edward E. Mason, M.D., Ph.D.

Objectives

1. To explain the effect of gastric bypass upon gastric secretion and the way in which stomal ulcer can be avoided by high division of the stomach.
2. To present the basis for weight loss following gastric bypass.
3. To present the various modifications of gastric bypass and gastroplasty and their advantages and disadvantages.
4. To present indications for use of gastric bypass.
5. To review the major factors in the risk of gastric bypass.

Gastric bypass was introduced as an operative treatment for obesity at a symposium held at the University of Minnesota in honor of Owen H. Wangensteen in December 1967 [1]. It appeared to be a more difficult operation than intestinal bypass. In addition, because it was a distal gastric exclusion procedure, it aroused fears that there might be a high incidence of stomal ulceration. Studies carried out with the help of Ito [1-3] supported the hypothesis that gastric bypass would actually suppress gastric acid secretion. Indeed, subsequent experience has shown that serum gastrin levels following a meal are suppressed [4]. Stomal ulcers have occurred in less than 2% of patients and have usually been due to division of the stomach at too low a level.

The defect in the obese patient is thought to be an absence of satiety rather than excessive and inappropriate hunger. Our experience supports this thesis in that patients are happy with a restriction of eating following gastric bypass. There are two principles for the success of all gastric procedures used for

---

Edward E. Mason, M.D., Ph.D., Professor of Surgery, University of Iowa College of Medicine, Iowa City.

control of weight: (1) the fundic segment must be 50 ml or less in volume with a pressure of 25 to 30 cm of saline measured intraoperatively with a nasogastric tube and (2) this segment should empty through a stoma that is 12 mm in diameter or less. If the stoma is an anastomosis, it is not safe to make it smaller than 12 mm. If the channel is being fashioned without a fresh anastomosis, then an 8 mm diameter is optimum. Revisions to reduce stoma size will fail unless the fundic segment of stomach is less than 50 ml in volume. A large pouch combined with a small stoma leads both to symptoms of retention and continued excess weight.

The modus operandi today is to staple the stomach without transection. This has been followed by occasional staple disruption probably caused either by the use of 3.5 mm staples instead of the recommended 4.8 mm or because the upper gastric segment was too large. It is also possible that the patient was allowed to overindulge too soon after operation. The law of Laplace is applicable in this situation and must be kept in mind. The distending force is related to pressure times diameter.

There have been enough staple disruptions that many of us are now using two applications of the TA90 or TA55 with 5 to 10 mm between in order to obviate the problem. Some are continuing to divide the stomach as originally described. Alden's operative procedure [5] is highly recommended in view of the fact that he has the lowest operative mortality and morbidity of anyone who has performed 350 or more of these operations. Weight loss in his series has been as great with gastric as with intestinal bypass.

A loop gastroenterostomy is sometimes difficult to fashion without tension. Also about 3% of patients complain of bile regurgitation or symptoms related to bile gastritis and esophagitis. This can be corrected by converting the anastomosis to a Roux-en-Y. A Roux-type anastomosis has been used by Griffen [6], Buckwalter [7] and Mason [8] as the initial operation. This has the drawback of a more complex and therefore riskier procedure and precludes subsequent fiberoptic examination of the duodenum and excluded stomach. For patients with esophageal reflux after gastric bypass the Roux-en-Y gastroenterostomy is preferable to Nissen fundoplication or other antireflux operations.

During 1971, gastroplasty was used in 53 patients. However, by the end of the year the data were conclusive that this operation was not providing adequate control of weight. In retrospect, the upper segment was made too large. Recently I have begun to use this procedure again at the suggestion of Cesar Gomez, who has performed 200 such operations during the last ten months. Gomez passes a 24 F Hurst dilator and then staples the stomach from the lesser curvature, placing two sets of staples a few millimeters apart. He then passes a 34 F dilator and with this in place he uses a 3-0 Prolene running seromuscular suture to invert the wall of the stomach so as to form a ring of tissue around the circumference of the passage. The dilator guarantees an accurate 12 mm diameter and the seromuscular nonabsorbable suture helps to guarantee that the stoma will remain at 12 mm diameter. If weight loss proves to be satisfactory at the end of the first year, our experience with the follow-up of such operations would lead us to believe that gastroplasty will be the operation of choice. There are several other surgeons studying the procedure, but I would discourage general use of gastroplasty until we have more assurance of its long-term efficacy. Even if gastroplasty becomes the operation of choice, gastric bypass, with a Roux-en-Y type of gastroenterostomy, may still be required for patients with decreased lower esophageal pressure and reflux. This is purely speculative since late results with gastroplasty are not yet available.

There are many lessons to be learned. Operative mortality should be less than 1% but will be higher if surgeons attempt to perform gastric bypass without proper selection and preparation. Patients should be more than twice the estimated ideal weight. They should be potentially vigorous, active people who have plans for a productive and rewarding life, but have the burden of fat, gallstones, hernias, edematous aprons, swollen legs, aching backs, sciaticas or other problems for which weight reduction is indicated.

Patients are usually intubated awake. After all the arterial, intravenous and monitoring equipment is in place, the arms are suspended with skin traction at the head of the table from poles used by the gynecologists for stirrups. A special retractor*

*Poly-Tract Retractor System as modified for obese patients is available through Pilling.

secured to the table used to elevate the rib cage, retract wound edges, retract the left lobe of the liver provides excellent exposure. A head light is of great help especially with the heaviest patients. Glucose is infused from the night before operation until oral intake is again established in order to suppress free fatty acids, which may contribute to thromboembolism [9]. Heparin and leg wrapping are not usually used. In older patients or patients whose care is complicated by prolonged operations, peritonitis and/or the need for respirator care, heparin may be indicated.

The functional residual capacity of the lungs must be maintained above closing volume to prevent hypoxia, hypercarbia, atelectasis and pneumonia. Patients should be ambulated early and required to deep breathe. They should not be allowed to breathe through an open endotracheal tube at atmospheric pressure without periodic sigh-type ventilation.

Nasogastric suction is of extreme importance. Gastric dilatation is not easily recognized and can be fatal if not treated (or preferably prevented). Unlike Billroth II gastrectomy, gastric bypass provides two segments each of which can become overdistended and leak. About half of leaks have occurred from the distal segment. If the pulse rate rises more than 1 SD above the mean (120 per minute on the first postoperative day; somewhat less on subsequent days) then reexploration is indicated, unless some other explanation can be provided. If acute gastric dilation is found at reoperation, a temporary gastrostomy should be placed in the excluded stomach. If there is a leak the abdomen should be freshened as described by Hudspeth [10]. I have participated in 220 gastric bypass operations, 42 gastroplasties, 13 conversions of gastroplasty to gastric bypass and 49 revisions of gastric bypass to make the pouch or stoma smaller. There have been ten leaks (3%) in these 324 operations. Ischemia has not been a cause. Of course, this does not mean that we ignore the anatomy or do not appreciate the need for preservation of blood flow high on the lesser curvature. Nevertheless, our leaks have been due to other causes, with overdistention being the most common.

As mentioned above, stomal ulcer incidence is less than 2% [11, 12]. Obstruction of the small passage is usually functional or due to food that is inadequately chewed.

Fiberoptic gastroscopy is the major diagnostic tool if there are problems. The major problem in gastric bypass has been a failure to perform the operation so as to produce a volume of less than 50 ml and a stoma of 12 mm or less. Consequently, revision has been necessary in about 20% of patients. This has been a difficult lesson for us and for our patients and must be learned by anyone who uses the procedure. You must measure the volume of the functional gastric segment intraoperatively.

Those who would like to undertake the care of morbidly obese patients should make sure that they have the needed facilities, equipment and the support of colleagues. These high gastric operations can be simple and easy in patients who are only twice the ideal weight. However, they can also be very difficult. There are too many problems in the hands of surgeons whose series are small. A national registry is being maintained in Iowa City for the use of those who wish to share their experience. A gastric bypass workshop was held in April 1977 and will be held again May 24 and 25, 1979.

There is also a growing volume of literature. These and other forms of communication plus the tremendous background of knowledge regarding the use of gastric resection have encouraged a rapid increase in the use of gastric operations as the initial treatment in the management of morbid obesity. Furthermore, they are becoming popular as replacements for intestinal bypass in patients who have developed renal stones, liver failure, arthralgia, intractable diarrhea or other problems. Proper preparation of patients with malnutrition secondary to intestinal bypass is important in those who require conversion to gastric bypass. This may require weeks of central venous feedings for the most seriously depleted individuals.

The weight loss to be expected from gastric bypass is comparable to that observed after intestinal bypass. The functioning stomach can be reduced to 50 ml or less without risk of producing either kwashiorkor or marasmus. The importance of a small fundic segment has been stressed by Hornberger who has participated in operations with me on several occasions. When I thought I was constructing a small volume passage between esophagus and intestine, he assured me his are smaller. His results [13] are excellent and his observations are appreciated.

Patients do not usually reach an ideal weight. Weight loss is improving, but currently the average loss is 30% of initial weight, 55% of excess weight or 40 kg. Like intestinal bypass, gastric bypass causes the greatest absolute weight loss in those patients whose initial weight is the greatest. There are ancillary benefits, reduced hypertension, easier management of diabetes, increased ability to work and improved social contacts. The risk-benefit ratio promises to be rewarding if patients are properly selected and the procedure appropriately applied.

References

1. Mason, E.E. and Ito, C.: Gastric bypass in obesity. Surg. Clin. North Am. 47:1345, 1967.
2. Ito, C. and Mason, E.E.: Gastric bypass and pancreatic secretion. Surgery 69:526, 1971.
3. Ito, C., Mason, E.E. and DenBesten, L.: Experimental studies on gastric bypass versus standard ulcer operations. Tohoku J. Exp. Med. 97:269, 1969.
4. Mason, E.E., Munns, J.R., Kealey, G.P. et al: Effect of gastric bypass on gastric secretion. Am. J. Surg. 131:162, 1976.
5. Alden, J.F.: Gastric and jejunoileal bypass. A comparison in the treatment of morbid obesity. Arch. Surg. 112:799, 1977.
6. Griffen, W.O., Young, V.L. and Stevenson, C.C.: A prospective comparison of gastric and jejunoileal bypass procedures for morbid obesity. Ann. Surg. 186:500, 1977.
7. Buckwalter, J.A.: Morbid obesity: Jejunoileal or gastric bypass? World J. Surg. 1:757, 1977.
8. Mason, E.E., Printen, K.J., Blommers, T.J. and Scott, D.H.: Gastric bypass for obesity after ten years experience. Int. J. Obesity 2:197, 1978.
9. Mason, E.E., Gordy, D.D., Chernigoy, F.A. and Printen, K.J.: Fatty acid toxicity. Surg. Gynecol. Obstet. 133:992, 1971.
10. Hudspeth, A.S.: Radical surgical debridement in the treatment of advanced generalized bacterial peritonitis. Arch. Surg. 110:1233, 1975.
11. Mason, E.E., Printen, K.J., Hartford, C.E. and Boyd, W.C.: Optimizing results of gastric bypass. Ann. Surg. 182:405, 1975.
12. Mason, E. and Ito, C.: Graded gastric bypass. World J. Surg. (In press.)
13. Hornberger, H.R.: Gastric bypass. Am. J. Surg. 131:415, 1976.

Self-Evaluation Quiz

1. Gastric bypass is an exclusion operation which has been followed by a 2% incidence of stomal ulcer because: *(Select the false completion(s))*

a) The vagus nerve remains intact and produces excessive acid secretion
b) There is usually so much parietal cell mass excluded as to suppress antral gastrin
c) Transection of the stomach at too low a level has allowed antral overactivity
d) Low transection leaves too many parietal cells above the gastroenterostomy
e) The food no longer passes through the distal stomach so that there is less mechanical and chemical stimulation of the antrum

2. Weight loss occurs following gastric bypass because: (*Select the least accurate*)
   a) The operation simulates subtotal gastrectomy which was largely abandoned for treatment of ulcer because of poor maintenance of weight
   b) The upper segment is fashioned so as to have a capacity of about 50 ml
   c) The gastroenterostomy stoma of 12 mm in diameter helps to prevent overeating
   d) Malabsorption results from rapid transit and from other manifestations of the dumping syndrome in 70% of patients
   e) A deficiency common to the obese is corrected in that they now recognize satiety or a sense of fullness
3. Which of the following is false?
   a) Gastroplasty was used in 1971 and was proven to be an unsatisfactory operation for production of weight loss
   b) Gastric bypass can be performed properly and successfully only by dividing the vessels along the upper greater curvature all of the way to the esophagus
   c) The law of LaPlace explains why large fundic segments are more likely to increase in size, or even to rupture, than small volume segments
   d) Staples placed across the undivided stomach have pulled through in some patients requiring reoperation to correct
   e) Reoperation has been necessary in about 20% of patients because the upper segment was not measured and was left too large and/or because the stoma was too large and the patient did not lose enough weight

4. Which of the following is *not* a reason for recommending weight reduction by gastric bypass?
   a) More than twice estimated ideal weight
   b) Failure of dietary weight loss under medical guidance
   c) Absence of myxedema, adrenal overactivity, or other endocrine diseases
   d) Presence of complications of obesity such as diabetes, varicose veins, degenerative arthritis, intertrigo, hypertension
   e) Presence of angina or history of myocardial infarction
5. Which of the following has not been important in the course of recognition and prevention of serious morbidity and potential mortality following gastric bypass? (*Choose one*)
   a) Pulmonary embolism
   b) Acute gastric dilation from poorly functioning nasal gastric tube
   c) Postoperative pulse rate of more than 120/minute
   d) Radical debridement in the treatment of peritonitis
   e) Acute pancreatitis
6. Which of the following is shared by both gastric and intestinal bypass?
   a) Liver failure
   b) Renal calcium oxalate stones
   c) Arthralgia
   d) Inadequate weight loss in some patients
   e) Enteritis
7. Which of the following cannot be expected to result from gastric bypass?
   a) A loss of 30% of initial weight on the average
   b) Improvement in exercise tolerance
   c) Tightening up of loose skin with exercise
   d) Loss of 55% of excess weight on the average
   e) Loss of 40 kg of initial weight on the average
   f) Lowering of insulin requirement for diabetics
   g) A lowering of blood pressure if it is high before operation
8. Reflux esophagitis before or after gastric bypass is best managed by
   a) Nissen fundoplication
   b) Not performing gastric bypass or restoring normal gastric continuity

   c) Braun type of enteroenterostomy
   d) Roux-en-Y gastroenterostomy
   e) Reduction of acid by vagotomy
9. Which of the following has *not* been of use in performing gastric bypass or gastroplasty?
   a) Watching others perform the operation
   b) Repetition
   c) Polytract Retractor System
   d) Surgeon's head mounted light source
   e) Stapling instruments
   f) Hegar 12 mm dilator
   g) Hurst dilators, numbers 24 and 36 F
   h) Nonabsorbable suture such as 3-0 polypropylene
   i) None of the above

Answers on page 721.

Comparison of Gastric Bypass and Jejunoileal Bypass

John F. Alden, M.D.

Objectives

The objective of this paper is to show the difference in the effects of the gastric bypass and the intestinal bypass on the patients and to indicate by the comparison which one is superior. In the systems, the gastric bypass is superior.

Experience with surgery for morbidly obese patients began with jejunocolic shunts which were disastrous operations. The 14-4 jejunoileal bypass popularized by Payne was a great improvement over the former operation; however, Arnold Kremen, who initiated this procedure, stopped doing it in 1954 after treating about 20 patients. He felt that the side effects were too severe to warrant its continued use. After 250 operations, using intestinal bypass, my enthusiasm waned, because so many of the patients had such severe side effects that they had become a tremendous burden to care for. Mason's gastric bypass was tried next. In its initial form, when the stomach was completely transected into a large and small pouch, the difficulty of the operation made it very unattractive. Modifying the operation simplified it and increased its safety so that it now has become quite acceptable.

After performing approximately 100 gastric bypass operations, it seemed that the procedure effected a reasonable weight loss with a minimum of unpleasant side effects. One hundred randomly selected patients from the intestinal bypass series were compared with the first 100 patients from the gastric

John F. Alden, M.D., Clinical Professor of Surgery, University of Minnesota Medical School, Minneapolis.

bypass series. All patients in both series met the usual criteria of being 100 or more pounds overweight for more than five years without lasting success from medical management. Most were in their thirties and most were females.

Figure 1 illustrates the intestinal bypass popularized by Payne and is the operation which has been most often performed in the United States. This is the operation done in most of the patients compared with the gastric bypass patients.

The modification of the gastric bypass operation is indicated in Figures 2-4. A midline incision running from the xiphoid to the umbilicus is used. The abdominal esophagus is encircled with a large penrose drain in order to outline the cardio-esophageal junction. The proximal third of the greater curvature of the stomach is completely freed, up to and including the esophagus. The small vessels are either tied with silk or controlled with hemoclips. A second smaller penrose drain is placed through the lesser omentum to serve as a guide for the TA 90 stapling instrument. This part of the dissection is kept close to the wall of the stomach so as not to injure the left gastric vessels or the nerves. The opening is about 2 cm below the esophagus.

A loop of jejunum is brought up antecolonically and tacked to the proposed gastric pouch with three silk stitches. The anastomosis is then made using a GIA instrument inserted to the 2-cm mark through small stab wounds made with electrocautery in the anterior wall of the stomach and in the jejunum. The anastomosis is completed with interrupted 3-0 silk sutures. A sufficient amount of cuff is turned in to make the stoma about 1.5 cm in diameter.

The nasogastric tube is placed into the efferent limb of the jejunum. The TA 90 is inserted from the patient's right side and a row of 4.8-mm staples is placed to divide but not transect the stomach. The pouch in the last several hundred operations has been reduced to about 5% of the original gastric volume. In fact, the pouch is really only a conduit from the esophagus to the jejunum. It is usually about the size of one's thumb. Finally, the jejunum is sutured to the greater curvature of the stomach for about 5 or 6 cm so there will be no kinking or twisting of the efferent limb. In both operations, the abdominal closure is made with interrupted stainless steel wire sutures. The sub-

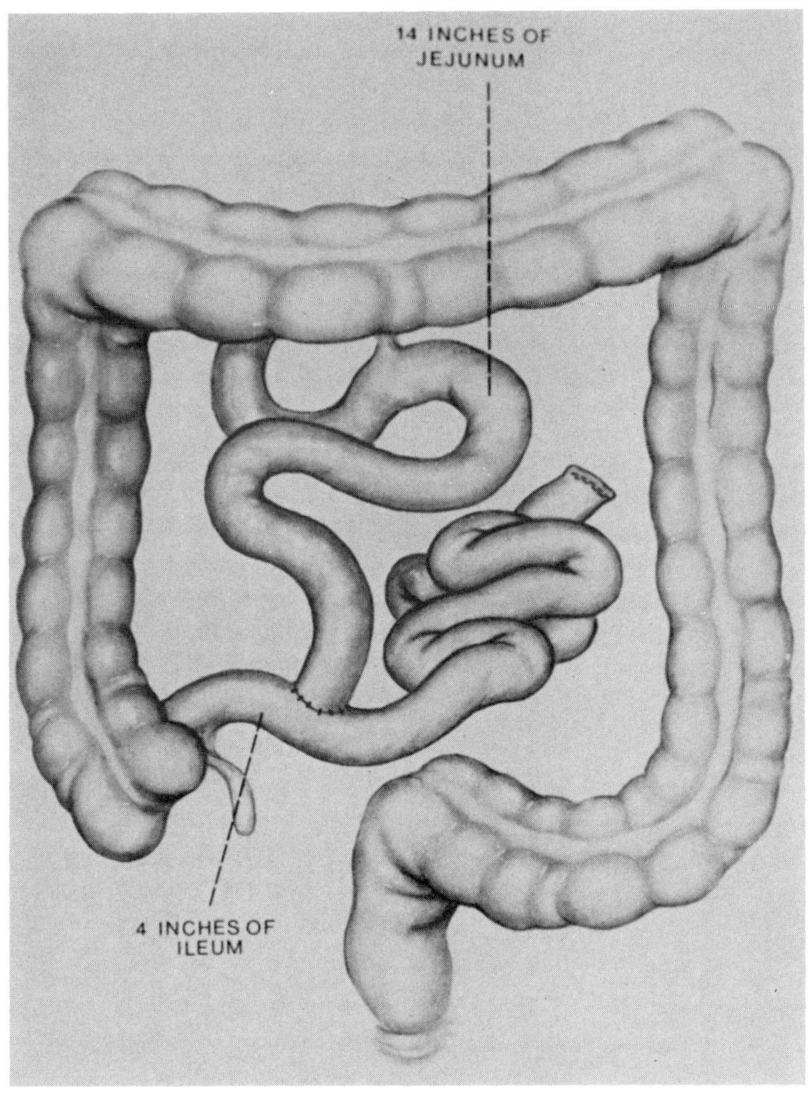

FIGURE 1.

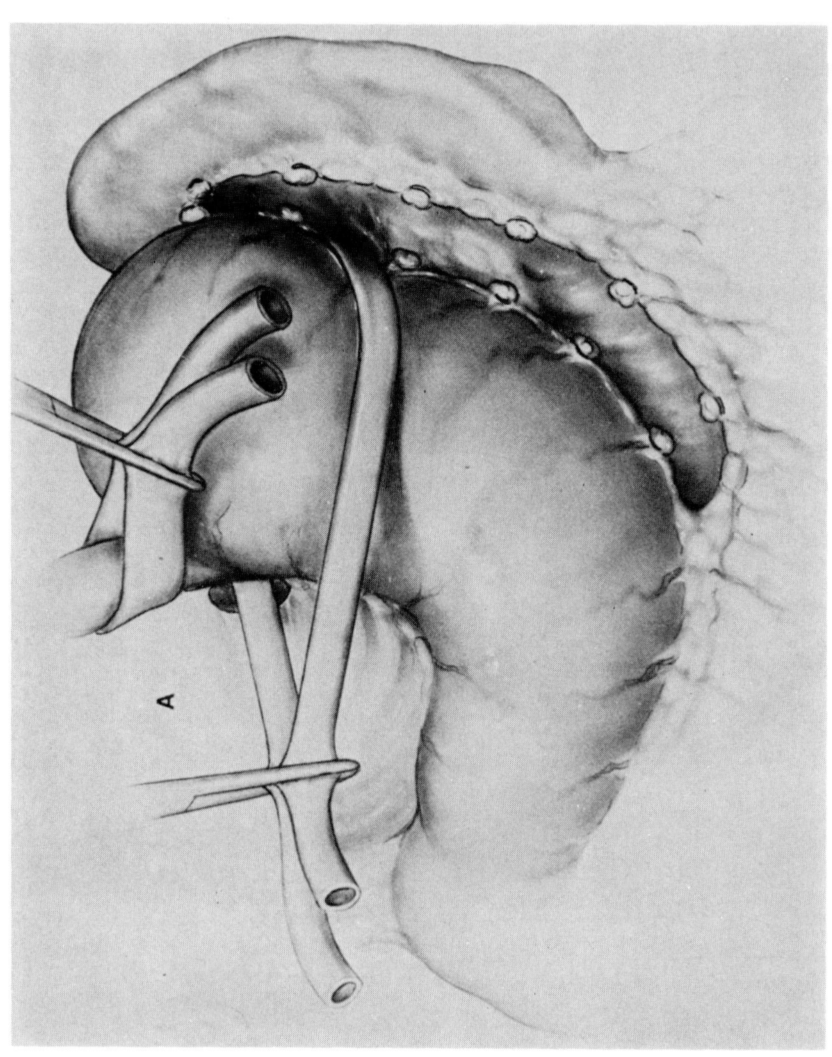

FIGURE 2.

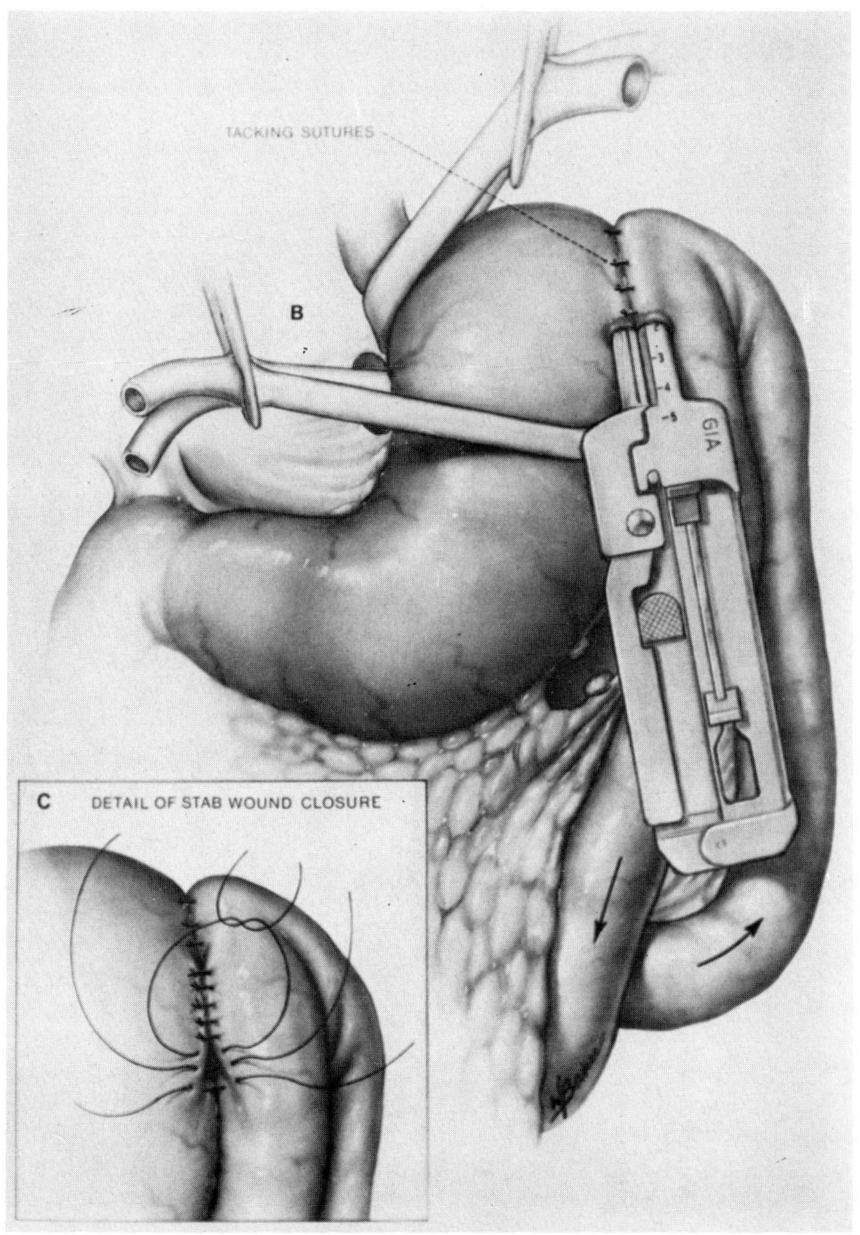

FIGURE 3.

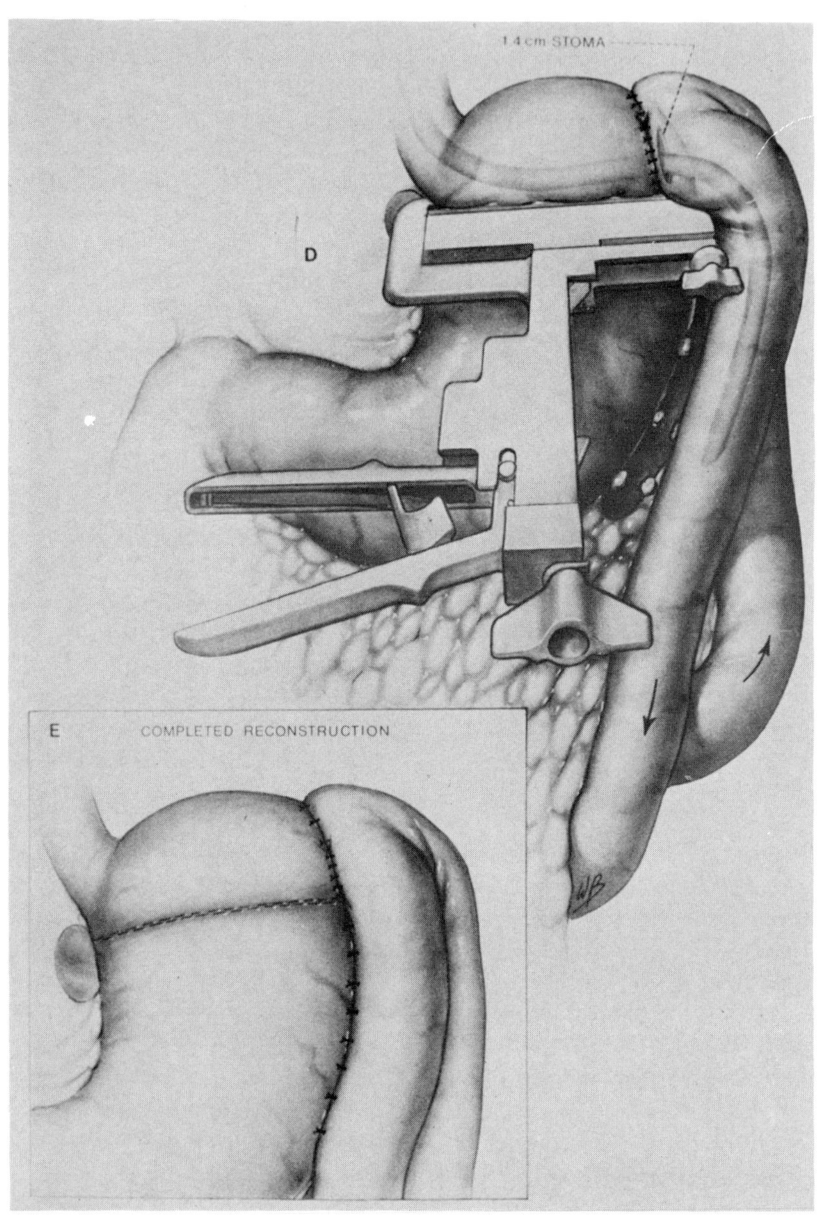

FIGURE 4.

cutaneous fat is irrigated with Kantrex solution. No sutures are used in the fat. The skin is stapled and no drains are used.

The average patient in the intestinal bypass series weighed 280 pounds. The intestinal bypass operation took an average of 60 minutes to perform. Fifteen of the 100 patients also had cholecystectomy. The average hospital stay was 8.6 days. Weight loss after one year averaged 89 pounds. This is a median percent weight loss of 31% for the intestinal bypass group. There were two wound infections and two wound dehiscences in this group. Seven patients developed incisional hernias.

The 100 gastric bypass patients weighed an average of 270 pounds, 10 pounds less than the intestinal bypass group. Otherwise, the preoperative vital statistics were similar. The average operating time for the gastric bypass was 68 minutes and 15 cholecystectomies were done. The average stay in the hospital was 8.2 days. At the end of one year, the average weight loss was 88 pounds. This is a median percent weight loss of 36%. In this group there were two wound infections, one dehiscence, and three incisional hernias.

The progression of weight loss was steady at first, but in the later months appeared to be rather spotty for the gastric group (Fig. 5). This is due to the fact that the earlier patients had pouches and stomas that were too large. Later experiences show an average weight loss of 95 pounds at one year among a group of patients weighing an average of 260 pounds. This represents a median one year weight loss of 37% for the gastric bypass group.

During the first three postoperative months, almost all of the intestinal bypass patients had severe diarrhea and anorectal problems. Additional complaints were fatigue, cramps, nausea, bloating and foul and excessive flatus which threatened the jobs of a few patients. Electrolyte problems, in particular hypokalemia, were common. Hypocalcemia seemed to appear later. The single early death was due to sigmoid diverticulitis. Both operations are about equally safe and the weight loss is similar. The big differences in the two operations become apparent when later side effects are examined.

Liver disease is the most serious complication of the jejunoileal bypass. Fortunately only one patient in this series died of liver failure. After becoming more aware of this

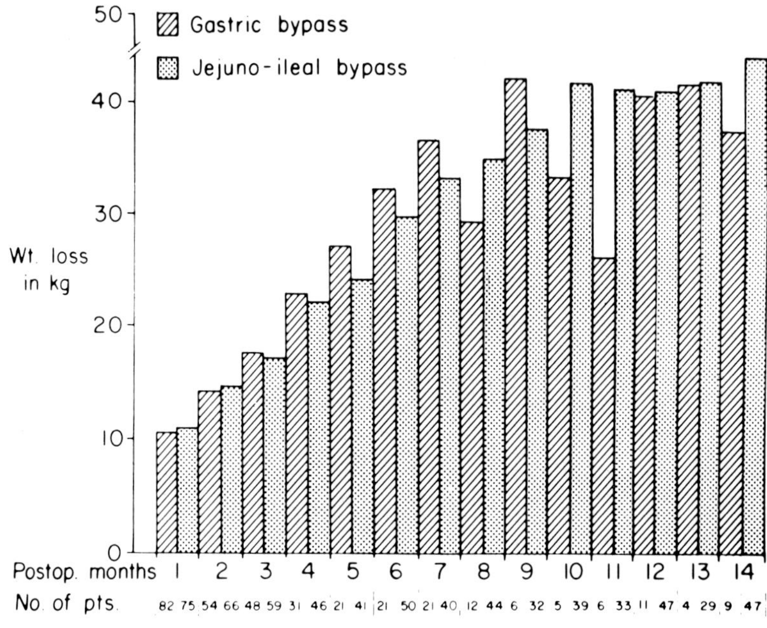

FIGURE 5.

problem, the intestinal bypass was taken down in two other patients because of severe liver disease. This complication seems to be unique to the jejunoileal bypass and has not been seen in the gastric bypass series.

In this patient with intestinal bypass, the initial biopsy specimen of the liver is on the left. Eighteen months later when the bypass was taken down, the liver histology was much worse and the weight loss was only 34 pounds (Fig. 6).

The initial biopsy in this gastric bypass patient is on the left. Eleven months later, after a weight loss of 80 pounds, a second biopsy was done at the time of a cholecystectomy. This is shown in Figure 7. The liver appeared normal.

Figure 8 shows a similar improvement of the liver a year after a gastric bypass with good weight loss. The initial biopsy is on the left. The one on the right is normal 11 months later. Thus, it seems that rapid weight loss alone does not explain the liver problem of intestinal bypass.

Ten patients in the intestinal bypass group developed calcium oxalate, urinary stones, most of which were passed

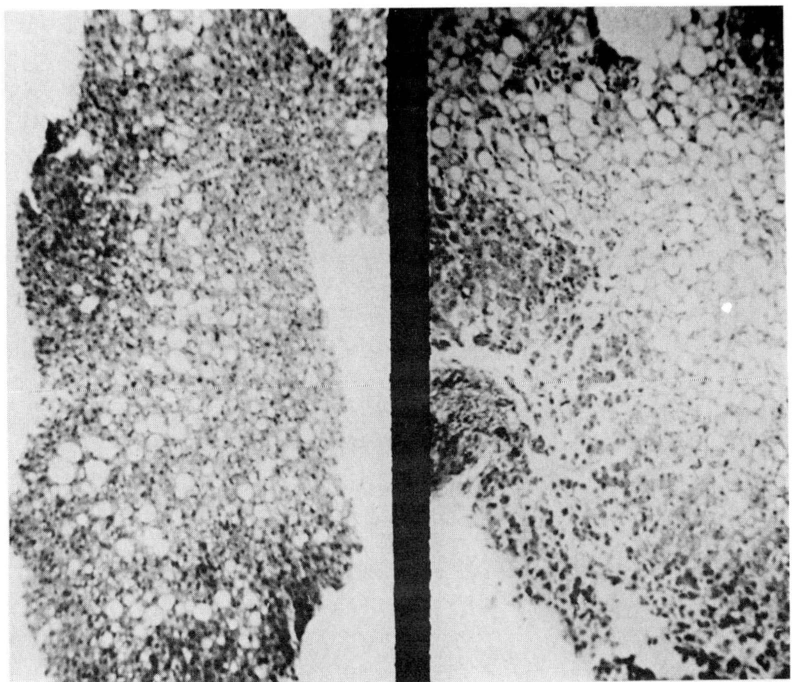

FIGURE 6.

spontaneously, although some were removed surgically. Recurrent stone formation made it necessary to take the bypass down in three patients. This number grows larger as more time passes. Prophylaxis with oral calcium carbonate to bind the oxalate is a great help in reducing stone formation and also helps to control the diarrhea, but unfortunately most of the patients did not receive this benefit.

Seven patients developed severe arthritis and four of these had the bypass taken down because of this. Steroids are useful in controlling the arthritis when it is not too severe for too long a period of time.

Diarrhea, bloating and fatigue have continued for long periods in many patients; some once thought to be among the best results are returning seven and eight years later requesting that the intestinal bypass be taken down.

In the first few postoperative weeks some of the gastric bypass patients experienced nausea and vomiting. This was mostly of a minor degree and improved after they learned to eat

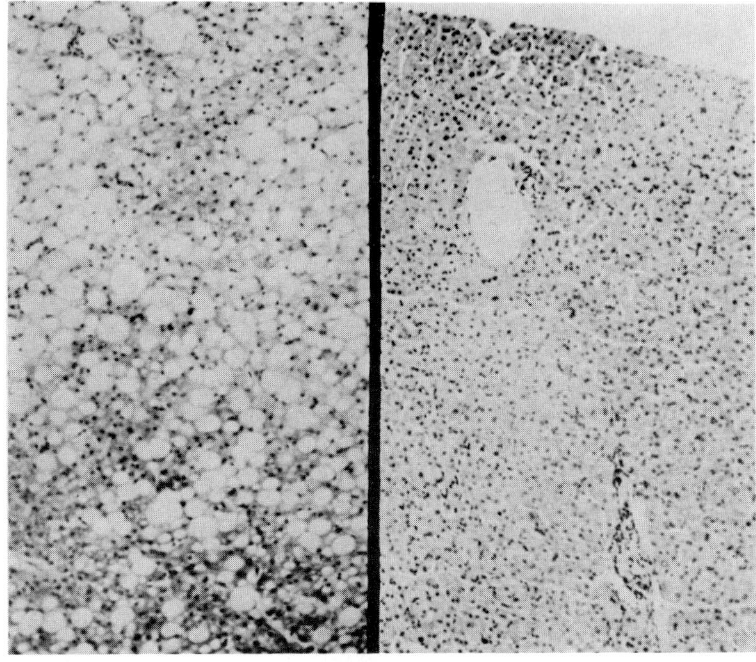

FIGURE 7.

less. Only one patient was hospitalized for vomiting. Meat is a particularly difficult food to digest after gastric bypass and beef seems to be the worst.

One gastric bypass patient developed an efferent limb obstruction which was corrected on the tenth postoperative day by a second operation. Another patient bled from a superficial erosion of the stoma on the fifth postoperative day. Several transfusions were given and the lesion healed spontaneously. Ten months after the gastric bypass another patient bled from an ulcer that developed in the 10% pouch. The serum gastrin level was low. No transfusions were needed and the lesion healed in three weeks under medical management.

Mild dumping has been seen in several patients and mild reflux esophagitis in a few more. No liver disease or kidney stones have been encountered in the gastric bypass patients.

A single late death occurred in a 53-year-old male, who died from a heart attack at home two months after the gastric bypass.

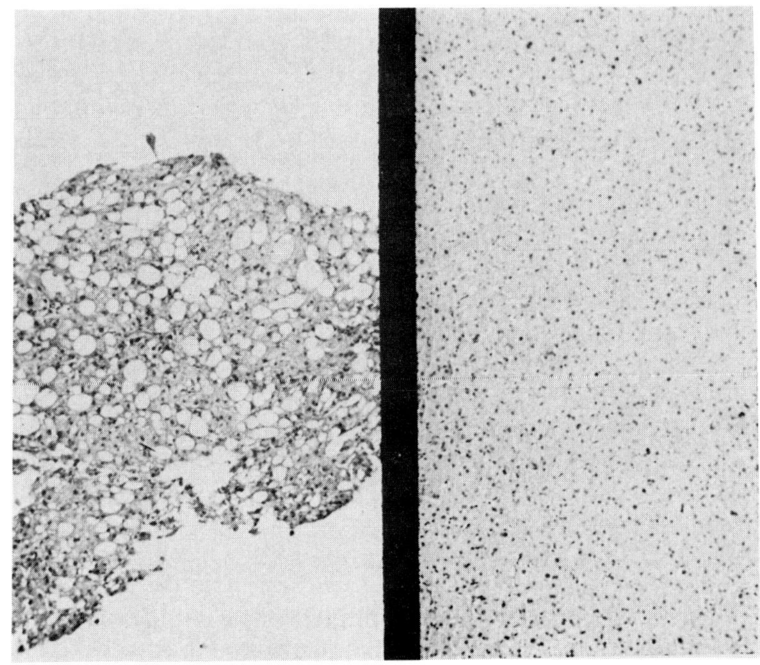

FIGURE 8.

During the first postoperative year, the rate of rehospitalization for all causes was 32% in the jejunoileal bypass group and 12% in the gastric bypass series. Despite this, patient satisfaction at one year was at the 90% level in both series, indicating that for these people anything beats being fat.

Several uneventful pregnancies followed both operations.

No diabetics were included in the intestinal bypass group. In the gastric bypass group, four diabetics taking 25 to 40 units of insulin per day were able to give up their insulin. Another patient dropped his insulin from 150 units to 25 units after gastric bypass.

Although gastric bypass is somewhat more difficult to do, it can be done in about the same amount of time as the jejunoileal bypass and with equal safety. The use of stapling instruments has reduced operating time and increased the safety of the procedure.

The patients in the gastric bypass series had a slightly greater weight loss than did the jejunoileal bypass patients. Yet they returned to energetic good health more rapidly and consistently. They have not experienced the persistent and often serious problems of diarrhea, fatigue, liver disease, urinary stones and arthritis. The incidence of peptic ulcer, dumping, vomiting and reflux esophagitis has been low in the gastric bypass group.

Experience with the two operations indicates that the gastric bypass operation is superior. It has become the procedure of choice. Having come to this conclusion, I now use it exclusively and have increased the size of the gastric bypass series to 478 patients. There have now been two deaths, both due to massive pulmonary embolism despite the routine use of low dose heparin.

There are a large number of dissatisfied intestinal bypass patients among whom perhaps 20%, or more, will need corrective surgery later. Restoring the intestine to normal permits rapid weight gain. Adding a few more inches of small intestine to the bypass has given good results in only about half of the patients so treated.

Gastric bypass has been combined with reconstruction of the intestine in one operation. This has been a most satisfactory method of handling side effects severe enough to justify an additional operation. This combined operation has been done 75 times with no operative deaths and few postoperative complications. Its use is reserved for the relatively healthy patients who are unwilling to put up with the side effects of the jejunoileostomy. Most commonly these have been severe diarrhea, bloating, arthritis, chronic fatigue, or urinary stones.

In order to make the combined operation of the gastric bypass and takedown of the intestinal bypass simple enough to be done in one stage, stapling instruments are needed. The procedure is illustrated in Figures 9 and 10.

The dilated 14-inch segment of the jejunum is detached from the ileum with the aid of the TA 90 using the 4.8-mm staples. The Kocher forceps on the jejunum are applied so as to leave a small opening in the bowel toward the antimesenteric border for the insertion of the GIA in the next step.

The dilated segment of the proximal jejunum and the narrowed segment of the defunctionalized intestine are placed in proper apposition and held there with stay sutures. A small

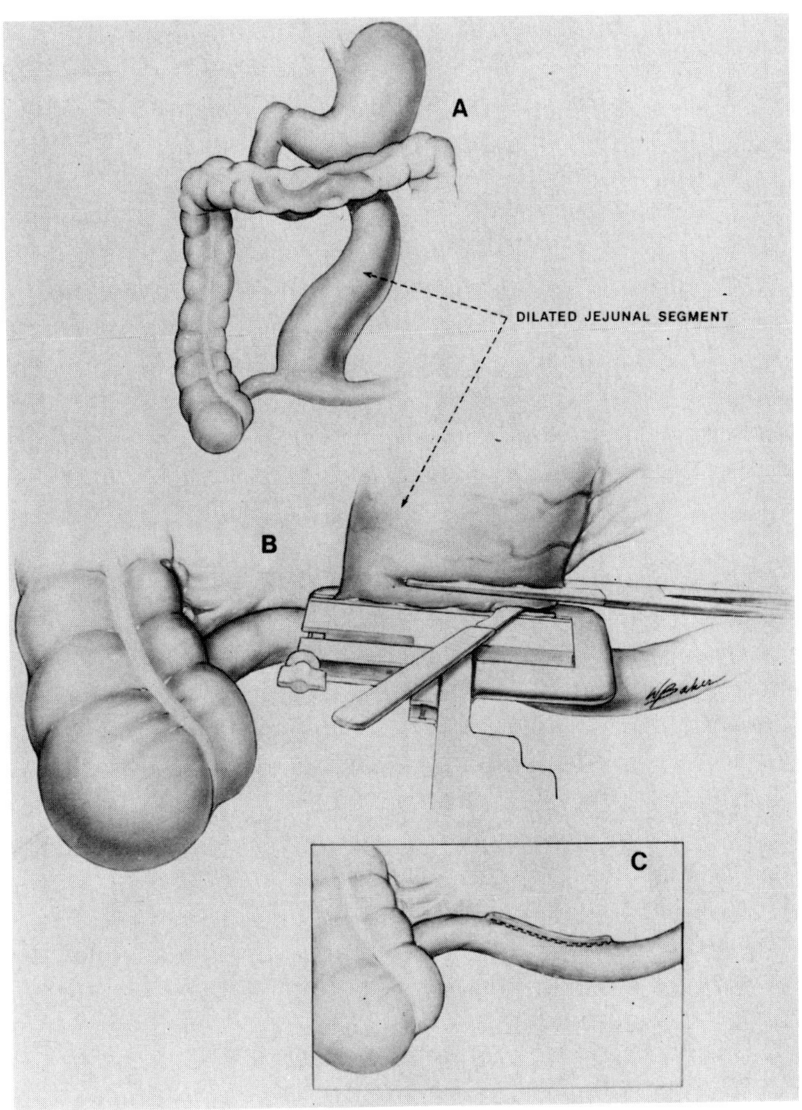

FIGURE 9.

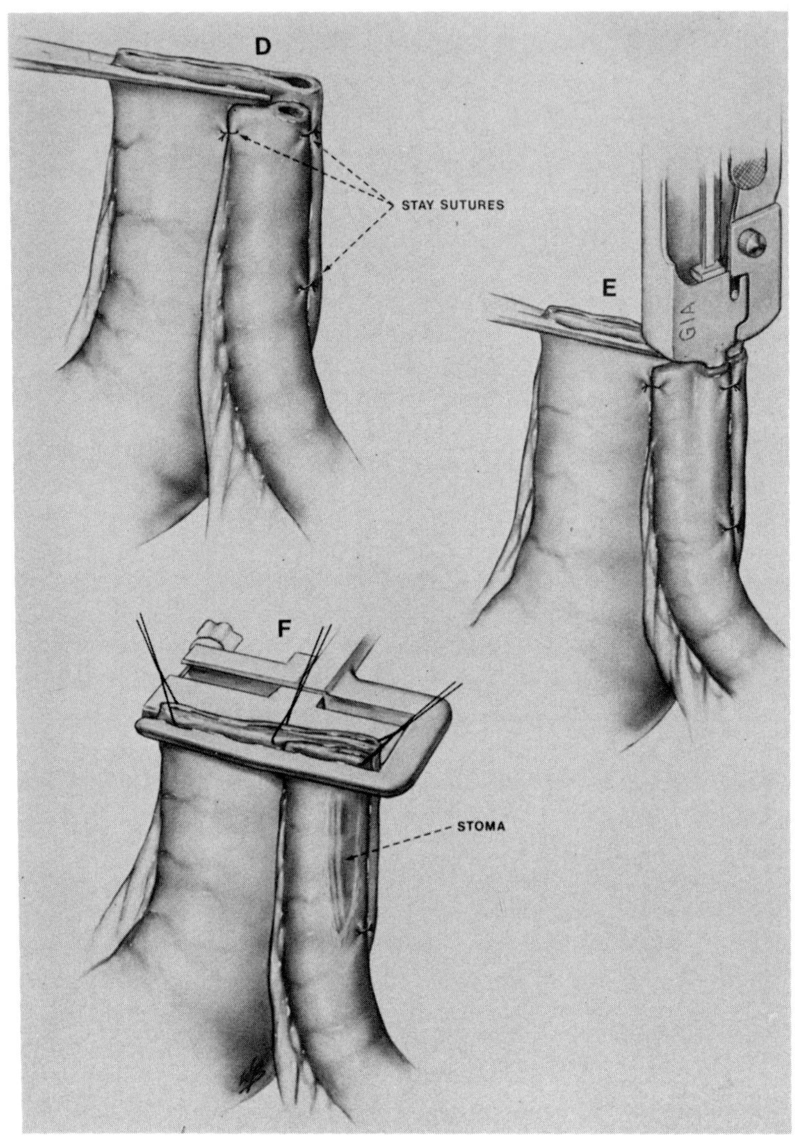

FIGURE 10.

opening is made in the end of the narrowed jejunum with the cautery. The GIA is inserted through these openings and fired leaving a wide stoma between these unequal segments of intestine. A single cartridge of 4.8-mm staples in the TA 90 closes the ends of the bowel and the anastomosis is completed. The anastomosis is covered with 4-0 silk Lembert sutures. This type of anastomosis makes a wide stoma between the atretic and the dilated segments of the jejunum. After the intestine has been re-anastomosed the gastric bypass is done as described earlier.

These operations have been performed as late as eight years after jejunoileostomy and the bypassed segment of the small intestine has functioned well.

The patients converted from the jejunoileal bypass to gastric bypass have offered us an opportunity to compare the two operations in the same person. These patients are much happier with gastric bypass than they were with jejunoileal bypass. Naturally they wouldn't have had the second operation if they were happy with the first.

In summary, intestinal and gastric bypasses were compared. The side effects of the gastric bypass are much easier for the patient to live happily with than those of the jejunoileal bypass. Weight loss has been a little better for the gastric bypass group. The risk of the operations and the time required to perform them are about the same. Finally, the gastric bypass has been used to rescue the relatively healthy patient from the side effects of the jejunoileal bypass. This has been done in a single stage consisting of dismantling the intestinal bypass and substituting the gastric bypass to control the obesity. Again, this is not done on critically ill patients. Stapling instruments have been a great help in reducing the risks of surgery.

Gastric bypass is the better of the two operations for control of morbid obesity.

Self-Evaluation Quiz

1. In order to be considered for a bypass operation, the patient must be:
   a) 50 pounds overweight
   b) 75 pounds overweight

c) 100 pounds overweight
d) 125 pounds overweight

2. The most dangerous sequela of the intestinal bypass is:
   a) Hepatic failure
   b) Hypokalemia
   c) Hypocalcemia
   d) Incisional hernia
3. Gastric bypass affects the liver by causing:
   a) Cirrhosis
   b) Fatty deterioration of the liver
   c) Portal fibrosis
   d) None of these
4. The prophylaxis of urinary stones following intestinal bypass is best accomplished by:
   a) Increased fluid intake
   b) Vitamin E
   c) Calcium carbonate orally
   d) High doses of vitamin C
5. The best method of handling the side effects of intestinal bypass which require additional surgery is:
   a) Takedown of the intestinal bypass
   b) Takedown of the intestinal bypass and shortening of the small intestine
   c) Revising the small intestinal anastomosis
   d) Gastric resection after takedown of the jejunoileal bypass
   e) Simultaneous gastric bypass and takedown of the jejunoileal bypass

Answers on page 721.

Discussion

Moderator: Richard C. Lillehei, M.D.

Moderator: I think all the surgical supply houses have the Leonard tube, and you can get them just by ordering. The questions I have received from the audience are predominantly on the gastric and jejunoileal bypass. Dr. Wangensteen, someone wants you to clarify when you would operate for bowel obstruction. Since you get such good results with intubation, at what point do you operate?

Dr. Wangensteen: In the series that Doctors Leonard, Edlich and I published in the late 1960s, where we substituted peroral intubation for early operation, we decompressed the majority of the patients solely by intubation, making enterotomy or enterostomy unnecessary. But we did operate upon all those patients usually within 12 hours after entry when the decompression was fairly complete. My understanding from Dr. Goodale is that he has decompressed quite a number of patients, guiding the Leonard tube down with a flexible gastroscope, and has not operated upon some of those patients. But experience dictates that in the presence of a mechanical obstruction, an operation is in order to remove the site of the obstruction.

Moderator: I shall ask each of the three speakers on the bypass procedure to answer this question, about the comparison of blood lipid changes between the jejunoileal bypass and the gastric bypass. Dr. Mason, do you have any information on the initial as well as the long-term effects on blood lipids?

Dr. Mason: I cannot give you the kind of information that Dr. Buchwald can. We have measured cholesterol and triglycerides in most of the patients initially, but we do not have follow-up data. A few patients have had very high levels. I remember one patient who was having repeated attacks of pancreatitis. With the weight loss, the cholesterol and triglycerides dropped down into the normal range and the patient has had no more pancreatitis. It is my impression that the vast majority of our patients do not have hyperlipidemia. The cholesterol levels do not really change much. This does not bother me because it is not a problem in the first place. I wonder about using that as an argument for intestinal bypass. I do not see how you can argue that an intestinal bypass should be used in preference to some other procedure for the treatment of obesity combined with hyperlipidemia, when the patient really does not have hyperlipidemia.

Moderator: Dr. Alden, have you made any comparison of the lipids between the two groups?

Dr. Alden: I have not made any comparisons. My feelings are very much the same as Dr. Buchwald's, who I think has the information on this. I would be very interested to hear what he has to say to this question.

Dr. Buchwald: I can offer some data in contrast to the other comments. Any weight-losing procedure will cause a marked reduction of the serum cholesterol during the period of weight loss. Once the weight levels off after the gastric bypass, the cholesterol level returns to the preoperative value and there is, therefore, no permanent reduction of the serum cholesterol level; whereas, after the jejunoileal bypass there is a permanent reduction of 40% to 50% in the plasma cholesterol level. With regard to triglycerides, weight loss lowers triglycerides, regardless of how it is achieved. Thus, triglycerides go down after either procedure. Now, how important is cholesterol? How important are the triglycerides? The newest data would seem to conclude that the triglycerides are a secondary factor for atherosclerosis, not a primary risk factor. That is, they are secondary to the plasma cholesterol concentration elevation. Thus, to reduce triglycerides per se does not seem to be a justification, really, for any procedure, be it drug or surgical. As to a reduced cholesterol, is this beneficial? Well, we do not precisely know the answer to that question. Therefore, one has to go by a gut reaction, if I may use that pun. If one believes that the average cholesterol in the United States is too high and that reducing it is beneficial, since 52% of our population dies of some sort of atherosclerotic complication, then the reduction that is achieved from even the preoperative levels that Dr. Scott discussed must be beneficial. We are gaining evidence to show that this will be true in the long run.

Moderator: I noticed in the presentations made by all those interested in the bypass problem that no one showed any longevity comparisons with the normal population. What evidence do you have that longevity is increased by the bypass procedure? I think you will concede that patients look better and that generally people feel better. But how about statistics for longevity? Dr. Mason, would you like to begin?

Dr. Mason: We do not have any control group.

Moderator: Quite often this is the case, but we may use the mortality curves for the normal population and that is better than nothing. After the jejunoileal bypass does the patient follow the normal curve of mortality? Dr. Alden, do you have any data?

Dr. Alden: We do not have any data as to the patients upon whom we operate so we have to extrapolate from other data. The most important is that of Ernst Drenick. He indicates that the morbidly obese patient will have no higher mortality up to the age of 35 years. At the age of 35 years, only one out of seven of those people will live a normal life span and have the mortality of the rest of the population. When they reach the age of 40 years, only one out of 11 of those people will live a normal life span. So you could say that ten out of 11 people will die too early. Then, if you turn to life insurance tables, you will find that people who had formerly been very obese and then lost weight have the same life expectancy as those who have maintained a normal weight all of their life.

Dr. Buchwald: Dr. Lillehei, we do not have a series in this country. No one has been able to do a randomized controlled study under the conditions in which we practice medicine in this country. If you compare any series with some sort of general population statistics, no statistician would accept it and probably very few clinicians would. In Denmark, however, they have done a two-year controlled study. They have patients who came in for jejunoileal bypass surgery and were randomized. The patients accepted this randomization, as under socialized medicine, they had no other choice. Two years later, the preliminary data seemed to conclude that having had the bypass, even with the resulting complications, they were better off in terms of life expectancy, complications of diabetes, complications of atherosclerosis and so on.

Moderator: Dr. McKhann, the *Proceedings of the Mayo Clinic* recently had an article on CEA. They were quite disappointed with it in most cases I believe. Is that correct?

Dr. McKhann: Yes, I think Dr. Mortel is pretty disappointed. I should point out that the studies I showed are the most optimistic potential uses for CEA that now exist.

Dr. Wangensteen: Just 30 years ago, I suggested the second look for lesions like cancer of the colon, for cancer of the ovary and retroperitoneal rhabdomyosarcomas. Dr. McKhann, since you do not seem to have much confidence in the carcinoembryonic antigen, what do you think of the criteria that my associates and I, Doctors Arhelger, Ward Griffin and John Lewis, proposed back 30 years ago?

Dr. McKhann: The problems with the blind second look procedures were the patients who had real morbidity and mortality from them. A number of times you got there and found that you could not do anything curative. The actual number of patients in whom you could operate and successfully resect tumor and prolong or save life was not very large. CEA studies may narrow down that population by helping to select those people who should have a second look. The most significant slide I showed was that of Martin. His study is still too early and too small, with only 25 patients entered, to say what is really going to come out. But perhaps five of those patients have been salvaged.

Dr. Wangensteen: Dr. McKhann, our conversion rate, however, on operation of the patients who were positive for tumor was 17% for cancer of the colon, 22% for cancer of the ovary and 30% for retroperitoneal rhabdomyosarcoma. It is a modest accomplishment, I agree, but yet something definite.

Dr. McKhann: Absolutely.

Moderator: Pancreatitis after gastric bypass — is that a problem?

Dr. Mason: I have not seen it. We had one patient early in the series who had pancreatitis before he was operated upon, and we thought maybe we should treat his obesity, and maybe if he could not drink as much and eat as much, his pancreatitis would be better. Well, he was not any better. When we did an intraoperative pancreatogram, we found that he had normal pancreatic ducts with normal passage into the duodenum. His pancreatitis was a fibrosing type which could be treated not by drainage but by resection.

Moderator: So you had only that one patient?

Dr. Mason: We really have not had any pancreatitis that we could say was due to the operation.

Dr. Alden: I have never seen pancreatitis associated with a gastric bypass.

Dr. Buchwald: I think we had two episodes of chemical pancreatitis immediately postoperatively. You do lean on the pancreas for part of the dissection. We have ignored it and it went away. We just happened to look for it.

Moderator: I have several questions from the members of the audience that are directly or indirectly aimed at the same area. The audience would seem to believe that gastric bypass, from what has been presented, has fewer problems postoperatively. Why should one continue to do jejunoileal bypass?

Dr. Mason: I did two intestinal bypasses at the suggestion of Dr. Kremen about 1955 and decided that there was not any place for it. I could not see why people were continuing to write papers about it.

Dr. Alden: It took me 250 patients to learn the same thing. I really do not have any reason to continue doing intestinal bypasses.

Moderator: You just do not do jejunoileal bypass anymore?

Dr. Alden: I think there may come a time when some man with a very high cholesterol who has had some coronary disease and who is exceedingly fat might make me think of doing this. But I have not yet encountered that patient.

Dr. Buchwald: I do both. I have not made up my mind. I actually place all the data as I see them before the patients when they come in and try to let them help make a selection of procedure. I talk to six, eight or ten new patients at once, giving them exactly the same talk, and then talk to each one privately. One week they all want a jejunoileal bypass, and the next week they all want a gastric bypass. I do not think that I change that much from one week to the next. I do not know what influences them. I think there is a lot of faddism. In our community jejunoileal bypasses were big. Now, gastric bypasses are big. I really do not believe we have the data to say one is better than the other. Basically, I think the jejunoileal bypass still causes the greatest weight reduction, in comparison to the gastric bypass. It comes down to the fact that a 300-lb person in our series with a jejunoileal bypass goes to 190 lb; whereas, in Dr. Mason's series, and using his statistics, he would weigh 225 lb postoperatively. The weight loss is greater, at least at this time, with the jejunoileal bypass. Then, there are other differences. Some people do not like diarrhea. Some people do not like to vomit. Some people do not want to give up eating. Some people do not like dumping. These things are very real. It cannot be denied that jejunoileal bypass has a higher rate of complications — 5% serious and maybe another 5% or 10% not so serious. But 85% to 90% of patients are extremely happy and are doing very well. With respect to Dr. Alden's experience of taking down jejunoileal bypasses and doing gastrics, yes, I have done that. I have also taken down gastrics, or left them alone, when they have been totally ineffective and I have added the jejunoileal. Patients can outeat the gastric. They cannot outeat the jejunoileal. I do not think this issue is settled. One can say good and bad about both procedures. It is premature to be dogmatic. Both the learning process and the best care for the obese patient predicates that at this time, both procedures have a role.

The Importance of Antibiotics in Bowel Preparation for Colonic Surgery

Robert E. Condon, M.D.

Objectives

To review evidence of efficacy, especially from controlled studies of antibiotics and antimicrobials in bowel surgery, for penicillin, cephalosporins, neomycin, erythromycin, kanamycin, sulfonamides, tetracyclines, aminoglycosides and metronidazole.

The first issue I will address is whether antibiotics should be used in colon surgery. Surgeons have been using antibiotics since the first antimicrobials, the sulfonamides, were introduced 40 years ago. Intuitively over the years, we recognized that this was an appropriate practice and, for most of us, it seemed to reduce the risk of infectious complications. It was a somewhat controversial issue until the 1960s, when it became a rather heated controversy; the reason, of course, was that there were little in the way of solid controlled investigative data to establish the efficacy of antibiotics. Over the last decade, we all have been the beneficiaries of a large number of controlled studies. This paper deals with the evidence from controlled clinical trials that bears on the use of antibiotics.

In control patients from clinical trials who received vigorous mechanical preparation but did not receive antibiotics, the septic complication rates varied from 25% to 63% and averaged around 40%. When this issue is considered under rigorous

---

Robert E. Condon, M.D., Professor, Department of Surgery, The Medical College of Wisconsin; Chief of Surgical Services, Veterans Administration Center, Milwaukee, Wisc.

conditions, there is no question that patients undergoing colon surgery have a considerable risk of developing one or another septic complication. That is the background risk. As we will see in a moment, the appropriate use of antibiotics reduces this risk.

Let us look first at the systemic administration of various antibiotics. Mr. Hughes in his 1970 paper reported on the use of penicillin-G. This was short-term, high-dose penicillin, 4 million units in a shot on the way to the operating room and again in the operating room, and again at the conclusion of the operation. Under those circumstances, Mr. Hughes and his colleagues were able to demonstrate that penicillin resulted in a significant reduction in the incidence of wound sepsis, from 27% down to 10%.

Should penicillin be used? In looking at its antibacterial spectrum, I really think that it is an inadequate drug. In high doses, it will cover many of the aerobic coliform organisms, but it is not very effective against *E. coli*. It also will cover most of the anaerobic fecal organisms, but it is really ineffective, even in these high doses, against *Bacteroides fragilis*.

What about the cephalosporins? Several years ago, we took a survey and it will not surprise you to learn that three out of four surgeons who responded to our survey indicated that they were using cephalosporins in their practice in preparation of patients for elective colon operations. Here are the controlled data available in the literature about the administration of systemic cephalosporins.

It began in 1969 with Hiram Polk's well-known paper in which he studied cephaloridine and was able to demonstrate that one could significantly reduce the risk of septic complications of colorectal operations with the use of that drug. That study was repeated a few years later by Evans and Pollack in Britain who looked at a whole variety of operations. In their subset of colorectal operations, they were not able to demonstrate a significant reduction in the incidence of septic complications with cephaloridine.

Burden and colleagues from Australia looked at cephalothin and reported their study in the *Archives of Surgery* in the fall of 1977. They were also unable to demonstrate a significant reduction in the incidence of sepsis with that particular cephalosporin.

At the infectious disease meetings in the fall of 1977, Panchrisospathos reported in abstract on a small group of patients to whom cefazolin had been administered, with a significant reduction in the incidence of wound complications.

For practical purposes, when appropriate dosages and appropriate intervals between dosing are chosen, cephalosporins all are equivalent to one another. Their antibacterial spectrum is identical. The evidence of their efficacy as prophylaxis for colorectal operations is a mixed bag.

We recently completed a controlled clinical trial that looked at the administration of systemic cephalothin, the most widely used antibiotic in surgical practice in this country, in connection with colorectal operations. This was a Veterans Administration Cooperative Study conducted in 16 hospitals, one of which was the Minneapolis Veterans Administration Hospital. In 67 patients who received IV cephalothin and a rigorous mechanical bowel prep, compared to 126 patients who received a vigorous mechanical bowel prep and oral neomycin-erythromycin base, with or without the IV drug, the incidence of septic complications was as follows: a 30% incidence of wound infection, as compared to 6%: an 18% incidence of peritonitis and intra-abdominal abscess, as compared to 2%; a 10% incidence of anastomotic leak, as compared to zero. That observation bears importantly on the notion of the cause of an anastomotic leak — is it a technical fault of the operating surgeon or is it the result of infection in the suture line that leads to its disruption? Continuing, 7% versus 1% for septicemia; and 6% versus 2% in terms of mortality; 48 septic complications in 26 patients receiving IV cephalothin, an over-all septic complication rate of 39%, as compared to 6% for those getting neomycin-erythromycin base; 39% really is not very different from the experience in patients who did not receive any antibiotics at all. So, in our study, cephalothin simply failed to control septic complications in colorectal operations. As a single drug, I could not recommend it to you and I would not recommend that any of the cephalosporins be used alone.

Let us look now at oral drugs. Oral sulfonamides were the first antimicrobials used in connection with colorectal operations. There are, however, only two prospectively organized controlled clinical trials available in the literature. Both of them are relatively recent: Rosenberg's study in 1971 and Niegard's study in 1972, both of which used sulfathalidine, probably the most commonly used sulfonamide in recent surgical practice. Both studies failed to demonstrate any reduction in the incidence of wound complications and other septic complications associated with colon operations. So it looks as though oral sulfonamides alone are not adequate to solve the problem.

Oral tetracyclines have been the subject of only one very recent study. This study, I would point out, used doxycycline, not the older varieties of tetracyclines. Doxycycline is effective against *Bacteroides fragilis*, at least currently. One hopes that it will remain effective. But, if past experience with other members of the tetracycline group of drugs is any guide to the future, what we will probably see is a slow but persistent increase in the incidence of resistance of *Bacteroides fragilis* to this newly introduced tetracycline. In any case, as of 1977, this drug significantly reduced the incidence of septic complications associated with elective colorectal operations, when administered by mouth.

Aminoglycosides have been very popular drugs used in association with bowel preparation. Summarizing all of the available controlled clinical trials in the literature gives a bit of a mixed bag but most of the studies have failed to demonstrate that aminoglycosides alone reduce the incidence of wound sepsis.

In 1965, Professor Rubbo in association with E. S. R. Hughes conducted an oral aminoglycoside study. It was very interesting to note that neomycin was associated with significant reduction of the incidence of wound sepsis, whereas kanamycin was not. Common sense says that that is not a reasonable conclusion. The aminoglycosides, like the cephalosporins, have some differences in pharmacologic kinetics but by and large, when dealing with fecal organisms, they are equivalent drugs if appropriate doses and dosing intervals are chosen.

There were a whole series of studies. Perhaps the one which most people know best was the recent study reported from the Mayo Clinic, where oral neomycin was one arm of a three arm study. Compared to controls, it failed to alter the incidence of septic complications, which were about the 40% level. The preponderance of evidence indicates that oral aminoglycosides given alone do not control the septic complications of colon operations.

Several years ago, we reported the results of a large scale controlled clinical trial that looked at combination oral antibiotics. I would emphasize that in administering oral drugs, combinations are essential to achieve control of the full microbial spectrum that inhabits the colon. The particular combination that we studied was neomycin plus erythromycin base. These drugs were chosen because they are cheap, readily available, have no particularly important in-hospital uses, and of the available drugs are the most poorly absorbed so that most of the drug acts within the colon lumen. In that study, which was reported to the American Surgical Association and was published in *Annals of Surgery* in September 1977, these were the septic complications: In the placebo-treated group, which received vigorous mechanical preparation but no antibiotics, among 60 patients, 2 deaths, 6 episodes of bloodstream invasion, 10 anastomotic leaks, 10 abscesses, 21 wound infections, septic complications in 26 patients, for a 43% incidence of sepsis related to colon operations. With oral neomycin-erythromycin base, the numbers were ten complications in five patients, for an incidence of 9%. The combination of neomycin-erythromycin was very effective in reducing the incidence of septic complications associated with elective colon operations.

Generally, oral combination chemotherapy, using drugs which are directed specifically at both the aerobic and the anaerobic components of the fecal flora, has been reasonably successful in reducing the incidence of septic complications.

Goldring and colleagues in Glasgow, Scotland, reported in *Lancet* in 1975 that a combination of kanamycin and metronidazole was effective in reducing the incidence of septic complications. Metronidazole has now become what amounts to a fad drug in England for the control of anaerobes. There are literally dozens of studies being published every month from England concerning the oral administration of metronidazole. It is effective in controlling the anaerobic component of the fecal flora. There may be some other problems that we do not yet fully appreciate, but it looks as though this drug is going to be an effective form of preparation.

A recent study by Taylor looked at sulfathalidine and metronidazole. This combination in this single study was effective. Sulfathalidine is effective against *E. coli* but practically nothing else in feces. Metronidazole seems to control most of the anaerobes, particularly *Bacteroides fragilis*, and so it is probably not an irrational combination, although it does leave more holes, particularly on the aerobic side of the fecal spectrum, than do the other combinations discussed above.

One of the objections often raised to antibiotic therapy among surgical patients and which has been raised in connection with the use of orally administered drugs to patients undergoing colon operations is the concern that the use of antibiotics results in the emergence of resistant organisms. We studied the first stool passed postoperatively in our study of neomycin-erythromycin base, compared to placebo. Among the placebo patients, who had not received any antibiotics at all, coliform organisms resistant to neomycin were recovered in 16 out of the 46 patients. Looking at the issue of the multiply-resistant organism, that is, an organism that is resistant to multiple antibiotics, there were two strains from the 46 patients also resistant to gentamicin; there were 5 resistant to *Staphylococcus aureus*. In 11 patients significant numbers of fungi grew from postoperative stool. Comparing those figures to the 39 patients who received oral neomycin-erythromycin base, there were 12 who postoperatively had organisms that were resistant to neomycin, 4 were resistant to gentamicin, 3 resistant to *Staphylococcus aureus* organisms, and 14 who grew fungi. There were no significant differences between the groups who did and who did not receive antibiotics. It appears, at least from these limited data, that the short-term intensive administration of oral antibiotics in the immediate preoperative period does not have an adverse impact on the bacterial ecology of patients receiving those drugs.

Another issue that sometimes arises is the matter of suture line recurrence. Twenty-five years ago, Vink, the Dutch surgeon, reported a study on rabbits, in which a V-2 carcinosarcoma cell slurry had been injected into the colon lumen and then a colon resection and anastomosis performed. The animals which had received tetracycline had essentially twice the incidence of suture line implantation of tumor as did animals which had received no antibiotics.

That experimental finding was subsequently confirmed by Isidore Cohn, using a different tumor model system, the

Brown-Pierce carcinosarcoma, and different antibiotics. That is where the matter stood for some time. The incidence of suture line implantation in the control animals in these studies was on the order of 45%, something which is totally outside general clinical experience. None of us experience suture line implantation or suture line recurrence rates of that order of magnitude.

Fortunately, there is clinical evidence which bears on the issue. It comes from Professor Hughes and his colleagues in Australia. You will recall from the preceding discussion that they had two groups of controlled prospective clinical trials, one looking at penicillin and one looking at aminoglycosides. Among antibiotic-treated patients compared with the placebo groups, the incidence of suture line recurrence with five years of follow-up was 10% and 8% versus 8% in the placebo group. There is no significant difference between the placebo-treated patients and patients receiving antibiotics. It appears that the experimental evidence does not bear on the clinical situation. For the time being this concern about antibiotic therapy can be set aside.

The evidence currently available from controlled clinical trials indicates that properly chosen oral antibiotic therapy significantly reduces the incidence of septic complications associated with colon operations. The evidence about systemic administration of antibiotics is very much more mixed and is not as clear-cut as is the evidence relating to oral administration. Oral, as compared with systemic administration, has a number of advantages. Oral administration puts the antibiotic in the colon lumen where it can directly reduce the numbers of bacteria. One can use drugs which really have no other important uses in the hospital, to get away from considerations about alteration of either the hospital bacterial ecology or the patient's bacterial ecology. Because we choose drugs which are poorly absorbed, there is a minimal risk of systemic reactions. Because you can employ drugs in a short intense course, you do not have the problem of emerging resistant organisms.

It will come as no surprise that other data that emerged from the survey we took several years ago indicated that the majority of surgeons around the country were using not only oral drugs but also systemic antibiotics concomitantly. That is, they were administering antibiotics via both routes. Whether that is a rational practice is at the moment unclear. We are currently engaged in a controlled trial which may shed light on that practice. It appears from the data that are available from our ongoing trial that there is no significant difference between the group which receives only oral drugs and the group which receives oral drugs combined with systemic drugs. But the numbers are too small yet to be certain. This is an important issue to settle. If there is an advantage to this kind of combination of routes of chemotherapy, we ought to know about it. If there is no advantage to adding systemic chemotherapy, there is no point to exposing patients to the risks of administering drugs systemically or to the costs involved, which, while tolerable, are not insignificant.

In summary, the present position is that one should administer oral drugs to patients undergoing elective colorectal operations. I would recommend the regimen of neomycin-erythromycin base, which we have developed, the details of which are available in the September 1977 issue of *Annals of Surgery*.

Self-Evaluation Quiz

1. In control patients who received vigorous mechanical preparation but not any antibiotics, the septic complication rates varied from:
   a) 10% to 20%
   b) 23% to 33%
   c) 25% to 63%
   d) 45% to 54%
2. Mr. Hughes and colleagues demonstrated that penicillin caused a reduction in wound sepsis from:
   a) 17% to 10%
   b) 27% to 10%
   c) 37% to 10%
   d) 37% to 16%
3. In high doses, penicillin:
   a) Is not very effective against *E. coli*
   b) Is very effective against *Bacteroides fragilis*
   c) Will not cover many aerobic coliforms
   d) None of the above

4. Rosenberg's 1971 study and Niegard's of 1972 both involved sulfathalidine, probably the least used sulfonamide in recent surgical practice.
   a) True
   b) False
5. For practical purposes, when appropriate dosages and intervals between dosages are used, cephalosporins:
   a) Are all equal
   b) Have different antibacterial spectra
   c) Are perfect for prophylaxis in colorectal surgery
   d) Are still useless
6. In a VA study of 67 patients who received cephalothin IV plus a rigorous mechanical bowel prep, compared with 126 patients who received a vigorous mechanical bowel prep and oral neomycin-erythromycin base with or without the IV drug, the incidence of wound infection was:
   a) 30% versus 6%
   b) 20% versus 10%
   c) 15% versus 14%
   d) 5% versus 36%
7. In 1965, Rubbo reported:
   a) Kanamycin reduced sepsis, but neomycin did not
   b) Both kanamycin and neomycin reduced sepsis
   c) Neomycin reduced sepsis, but kanamycin did not
   d) Neither neomycin nor kanamycin reduced sepsis
8. Evidence indicates that oral aminoglycosides:
   a) Alone control septic complications
   b) Alone do not control septic complications
   c) None of the above
9. Goldring reported in *Lancet* (1975) that:
   a) Kanamycin + metronidazole reduced septic complications
   b) Kanamycin + neomycin reduced sepsis
   c) Kanamycin + metronidazole increased septic complications
   d) Kanamycin + neomycin increased sepsis
10. Vink reported that in animals which received tetracycline, compared with animals not receiving any antibiotics, the incidence of suture-line implantation of tumor was:

a) Lower
b) Two times higher
c) Four times higher
d) The same

Answers on page 721.

Management of the Obstructed Colon

John Alexander-Williams, M.D.

Objectives

1. To review the diagnosis of obstruction, particularly the use of x-ray contrast studies.
2. To review three operations for the obstructed colon.
3. To review three operative options once resection of the obstructing lesion is accomplished.

Introduction

Patients presenting with the clinical picture of acute large bowel obstruction must always have the precise site and cause of the obstruction determined before operation. The phenomenon of pseudo-obstruction of the large bowel is well described but, even today, is often missed. Patients with obstipation, colicky pain, distention and flat-plate evidence of grossly dilated large bowel may not have an organic obstruction. In our institution an x-ray contrast study is mandatory to exclude pseudo-obstruction. Furthermore, the x-ray will usually differentiate intrinsic malignant obstruction from obstruction due to external pressure, volvulus or peridiverticular inflammatory disease. The common site of malignant obstruction of the colon is close to the rectosigmoid junction. In such patients, a precise diagnosis can be made on sigmoidoscopy. Operative treatment of rectosigmoid obstruction is rarely so urgent that histological confirmation cannot be obtained.

Once the presence of an organically obstructed colon has been substantiated and the probable etiological agent deter-

---

John Alexander-Williams, M.D., Chairman of Gastroenterology Group, University of Birmingham, Birmingham, England.

mined, it is possible to plan therapy. Obstruction due to intrinsic carcinoma is generally progressive and unremitting. Usually, it is not possible for the obstruction to be relieved, but occasionally it is worthwhile attempting to soften the colonic contents so that they may pass the malignant stricture and allow an emergency operation to be superseded by a safer elective operation. On the other hand, obstruction due to volvulus may be decompressed and that due to inflammatory edema associated with peridiverticular inflammatory disease will resolve on conservative therapy so allowing later elective operation. Obligatory emergency surgical treatment of the obstructed colon is therefore usually in patients with carcinoma. The most common site of such a malignant obstruction is the sigmoid colon, but may occur elsewhere throughout the large bowel.

Operative Options

1. A loop colostomy of the transverse colon well proximal to the obstruction is the safest operation, particularly in the ill, frail and the elderly. However, it is not ideal in the management of patients with obstruction due to diverticular disease since this is usually associated with a peridiverticular abscess that does not necessarily resolve with simple proximal diversion.

When a patient has a transverse colostomy performed for malignant obstruction of the sigmoid colon, he or she is committed to a three-stage operation; the next stage being resection of the segment of bowel containing the obstructing carcinoma and the third stage the closure of the colostomy. Although the three-stage operation usually appears to be the safest course of action, it is an ordeal that many frail, old patients fail to survive. This is an important consideration because if the patient is not fit for the second stage of the operation, a permanent transverse colostomy is difficult to manage because the stoma may be sited inconveniently high in the abdomen. Furthermore, the amount of functioning colon proximal to the colostomy may be insufficient to dehydrate the stool and so a “wet colostomy” results. In my opinion, a transverse colostomy is unsuitable as a permanent arrangement, although technical difficulties sometimes make it the practical site.

2. A loop colostomy immediately proximal to the lesion. If the colostomy to relieve the obstruction is sited immediately proximal to the obstruction, the second operation can resect both the stoma and the obstructing lesion. As an elective procedure, it should be safe to perform this second operation with a primary anastomosis, so permitting a two-stage procedure. The theoretical attractions of a two-stage operation tend to be marred by the technical difficulties of mobilization of the descending colon in patients with an obstructing sigmoid lesion. The immediately proximal loop colostomy is best reserved for those patients having obstructing carcinomas in the region of the sigmoid flexure or descending colon. In these sites the en bloc resection of the obstructing carcinoma is a straightforward surgical exercise.

3. Primary resection. Primary resection of the obstructing lesion is the best operation under optimum circumstances and is always the operation of choice in obstruction due to diverticular disease. The advantages of primary resection for carcinoma are obvious. There is an immediate removal of the tumor and any peripheral malignant cells, whereas in multiple stage procedures the tumor may remain for several weeks or months before a definitive resection can be performed.

Once the resection of the obstruction is achieved, three options remain.

a. Primary anastomosis. It is relatively uncommon for lesions of the right side of the colon to obstruct. However, if and when they do, primary resection and primary anastomosis is feasible and should always be performed. Elsewhere in the colon primary resection with end-to-end anastomosis is a reasonable goal provided that there is healthy bowel to anastomose and provided that there is no gross proximal fecal retention. In patients with acute obstruction of the sigmoid colon who have gross fecal obstruction of the transverse and descending colon it is often best to perform a primary resection of the majority of the large bowel containing the grossly impacted feces and perform an anastomosis between the cecum and the sigmoid or rectum distal to the obstruction. Patients with obstructing carcinoma usually have healthy large bowel mucosa and in them the retention of the cecum and the rectum is sufficient to insure that subsequently they pass moderately well-formed stools with complete continence. The added advantage of subtotal colonic resection for sigmoid lesions is that it removes a large bowel that might be the site of synchronous carcinoma and also it permits regular sigmoidoscopic review of the remaining bowel that might later become affected by a second primary.

If gross fecal loading proximal to the anastomosis is present and subtotal colonic resection is judged inadvisable, then it is safer to avoid a primary anastomosis.

b. Resection of the lesion with an end colostomy and a mucous fistula is often the quickest and safest operation in the elderly, the frail and the ill. It is the optimal operation in obstructing diverticular disease provided that there is sufficient large bowel distal to the obstruction to permit the creation of a mucous fistula. The disadvantage of the procedure is that a mucous fistula inevitably discharges mucus and purulent material. This may be malodorous and copious and may necessitate the wearing of a second stomal appliance. It is reasonable to argue that if sufficient mobility remains in the sigmoid to bring to the surface to make a mucous fistula, then there is sufficient mobility to permit a primary anastomosis, protected if necessary by a proximal defunctioning stoma.

After creating a defunctioning colostomy and a separate mucous fistula, it is a major surgical exercise to later restore intestinal continuity by anastomosis of the colostomy at, or distal to, the mucous fistula. It is certainly much greater than the simple closure of a defunctioning colostomy used to protect an initial primary anastomosis.

c. Closure of the rectal stump. If there is insufficient sigmoid colon to permit the creation of a mucous fistula, the rectum may be closed. If it is to be closed with the hope of later reconnection, it is important not to resect too much of the rectum. It is not necessary to bury the closed rectal stump extraperitoneally; the closure with black nonabsorbable sutures facilitates the identification of the site of the stump when reconstruction is attempted. This maneuver is particularly useful when operating on obstructive diverticular disease when there is a reasonable hope of a long-term survival and every incentive to restore normal continuity.

The optimum time for attempted restoration of intestinal continuity is as soon as the patient has regained full health, which is usually at about three months.

A useful tip that I can offer to aid the identification of the rectal stump is to insert through the anus a balloon catheter. Once the pelvis is exposed via the abdomen, the rectum is distended intermittently with an antiseptic or antibiotic solution. This enables the fundus of the rectal stump to be identified with accuracy and stay sutures to be inserted.

Bowel preparation is virtually impossible when operating on the acutely obstructed colon. When it is possible to delay surgery for 48 hours, oral prophylaxis should be given. However, in all cases, adequate parenteral prophylaxis is given, active against aerobic and anaerobic microorganisms. We currently use metronidazole and kanamycin.

Self-Evaluation Quiz

1. Organic obstruction is always present if there is colicky abdominal pain, distention and flat-plate evidence of a dilated proximal large bowel with an empty rectum.
   a) True
   b) False
2. In the emergency contrast x-rays will usually differentiate all but one of the following:
   a) Pseudo-obstruction
   b) Intrinsic malignant obstruction
   c) Obstruction due to external pressure
   d) Aganglionosis
3. In one of the following causes of acute large bowel obstruction, operative therapy is obligatory:
   a) Peridiverticular inflammatory disease
   b) Volvulus of the sigmoid colon
   c) Ischemic disease of the colon
   d) Carcinoma of the sigmoid colon
4. The most common site for malignant obstruction of the large bowel is the:
   a) Rectum
   b) Sigmoid

c) Descending colon
d) Transverse colon

5. In the frail ill patient with acute malignant obstruction of the sigmoid colon, the safest operation is:
   a) Loop colostomy of the transverse colon
   b) Mobilization and exteriorization of the sigmoid, including the tumor
   c) Resection of the obstruction with end colostomy and mucus fistula
6. The best operation for obstructing diverticular disease that does not respond to conservative management is:
   a) Transverse loop colostomy
   b) Exteriorization of the sigmoid colon, including the mass
   c) Resection with primary end-to-end anastomosis
   d) Resection of the sigmoid with end ileostomy and closure of the rectal stump
7. All but one of the following are reasons why an emergency transverse loop colostomy is not suitable as a permanent ileostomy:
   a) It is likely to be situated too high on the abdomen for the fitting of a colostomy bag
   b) The colonic contents may be too fluid and excoriate the skin
   c) It is more likely to prolapse than stomas in other sites
8. After resection of obstructing primary carcinoma end-to-end anastomosis is best for:
   a) Right-sided colonic lesions
   b) High rectal carcinoma
   c) When there has been peritonitis due to perforation
   d) Proximal fecal loading
9. After resection of a sigmoid carcinoma without primary anastomosis a mucus fistula may be formed. One of the following is not a disadvantage of the technique:
   a) The bowel may be too short to bring to the surface without undue tension
   b) Malodorous mucus discharge may necessitate the wearing of a second appliance
   c) The re-establishment of intestinal continuity at a second operation will be a major surgical exercise
   d) It may cause tenesmus

10. All but one of the following are considered to be useful tips to the identification of the rectal stump when restoring bowel continuity when the patient has fully recovered from a sigmoid or upper rectal resection and a Hartmann's procedure:
    a) Leave as long a rectal stump as possible
    b) Close it with nonabsorbable black silk sutures
    c) Fill it with contrast and take a lateral x-ray
    d) Insert a balloon catheter and distend with an antiseptic solution after the pelvis is exposed at operation

Answers on page 721.

Colonic Polyps: How Long Should They Be Followed?

Robert E. Condon, M.D.

Objectives

The author raises and attempts to answer these questions: (1) What is the frequency and duration of follow-up for colon polyps? (2) What should the management be besides removal? (3) What predicts recurrence? (4) What is the incidence of subsequent cancer? (5) What distinguishes the histology of excised polyps?

The issue is a common problem which we all face. When you find a colon polyp, how long should you follow it? Other than removing it, what needs to be done? I am not sure that we have a final answer, but we do have some information that bears on the issue and may help in making judgments about follow-up of colon polyps.

I have seen a single colon segment which contained a perfectly benign adenoma along with hyperplastic polyps, which really amount only to focal mucosal edema and are not polyps and need no treatment at all, a villous adenoma which does contain several foci of carcinoma in situ but no invasive cancer and an ulcerated invasive cancer. Patients who develop this kind of neoplasm (benign adenoma) seem to be at excess risk for developing cancer. That the benign adenoma is often associated with cancer may be a harbinger of a diffuse capacity of the colon mucosa to undergo neoplasia. There is also another issue, which will probably never be settled, and that is whether an adenoma becomes cancer at some time in the course of its

---

Robert E. Condon, M.D., Professor, Department of Surgery, The Medical College of Wisconsin; Chief of Surgical Services, Veterans Administration Center, Milwaukee, Wisc.

biology. That is a chicken and egg argument, and I do not know how to solve it.

At the Wood Veterans Administration Hospital, my predecessor, Dr. Forrester Raine, some years ago started a policy by which every patient identified as having a colon polyp was entered into a program of follow-up in which he would get a proctosigmoidoscopic examination every six months and a barium enema. As this program progressed, it developed a life of its own. Some patients have had large numbers of proctosigmoidoscopic and barium enema examinations following up on an initial colon polyp. This study allowed me to look at what had been found during the course of this follow-up. There were 268 patients who had initially been entered. We eliminated from the study population those who had co-existing carcinoma, those who had multiple polyposis, a single patient with Crohn's disease who had initially presented with what appeared to be a benign polyp in the rectum, 15 patients in whom there was no histologic confirmation of the nature of the polyp and 41 patients who were lost to follow-up. That left us with 154 patients who had been followed up, in one case, 24 years, and the median follow-up approached 10 years.

The questions we asked were: What predicts recurrence, if anything? Is there any time during which recurrence is more or less likely? How often do we really need to reexamine patients and for how long? What is the incidence of subsequent cancer, the major worry in connection with benign colon polyp disease?

We divided the patients into two groups (1) those who never developed a recurrence and (2) those who did develop a polyp recurrence. We looked at things such as age, which was not different, the complaints with which they presented. We had a rather excessive incidence of lower GI bleeding in comparison with the usual relatively asymptomatic state of colon polyps, change in bowel habits and other GI symptoms. There were no differences between the two groups in these features. What about the site? If the initial polyp was located within the rectum, rectosigmoid and distal sigmoid, within reach of the standard sigmoidoscope, there was no difference there. As for size, there was a slight increase in the incidence of recurrence with an initially big polyp, but the difference was not statistically significant.

We then looked at the number of polyps that had been removed at the initial episode. As you might suspect, most patients had a single polyp removed, and there was no difference between the two groups. The same was true if two polyps were removed. There seemed to be a difference if three polyps were removed at the initial examination, but the numbers were so small that it does not achieve statistical significance. Clearly, if more than three polyps were harvested at the initial examination, there was a statistically significant increase in the probability of recurrence. So this identifies one group of patients, one subset, that is at risk of recurrence, patients who have had more than three polyps removed at the initial examination.

What about the histology of the initially excised polyp? It did not make any difference, with the exception that patients who had presented initially with a villous adenoma had a higher incidence of recurrence. That does identify a second subset of patients, those with an initial villous adenoma, who have a significantly increased risk of subsequently developing recurrent crops of polyps.

That leaves us, then, with the large majority of patients who had three or fewer initial polyps who did not have a villous adenoma. What happens to that group? If you follow that group, in terms of polyp recurrences, if you look at the first episode of recurrence, that is, the first recurrent polyp after the initial excision, you see that in the first year 18 patients developed a second polyp, and then the incidence begins to fall, so that by the fourth year, a relatively low incidence prevails.

If you then take these patients who had had a first recurrence and look for the time of the second recurrences, it is scattered. It appears that the risk of first recurrence is a time-dependent phenomenon but, if a second recurrence, is not clearly time-dependent and may represent a prolonged or perhaps permanent tendency of colon mucosa to undergo neoplasia.

The risk in the general population is about 0.7% per year. If you take a population of adults and follow them over the course of time, you will get a cumulative incidence of about 7% of them having polyps over the course of a decade. In our patient population, with known polyp disease, we found that there is an initial high rate of recurrence which persists for about 2 or 2½ years and then there is a break. After four years, the continued incidence of recurrence really only parallels the incidence in the general population. So it seems that the maximum risk of recurrence is early. Most recurrences turn up within a few years, and after four years there is no further excess risk of polyp recurrence in this study population, as compared with the risk of the incidence of polyps in the population as a whole.

What about cancers? We compared the location of the initial polyp and of the subsequent cancer in four patients in whom cancer occurred during follow-up. An initial polyp in the rectum, a subsequent cancer in the proximal sigmoid. An initial polyp in the sigmoid, followed three months later by the diagnosis of a carcinoma at the same site. This obviously is a diagnostic miss on the part of the operator who performed the first proctosigmoidoscopic examination. Another polyp in the rectum, followed subsequently by a sigmoid cancer. Another polyp in the rectum, followed subsequently by a cecal carcinoma. The time sequence, with the exception of this diagnostic miss, was that the cancers followed the polyps within four years. It does not appear that this group of patients had any more risk of developing cancer than would be found in the population as a whole, if you took 150-odd patients and followed them for two decades.

So we found that one third of the patients with a benign colon polyp not associated with more than three polyps at the initial examination or with a villous adenoma, that one-third developed a recurrence of a benign polyp. The presence of a villous adenoma or more than three polyps predisposed to recurrence and these patients obviously need continuous follow-up because of their persisting predisposition. But, for the other patients, the excess risk of polyp recurrence and cancer is in the four years following removal of the first polyp. This has some interesting implications about the biology of colon polyp disease. In the majority of patients, it appears to be a time-dependent and a time-limited phenomenon, indicating that whatever influence, probably environmental, acting on the colon mucosa does not necessarily persist in all patients. It does in the subset with villous adenomas. It apparently does in the subset with large numbers of polyps initially and also does in the subset that gets second recurrences. But, for most patients who have a single benign colon polyp removed, the excess risk of recurrence is limited to the subsequent four years.

What does that mean in terms of patient management? Obviously, it means that for that four-year period, regular follow-up of patients presenting with benign colon polyps is indicated. What does it mean after four years? It means the same thing that you would do for the population as a whole. One half of the people in this country are over 40 years of age and in the population group that is at risk for development of colon polyps. If we are to do proctosigmoidoscopic examinations as frequently as once annually, that is a significant number of proctosigmoidoscopies — 100 million per year. I am not sure that we have the resources to do that.

The point I would like to leave you with is this: Having seen a patient with a polyp and having followed him for four years without recurrence, what you should do in terms of management after that point is what you would do for any other patient who is over 40 years of age. That may not be a very clear answer because I do not think there is necessarily a very clear and solid answer to this particular problem of patient management. I suspect in this country most patients over 40 do not undergo annual proctosigmoidoscopic examination, however desirable that might be. In terms of public health and patient management, the implications of the findings of our little study are that patients who are followed for four years intensively but not subsequently will be no worse off than the population as a whole in the management of polyp disease and colon cancer.

Self-Evaluation Quiz

1. Patients who develop benign adenoma seem to be at:
   a) Greater risk of developing cancer
   b) Less risk of developing cancer
   c) The same risk of developing cancer as the average population
2. Every patient in the Wood VA study with a colon polyp was scheduled for proctosigmoidoscopy every:

a) Seven months
b) Eight months plus barium enema
c) Year
d) Six months plus barium enema

3. Of the series of 268 patients at Wood VA, median follow-up time was:
   a) 5 years
   b) 6 years
   c) 10 years
   d) 15 years
4. In two subgroups of the above study, if the initial polyp was in the rectum, rectosigmoid and distal sigmoid within reach of the standard sigmoidoscope, recurrence differences between the two groups were:
   a) Nil
   b) 10%
   c) 30%
   d) 82%
5. When dealing with an initially large polyp, the incidence of recurrence in the above study was:
   a) Slightly increased
   b) Slightly decreased
   c) Greatly increased
   d) Greatly decreased
6. For most patients who have a single benign colon polyp removed, the excess risk of recurrence is limited to the subsequent four years.
   a) True
   b) False
7. The author found that one fourth of the patients with a benign colon polyp not associated at the initial exam with more than three polyps or with a villous adenoma developed recurrence of a benign polyp.
   a) True
   b) False
8. The risk of first recurrence is a time-dependent phenomenon.
   a) True
   b) False
9. If more than three polyps were harvested at the initial exam, there was:

   a) Nothing noteworthy
   b) A drop in the probability of recurrence
   c) An increase in the probability of recurrence
   d) The patient did not live long enough to be followed

10. Patients who presented initially with villous adenoma:
   a) Had higher incidence of recurrence
   b) Had lower incidence of recurrence
   c) Had the same incidence of recurrence
   d) Were not in the author's paper

Answers on page 721.

Massive Lower Gastrointestinal Hemorrhage: Diagnosis and Management

William R. Johnson, M.B., F.R.A.C.S., F.R.C.S. and
Stanley M. Goldberg, M.D., F.A.C.S.

Objectives

1. To discuss the management of a patient with massive lower gastrointestinal hemorrhage.
2. To consider the various etiologic factors that have been advocated as the cause of lower gastrointestinal hemorrhage.
3. To delineate the role of colonic surgery in massive lower gastrointestinal surgery. At the end of the paper the reader should have a knowledge of the appropriate, immediate approach to the patient with massive lower gastrointestinal hemorrhage and a current understanding of the etiology of lower gastrointestinal hemorrhage.

Introduction

The whole concept of the etiology, diagnosis and management of massive lower gastrointestinal hemorrhage has undergone a radical change following the increased use of selective visceral angiography.

The need for a multidisciplinary approach is crucial. A clinical team composed of surgeon, radiologist and internist with an interest in, and understanding of, the disease and the therapeutic expectations significantly increases the chances of a successful outcome.

W. R. Johnson, M.B., F.R.A.C.S., F.R.C.S., Medical Fellow, Division of Colon and Rectal Surgery, University of Minnesota Medical School, Minneapolis and S. M. Goldberg, M.D., F.A.C.S., Clinical Professor of Surgery; Director, Division of Colon and Rectal Surgery, University of Minnesota Medical School, Minneapolis.

Etiology

By association, diverticular disease was convicted as the most common cause of massive lower gastrointestinal hemorrhage. The extensive reviews of Noer [1] and Rushford [2] of patients with diverticular disease reported the incidence of macroscopic bleeding as being 11% and 17%, respectively. Severe bleeding can be expected in 2% to 6% of patients with diverticular disease [3]. The disconcerting features were that it was unrelated to inflammation, and blind segmental resection of the left colon, which was predominantly involved in the diverticular disease process, was associated with a rebleeding rate of up to 50% [4, 5].

With the use of angiography the majority of demonstrated hemorrhages were found to be located to the right of the splenic flexure, predominantly in the cecum and ascending colon [6, 7]. Of patients presenting the combination of diverticular disease and hemorrhage, 70% were above 70 years of age [3].

Meyers et al described the angioarchitecture of the diverticulum and proposed a pathogenesis of the bleeding [8, 9]. This appeared to confirm the diverticular-hemorrhage story and to conclude the debate on the predominant cause of hemorrhage in the lower gastrointestinal tract.

Angiodysplasia and congenital vascular abnormalities had long been known to be associated with chronic gastrointestinal bleeding. There were isolated reports of significant hemorrhage from this source. Boley [10] defined an acquired lesion, which he termed "vascular ectasia." He felt this occurred as part of the aging process. The lesions are found predominantly in the cecum and ascending colon of elderly people. These may play an increasingly dominant role in the etiology of massive lower gastrointestinal bleeding, particularly in the elderly patient. The right colon predominance was felt by Boley to be related to the wall tension which, because of the greater diameter of the right colon and cecum, was higher at a given pressure than that of the sigmoid colon. On this basis he proposed his theory for the formation of these ectasias.

In both diverticular disease and vascular ectasias, rises in colonic pressure are implicated. In the case of vascular ectasias the additional factor is the increase in wall tension and the response of the muscular layer to this, affecting the venous drainage from the submucosa of the colon. In neither was it clear what causes the mucosal breakdown and subsequent bleeding, and in the case of diverticular disease there is no satisfactory explanation for the right side being the predominant source of bleeding.

Diagnosis and Management

With the multidiscipline approach to these patients, diagnosis and management are integrated in a therapeutic flow chart. When first seen in the emergency room the history is usually typical. A middle-aged to elderly patient, previously healthy, presents with the history of an abrupt onset of significant rectal hemorrhage. There is usually a history of a sudden call to stool with an intense desire to defecate which is followed by the passage of a large dark red stool recognized by the patient as blood; the patient at this stage often faints. The time sequence suggests that the syncope is predominantly vasovagal in origin with a secondary hypovolemic phase if bleeding continues. It is estimated that 90% to 95% of these patients will have stopped bleeding at the time of presentation or will stop spontaneously within the first 24 hours. Five percent will rebleed in the first week [11], and 25% will re-present with bleeding at some time in the future [5]. This latter re-presentation need not be with massive hemorrhage.

Assessment

The hemodynamic status of the patient must be assessed accurately. If hypovolemia is significant or continued bleeding suspected, resuscitation is begun. Blood is drawn for typing, crossmatching, a blood count, electrolytes and a coagulation profile.

In addition to general physical examination, a sigmoidoscopic examination should be added. Although this is difficult under the circumstances of a large amount of blood in the rectum, with the use of good suction apparatus it is possible to at least view the rectal mucosa. This is useful to exclude ulcerative colitis or ischemic colitis, if it involves the rectum, from the diagnosis. In addition, it must be remembered that local rectal causes for significant hemorrhage occur and they may be detected at this examination.

If continued bleeding is suspected, a nasogastric tube should be passed as a simple test of an upper gastrointestinal source of hemorrhage. Adequate sedation should be administered and in the circumstance of hypovolemia the intravenous route should be used as a means of titrating the patient to an adequate level of sedation.

Hemodynamic stabilization should be achieved rapidly, but care should be exercised lest overinfusion aggravate the colonic bleeding. The aim of resuscitation is not to normalize the blood volume, but to get it to a safe level which allows maximum chance for hemostasis to occur and at the same time a margin for continuation of blood loss without danger.

Bleeding Continues

If, despite adequate sedation, bleeding continues, a factor assessed on the basis of fluid requirement and hemodynamic changes occurring in the patient, two investigations should follow:

1. *Upper gastrointestinal endoscopy.* Upper gastrointestinal endoscopy should be performed to exclude the esophagus, stomach and duodenum as a source of bleeding. If active bleeding is occurring, then the accuracy of determining this fact approaches 95%. The 5% negative rate is related to failed studies and distal duodenal bleeding.

2. *Selective visceral angiography.* With a negative upper gastrointestinal study the patient should proceed to have selective visceral angiography. It is a mistake at this stage to administer a sedative with the aim of achieving that state of sedation which should have been aimed at initially, because as one achieves success with the sedative, bleeding may be arrested and the angiography negative.

There have been many reports about the techniques of selective visceral angiography. A few points are worth emphasizing. As recommended by Baum [12], the sequence of catheterization should be (a) superior mesenteric artery, (b) inferior mesenteric artery and (c) celiac axis. The emphasis should be on selective or subselective angiography. The angiographic appearance of extravasation is absolute proof that the source has been identified. We accept Boley's concept that early venous filling is seen in well-developed vascular ectasias and that the earliest angiographic appearance of their presence is delayed venous emptying.

There are other conditions which can present as massive lower gastrointestinal hemorrhage. Any lesion capable of causing significant hemorrhage into the gastrointestinal tract can be included in the differential diagnosis [13]. Many will have a characteristic appearance on angiography and often an associated history.

Bleeding Site Identified

If a bleeding site is identified, and this means extravasation, or a suspicious area of ectasia or vascular abnormality, then vasopressin infusion should be commenced. We follow the protocol of Baum [12]. Infusion of vasopressin is begun at the rate of 2 units/minute; if this holds the bleeding, it is continued for 12 hours, then reduced to 1 unit/minute for a further 12 to 24 hours. If no bleeding is evidenced at this stage, the infusion is discontinued, but the catheter is left in situ for a further 12 hours. By this method 22 of 24 patients were controlled in the series reported by Athanosoulis [7].

If bleeding is not controlled by this technique or if breakthrough bleeding occurs during vasopressin infusion, then angiographic localization is again recommended. If facilities are available and the radiologist experienced, an attempt at embolization would appear to be a reasonable approach. The technique [14] requires subselective cannulation of the tertiary mesenteric vessels and the installation of Gelfoam or Oxycel to achieve permanent vascular occlusion. Pathological study of colectomy specimens removed following successful arrest of hemorrhage by this technique has demonstrated no ischemic damage to the organ [14]. However, there are complications associated with this technique, especially in inexperienced hands.

Failure To Locate Bleeding Site

This can occur in two situations. The first is a totally negative angiogram, the second is the demonstration of vascular ectasia or abnormality in the right colon but no extravasation. Clearly, if angiography demonstrates a vascular tumor and extravasation is not seen, the examiner can be fairly confident that this will be the source. Ectasia and minor vascular abnormalities do not hold this surety.

In the situation of a negative angiogram or one with ectasias demonstrated without extravasation, the catheter should be left in situ and the study repeated in 30 to 60 minutes. If the study is still negative for active bleeding but bleeding is continuing, then blind infusion of vasopressin has been recommended. While some suggest that this should be done into the superior mesenteric artery, we would favor peripheral intravenous infusion. The work by Swan et al [15] suggests that the long half life of vasopressin together with the failure of autoregulatory escape of the mesenteric vessels should make this a successful technique. In addition, it prevents the theoretical problem of vasoconstriction in the wrong area with increased perfusion and, hence, bleeding from an adjacent involved segment. The mesenteric catheter in either case should be left in situ.

Bleeding Continues Despite Angiographic Therapeutic Maneuvers

If bleeding has continued despite the angiographic maneuvers whether or not extravasation has been demonstrated, a barium enema should be performed. The results reported by Adams [11] with the use of barium enema alone as a therapeutic agent justifies its use in this situation. Although we are skeptical of its real effectiveness in producing hemostasis, the results are impressive. It may stop the bleeding and will also give more information about related pathology. The hemostatic potential is felt to be due to tamponade caused by the hydrostatic pressure of the barium or saline enema.

When bleeding has stopped either by therapeutic manipulations or spontaneously, a barium enema should be performed at an early date to identify associated pathology. It should always be performed before surgery. If colonoscopy is not available, an air contrast barium enema should be requested.

Colonoscopy

If the colon can be cleared, then colonoscopy can be performed. A high pick-up rate of significant lesions not seen on the barium enema has been reported [16].

Surgery

It must be emphasized that without preoperative diagnosis laparotomy in an attempt to diagnose the problem can be a soul destroying experience.

Site Identified

If active bleeding (extravasation) has been demonstrated, and this will be the case in about 50% of all angiographic studies, then segmental resection is the treatment of choice. This will depend upon the barium or colonoscopic examination which is necessary to exclude associated pathology which could modify the extent of resection.

Ectasias Only

When vascular ectasias in the right colon are the only abnormality demonstrated then, unless bleeding has been recurrent, this alone should not precipitate surgical intervention. If the bleeding continues or is recurrent, and vascular ectasias are the only abnormality demonstrated, surgery should be performed. The surgeon must be aware that if vascular ectasias are the source of bleeding, there will be no external abnormality visible on the colon nor will there be anything to feel or, in all likelihood, to see were a colotomy performed. This is why the team approach is so important. Confidence in our radiological colleagues allows the decision for segmental resection to be made.

Ectasias Associated With Other Colonic Pathology

If the only other abnormality is diverticular disease in the left colon and bleeding is continuing or has been recurrent, then following exclusion of other sites at the time of laparotomy, a subtotal colectomy and ileoproctostomy is the treatment of choice.

The "Diagnostic" Laparotomy

When all studies have been negative and bleeding is continuing, then laparotomy may be forced. Again, it must be emphasized that blind laparotomy is seldom rewarding. Despite this fact, there is little doubt that this situation is a reality.

Again, the team approach is emphasized. A careful study of all intraabdominal organs is essential. The facility for on-table selective mesenteric infusion should be available. Although the evidence thus far is only experimental, infusion of toluidine blue may have a role when attempting to locate the site of bleeding [17]. The opportunity for a repeat of the upper gastrointestinal endoscopy should be taken even if this area does not appear suspicious. It is possible at operation to feed the scope down into the third portion of the duodenum and into the upper part of the small bowel.

Examination of the small bowel by palpation and transillumination should be performed. Special note of the symmetry of the vascular arcades may show a change in pattern suggesting a vascular abnormality. Likewise, the colon should be examined in detail. If a significant arteriovenous abnormality exists, the venous blood draining the site can have a PO_2 10 mm Hg above that of venous blood elsewhere. This, together with an elevated venous pressure in such a vein, suggests the presence of an arteriovenous communication [18].

It must be remembered that blood moves both retrograde and antegrade within the bowel and this gives an erroneous impression of the level at which bleeding is occurring.

If the ileocecal valve is continent and bleeding is localized to the colon, the only procedure which can be offered is a subtotal colectomy. Multiple colotomies are contraindicated and do nothing but contaminate the surgical field. If the sigmoid colon and rectum are clear, then ileosigmoid anastomosis can be performed.

When all on-table attempts at localization have failed to define a site of bleeding, the patient should be returned to the ward and studies repeated. It is rare that massive hemorrhage will remain unlocalized. It is when the bleeding has stopped or is of small volume that difficulty is encountered and this is not a "life-threatening" situation.

Summary

A combined multidisciplinary approach to massive lower gastrointestinal hemorrhage is essential. Diagnosis and management are integrated toward a successful conclusion. The majority of patients stop bleeding before admission or shortly thereafter, and overtransfusion must be avoided. Upper gastrointestinal causes must be excluded, because these are the most common cause of massive gastrointestinal bleeding. Sigmoidoscopy should be performed on all patients, for despite the difficulties, a view of the rectal mucosa will be possible to determine its normality and, in some instances, identify a local bleeding source.

Angiography provides a powerful weapon for diagnosis and with the use of vasopressin or embolization, a therapeutic modality.

Barium enema is necessary to define gross associated pathology and colonoscopy will add finer detail. In addition, barium enema may have a therapeutic role.

When the bleeding site has been identified, segmental resection is the treatment of choice. When the exact site is uncertain but the hemorrhage can be localized to the colon, subtotal colectomy is the operation of choice. The point of distal anastomosis will depend upon the state of the rectum and sigmoid.

Laparotomy for diagnosis is seldom rewarding. Gross pathology may be identified and some techniques for the localization of bleeding have been discussed. The most common etiologies for lower gastrointestinal hemorrhage, when a source has not been identified preoperatively, give no obvious markers on the colonic serosa, nor can they be palpated and often are not even identifiable following resection unless special techniques are used.

The team, composed of an interested group of clinicians, an internist, radiologist and surgeon who understand the problems and therapeutic expectations is essential.

References

1. Noer, R.J.: Hemorrhage as a complication of diverticulitis. Ann. Surg. 141:674, 1955.

2. Rushford, A.J.: The significance of bleeding as a symptom in diverticulitis. Proc. R. Soc. Med. 49:577, 1956.
3. Genarro, A.R. and Rosemond, G.P.: Colonic diverter and hemorrhage. Dis. Colon Rectum 16:409, 1973.
4. Ramonath, H.K. and Hinshaw, J.R.: Management and mismanagement of bleeding colonic diverticular. Arch. Surg. 103:311, 1971.
5. Parsa, F. and Wilson, S.E.: Bleeding diverticulosis of the colon. Am. J. Surg. 127:708, 1974.
6. Casarella et al: Lower gastrointestinal tract hemorrhage. Am. J. Roentgenol. Radium Ther. Nucl. Med. 121:357, 1974.
7. Athanosoulis, C.A. et al: Mesenteric arterial infusion of vasopressin for hemorrhage from colonic diverticulosis. Am. J. Surg. 129:212, 1975.
8. Meyers, M. et al: The angioarchitecture of colonic diverticula. Diag. Rad. 108:249, 1973.
9. Meyers, M. et al: Pathogenesis of massively bleeding colonic diverticulitis: New observations. Am. J. Roentgenol. Radium Ther. Nucl. Med. 127:901, 1976.
10. Boley, S.J. et al: On the nature and etiology of vascular ectasias of the colon. Gastroenterology 72:650, 1977.
11. Adams, J.T.: The barium enema as treatment for massive diverticular bleeding. Dis. Colon Rectum 17:439, 1974.
12. Baum, S.: Angiographic diagnosis and control of large bowel hemorrhage. Dis. Colon Rectum 17:447, 1974.
13. Welch, C.E. et al: Gastrointestinal hemorrhage. Adv. Surg. 7:95, 1973.
14. Goldberger, L.E. and Bookstein, J.J.: Transcatheter embolization for treatment of diverticular hemorrhage. Diag. Rad. 122:613, 1977.
15. Swan, K.: Experimental observations and clinical recommendations on vasopressin control of gastrointestinal hemorrhage. Am. Surg. 9:545, 1977.
16. Waye, J.: Colonoscopy in rectal bleeding. S. Afr. J. Surg. 14:143, 1976.
17. Rigas, A. et al: Toluidine Blue O used to identify bleeding points and minute ulcerations of the stomach during surgery. An experimental study in dogs. Int. Surg. 62:391, 1977.
18. Evans, W.A. et al: Localization of intestinal arteriovenous malformations. Am. J. Surg. (In print.)

Self-Examination Quiz

1. In the treatment of massive lower gastrointestinal hemorrhage of colonic origin:
   a) Sigmoid colectomy cures the patient because most bleeding is associated with left sided diverticula
   b) Hemorrhoidectomy cures most patients
   c) Left sided colectomy as a blind procedure is associated with a rebleed rate of approximately 50%

   d) All of the above are incorrect
2. Massive diverticular hemorrhage:
   a) Is associated with episodes of acute diverticulitis
   b) Occurs in the absence of inflammation
   c) Is most commonly associated with portal hypertension
   d) Is common in the third and fourth decade
3. Vascular ectasias as described by Boley:
   a) Are congenital in origin
   b) Are related to fecal damage to the colonic wall
   c) Are due to autodigestion of the colonic mucosa
   d) Are probably a phenomenon of the aging process
4. Positive visceral angiography demonstrates that bleeding occurs most commonly:
   a) In the cecum
   b) In the rectum
   c) In the sigmoid colon
   d) To the right of splenic flexure
5. The right colon predominance of vascular ectasia is felt by Boley to be related to:
   a) Bacterial flora of the right colon
   b) Unusual vascular supply to the right colon
   c) Ischemia of the right colon
   d) Colonic wall tension which because of the diameter of the right colon was higher at a given pressure than the left
6. Sigmoidoscopy is useful:
   a) To confirm massive rectal hemorrhage
   b) In no patients with massive rectal hemorrhage
   c) Only when all other investigations are negative
   d) To examine the rectal mucosa
7. Sedation is administered intravenously:
   a) Because sedatives cannot be given intramuscularly
   b) Because they have a rapid action
   c) Because muscle blood flow is low in hypotensive shock and the intravenous route is the safest way to deliver an accurate dose in these patients
   d) Is dangerous
8. Upper gastrointestinal endoscopy:
   a) Has no place in the management of lower gastrointestinal hemorrhage

b) Should be used after colonoscopy
c) Is recommended to exclude an upper gastrointestinal cause of hemorrhage early in the diagnostic work-up
d) Is no more useful than nasogastric aspiration

9. Vasopressin infusion:
a) Should be used only when surgery is contraindicated
b) Has many side effects and should not be used
c) Should be used routinely in young patients
d) Should be used in all patients before surgery either as a selective infusion or as a systemic infusion

10. If a bleeding site cannot be located and a diagnostic laparotomy is necessary the following may be useful:
a) Asymmetry of the vascular arcades
b) Transillumination of the bowel
c) Arteriovenous oxygen differences
d) All of the above may be useful

Answers on page 721.

Discussion

Moderator: J. Englebert Dunphy

Moderator: Dr. Condon, I have many questions for you from the members of the audience. First, if a patient has a family history of carcinoma and has one or two or three polyps, does this alter your follow-up program?

Dr. Condon: If you suspect that this may be one member of a cancer family, that is, there really is an excess incidence of cancer in other relatives, obviously it does. I am really not sure that the single occurrence of cancer in another family member necessarily indicates a change in management plans, however.

Moderator: Why do you discount systemic antibiotics? Do you feel that the key has to be oral preoperative prep?

Dr. Condon: I do not want to be misunderstood in this regard. I do not discount them; it is just that at the present time the evidence is not very clear. It is mixed, particularly as regards the use of the cephalosporins systemically. The evidence available about the other drugs that are commonly used, the aminoglycosides, is clearer. The weight of evidence indicates that aminoglycosides systemically alone are not any more effective than when given orally alone. As I mentioned, we are studying a combination of cephalosporins plus oral drugs. But the evidence is not all in. Only one study of which I am aware has been published on this matter and that is Harlan Stone's study, where he showed that a combination of oral neomycin-erythromycin and systemic cephalothin resulted in a decrease in infections, as compared with the oral drugs alone. But the infection rates with the oral drugs alone were relatively high, much higher than in our experience.

Moderator: If one goes back to earlier days, there were many studies of colonic surgery in patients who had simply mechanical prep of the bowel and then systemic antibiotics with really quite a reasonable incidence of septic complications. Would you like to comment on this, Dr. Alexander-Williams?

Dr. Alexander-Williams: There is much to be said for giving parenteral antibiotics. Obviously, in a patient having an operation for an obstructed colon, it is essential. Currently, we are conducting a trial comparing oral with systemic prophylaxis. However, many of the oral drugs are absorbed. Even erythromycin has quite a reasonable absorption, does it not?

Dr. Condon: Yes it is not ideal.

Dr. Alexander-Williams: So with many oral drugs you are getting a systemic effect as well.

Dr. Condon: Yes, probably.

Dr. Alexander-Williams: What about aminoglycoside-resistant strains of coliform bacteria? We are employing metronidazole and kanamycin as our standard preparation and are comparing parenteral with oral. So far there is no significant difference between the two, but the trial is not finished yet. The trouble we are finding is that we have still about a 15% wound infection rate due to kanamycin-resistant coliform bacteria. Is that your experience as well?

Dr. Condon: No, that has not been our experience. The wound infections in both of the colon studies which we have reported were mixed and fell essentially into two groups: (1) those who got infections with *Staphylococcus aureus* and (2) those who got infections with aerobic *E. coli.* The incidence of resistant organisms of both types was not different between patients who in the first study had received no antibiotics versus oral drugs and in the second study who had received oral drugs versus systemic drugs.

Moderator: What about the emergency operation — obstructed colon, perforated colon? You cannot prep the bowel. Dr. Alexander-Williams and Dr. Condon?

Dr. Condon: There are two considerations: (1) If I need to choose antibiotics which are effective against the full fecal spectrum I currently use gentamicin and clindamycin in full doses systemically, begun several hours before the operation; (2) I am reluctant to do an anastomosis under those circumstances. When dealing with obstructed bowel, it is really unusual that the bowel proximal to that obstruction is not edematous or otherwise unsuitable for anastomosis. So I turn the ends out and go back ten days later and do the anastomosis.

Moderator: Dr. Goldberg, do you do the same thing?

Dr. Goldberg: I was going to change the subject. Dr. Alexander-Williams, do you ever decompress the ileum with a large tube? When you are doing a primary resection for obstructive carcinoma, do you place a large bore tube into the ileum and pass it up into the colon in order to decompress it before you do an emergency resection for the obstructed colon?

Dr. Alexander-Williams: No, I do not. I think one very rarely sees a patient that bad nowadays. I think modern anesthesia enables one to close the abdomen perfectly satisfactorily without decompressing the bowel. I think it is a rather messy procedure and I am against decompression.

Dr. Goldberg: We have done six in that way. It has proven handy. In the patient with an obstructing carcinoma of the splenic flexure, let us say, a dilated transverse and right colon and an incompetent ileocecal valve, we place a large bore chest tube through the terminal ileum, feed it up into the right colon and decompress the right side. We then do an ileo-descending anastomosis primarily. We have just done six in this way and are pleased with what it has accomplished.

Moderator: That sounds like a lot of gadgetry to me. Dr. Condon, there are studies in which the parenteral antibiotic control group incidence of infection is similar to your oral antibiotic group. Why do you have such a high infection incidence in your control group? I would merely suggest that in your population the antibiotics served to reduce the infection rate to a level that many experience without the technique that you use.

Dr. Condon: I hear many stories from Dr. Dunphy as well as others about the fact that he does not get any infections to speak of. I challenge anyone who makes such a statement to let somebody else rigorously review their experience. You have more complications than you think you do. When this issue has been looked at rigorously, in the hands of a variety of very competent surgeons around the world, the wound infection and other septic complication risks associated with elective colon operations appear to run about 40% without antibiotics. That is a fact. The rest is pure speculation. Now, why is the infection incidence still as high as 10% when we are using antibiotics? I do not really have a good explanation.

Moderator: The reason, of course, is that they smear the feces all over the wound during the operation. If you use good surgical technique and do not spill feces, I do not believe you would have a 40% infection rate. I have been very much interested in this. We have had a very close control in our department. I go back to the early days of the Brigham, and I can tell you that if I had a 40% incidence of wound infection after colonic surgery, I would quit operating.

Dr. Alexander-Williams: I would like to say that it is fortunate that none of your residents had the nerve to check and find out what your infection rate actually was because you might have had to quit early. Dr. Condon once told me how dirty and sloppy the English surgeons were and I said, "I do not have a high infection rate." I went home and checked and our rate was 60% in patients operated upon with an unprepared bowel. Before Dr. Condon alerted me I did not think infection was a problem. You just have to have an independent investigator look at your results.

Moderator: Now, wait a minute. We are not including systemic antibiotics. We are talking about oral antibiotics. Everybody has used systemic antibiotics for years. In the pre-antibiotic era, I made a study at Peter Bent Brigham Hospital. We had a 60% incidence of overall infections with no antibiotics whatsoever. That subsequently fell to a level of 6%. We are only arguing about the crucial fact of oral administration.

Dr. Condon: Let me respond to that, if I may. The overall sepsis rate was 9% in the first study and 6% in the second study. That is probably not a significant difference. The overall sepsis rate in my personal cases is 3%. I think there are differences in the patient populations. The populations that have often been studied have been in Veterans Administration hospitals and other public institutions, with a higher incidence of late disease, general malnutrition and other kinds of problems that do influence the patient's ability to withstand infection. Under optimal circumstances, dealing with optimal patients, as Dr. Dunphy apparently has, you can get down to quite reasonable figures.

Moderator: Dr. Condon, do you personally have a yearly proctosigmoidoscopy or colonoscopy?

Dr. Condon: No, I have no colon symptoms and so I have no colon investigations.

Moderator: Would you recommend it for the panel?

Dr. Condon: No, I would not recommend it for the panel. As a matter of fact, I would not recommend routine proctosigmoidoscopy for patients over 40 years of age. One of my internist friends does that and says that he has never had a patient lose his rectum because of cancer. But, as a practical recommendation, we would be up to our ears in sigmoidoscopes if we were to try to do this on an annual basis for everybody who is at risk, ie, people over 40 years of age. I do not think it is a practical solution to a real problem. Other screening methods, perhaps the screening methods that look for occult blood, may be as effective and certainly are more economical and within our manpower capabilities.

Moderator: Let us move on to the problem of perforated carcinoma of the colon. Dr. Alexander-Williams, how do you manage the problem of the patient who comes in with an acute perforated nonobstructed carcinoma of the colon?

Dr. Alexander-Williams: Perforated colonic carcinoma is a fairly rare event. I am trying to recall whether I ever met the problem clinically. I have seen patients with paracolic abscesses that have ruptured, but not a simple rupture of a carcinoma. If I were to see one I would undoubtedly perform a primary resection and I would not perform a primary anastomosis.

Moderator: You would do a resection without an anastomosis.

Dr. Alexander-Williams: Yes, without an anastomosis.

Moderator: What about diverticulitis?

Dr. Alexander-Williams: That is a much more common problem. I have come around to the view that you should always resect perforated diverticular disease at the first operation, particularly if there is fecal peritonitis. I do not mean a tiny paracolic abscess, you probably should not operate on that. But if it is perforated diverticular disease and there are feces in the peritoneum, a primary resection is life-saving. The worst thing you can possibly do is perform a defunctioning transverse colostomy. That is to be condemned.

Moderator: I would agree completely that the transverse colostomy for diverticular disease is really a thing of the past. Do you agree with that, Dr. Goldberg?

Dr. Goldberg: I could not agree more. I think you must get the disease out, make a nice end-on colostomy and then come back and fight on another day.

Moderator: It must have been about 20 years ago that Alan Boyden in Oregon first advocated this approach. It seemed so radical at the time that it took a little while to catch on. There is no question that this was the right procedure.

Dr. Alexander-Williams: The reason people do not do it is because it is technically difficult to resect the diverticular disease at the first operation. It is technically easier to do it at the first than at the second operation.

Moderator: When you have done this subtotal colectomy and you are anastomosing the cecum to the sigmoid, are there any special methods of anastomosis?

Dr. Alexander-Williams: The main thing is to make sure that you do not rotate it through 360 degrees. Most of my anastomoses seem to find themselves rotated through 180 degrees, but 360 degrees is bad.

Moderator: As a matter of fact, it is not too difficult to do. It sounds a bit difficult, but it is very easy to rotate the cecum.

Dr. Alexander-Williams: Obviously, we have both done it!

Moderator: Let me say that the resident recognizes it.

Dr. Alexander-Williams: But otherwise just use a standard anastomosis. I usually use a two layer anastomosis.

Dr. Goldberg: May I ask Dr. Alexander-Williams a question? Do you really feel strongly about the cecum? You want to save the ileocecal valve, is that why you are using the cecum?

Dr. Alexander-Williams: I am becoming less keen than I was. I have performed a cecorectal anastomosis two or three times. However, I am not convinced that diarrhea is significantly less than if one does an ileosigmoidostomy, which technically is much easier.

Dr. Goldberg: It is far better plus you have two good muscular layers to work with.

Dr. Alexander-Williams: Dr. Ward Griffen always used to tell us that we should preserve the ileocecal valve. He thought it was the third most important sphincter in the body.

Moderator: Dr. Dehner, do you like to receive the specimen in one or two pieces?

Dr. Dehner: I have always been struck by the fact that surgeons like to go at each other and I do enjoy listening to the open confessions of surgeons. We usually get this once a week at our Saturday morning conference, but this larger forum makes it even more interesting. I am not certain whether you are referring to colonic biopsies or what? If you are talking about the problem of dysplasia of the colon, it is important for the surgeon and pathologist to have some idea about where the dysplasia is taking place. It is felt that there is a relationship between the dysplasia and the occurrence of cancer but also a spatial one. Therefore, we like to have the biopsies properly labeled. However, we appreciate even more a clinical history once in a while. It is very interesting to note that sometimes, I suppose none of you here ever do this; we will get specimens submitted to the laboratory labeled: "This is a liver biopsy" or "biopsy of the colon." That is the one fact we can derive rapidly from the histological examination. The ideal, of course, is to have properly labeled biopsies.

Dr. Goldberg: Dr. Dehner, you made a point about the fact that we are seeing more carcinoma in patients who have Crohn's disease. Did not most of those cases occur in bypassed segments?

Dr. Dehner: Not in all cases but certainly in a high percentage. I believe one of the reasons we have not seen carcinoma in Crohn's disease as often is the fact that many of these patients have had segments of the inflamed bowel removed, whereas there is much more temporizing with ulcerative colitis. It is true that those segments of inflamed bowel which are left in is where the cancers arise. The fact is that segments of inflamed bowel in Crohn's disease are removed more often from the patient. If you treated patients with Crohn's disease in the same fashion that you did ulcerative colitis, in other words, managing them for prolonged periods of time with medical therapy, it may be that the cancer figure would be as high as it is with ulcerative colitis.

Moderator: Dr. Najarian told me earlier at this course that you are the best surgical pathologist in the world and the reason he never bothered to send you any history is because you could figure it out anyway.

Dr. Dehner: There are limitations even to the greatest surgical pathologist in the world.

Moderator: In relation to the question of toxic megacolon, what do you recommend to make sure that you are not dealing with acute amoebic dysentery?

Dr. Dehner: The most important thing is to think about that as a diagnostic possibility. At my previous institution, we had a few cases in which the patient had amoebic colitis and was treated with steroids for a period of time. It is interesting how amoebic colitis does *not* respond to steroids. I suppose if you are along the Gulf coast, with individuals coming from ships, that one would think about that diagnosis. As you move inland and northward, it is less often considered. In the last case of amoebic colitis we saw, the clinical diagnosis was acute idiopathic ulcerative colitis and the clinician was rather horrified to find out that in fact the patient had amoebic colitis. Like anything else, you must think about the diagnosis before you can make it. As you know, terrible complications and even life-withdrawing ones can occur if the diagnosis is not recognized.

Dr. Goldberg: I was stung by just such a case. I had a man from Springfield, Minnesota, and Minnesota is not exactly an endemic area for amoebic colitis. The cultures were all negative. The diagnosis was not made until we were at the operating table and realized that we were dealing with something other than Crohn's disease. For a change we were smart enough not to put the bowel back together again. That patient happened to make it. I think maybe we should consider treating some of our patients with inflammatory bowel disease with Flagyl like we formerly did. In some of the older literature, they reported they treated them routinely with anti-amoebic therapy. Dr. Alexander-Williams, do you see amoebic colitis?

Dr. Alexander-Williams: Perhaps that is good sense in the medical treatment of fulminating ulcerative colitis. To add metronidazole as part of the 24- to 48-hour active therapy might differentiate amoebic from ulcerative colitis because it is so difficult to make an accurate diagnosis. Metronidazole is good treatment for ulcerative colitis anyway, so why not make it obligatory?

Dr. Goldberg: It is a treatment that does not hurt them very much.

Moderator: What about sigmoidoscopy?

Dr. Goldberg: Well, when I sigmoidoscoped this patient, I saw the oddest-looking yellow ulcers I had ever seen. I did not know what I was looking at. I just thought it was a fulminant form of Crohn's disease.

Moderator: Do you not think that is a clue when you see those yellow ulcers the next time?

Dr. Alexander-Williams: It is not easy to make the diagnosis of amoebic colitis on sigmoidoscopy.

Moderator: It may not be but sometimes it is quite obvious.

Dr. Dehner: In a patient with active acute colitis a rectal biopsy may not differentiate idiopathic ulcerative colitis from Crohn's disease. When either of these diseases is in a very active inflammatory and ulcerating stage, it is sometimes impossible for the pathologist to give you any help in distinguishing these two diseases. In the majority of cases, it is uncommon to find granulomas in the rectal biopsy. The optimal time to make the diagnosis is when the disease has quieted down. At that stage the differentiating features begin to segregate out. For instance, it is very difficult to tell about goblet cell depletion, which is important in the diagnosis of ulcerative colitis when there is no colonic mucosa. You may be frustrated by the fact that the pathologist cannot help you in this situation but that happens to be a fact of life.

Moderator: Dr. Alexander-Williams, I have several questions from the audience, asking you to explain the Turnbull blow hole colostomy.

Dr. Alexander-Williams: They want to try to convert me back to it, do they?

Moderator: They would like to know what happened when you did it. Are you condemning it out of hand because it was an older American surgeon who did it?

Dr. Alexander-Williams: We only tried it a few times. It worked dramatically the first time. But when we came to do the subsequent colectomy, it was extremely difficult. It was a very messy colectomy associated with a great deal of sepsis. The second time we did a blow hole, it did not isolate the sepsis. The bowel was necrotic and it ruptured subsequently. That was only the first two cases, but that was enough to make me give it up.

Dr. Goldberg: I would like to comment on blow hole colostomy. We never took it up. I must admit that when reports started coming out of Cleveland, we considered it. But as we thought about it, we did not have any desire to get involved with an operation that left the disease in place. One thing I am curious to know is: Where are all the toxic megacolons going?

We are seeing a tremendous decrease in this entity. We formerly saw them right along. Now we rarely see a patient who presents with a classic picture of toxic megacolon. Do you have that same situation?

Dr. Alexander-Williams: Toxic megacolon represents neglected disease. If colitis is treated properly medically, it does not occur.

Moderator: I think that is a good point. I think there is so much better cooperation between gastroenterologists and colonic surgeons. Also, they have become aware of the tragedies which have been encountered when they have followed patients often with very minimal signs but a chronically distended belly. I remember a patient who was presented at rounds at one of our hospitals in San Francisco. The patient was examined by a professor of medicine who discussed the progress and how it was getting on. He had already had a significant perforation of a toxic megacolon and went into shock a few hours later. I do think the incidence has dropped substantially.

What about obstruction of the right colon, not common, but it does occur?

Dr. Alexander-Williams: It is not a problem, really, just perform a right hemicolectomy. There is no need to worry, the anastomoses will heal well.

Moderator: And primary anastomosis?

Dr. Alexander-Williams: I advise a primary anastomosis for all right-sided obstructive lesions.

Moderator: That is a very interesting point because colocolonic anastomoses are much more vulnerable to break down than small bowel-colonic anastomoses.

I have many questions in relation to the management of the posterior wound. You have described the omental pad and vaginal communication. Dr. Goldberg, how do you manage the posterior wound?

Dr. Goldberg: I have to disagree with Dr. Alexander-Williams. I happen to be a packer. I happen to think that packing the posterior space stimulates healing.

Dr. Alexander-Williams: I do not think it stimulates anything.

Dr. Goldberg: Obviously, you do not. Yet, I have nothing else to offer these patients with draining wounds. If you will work at them with packing and with curetting a little hydrogen peroxide to clean these things up, that is the best way we can handle them.

Dr. Alexander-Williams: You have forgotten all I have taught you!

Moderator: I must say that I started closing the posterior wound in 1947 with a small drain. Do you stick your head in?

Dr. Goldberg: No, no, now wait a minute! I am talking about the wound that is persistent. I thought you were talking about the persistent unhealed wound and the treatment of that.

Moderator: No, no.

Dr. Goldberg: Are you talking about primarily at the operating table?

Moderator: Yes.

Dr. Goldberg: Primarily at the operating table, we close them. I must admit I was one of the last people to give in to that practice. I am interested to hear that the persistent sinus rate is still pretty high even when that is done. But I agree with Dr. Alexander-Williams, I think we end up with smaller sinuses that are less troublesome to the patient.

Moderator: I am glad you clarified that. So you close the posterior wound with a suction catheter?

Dr. Goldberg: Yes. We use suction catheters. We either put them through the wound or we put them in through stab wounds on either side.

Dr. Alexander-Williams: Why on earth do you bring them out through the perineum if you are using suction? The perineum is an uncomfortable area to have drains. Why not bring them out through the abdomen?

Dr. Goldberg: I think you have a good point. However, recently, we introduced the use of a very soft Silastic tube called the Jackson Pratt. It is a soft Silastic tube that we picked up from the plastic surgeons. It is very malleable and very comfortable for the patient.

Moderator: Actually, if you have a tight space and you put something on it, you can create fluid. This is true in closing breast wounds. I have closed breast wounds primarily for years without any suction. You can use a little suction to get the flap to settle down. We do have a collection of fluid here and there, but it is very simple for the patient. You make a little incision and evacuate the fluid. I think if you put a catheter in the posterior wound, on continuous suction, you actually fool yourself. Suction will get it clear for a while, and then I think simple drainage is in order. I do not think it is a wise idea to close the space primarily.

Now I shall come back to what you thought I asked earlier, the treatment of the nonhealing posterior wound. You simply put a pack in it, is that correct?

Dr. Goldberg: I have been treating them with curettement at the clinic and also with hydrogen peroxide and having the patient pack these with one-half inch gauze in order to stimulate healing. Another little trick was alluded to — the placement of omentum down into the posterior space. We tried that on two occasions. Both patients told me that they felt like they were sitting on a tennis ball. But I must agree it healed up. I just recently heard about another technique that will be reported shortly from a group in Texas at one of the United States Air Force hospitals. They are using a gluteus muscle graft, sliding it in and closing them primarily. So those are some of the tricks you can try. But you must be persistent.

Dr. Alexander-Williams: Could I make a point? I think a sinogram is invaluable in the assessment. Some of the tracks are just slow healing, well-draining wounds. That is no great problem. But if on a sinogram you find a flasklike cavity with a narrow neck, it will never heal. Once you identify the narrow neck, then you have to open it. I would reiterate the advice about nibbling the sacrum. I take a pair of bone nibblers and go up until the feet start to twitch and then I quit!

Moderator: This is good, solid, old-fashioned technique. If you have a cavity with a small hole, it will never heal. It must be totally unroofed. If it is a relatively fresh cavity, and the walls are somewhat mobile, with just simple packing it closes progressively and rapidly. The problems are in those patients who were closed originally or partially closed, had a major infection, then broke down. Then you have a rigid cavity, and that is the one everyone struggles with. We have laid them open and packed them. They have not healed. We have skin-grafted them. We have done all kinds of maneuvers.

Dr. Dehner, back to you, the pathologist. How do you feel about Morson's atypia? How reliable is it? Can you just biopsy the rectum? Or should you try to get a biopsy through a colonoscope in the area of a questionable lesion?

Dr. Dehner: I think that it is extremely important to go above the point which you would ordinarily reach with the sigmoidoscope. I think in those patients who have the chronic continuous form of ulcerative colitis that it is an extremely important way of following those patients. Patients who have the intermittent form of the disease, we know, have a much lower cancer risk. It is not only Morson. Morson and Pang's original observation (*Gut* 8:423, 1967) about the significance of dysplasia has been corroborated by Riddell (*Curr. Top. Pathol.* 63:179, 1976) and the group at the University of Michigan (*Arch. Surg.* 111:326, 1976). They have also reported that dysplasia is apparently an extremely important progenitor lesion in the development of cancer in these patients. Histopathologically, the individual glandular changes if you did not know that they had come from a patient with ulcerative colitis resemble a biopsy from a large adenomatous polyp. It would be extremely risky, given the available information, to disregard the finding of dysplasia. What Riddell and Morson and others have emphasized, however, is that there is dysplasia and then there is regenerative atypia. It is important for the pathologist to differentiate these. Given a site of active ulcerative colitis, mucosa is regenerating and there is a great deal of mitotic activity. Regenerative atypia will eventually subside when the disease has quieted down. On the other hand, dysplasia, a preneoplastic alteration of the mucosa, will remain as a fixed change in the tissue after the disease has quieted down. It is important, therefore, to follow up a histologic diagnosis of atypia in the acute stage of the disease with later biopsies to determine the significance of the changes. Then you and the patient have to decide what route to take. It is incumbent upon you to tell the patient that changes are present in the mucosa and that they may represent the progenitor of cancer.

Moderator: Is there any place for delayed wound closure, leaving the skin and subcutaneous tissue open, in colonic surgery, particularly in a contaminated field?

Dr. Alexander-Williams: Yes, there is an important place.

Moderator: We would all agree to that. It is probably the most important factor initially. If one does close those wounds, that is where a high incidence of infection occurs; whereas, if you leave a significant proportion open, you decrease your septic wound complications enormously.

Dr. Alexander-Williams: I wanted to comment on what has been said about dysplasia. I quite agree with you. You must not disregard it, heaven forbid! But you do not necessarily have to take the colon out just because it is present. I agree you must biopsy the colon frequently but there are many cases both at St. Mark's Hospital and at our institution where there is no doubt about there being dysplasia on biopsy and the patients remain for years with dysplasia but without developing carcinoma. Furthermore, dysplasia is a patchy abnormality. Even in patients who have a cancer, there are patches where there is no dysplasia and patches where there is dysplasia. So we cannot rely on the absence of dysplasia as representing absolute safety from developing cancer.

Dr. Dehner: That is right. But in the patient who has dysplasia, it is important to take cognizance that there is mild dysplasia, moderate dysplasia and severe dysplasia. There are grades of dysplasia. Initially, if one finds dysplasia in one of 20 biopsies, and the second time around it is in 5 biopsies of 20, the trend is obvious. To wait may subject your patient to a very risky game.

Dr. Alexander-Williams: Agreed!

Continuing Controversy Over Carcinoma and Polyps of the Colon

Patrick C. J. Ward, M.D.

Objectives

1. To present current views on de novo origin of carcinoma of the colon versus origin in polyps.
2. To list and describe the common colonic polyps which undergo malignant transformation.
3. To review current concepts of therapy for tubular (adenomatous) polyps containing carcinoma.

Q. *Do carcinomas of the colon arise de novo in flat mucosa?*

A. There is presently no good evidence that they do (except in the special circumstance of ulcerative colitis). If in fact they did, by now minute carcinomas less than 5 mm in diameter would have been occasionally found by chance alone during colonoscopy, in colectomy specimens or at autopsy. The acknowledged extreme rarity of such lesions militates against origin de novo in flat mucosa [1-3]. This implies, therefore, that carcinomas arise in polypoid lesions.

Q. *What polypoid lesions might give rise to carcinoma?*

A. There are four candidate lesions: (a) hyperplastic, (b) villous, (c) tubulo-villous and (d) tubular (adenomatous) polyps. Of these, hyperplastic polyps are by far the most common. They constitute 90% of all colonic polyps [4]. Of the remainder, 10% are villous, 10% are tubulo-villous and 80% are tubular (adenomatous) [5]. If a carcinoma is present in a polypoid lesion, it should be possible to demonstrate specific

Patrick C. J. Ward, M.D., Associate Professor, Department of Laboratory Medicine and Pathology, University of Minnesota Hospital and Director of Clinical Laboratories, Mount Sinai Hospital, Minneapolis, Minn.

polyp epithelium at the perimeter of the carcinoma. The lesion is then defined as a carcinomatous polyp. In contrast, a polypoid carcinoma is defined as a malignant polypoid lesion with no residual benign foci [6]. Specific polyp epithelium cannot be demonstrated in juxtaposition to the carcinoma. Possibilities as to the pathogenesis of a polypoid carcinoma would include (a) total destruction of original polyp epithelium by tumor and (b) pedunculization of a de novo flat mucosal carcinoma. There is little evidence for the existence of the latter entity.

Q. *Do carcinomas arise in hyperplastic polyps?*

A. Probably not. Although they constitute the largest percentage of colonic polyps, there is no substantial evidence that hyperplastic polyps undergo malignant transformation. One proponent of malignant potential argues that some hyperplastic polyps may develop concave depressions with less differentiation than usual and ultimately transform into ulcerated carcinomas simulating de novo origin [7]. It might just as easily be argued, however, that stellate glands in the colonic mucosa surrounding a carcinoma reflect a secondary or reactive phenomenon. Thus, although the issue is not quite dead, most authorities agree that hyperplastic polyps play little or no role in colonic carcinogenesis.

Q. *Do carcinomas arise in villous polyps?*

A. There is almost universal agreement that carcinomas do in fact occur in association with villous polyps. Whether carcinomas arise in villous polyps or, as some authorities imply, villous polyps harbor carcinomas, is moot: the net effect is the same [8]. The average size of a villous tumor when carcinoma is present is 4.5 cm. About 40% of villous tumors eventually go on to develop carcinoma. This contrasts with the roughly 5% of tubular (adenomatous) polyps which undergo malignant transformation [5]. The potential for malignancy in a tubulo-villous polyp depends to an extent upon the quantity of villous epithelium present. The incidence of malignancy is therefore intermediate between that of villous and tubular polyps. In general, tubulo-villous polyps behave more like villous than tubular polyps [5].

Q. *Do all carcinomas arise in polyps?*

A. There is now almost universal agreement that most, if not all, carcinomas of the colon and rectum arise in preformed polyps [9-11]. With regard to the tubular (adenomatous) polyp as precursor to carcinoma, most authorities now believe that malignant transformation does indeed take place, especially in larger lesions [4, 5]. Invasive carcinoma is uncommon in pedunculated tubular (adenomatous) polyps less than 1.5 cm in diameter but occurs in 10% of those larger than 1.5 cm in diameter [4].

Q. *What are the stages of carcinoma in villous or adenomatous polyps?*

A. Stage 0 is carcinoma-in-situ. This term refers to frankly malignant changes within mucosal glands without breach of basement membranes. This is a rather rare lesion. Stage I is superficial carcinoma. Here, there is extension of malignant glandular cells into the lamina propria but not through muscularis mucosae. Stage II is superficially invasive carcinoma, ie, the carcinoma penetrates the muscularis mucosae and extends into the submucosa. Stage III carcinoma implies invasion of the stalk (see below). In stage IV carcinoma, the tumor penetrates the muscularis propria, eventually becoming the familiar encircling napkin-ring lesion [2]. The degree of differentiation may vary considerably.

Q. *What clinical decisions must be made following removal of a carcinomatous polyp at colonoscopy?*

A. There are basically two options: (a) to cease and desist from further surgical activity (b) resect. These decisions in turn rest on the staging of carcinoma in a well-sectioned polyp. The anatomy of an adenomatous polyp is shown in Figure 1. The small circles on the left reflect carcinoma confined to glands, ie, carcinoma-in-situ (stage 0). The shaded area on the right shows superficial carcinoma (stage I). In the apex is a superficially invasive carcinoma (stage II). In the center of the upper stalk is a deeply invasive carcinoma (stage III). The X-Y line is an arbitrary line drawn between the points of junction of normal and adenomatous mucosa. Two lymphatics are shown in the submucosa of the head.

Following polypectomy, no further surgical activity is indicated when carcinoma is either in situ or superficial (lymphatics are absent from the lamina propria in a fully developed pedunculated adenomatous polyp [12]). In the case of superficial invasion, several factors may influence the decision to resect. When the tumor is superficially invasive (but

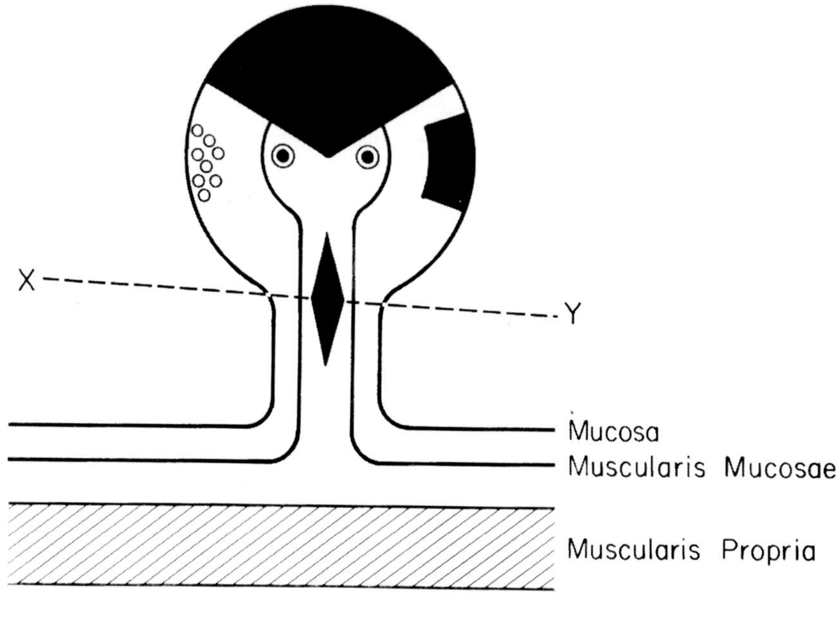

FIGURE 1.

distal to the X-Y line), well differentiated and at the end of a 1.0 cm stalk (or longer), no further treatment may be necessary. Very few such tumors have metastasized. Such conservatism is especially appropriate in cases where surgical morbidity might be anticipated. On the other hand, resection is indicated when the tumor crosses the X-Y line (reflecting stalk invasion), is poorly differentiated, occurs in a polyp with a short stalk (less than 0.5 cm) or is present in submucosal lymphatics in the head of a polyp [13].

Q. *What factors might influence the transformation of a benign polyp to a carcinomatous polyp?*

A. It has recently been suggested that certain individuals have a genetically determined proneness to develop polyps [14]. In such individuals it has been hypothesized [15] that an environmental agent A would allow the expression of this genetic proneness resulting in the appearance of a small polyp. The polyp would then grow under the influence of agent B, a growth factor possibly deriving from the action of bacteria on bile acids. At a certain size, a third agent C would induce malignancy. This hypothesis remains to be tested.

References

1. Lane, N., Kaplan, H. and Pascal, R.R.: Minute adenomatous and hyperplastic polyps of the colon: Divergent patterns of epithelial growth with specific associated mesenchymal changes. Gastroenterology 60(4):537-551, 1971.
2. Waye, J.D.: The development of carcinoma of the colon. Am. J. Gastroenterol. 67:427-429, 1977.
3. Fenoglio, C.M. and Lane, N.: The anatomic precursor of colorectal carcinoma. Cancer 34:819-823, 1974.
4. Rawson, W.: Colonic polyps: Antecedant or associated lesions of large bowel cancer. Semin. Oncol. 3(4):361-367, 1976.
5. Morson, B.C.: Evolution of cancer of the colon and rectum. Cancer 34:845-849, 1974.
6. Silverberg, S.G.: Focally malignant adenomatous polyps of the colon and rectum. Surg. Gynecol. Obstet. 131:103-114, 1970.
7. Bussey, H.J.R.: Familial Polyposis Coli. Baltimore, Md.:The Johns Hopkins University Press, 1973.
8. Horn, R.C.: Malignant potential of polypoid lesions of the colon and rectum. Cancer 28(1):146-152, 1971.
9. Morson, B.C.: Polyp cancer sequence in the large bowel. Proc. R. Soc. Med. 67:451-457, 1974.
10. Muto, T., Bussey, H.J. and Morson, B.C.: The evolution of cancer of the colon and rectum. Cancer 36:2251-2270, 1975.
11. Enterline, H.T.: *In* Morson, B.C.: Pathology of the Intestinal Tract. Berlin, 1976, p. 95.
12. Fenoglio, C.M., Kaye, G.I. and Lane, N.: Distribution of human colonic lymphatics in normal, hyperplastic and adenomatous tissue: Its relationship to metastasis from small carcinomas in pedunculated adenomas, with two case reports. Gastroenterology 64:51, 1973.
13. Shatney, C.H., Lober, P.H., Gilbertson, V. and Sosin, H.: Management of focally malignant pedunculated adenomatous colorectal polyps. Dis. Colon Rectum 19(4):334-341, 1976.
14. Lovett, E.: Family studies in cancer of the colon and rectum. Br. J. Surg. 63:13-18, 1976.
15. Hill, M.J., Morson, B.C. and Bussey, H.J.R.: Aetiology of adenoma-carcinoma sequence in large bowel. Lancet 1:245-247, 1978.

Self-Evaluation Quiz

1. Most colorectal carcinomas arise de novo from flat mucosa.
   a) True
   b) False
2. All of the following polypoid lesions may undergo malignant transformation: a) tubular, b) villous, c) tubulo-villous.
   a) True
   b) False

3. Hyperplastic polyps constitute a certain percentage of all colorectal polyps:
   a) 10%
   b) 30%
   c) 50%
   d) 70%
   e) 90%
4. The association between villous polyps and carcinoma of the colon remains highly controversial.
   a) True
   b) False
5. Invasiveness is uncommon in pedunculated tubular (adenomatous) polyps less than 1.5 cm in diameter.
   a) True
   b) False
6. Stage II carcinoma in an adenomatous polyp of the colon implies:
   a) Invasion of the muscularis mucosae in the head of the polyp
   b) Carcinoma confined to the lamina propria of the head
   c) In situ changes only
   d) Invasion of the stalk, across the X-Y line
   e) Invasion of the muscularis propria
7. One of the following findings does not belong to the group:
   a) Superficial invasion
   b) Involvement of lymphatics
   c) Well-differentiated
   d) Long stalk
   e) Conservative approach

Answers on page 721.

Colonoscopy

Santhat Nivatvongs, M.D.

Objectives

The objectives of this paper are to present the current applications of colonoscopy in diagnosis and treatment of colon and rectal diseases, and to present the results of colonoscopic polypectomy.

Introduction

Colonoscopy is not a routine procedure although its indications have been greatly broadened during the past few years. For most colonoscopists, barium enema is still the first line procedure and colonoscopy is used to complement or to double check the study. Our overall success to pass the scope all the way to the cecum is about 70%. Table 1 shows a list of conditions not suitable for colonoscopy. These are not absolute contraindications, but may force one to discontinue the procedure before reaching the cecum.

I will discuss a few conditions in which colonoscopy is helpful.

Table 1. Conditions Interfering with Successful Colonoscopy

Fixation of colon from previous operation, diverticular disease, irradiation
Acute inflammatory bowel disease
Inadequate bowel preparation
Large aortic or iliac aneurysms
Pregnancy, second and third trimester
Partial colonic stricture
Uncooperative patient

Santhat Nivatvongs, M.D., Assistant Professor, Division of Colon and Rectal Surgery, Department of Surgery, University of Minnesota Medical School, Minneapolis.

Occult Blood in Stool

This is the most common indication for colonoscopy at the present time. Dr. Victor Gilbertsen has provided the results of the Hemoccult test proving that colonoscopy is essential for a complete colonic examination. Numerous small early colon cancers missed by barium study were identified by colonoscopy.

Suture-Line Recurrence

Many suture-line recurrences present as a shallow ulceration and may not show well on the barium enema. Colonoscopy is ideal in this situation. It is our practice to follow patients who have had colonic resection for carcinoma by barium enema alternated with colonoscopy every 6 to 12 months for the first two years and less often thereafter.

Ischemic Colitis

In the past, the diagnosis of ischemic colitis relied entirely on the clinical symptoms of sudden onset of crampy abdominal pain, the passage of bloody stool and the thumbprinting appearance of the involved segment of the colon on barium enema. More recently colonoscopy has been successfully used to diagnose this condition. The colonoscopic features ranged from mucosal hemorrhage and edema in a mild case to necrosis and gangrene in a severe one [1].

Colonoscopy is also useful to detect ischemic colitis following the abdominal aortic reconstruction. In the prospective study of 50 patients with nonemergency aortic reconstructive procedures, Ernst and co-workers [2] found a 6% incidence of colonic ischemia.

Examination of Stricture or Narrowing of the Colon

An "apple-core" lesion seen on barium enema study is typical for carcinoma of the colon but a smooth narrowing or a stricture especially in the sigmoid is a common differential diagnostic problem to the radiologist. Colonoscopy is most useful for providing the diagnosis and has saved a number of patients from unnecessary laparotomy and colon resection.

We have examined 37 patients (Table 2) with stricture or narrowing of the colon seen on barium enema (Fig. 1). Typical apple-core lesions were excluded. We were successful in making a diagnosis in about two out of three patients. The causes of the strictures are shown in Table 3.

Massive Colonic Bleeding

Colonoscopy has no place in patients who are having massive and active colonic bleeding. Selective arteriogram is more appropriate. However, when the bleeding has ceased or

Table 2. Examination of Strictures of the Colon

Number	*Successful*	*Unsuccessful*
37	25	12

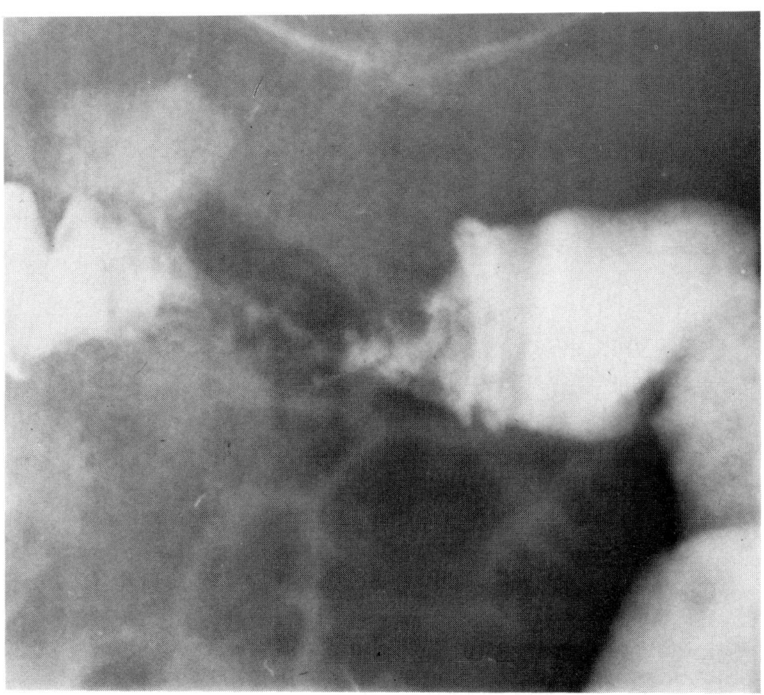

FIG. 1. Stricture of sigmoid colon from diverticular disease.

Table 3. Causes of Colonic Stricture Diagnosed by Colonoscopy

Diagnosis	*No. of Patients*
Diverticular disease, or spasm	10
Anastomotic spasm or scar	5
Carcinoma	3
Extrinsic compression	3
Radiation colitis	2
Suture-line recurrence	1
Crohn's colitis	1
Total	25

slowed and the colon can be adequately prepared, colonoscopy can be useful to identify the source [3]. We have seen two patients with angiodysplasia (Fig. 2) of the right colon, causing severe chronic blood loss, diagnosed by colonoscopy after failures of other repeated studies including arteriogram.

Reduction of Colonic Volvulus

Sigmoid Volvulus

Sigmoid volvulus is best reduced by sigmoidoscopy and rectal tube. However, this is successful only about 70% of the time. More recently, colonoscopy has been successfully used to reduce the sigmoid volvulus [4,5] either as the primary approach or when sigmoidoscopy and rectal tube have failed.

Cecal Volvulus

In the past almost all patients with cecal volvulus required urgent operative intervention. Recently, Anderson et al reported three out of four cases of cecal volvulus successfully reduced by colonoscopy [6].

Unrelenting Colonic Dilatation Caused by Ileus (Pseudo-obstruction)

Colonoscopy is also a new mode of treatment for this difficult high mortality problem. We successfully decompressed one patient with postoperative colonic ileus (Figs. 3 and 4). Kukora and Dent [7] reported success in five of six patients.

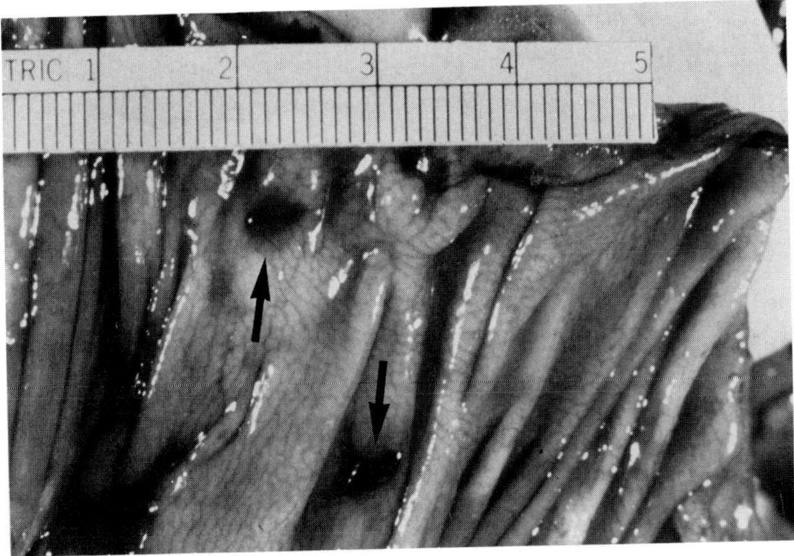

FIG. 2. Small ulcer (*arrow*) in angiodysplasia.

Obviously, successful colonoscopic decompression of colonic dilatation is limited to those patients with a reasonably clean colon.

Inflammatory Bowel Disease

Colonoscopy should not be performed in an acutely inflamed bowel because of the danger of perforation, nor should it be done in patients who are too sick to have an adequate bowel preparation. Colonoscopy is invaluable to detect early or mild disease which does not show on barium enema. The extent of the disease, evaluation of strictures, detection of mucosal dysplasia in chronic ulcerative colitis, differentiation between chronic ulcerative colitis and Crohn's disease, are all best accomplished by colonoscopic examination.

Chronic Ulcerative Colitis

The rectum is almost always involved although occasionally the rectal mucosa, especially in patients receiving steroid enemas, appears grossly normal; only biopsy will show signs of residual disease. In the typical case of chronic ulcerative colitis

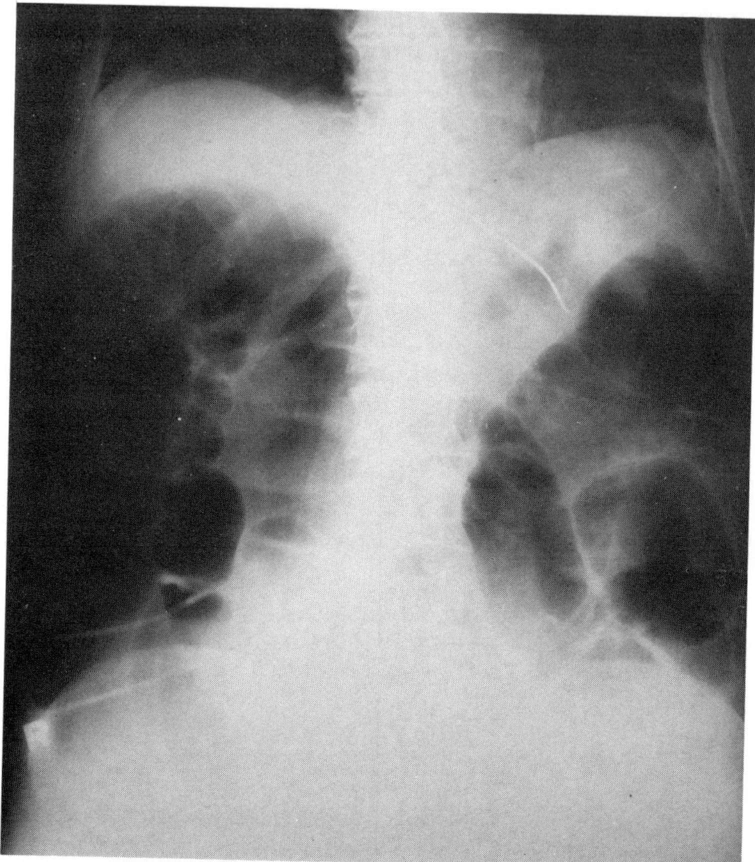

FIG. 3. Colonic dilatation from ileus.

the mucosa shows granularity, friability, erythemia and continuity from the rectum.

Morson and Pang [8] in 1967 studied 23 colectomy specimens removed for colitis in which one or more invasive carcinomas were found. They found that severe mucosal dysplasia was present both near and remote from the site of the carcinoma in all. They then proposed using rectal biopsy to identify the individual patients with chronic ulcerative colitis destined to develop carcinoma. Their original work has been supported by Lennard-Jones et al [9] and others [10-13]. The development of colonoscopy has enabled biopsies to be

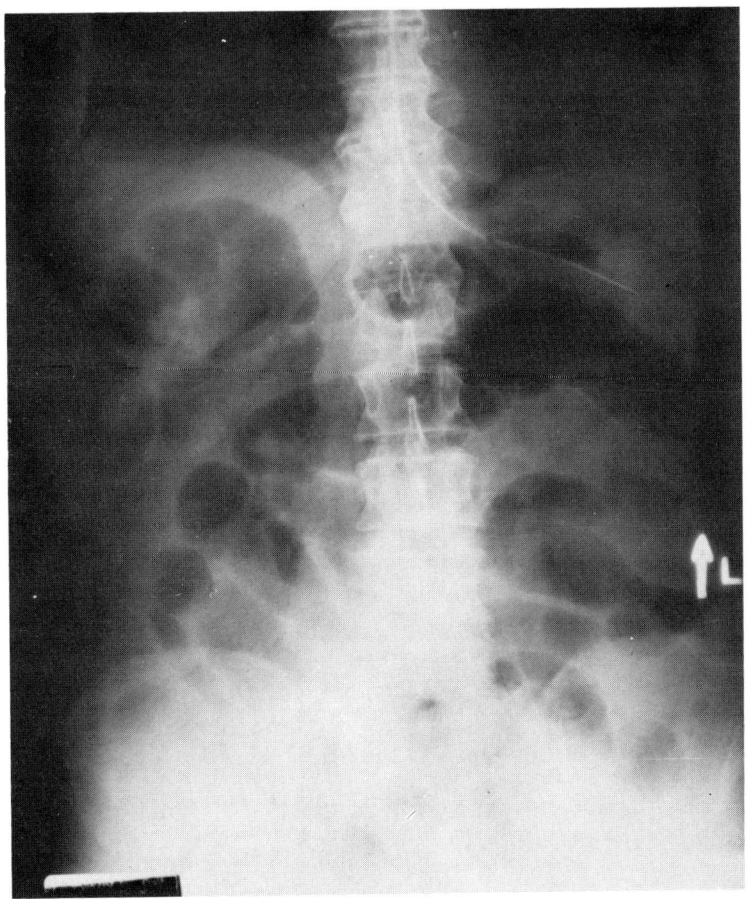

FIG. 4. After colonoscopic decompression.

obtained from all parts of the colon and has further increased the accuracy of this approach. Since severe mucosal dysplasia is rare in chronic ulcerative colitis with a history of less than ten years, it is recommended that patients with chronic ulcerative colitis of longer than ten years duration should have colonoscopy and multiple biopsies once a year. If severe dysplasia is present, total proctocolectomy should be considered. Using severe mucosal dysplasia from rectal or colonic biopsy as an indication for total proctocolectomy, carcinoma was found in 59% of the specimens (Table 4). If severe mucosal dysplasia is

Table 4. Using Severe Mucosal Dysplasia As an Indication for Operation

Author	*No. of Patients With Colectomy*	*No. of Patients With Cancer*
Morson [8]	9	5
Yardley [12]	3	2
Lennard-Jones [9]	7	4
Fuson [13]	8	5
Total	27	16

absent, a patient can be reassured that the short-term risk of carcinoma is low. Among 196 patients who showed no evidence of dysplasia in biopsy specimens, no carcinoma was observed in 941 patient-years of follow-up [9].

Crohn's Colitis

The colonoscopic appearance of Crohn's colitis is different from chronic ulcerative colitis. Crohn's colitis is asymmetric in distribution and patchy rather than continuous. Cobble stoning and longitudinal fissures, if present, are characteristic. In an early or mild Crohn's one often sees only multiple scattered areas of aphthous ulcers. Biopsies of these ulcers are helpful if granulomas are present but usually they show only nonspecific inflammation.

Colonoscopic Polypectomy

Colonoscopic polypectomy has become the standard treatment for clinically benign polyps anywhere in the colon. Between August 1972 and May 1978 we removed 800 polyps (Fig. 5), the size ranging from 5 mm to 5 cm (Fig. 6). Eighty-three percent of the polyps removed were in the left colon, 10% in the transverse colon and 7% in the right colon. The pathology of these polyps is shown on Table 5.

Almost all pedunculated polyps can be safely excised via the colonoscope, since the stalk diameter is rarely larger than 1.5 cm. Many sessile polyps are removed piecemeal, occasionally in more than one session. Flat polyps which are firm or have bases larger than 2 cm should be dealt with by colonic resection.

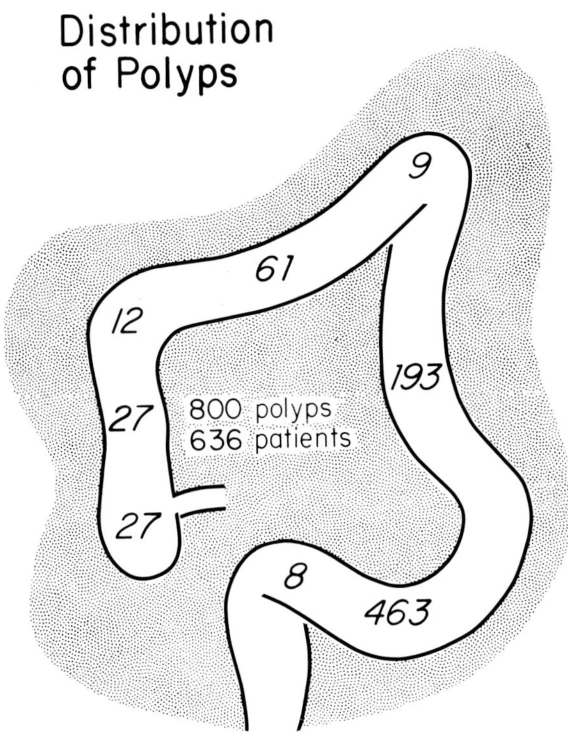

Pedunculated 645 ; Sessile 155

FIGURE 5.

Complications

1. Colonoscopy — 1503 examinations
   1 respiratory arrest; recovered after a brief resuscitation.
2. Electrocoagulation — 100
   2 free perforations; 1 had laparotomy with closure of the perforation; the other was treated nonoperatively.
3. Colonoscopic Polypectomy — 800 polyps

Bleeding (not requiring blood transfusion)	3
Pneumatosis of ascending colon, fever	1
Peritoneal signs, fever	1
Free perforation	0

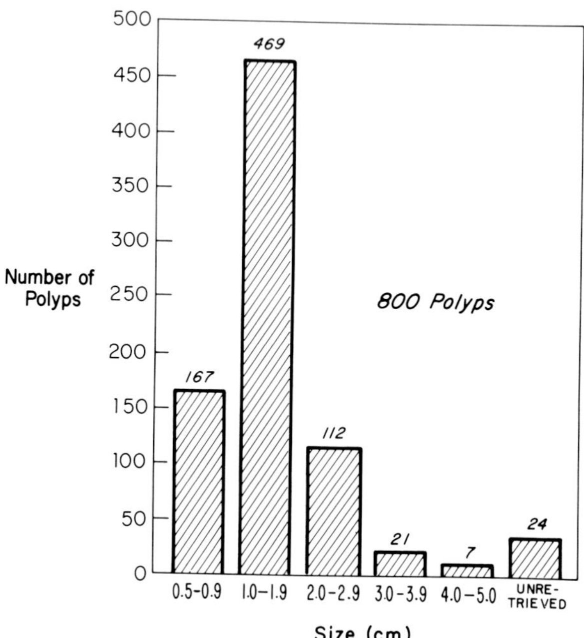

FIGURE 6.

All of the complications occurred during the first 150 polyp removals.

Management of Polyps With Invasive Carcinoma

Thirty-four patients had polyps removed which contained an invasive carcinoma. Almost all of the tumors were in the sigmoid colon and none were in the right colon (Fig. 7). It is of utmost importance to know the histologic details of invasion and the grade of the carcinoma in order to decide the appropriate treatment [14]. In general, a pedunculated polyp with the invasion limited to the head of the polyp requires no further treatment. But if it is an undifferentiated carcinoma or the lymphatics and venules in the head of the polyp contain cancer cell emboli, then colon resection should be considered. Sessile polyps with invasive carcinoma and pedunculated polyps with invasion into the stalk require colonic resection.

Table 5. Pathology

Benign adenomatous or villoglandular polyp	619
Villous adenoma	13
Polyp with superficial carcinoma	22
Polyp with invasive carcinoma	34
Juvenile polyp	23
Hamartoma (Peutz-Jeghers syndrome)	2
Hyperplastic polyp	29
Lipoma	6
Lymphosarcoma	1
Miscellaneous	27
Unretrieved	24
	800

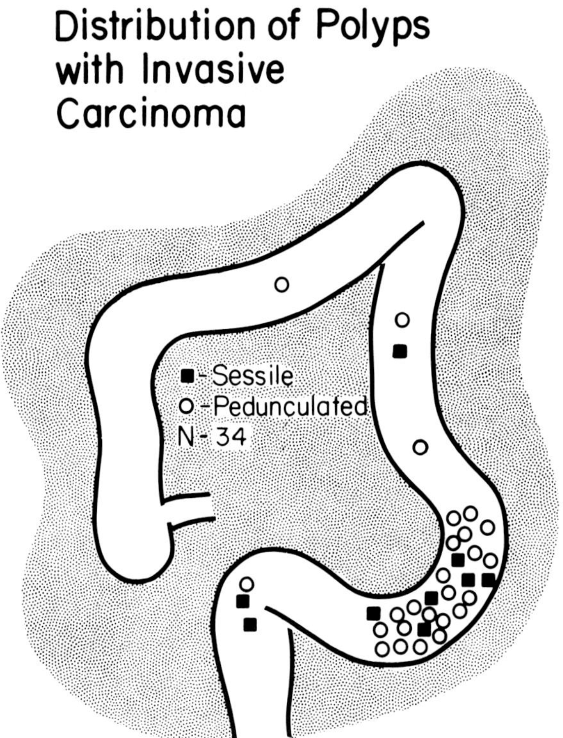

FIGURE 7.

References

1. Hagihara, P.F., Parker, J.C. and Griffin, W.O.: Spontaneous ischemic colitis. Dis. Colon Rectum 20:236, 1977.
2. Ernst, C.B., Hagihara, P.F., Daugherty, M.E. et al: Ischemic colitis incidence following abdominal aortic reconstruction: A prospective study. Surgery 80:417, 1976.
3. Wolff, W.I., Grossman, M.B. and Shinya, H.: Angiodysplasia of the colon: Diagnosis and treatment. Gastroenterology 72:329, 1977.
4. Ghazi, A., Shinya, H. and Wolff, W.I.: Treatment of volvulus of the colon by colonoscopy. Ann. Surg. 183:263, 1976.
5. Sanner, C.J. and Saltzman, D.A.: Detorsion of sigmoid volvulus by colonoscopy. Gastrointest. Endosc. 23:212, 1977.
6. Anderson, M.J., Okike, N. and Spencer, R.J.: The colonoscope in cecal volvulus: Report of three cases. Dis. Colon Rectum 21:71, 1978.
7. Kukora, J.S. and Dent, T.L.: Colonoscopic decompression of massive non obstructive cecal dilation. Arch. Surg. 112:512, 1977.
8. Morson, B.C. and Pang, L.S.C.: Rectal biopsy as an aid to cancer control in ulcerative colitis. Gut 8:423, 1967.
9. Lennard-Jones, J.E., Morson, B.C., Ritchie, J.K. et al: Cancer in colitis: Assessment of the individual risk by clinical and histological criteria. Gastroenterology 73:1280, 1977.
10. Gewertz, B.L., Dent, T.L. and Appelman, H.D.: Implications of precancerous rectal biopsy in patients with inflammatory bowel disease. Arch. Surg. 111:326, 1976.
11. Myrvold, H.E., Kock, N.G. and Ahren, C.H.R.: Rectal biopsy and precancer in ulcerative colitis. Gut 15:301, 1974.
12. Yardley, J.H. and Keren, D.F.: "Precancer" lesions in ulcerative colitis. A retrospective study of rectal biopsy and colectomy specimens. Cancer 34:835, 1974 suppl.
13. Fuson, J.A., Sullivan, B.H. Jr., Hawk, W. and Farmer, R.G.: Endoscopic cancer surveillance in chronic ulcerative colitis. Abstract. Gastrointest. Endosc. 24:196, 1978.
14. Nivatvongs, S. and Goldberg, S.M.: Management of patients who have polyps containing invasive carcinoma removed via colonoscope. Dis. Colon Rectum 21:8, 1978.

Self-Evaluation Quiz

1. Colonoscopy is at present a routine procedure.
   a) True
   b) False
2. Barium enema with air contrast could detect almost all colonic polyps and carcinomas, colonoscopy is unnecessary.
   a) True
   b) False

3. As in upper gastrointestinal hemorrhage, colonoscopy should be done immediately in massive and acute colonic bleeding.
   a) True
   b) False
4. Colonoscopy is the treatment of choice in sigmoid volvulus.
   a) True
   b) False
5. Pseudo-obstruction of the colon may be successfully decompressed by colonoscopy.
   a) True
   b) False
6. In patients with acute colitis:
   a) Colonoscopy should be done as soon as possible to establish the diagnosis
   b) Should have barium enema to confirm the diagnosis
   c) Should have sigmoidoscopy and biopsy
   d) Colonoscopy is contraindicated
7. Strictures of the colon are all from carcinoma, and colon resection is indicated:
   a) True
   b) False
8. Ischemic colitis is characterized by:
   a) Crampy abdominal pain
   b) Passage of bloody stool
   c) Thumbprinting appearance on barium enema
   d) Colonoscopic picture of inflammation, congestion, or necrosis
   e) All of the above
9. Suture-line recurrence of colon cancer is best detected by:
   a) Barium enema
   b) Arteriography
   c) Explorlaparotomy
   d) Colonoscopy
10. The colonoscopic appearance of Crohn's colitis:
    a) Patchy involvement and asymmetrical
    b) Aphthous ulcer
    c) Mucosal and submucosal edema
    d) Longitudinal fissures
    e) All of the above

Answers on page 721.

Modern Trends in Sphincter-Saving Operations for Carcinoma of the Rectum

John C. Goligher, M.D.

Objectives

To review various resection techniques (anterior, abdomino-anal pull-through and abdominosacral), the stapler gun for rectal and anal anastomosis procedures and the place of local excision or fulguration in the treatment of rectal carcinoma.

To most surgeons, the phrase, sphincter-saving resection of the rectum, means one thing and one thing only — anterior resection. It might be appropriate to remind some of the younger members of this audience that this operation is a Minnesota procedure which originated with Dr. Fred Dixon of the Mayo Clinic and his colleagues, John Waugh, Charles Mayo and Marden Black. It enjoyed the very influential support of that great surgeon, Owen Wangensteen, in Minneapolis. This attitude of the average surgeon toward anterior resection is entirely realistic because, of the various sphincter-saving operations that have been suggested for rectal cancer, it is the only one that has secured universal acceptance. There are other methods which sometimes work quite well, but they seem to have numerous complications, and the functional result is not always entirely satisfactory.

John C. Goligher, M.D., Consultant in General and Colorectal Surgery, Leeds, England; Emeritus Professor of Surgery, University of Leeds; formerly Surgeon, The General Infirmary at Leeds; Consulting Surgeon, St. Mark's Hospital for Diseases of the Rectum and Colon, London, England.

When one considers carcinomas in the various segments of the rectum, for lesions of the rectosigmoid or the upper third, anterior resection would seem to be the natural procedure for their treatment. Indeed, with all the wisdom that goes with hindsight, it is remarkable that it took so long for anterior resection to become the standard procedure for cancers in these locations.

But turning to carcinomas of the middle third, if one is not a surgeon but a medical student or a nonsurgical doctor, one might be excused for wondering if there could be any place at all for a sphincter-saving operation — anterior resection or any other — for a lesion at 7 or 8 cm from the anal verge. If one takes a distal margin of clearance of 4 or 5 cm, which seems to be generally accepted as necessary, it would mean that the distal line of resection is in the upper part of the anal canal, which would not augur well for a satisfactory functional result. But, of course, as surgeons, we know that at operation when the rectum is mobilized by dividing the lateral ligaments, it loses its anterior and posterior curves, straightens out and lengthens. So the lesion that lay at about 8 cm on preoperative sigmoidoscopy may move up to about 12 cm. It is quite possible, then, to do a resection with a 5 cm distal clearance and still be left with a very respectable anorectal remnant.

Whether or not the surgeon will be able to join the colon to that remnant by anastomosis from above will depend upon certain factors, of which the most important is the sex of the patient. Wide female pelves are far more conducive to difficult low anastomoses. Another consideration is the general physique of the patient. These operations are much easier in thin subjects. A third consideration is, of course, the expertise of the surgeon. It is not at all unreasonable to expect that the average surgeon with a good deal of experience in rectal surgery should be able to do a radical anterior resection for a growth at 8 cm in a thin female. In a thin male he would be quite lucky to be able to handle a growth at 10 cm by anterior resection. In obese subjects, the lower limit for growths for treatment by anterior resection would be 11 or 12 cm or higher.

This means that if the only sphincter-saving operation the surgeon has in his repertoire is anterior resection, a certain number of the patients with growths in the middle third, particularly males, will not be given a sphincter-preserving operation. They will instead be relegated to combined excision and a permanent colostomy. Clearly, it is for this group of patients that we must think of alternative forms of sphincter-saving resection, which would be substitutes not for anterior resection, but for combined abdominal-perineal rectal excision.

What are the alternatives? The first is not really an alternative operation at all. It is just anterior resection with the anastomosis done by a different technique, that is, stapling instead of conventional suturing. Dr. Mark Ravitch is the father of stapling in this country, and I do not want you to be overexposed to this subject, but I have had a good deal of practical experience with stapling in connection with anterior resection. I have mostly used the original Russian machine, upon which the more recent American E-E-A machine is modeled.

The Russian machine we call the suture gun because it looks very much like a Thompson submachine gun but with a rather expanded terminal part of the barrel. This terminal part of the barrel is composed of a head and a shoulder piece, which can be separated. The shoulder piece contains a circumferential row of staples. There is a central circular or trephine knife. The staples and knife are advanced when the handles of the pistol grip C are compressed.

In using this instrument, it is preferable that you should put the patient in the lithotomy-Trendelenburg position, which is in any event employed routinely for rectal incision of any kind in Britain. With the patient in this position, the gun can be got to the intended site of the anastomosis by inserting it through the anus from below during the procedure. But if one prefers, it is possible to deliver the instrument to the anastomosis from above by making a side opening in the colon and passing the gun through it and down into the rectal stump. But this might be rather traumatic to the colon which is normally much narrower than the rectum. It seems to be much better to introduce the instrument from below.

The resection itself is conducted exactly as in any ordinary anterior resection. I want to emphasize the technique for inserting the pursestring sutures. Dr. Ravitch has showed a device composed of a double Furniss clamp for placing these sutures. It is quite good for the colon stump, but totally impossible to use on the rectal stump deep in the pelvis. Even when it is feasible, I am not sure that it is as reliable as a simple free hand pursestring suture. When you tie the suture it turns the mucosa in so that there is no tissue above the pursestring suture on the central shaft of the gun. This is very important; otherwise, the circular knife might not be able to circumscribe that wad of tissue.

The colon is slipped over the head of the instrument; this is often rather difficult to do because the colon is much smaller than the rectum. One of the advantages of the Russian machines is that they are supplied with four sizes of heads. You can interchange these heads, depending upon the size of the bowel, and by that I mean the size of the colon, for the rectum is virtually always quite capacious. The American machine has only one head. But I am sure it is only a matter of time before smaller heads are made for different cases, such as ileorectal anastomoses. The two stumps are apposed until finally a gap of 1.5 mm or so remains between the head and shoulder piece of the gun. Now is the time to fire the gun by apposing the arms of the pistol grip.

The effect is to put the staples through the tissues, and simultaneously to advance the knife and cut off the tissue that is attached to the central shaft. Then the instrument is opened a few millimeters and gently wiggled out by a delicate maneuver.

One of the reasons why you can get lower with this machine than you can with a hand sutured anastomosis is that after putting the pursestring suture in, another 1.5 cm is removed with the machine, which takes the anastomosis still lower. One can allow for that in the margin of clearance in the original resection.

What sort of reliability have we had with this machine? I do not have any controlled trials to report now. But I can tell you how our current results with the gun compare with the results we have had with hand suture in various controlled trials that I have done in the past. About a year ago, I published a report on a comparison of one- and two-layer hand suture for anterior resections, high and low anterior resections, and if we just lump together these one- and two-layer anastomoses, we see that of the 84 high anterior resections, 27% leaked; notice that these were nearly all radiological leaks, only one clinical. With low anterior resections, we have nearly 50% leaks but most of these were radiological and only eight were clinical.

For comparison, let me tell you about the first 35 that we did with the gun. With the high anterior resection, the results were really very good. With the low anterior resection, we had some leaks, mostly radiological. This is not a controlled comparison. One must be very careful in drawing conclusions from it but there are no real differences between the sort of cases that I am doing now and those I did with hand suture. Our results suggest that the anastomoses one gets with this machine are just as good as those one makes with hand sutures. But more important is the question whether this machine enables one to go lower with one's anastomoses than one can go with hand suture. In other words does the gun enable us to extend the range of anterior resections to take on those difficult growths in the middle third that we could not manage by an anterior resection with hand sutured anastomosis? I think it does help in that respect because one of the things that makes those results I have just described more credible is that the series includes some very low anterior resections which I could not have done by hand.

One could not get a hand anastomosis just above the anal canal. But the gun enabled me to do so. There are ways, indeed, of using this machine and putting the pursestring suture in the lower stump, not from above, but through the anal canal from below, using a bivalve anal dilator to open up the anal canal, and I have done some cases like that. So I think there are quite a number of possibilities for this instrument for extending the range of anterior resection.

Some of these anastomoses were at 4 cm, 4.5 cm, 5 cm, 5.1 cm. Six centimeters is usually about the lowest limit for hand sutured anastomoses under the most favorable circumstances. I think I have made my point with regard to possible usefulness of this instrument to increase the range of anterior resection. Whether or not it will succeed in replacing the other operations I am not prepared to say at this time. I think it will probably enable one to make anterior resections as low as one ever would want to go with a sphincter-saving procedure in female patients, certainly in all but very obese female patients. But in male patients, certainly more obese male patients, I think there will continue to be a significant place for the other maneuvers which I am going to discuss.

The first maneuver is the abdomino-anal pull-through resection. I am merely going to mention but not describe it. It has been used extensively in the United States with rather mixed results. Some surgeons claim excellent results, others much less satisfactory ones. The main objection is that function is often rather poor. At the Mayo Clinic, where many of these operations were done, nobody seems to be doing them now, which rather suggests that they were not as good as some of its former advocates suggested. I did quite a number of pull-through operations some years ago using the Turnbull technique, but I must say I was disappointed with the functional results and eventually abandoned the method.

A new operation that is now being used a good deal in England is that known as the abdominotransanal. Instead of pulling the colon through, the anastomosis is done from below, sutures being inserted between the colon stump and the anorectal remnant from below, working through the anal canal held open by a bivalve anal retractor. The bowel is clamped very low down in the sagittal plane and divided just below the clamp. Then the surgeon goes below and passes a bivalve speculum, which exposes the end of the anorectal stump and allows an anastomosis to be constructed between it and the end of the colon. Some will say that it looks like an awfully tricky maneuver. It is quite difficult. In fact, Parks, who originated this method, has recently given up using the method and instead he uses the Soave technique for doing the anastomosis. He blows up the submucosa with weak adrenaline solution on the posterior sector of the anal canal and then dissects out that mucosa and leaves it with a completely bared circular muscle coat and internal anal sphincter. Then he rotates the retractor around and does the same on the right lateral wall. Then the anterior wall. Then the left lateral wall. And then finally he has a completely denuded stump and he brings the colon down through that. An anastomosis is now constructed between the cut edge of the colon and the remnant of anal mucosa. He may put a few sutures between the serosa of the colon and the top edge of the anorectal muscle coat.

Again, this is quite a tricky anastomosis, but it can be done. We have used this method in about ten or so cases. It works quite well as a rule. We do get occasional leaks, occasional separations, occasional stenoses. As for function, you might say the idea is to preserve nerve endings in the muscle. Actually, Parks believes that the nerve endings are not in the muscle but in the puberorectalis muscle and levators. He claims that the results functionally are very good. All I can say from my experience is that for six months or so the patients pass through a very rough phase of partial incontinence, but eventually most of them seem to acquire a rather precarious continence. So this is an operation that is now being extensively tried in England and it will be interesting to see how it gets on.

Another operation is the abdominosacral resection. This operation was originated by a German surgeon, Kraske, who practiced in Freiburg. Then it was taken up by Finsterer in Vienna. But the person who has made most of it in recent years has been Arthur Localio in New York, who did a lot of cases by this method, using an ingenious technique. He does the whole operation as a synchronous procedure, a two team operation, in the sense that he has the patient on the right side throughout and does the abdominal resection through this long oblique incision. Then while the incision is still open, he moves to the back and makes a transverse cut, takes out the coccyx, and does the resection from below and completes the anastomosis.

I tried this operation some years ago for a trial period. I have done so many abdominal dissections of the rectum with the patient flat that I was reluctant to adopt the side position. So I used the classical method of doing the abdominosacral, which is to have the patient flat for the abdominal phase and then to turn him on his right side for the sacral phase. On the long colon stump the distal limit of viability is marked by tying a gauze swab to the bowel at that point, then pushing that part of the bowel down behind the mobilized rectum, and turning the patient on his side, doing a transverse incision, which can be extended, taking out the coccyx, and then going through the fascia of Waldeyer, taking out the loop of bowel with the gauze swab attached, then clamping the rectum below the growth and irrigating through the double channel anal tube and cutting the bowel below the clamp.

One surgeon who uses this method in England is York Mason. He has introduced a method of dealing with certain tumors of the rectum where one divides the sphincter posteriorly and goes through the levator muscles. The method was really originated by an American surgeon, named Dean Bevin, in Chicago, in 1916. But Aubrey York Mason has developed this method, I think, without any knowledge of that previous description. He has now married that operation to the abdominal phase. So it really means he does a sort of Localio operation except that, for the sacral phase, he does not remove any of the bone. He does the posterior phase of the operation with the patient in the jack-knife position.

The incision goes through the levators and the external sphincter. Then the growth is mobilized and excised. Then the anastomosis is made very low down. Finally, the sphincters and the levators are reconstituted.

One of the snags I have found in doing the abdominosacral or abdominotransphincteric operation is that, having done the abdominal dissection including the establishment of a covering transverse colostomy (as I always do with this sort of operation), one may find, when one has the patient turned round, that one cannot complete the operation as a sphincter-saving resection and has instead to do an abdominoperineal incision. Accordingly, one has to turn the patient on his back again, open up his abdomen, get rid of the transverse colostomy, and give him an end iliac colostomy. That is one reason why I am much happier to have the patient in the lithotomy-Trendelenburg position, and to do everything I can in that position without any turns at all and therefore to use anterior resection to the limit with hand suture or with the staple gun or to use the abdominotransanal resection.

Is it worthwhile? Does the quality of function justify the trouble? One must decide that for one's self. Your patients certainly will have a rough time, as I have explained, for quite a while before they get really normal continence after most of these extremely low operations, but I reckon that they usually are worth doing.

In summary, so that you can get your perspectives right, I want to tell you what happens to, say, 100 patients who come to me for rectal excision. It is fair to say that 45 of them with big growths in the anal canal or lower rectum cannot avoid an abdominoperineal excision. Another 40-45 will certainly be done by anterior resection. If one adds these two groups, 45 and 40-45 together, one is left with 10-15 patients for whom the decision about the form of operation is more doubtful and the alternative methods need to be considered. Finally, I would mention that there is also a small place for local excision or fulguration in the treatment of rectal carcinoma. Just how many cases should be so treated is debatable. The cases for this form of treatment are those with Dukes' A growths, if one can pick these out with reasonable accuracy on clinical examination.

Self-Evaluation Quiz

1. The major problem with sphincter-saving operations for rectal carcinoma is:
   a) Postoperative pains
   b) Local recurrence
   c) Poor sphincter control
   d) Risk of hemorrhage
2. Low anterior anastomoses are easier in men than women.
   a) True
   b) False
3. Hand-done anastomoses in low anterior resections have a lower leak rate than those performed with the EEA instrument.
   a) True
   b) False
4. What percentage of anorectal carcinomas will continue to require abdominoperineal resection despite the availability of the EEA?
   a) 5%
   b) 25%
   c) 45%
   d) 75%
   e) 90%

5. The nerve endings important in continence are located in the:
   a) Rectal mucosa
   b) External sphincter
   c) Wall of rectum and internal sphincter
   d) Puborectalis and levator muscles

Answers on page 721.

Nonocclusive Intestinal Infarction

William Silen, M.D.

Objectives

To review (1) theoretical studies on the mechanism of nonocclusive intestinal infarction, (2) diagnostic guidelines (especially on the use of angiography and the evaluation of symptomatology) and (3) treatment with intra-arterial papaverine or glucagon, and the discontinuance of digitalis and diuretics.

Introduction

Nonocclusive intestinal infarction has recently emerged as the most frequent form of intestinal vascular insufficiency, representing at least 50% of all cases of intestinal infarction [1, 2]. We have the distinct impression that nonocclusive ischemia is continuing to increase in relative frequency. It appears to be the most lethal form of intestinal vascular insufficiency with a mortality approximating 100% [1-4]. It would seem that a better understanding of the pathogenesis of nonocclusive ischemia will lead to an improved outcome.

Pathogenic Mechanisms

A decrease in mesenteric blood flow of either cardiogenic origin (paroxysmal arrhythmias, myocardial infarction, severe congestive failure) or from hypovolemia caused by hemorrhagic shock has been implicated in the causation of nonocclusive ischemia [1-3]. Recent studies have shown very clearly that digitalis glycosides have strong vasoconstrictive effects on the splanchnic circulation [5-7], an action which had previously

---

William Silen, M.D., Johnson & Johnson Professor of Surgery, Harvard Medical School; Surgeon-in-Chief, Beth Israel Hospital, Boston, Mass.

been suspected on clinical grounds [8-10]. Profound dessication induced by diuretic agents has also been implicated in the pathogenesis of nonocclusive ischemia [11].

The experimental studies I am describing are those of Adar and Salzman [12-14], working in our department to ascertain the mechanisms which perpetuate the spasm of the mesenteric vessels in this condition. They used dogs with flow meters placed on the descending thoracic aorta and the superior mesenteric (SMA) and renal arteries. The experimental groups consisted of animals subjected to profound dehydration caused by withholding of fluids and the administration of furosemide or subjected to a 50% reduction in aortic flow produced by instillation of mineral oil into the pericardial sac. These maneuvers were found to cause a selective decrease of blood flow in the SMA relative to changes in flow in the renal arteries. At the same time, mesenteric vascular resistance increased markedly whereas renal vascular resistance was altered only minimally. Adar and Salzman tested the hypothesis that angiotensin might be responsible for these phenomena by infusing angiotensin while SMA and renal artery flow and resistance were measured. They found that angiotensin II mimicked the effects of profound dessication and cardiac tamponade. In addition, saralasin, an inhibitor of angiotensin II, and SQ 20881 [13], an agent which prevents conversion of angiotensin I to angiotensin II, both ameliorate the changes in SMA flow and resistance produced by dessication. It is entirely possible that the use of these agents may hold considerable promise in the treatment of nonocclusive ischemia in the future.

Recent studies in Europe suggest that agents which bind calcium may reverse the vasoconstrictive effects of digitalis glycosides on the splanchnic circulation.

Diagnosis

Any patient with cardiac disease, especially congestive failure, who complains of diffuse abdominal pain has intestinal ischemia until proved otherwise. This aphorism is extremely useful and should lead to a very careful evaluation of such patients. The pain may be extremely mild. It is usually poorly localized and is most often cramping in nature. Diarrhea is common while nausea and vomiting tend to be less prominent.

The abdomen is usually somewhat distended with mild diffuse tenderness. The picture is initially one which causes little alarm and which scarcely conveys a hint of the serious nature of the underlying condition. The stools are usually found to have occult blood, and leukocytosis is frequent. The plain film of the abdomen is nonspecific, with mild to moderate distention of both the small and large intestine.

In a patient on digitalis glycosides who has been subjected to profound diuresis, these findings are virtually pathognomonic of nonocclusive ischemia and deserve detailed investigation. It is the opinion of this author that at this stage, angiography is indicated, not only for diagnostic purposes but also for therapy. Angiography will help ascertain whether occlusive ischemia or nonocclusive ischemia is responsible for the symptoms. Occasionally, neither will be found, in which circumstances angiography will often disclose the presence of another lesion [15]. The presence of nonocclusive ischemia is characterized by severe spasm of the medium- and small-sized arteries, but no obvious organic occlusive lesions of the blood vessels are observed. Occasionally, a slight narrowing of the superior mesenteric artery or an occlusion of the inferior mesenteric artery is found in association with the spasm, but the latter is clearly the dominant lesion.

Treatment

When nonocclusive ischemia is encountered, it is imperative that the physician caring for the patient be in a position to monitor very carefully the fluid balance and hemodynamic changes which are of such importance in these seriously ill patients with severe heart disease. For this reason a Swan-Ganz catheter and a urethral catheter are virtually indispensable. Large volumes of fluid should be given, under cover of careful monitoring, to the point at which the patient is maximally loaded without the induction of congestive failure. Digitalis and diuretics should be discontinued.

If nonocclusive ischemia is found by angiography, the preference of this author is for the continuous intra-arterial injection of either papaverine (1 mg/min) or glucagon (50 μg/min) into the superior mesenteric artery for 12 to 24 hours. Perhaps in the future this step will be unnecessary if inhibition of angiotensin II or chelation of calcium to reverse the effects of digitalis can be accomplished by the intravenous route. The purpose of a preliminary period of nonoperative treatment is to achieve maximal reversal of the vasospasm so that the true extent of involvement of the intestine can be ascertained by gross observation at the time of subsequent operation. This policy avoids so-called second-look operations in very ill patients. Intra-arterial glucagon or papaverine is continued during operation and for 24 to 48 hours postoperatively. Using rather similar techniques, Boley and his colleagues [15] have been able to salvage as many as 50% of patients with nonocclusive ischemia.

Summary

The relative incidence of nonocclusive intestinal infarction is increasing. Digitalis glycosides and powerful diuretics probably contribute significantly to this phenomenon. Recent studies suggest that the renin-angiotensin system may be responsible for the intense mesenteric vasospasm in these patients. Only early diagnosis and aggressive treatment will improve the usually dismal outcome of this serious problem.

References

1. Ottinger, L. and Austen, G.: A study of 136 patients with mesenteric infarction. Surg. Gynecol. Obstet. 124:251-261, 1967.
2. Pierce, G. and Brockenbrough, E.: The spectrum of mesenteric infarction. Am. J. Surg. 119:233-239, 1970.
3. Fogarty, T. and Fletcher, W.: Genesis of nonocclusive mesenteric ischemia. Am. J. Surg. 111:130-137, 1966.
4. Williams, L.: Vascular insufficiency of the intestines. Gastroenterology 61:757-777, 1971.
5. Shanbour, L. and Jacobsen, E.: Digitalis and the mesenteric circulation. Am. J. Dig. Dis. 17:826-828, 1972.
6. Shanbour, L. et al: Effects of ouabain on splanchnic hemodynamics in the rhesus monkey. Am. Heart J. 81:511-515, 1971.
7. Harrison, L. et al: Effects of ouabain on the splanchnic circulation. J. Pharmacol. Exp. Ther. 166:321-327, 1969
8. Ferrer, M. et al: The effect of digoxin in the splanchnic circulation in ventricular failure. Circulation 32:524-537, 1965.
9. Gazes, P. et al: Acute hemorrhage and necrosis of the intestine associated with digitalization. Circulation 23:358-364, 1961.

10. Polansky, B., Berger, R. and Bryne, J.: Massive nonocclusive intestinal infarction associated with digitalis toxicity. Circulation 30 (suppl. 3):141, 1964.
11. Sharefkin, J.B. and Silen, W.S.: Diuretic agents: Inciting factor in nonocclusive mesenteric infarction? JAMA 229:1451-1453, 1974.
12. Adar, R., Franklin, A. and Salzman, E.W.: Further observations on the effect of furosemide on mesenteric blood flow in dogs. Pharmacol. Res. Commun. 6:565-569, 1974.
13. Adar, R., Franklin, A., Spark, R.F. et al: Effect of dehydration and cardiac tamponade on superior mesenteric artery flow: Role of vasoactive substances. Surgery 79:534-542, 1976.
14. Adar, R., Franklin, A. and Salzman, E.W.: Disproportionate reduction in superior mesenteric artery flow during dehydration and cardiac tamponade. Surg. Forum XXVI:295-297, 1975.
15. Boley, S.J., Sprayregan, S., Siegelman, S.S. et al: Initial results from an aggressive roentgenological and surgical approach to acute mesenteric ischemia. Surgery 82:848-855, 1977.

Self-Evaluation Quiz

1. Of all intestinal infarction, nonocclusive intestinal infarction represents at least:
   a) 30%
   b) 40%
   c) 50%
   d) 60%
2. Mortality from nonocclusive ischemia approaches:
   a) 25%
   b) 50%
   c) 75%
   d) 100%
3. Etiology of nonocclusive ischemia involves:
   a) Increased mesenteric blood flow of cardiogenic origin
   b) Hypovolemia caused by hemorrhagic shock
   c) Only mild congestive failure
   d) Quite a few causes except myocardial infarction
4. Digitalis glycosides:
   a) Do not show strong vasoconstriction on splanchnic circulation
   b) Show strong vasodilation on splanchnic circulation
   c) Show strong vasoconstriction on splanchnic circulation
   d) Show only mild vasoconstriction on splanchnic circulation

5. European studies show that the vasoconstrictive effect of digitalis on splanchnic circulation may be reversed by agents that:
   a) Bind magnesium
   b) Precipitate oxides
   c) Release calcium
   d) Bind calcium
6. Diffuse abdominal pain in a patient with cardiac disease:
   a) Definitely means intestinal ischemia
   b) Hardly means intestinal ischemia
   c) Must be severe to indicate intestinal ischemia
   d) Must be assumed to be associated with intestinal ischemia
7. In a cardiac patient with intestinal ischemia:
   a) Only nausea is a consistent finding
   b) Diarrhea is a common finding
   c) Nausea and vomiting are common
   d) Diarrhea plus nausea and vomiting are common
8. In cardiac patients with intestinal ischemia:
   a) Occult blood may occur in the stools
   b) Leukocytosis may occur in the stools
   c) Occult blood in the stools plus leukocytosis may occur
   d) Distention is hardly present

Answers on page 721.

The Earlier Detection of Colorectal Cancers

Victor A. Gilbertsen, M.D., Stanley E. Williams, M.S. and Leonard Schuman, M.D., Ph.D.

Objectives

To appreciate the low cure-rate of one of the most common visceral cancers in America and to consider the diagnostic value of testing for occult blood in the stools and its importance in earlier detection of cancers of the intestine.

Introduction

Cancer of the large intestine continues to be one of the most common visceral cancers. More Americans have died of this disease during the past 50 years than from any other cancer. The rate of cure remains relatively low — only about one third of those throughout the country who develop the disease are cured.

For many years it has been recognized that most intestinal cancers bleed eventually during the course of their development. Rather simple tests have been available for some time to test for occult or hidden blood in the stool, the simplest and most reliable perhaps being the guaiac test.

A number of case reports, testimonials and small series of cases have appeared in the literature suggesting that testing for

---

Victor A. Gilbertsen, M.D., Associate Professor, Surgery, Stanley E. Williams, M.S., Executive Director, Colon Cancer Control Study and Leonard Schuman, M.D., Ph.D., Professor and Head, Department of Epidemiology, University of Minnesota Health Sciences Center, Minneapolis.

This study was supported in part by Contract No. NO1-CB-53862, National Cancer Institute, Bethesda, Md., and by the Fraternal Order of Eagles Cancer Research Fund.

occult stool blood may lead to earlier diagnosis of intestinal cancer and possibly to improved prognosis for patients with the disease. No large-scale controlled study, however, has been done.

Several years ago with the funding of the National Cancer Institute we began enrolling participants in a study designed to evaluate the merit of testing for occult blood in the stool as a means of improving the prognosis for patients with cancers of the intestine.

Forty-eight thousand participants have been enrolled. Each is in the high-risk group, ie, 50 years of age or older, and each has agreed to randomization following enrollment into one of three study groups. One group is screened yearly with a series of six Hemoccult slides, agrees to undergo careful examinations at the University of Minnesota Medical Center in the event of blood in the stool and agrees to continue with testing for five years plus another five years of follow-up. The second group is tested the first year, then every other year. The third group serves as "controls" and participates in the follow-up studies (Fig. 1).

Results of the Study

As seen in Figure 2, 23,500 participants have returned the Hemoccult slides: 525 participants have had one or more slides positive for occult blood in the stool, and 475 patients have come to the University of Minnesota Medical Center for

COLON CANCER CONTROL STUDY

48,000 PARTICIPANTS
+ 50 YEARS OF AGE

THREE STUDY GROUPS

1) CONTROL GROUP
2) YEARLY TESTING
3) Q 2 YEARS TESTING

FIGURE 1.

COLON CANCER CONTROL STUDY

23,500 PARTICIPANTS RETURNED SLIDES
525 ONE OR MORE POSITIVE
475 PATIENTS EXAMINED

FIGURE 2.

diagnostic evaluations. Fifty participants have chosen not to undergo examinations at the University.

The examination protocol includes a general physical examination, proctosigmoidoscopy, several blood tests, chest x-ray, barium enema, upper gastrointestinal x-rays and/or gastroduodenoscopy, and colonoscopy. Lesions found on colonoscopy are biopsied, if possible, by excision (Fig. 3).

Of the 475 patients examined, 54 cancers have been detected, including 47 gastrointestinal cancers (Fig. 4). Seven cancers other than gastrointestinal were found. The 47 gastrointestinal cancers were found in 45 patients (9.5%) (Fig. 5).

COLON CANCER CONTROL STUDY

EXAMINATION PROTOCOL

PHYSICAL EXAMINATION

PROCTOSIGMOIDOSCOPY

BLOOD WORK

CHEST X-RAYS

BARIUM ENEMA X-RAYS

UPPER G.I. &/OR GASTROSCOPY

COLONOSCOPY
EXCISION - BIOPSY

FIGURE 3.

COLON CANCER CONTROL STUDY

475 PATIENTS EXAMINED

54 CANCERS DETECTED (11.4%)

47 G.I. CANCERS

33 COLON

10 RECTUM

2 STOMACH

1 PANCREAS

1 SECONDARY COLON

7 OTHER CANCERS

2 BREAST

2 BONE MARROW

1 MULTIPLE MYELOMA

1 LUNG

1 SKIN

FIGURE 4.

COLON CANCER CONTROL STUDY

475 PATIENTS

47 G.I. CANCERS	**(10%)**
45 G.I. CANCER PATIENTS	**(9.5%)**

FIGURE 5.

Forty-five of the 47 gastrointestinal cancers were primary in the stomach, colon or rectum. Seventy-three percent of these cancers were found to be confined to the wall of the stomach or intestine at the time of therapy (Dukes A lesions). Another 11% had involved the connective tissue but not lymph nodes, for a total of 84% not involving nodes or additional tissues (Fig. 6). Of course, this is in contrast to the usual observation that about one third of such lesions are confined to the wall of the bowel.

Of interest is the observation that a number of cancers of the colon — those above the proctosigmoid area — were not

COLON CANCER CONTROL STUDY
45 PRIMARY CANCERS
STOMACH - COLON - RECTUM

DUKES A	33	73 %
DUKES B	5	11 %
DUKES C	4	9 %
DUKES D	3	7 %

FIGURE 6.

detected on barium enema examination and were found only on colonoscopy (Fig. 7). Of the 33 primary colon cancers detected, 14 (42%) were found only on colonoscopy. For women, of 14 colon cancers, nine (64%) were not found on barium enema and were detected only on colonoscopy.

The highest risk group was found to be those persons 63 years or older with four or more of the six Hemoccult specimens positive for occult blood (Fig. 8). In this group of patients, 20% were found to have gastrointestinal cancers with

COLON CANCER CONTROL STUDY
33 PRIMARY COLON CANCERS DETECTED

	BARIUM ENEMA X-RAYS	COLON-OSCOPY ONLY
MEN	14 (74 %)	5 (26 %)
WOMEN	5 (36 %)	9 (64 %)
ALL	19 (58 %)	14 (42 %)

FIGURE 7.

COLON CANCER CONTROL STUDY
63+ YEARS
4 OR MORE + HEMOCCULTS

CANCERS	14	20 %
POLYPS	29	42 %
POLYPS &/OR CANCERS	43	62 %
ALL	69	

FIGURE 8.

another 42% having polyps of the intestine, for a total of nearly two thirds with neoplasms of the gastrointestinal tract.

Summary and Conclusions

Intestinal cancer continues to account for a substantial proportion of all cancer deaths. Throughout the country, most persons who develop colorectal cancer continue to die of the disease.

The present study is designed to evaluate testing for occult blood in the stool as a method of earlier detection of cancers of the intestine. Preliminary results appear encouraging, but long-term follow-up results must be awaited.

Self-Evaluation Quiz

1. About one third of people who develop cancer of the large intestine are cured.
   a) True
   b) False
2. Testing for occult blood in the stools:
   a) Is useless
   b) Is a proven way to prevent cancer
   c) Is useful, but must await long-term results
3. More primary colon cancers in women were detected by colonoscopy than by barium enema.
   a) True
   b) False
4. The highest risk patients were:
   a) 50 years old or older with 6 positive Hemoccult slides
   b) 63 years old or older with 4 or more positive Hemoccult slides
   c) 70 years old or older with 4 or more positive Hemoccult slides
   d) Those who admitted a constant diet of convenience foods
5. Of patients with colorectal cancers detected by Hemoccult stool testing, what percentage had no metastases?
   a) 25%
   b) 50%
   c) 71%
   d) 84%
   e) 95%

Answers on page 721.

Local Treatment of Rectal Cancer

Jerome J. DeCosse, M.D., Ph.D.

Objectives

A small proportion of patients with rectal cancer can be treated by local excision or destruction. Safety depends upon accurate microscopic assessment of the specimen. Treatment may be accomplished by local excision, electrocoagulation, or contact radiation therapy. The discussion will center on the indications, strategies and methods for local excision and destruction of rectal cancer.

Introduction

"No two patients with rectal cancer are ever exactly alike" [1]. An important principle of surgery is adaptation of the treatment to fit the patient and disease, and the principle should be applied with equal rigor to patients with rectal cancer.

Local treatment alone provides useful therapy for selected patients with curable rectal cancer and for some with advanced rectal cancer. Rectal tumors labeled histologically as carcinoma in situ, noninvasive cancer, or focal atypia do not invade the muscularis mucosa, which are widely acknowledged as effectively treated by local methods are not considered here.

Local Treatment for Cure

About 15% of all rectal cancers have Dukes' A level of invasion, that is, cancer does not penetrate beyond the muscularis propria and lymphatic metastases are absent. In theory, all 15% should be curable by local treatment alone. In

---

Jerome J. DeCosse, M.D., Ph.D., Professor and Chairman, Department of Surgery, Medical College of Wisconsin, Milwaukee.

practice, that proportion is considerably less, and the chief difficulty is inaccuracy in preoperative staging of rectal cancer.

In a recently reported series, 91 small primary rectal cancers were treated by local excision and regarded as completely excised by both initial and subsequent histological review [2]. Only three patients sustained a recurrence, and the five-year survival rate for all was 100%. Most of the cancers were less than 3 cm in size and some were so-called malignant polyps. Even if removal was regarded as incomplete, only five of 14 recurred, probably because the base of the excised tumor had been electrocoagulated. In another series of 28 patients with malignant polyps, with carcinoma invading the stalk, treated at the University of Minnesota, eight were treated by local excision alone, and all were alive at a median follow-up of 87 months [3].

The main argument for local treatment of small curable primary rectal cancer is that if the patient can be selected properly, the small expected recurrence rate is exceeded considerably by the mortality of abdominal perineal resection which approximates 3% to 5%.

The chief deterrent to more frequent local excision or destruction of small rectal cancers is realization that some small rectal cancers, apparently limited to the bowel wall, in fact have lymphatic metastases. If a primary large bowel cancer is limited histologically to the mucosa and submucosa, 10.9% may be expected to have lymphatic metastases. If beyond the submucosa but confined to the bowel wall, 12.1% have lymphatic metastases. If tumor invades through the bowel wall, 58.3% are associated with lymphatic metastases [4]. An important point, however, is recognition that the small primary cancers associated with lymphatic metastasis often had a poorly differentiated histology.

The hallmarks of a Dukes' A cancer are a small size, nonulcerated polypoid configuration, uniformly soft texture and, in particular, mobility of the tumor by palpation against the adjacent rectal wall. Mobility to the examining finger means that the loose connective tissue space between muscularis mucosae and the circular muscle coat has not been invaded. In addition, the lateral pelvic wall should be palpated during rectal digital examination to assure absence of enlarged lymph nodes.

If a Dukes' A cancer is seemingly present, local treatment is appropriate when the following additional criteria are fulfilled: (1) The patient has an excessive risk for abdominal perineal resection from cardiopulmonary disease or other factors, or the patient cannot manage a colostomy due to faulty vision, obesity, neurological disorders or other impairment. (2) The rectal cancer is less than 5 to 6 cm in diameter and is located less than 10 cm from the anal verge. Rectal cancer above this level should be treated by anterior resection, and some cancers below this level can be removed by transsacral resection or, particularly in the thin female patient, by anterior resection. (3) Histology of the biopsy shows a well-differentiated adenocarcinoma and absence of spread in lymphatic channels; Broder's grade III and IV, or poorly differentiated, cancers account for a substantial proportion of small primary cancers associated with lymphatic metastasis.

If these criteria for selection are met, total excision or total destruction is appropriate therapy. Nothing is lost by total biopsy except waiting for microscopic analysis of the specimen. Since histology and depth of spread are the most important prognostic determinants, should subsequent microscopic examination show extramural extension, incomplete excision or undifferentiated carcinoma, the patient must then be subjected to a more extensive resection. If these determinants are absent, the patient can be followed safely with almost complete assurance of cure.

A small rectal cancer can be handled in several ways.

Excision

Often, local full-thickness sharp excision can be accomplished by the transanal approach with or without division of the anal sphincter. After insertion of anal retractors, very distal or caudad tumors can be excised and more cephalad rectal tumors can be brought to the anal orifice with a series of traction sutures and full-thickness local excision accomplished. An advantage of local excision is availability of the entire specimen for microscopic scrutiny.

Posterior approaches — namely, the Kraske approach with excision of the distal sacrum and coccyx, or the York Mason approach with a parasacral incision — can be applied to excise larger rectal tumors and achieve primary closure of the rectum. Either can be combined with a synchronous abdominal exploration, mobilization of the colon and excision of regional lymphatics. Risk and morbidity of these posterior approaches are higher than those of transanal procedures, and they are probably less desirable as operations for small distal rectal cancers.

Electrocoagulation

Diathermy may be the ideal treatment for the very caudad, easily movable polypoid rectal cancer in an elderly poor risk patient. Electrocoagulation provides some advantage over those operative techniques that require a perianal incision or divide the sphincter. Morbidity is clearly less, the technique is simpler and there might be some advantage by induction of antitumor immunity. In rodents, local destructive methods, either diathermy or cryotherapy, induced more systemic immunity than excision alone [5, 6], but there is no parallel evidence in human neoplasia. During the past decade, the virtues of electrocoagulation have been extolled by several authors [7-12].

The equipment necessary for electrocoagulation is widely available. A Bovie unit, Cameron unit or Hyfrecator provides the necessary bipolar high frequency electrical current. In addition, an operating anoscope or right angle retractors, suction equipment and an operating headlight are required. Ordinarily, the Bovie unit is placed on a current selection of two and a power control knob at 40 for coagulation. A needle point electrode, ball point tip and loop tips are applied successively followed by curetting, and the sequence is repeated several times to destroy tumor until a soft gray base is finally reached and coagulated.

The procedure should be performed in the operating room under regional anesthesia in patients whose bowel has been prepared mechanically and by oral antibiotics. In some poor risk patients intravenous analgesia is satisfactory. A lithotomy position may be used for posterior tumors, the prone position for anterior tumors and the Sims position for lateral tumors. In performing electrocoagulation, the anatomic relationship of the parietal peritoneum to the anterior wall of the rectum must be kept in mind. One can safely electrocoagulate in the extraperitoneal rectum. In the multigravida patient, the rectovaginal pouch may descend anteriorly to 4 cm from the anal verge. Patients are kept in the hospital about two days and are discharged on a low residue diet and stool softeners.

One or more repeat examinations and diathermies are usually necessary before complete removal of the tumor can be assured. Patients who respond satisfactorily to electrocoagulation do so within a period of several months. As a rule, one should not persist in treating with electrocoagulation beyond six months. If response has not occurred, an abdominal perineal resection should be performed.

Radiation Therapy

A third technique is that of endocavitary contact radiation therapy [13]. Up to 15,000 R may be administered by a 50 kv unit through a specially designed proctoscope with the radiation being placed directly on the tumor. Radium applications have also been used [8]. Results in selected patients have been excellent.

With appropriate choice of patients, anticipated cure rates equal or exceed that found after abdominal perineal resection, and any loss from unexpected lymphatic metastasis will be less than the anticipated mortality of abdominal perineal resection. It is possible that local treatment only should be extended to a larger group, but at present that concept should be regarded as investigative.

Local Treatment of Advanced Cancer

In patients with advanced and incurable rectal cancer, there is a tendency among some surgeons to promptly perform a palliative sigmoid colostomy. However, a sigmoid colostomy in a terminally ill patient is poor palliation. A palliative abdominal perineal resection shares not only the same functional limitations but also a substantial mortality.

Electrocoagulation and radiation therapy can be valuable substitute palliative modalities in these patients. Even though rectal cancers seem forboding, intestinal obstruction rarely results from cancer in the distal rectum. By judicious application of these techniques a sigmoid colostomy can be deferred, or even avoided, and rectal symptoms relieved. Initially, bleeding, diarrhea and tenesmus can be controlled by electrocoagulation using the same techniques that have been described, and, with subsequent benefits of radiation therapy administered concomitantly, prolonged relief of symptoms can be achieved.

References

1. York Mason, A.: Rectal cancer: The spectrum of selective surgery. Proc. R. Soc. Med. 69:237-244, 1976.
2. Morson, B.C., Bussey, H.J.R. and Samoorian, S.: Policy of local excision for early cancer of the colorectum. Gut 18:1045-1050, 1977.
3. Shatney, C., Lober, P.H., Gilbertson, V. and Sosin, H.: Management of focally malignant pedunculated adenomatous colorectal polyps. Dis. Colon Rectum 19:334-341, 1976.
4. Morson, B.C.: Factors influencing the prognosis of early cancer of the rectum. Proc. R. Soc. Med. 59:607-608, 1966.
5. Neel, H.B., III, Ketcham, A.S. and Hammond, W.G.: Experimental evaluation of in situ oncocide for primary tumor therapy: Comparison of tumor-specific immunity after complete excision, cryonecrosis and ligation. Laryngoscope 83:376-387, 1973.
6. Sobel, S.H. and Patterson, W.B.: Electrocoagulation vs. excision: Comparison of degree of immunity engendered by treatment of induced tumors in syngeneic mice. Surg. Forum 23:85-87, 1972.
7. Crile, G., Jr. and Turnbull, R.B., Jr.: The role of electrocoagulation in the treatment of carcinoma of the rectum. Surg. Gynecol. Obstet. 135:391-396, 1972.
8. Jackman. R.J.: Conservative management of selected patients with carcinoma of the rectum. Dis. Colon Rectum 4:429-434, 1961.
9. Kratzer, G.L.: Technique in fulguration of carcinoma of the rectum. Surg. Gynecol. Obstet. 137:673-674, 1973.
10. Madden, J.L. and Kandalaft, S.: Electrocoagulation in the treatment of cancer of the rectum. Ann. Surg. 174:530-540, 1971.
11. Salvati, E.P. and Rubin, R.J.: Electrocoagulation as primary therapy for rectal carcinoma. Am. J. Surg. 132:583-586, 1976.
12. Swerdlow, D.B. and Salvati, E.P.: Electrocoagulation of cancer of the rectum. Dis. Colon Rectum 15:228-232, 1972.
13. Papillon, J.: Resectable rectal cancers: Treatment by curative endocavitary irradiation. JAMA 231:1385-1387, 1975.

Self-Evaluation Quiz

1. In a classical Dukes' A level of invasion, the limit of penetration of tumor:
   a) Is confined to the mucosal surface (intraepithelial carcinoma)

Discussion

Moderator: John S. Najarian, M.D.

Moderator: Do the other members of the panel agree with Dr. Ward's interpretation that adenomatous polyps of the colon are premalignant lesions? Dr. Goligher, do you agree?

Dr. Goligher: Yes, I agree.

Moderator: Dr. DeCosse, do you?

Dr. DeCosse: Yes, I agree.

Moderator: Dr. Ward, would you define exactly where the XY line is?

Dr. Ward: The line is drawn between the points of junction of normal and neoplastic (adenomatous) mucosa on both sides.

Moderator: If the lesion is above the muscularis mucosa, but past the XY line, do you think it is adequately treated by polypectomy?

Dr. Ward: I think the questioner is asking about a superficial malignancy close to the resection margin. This would make everybody a little nervous but I have not seen any published data on this lesion. Since there are no lymphatics above the muscularis mucosa, polypectomy should be adequate therapy. Perhaps one of the other panelists would care to address this question based on his own experience.

Dr. Nivatvongs: We would consider the histology. If the lesion is undifferentiated or mucinous carcinoma, we would recommend colon resection.

Moderator: Dr. Goligher, would you comment.

Dr. Goligher: I would be influenced by the activity of the growth, as just stated. If well differentiated with a little margin of clearance, I would be conservative. Certainly, with a rectal lesion I could watch the site afterwards. Admittedly, that would not tell if there were lymphatic metastases. If it were poorly differentiated, I would be inclined to go for a resection whatever the local situation.

Moderator: Somebody wants to pass some information along to you, Dr. Ward. They say: You told us that the cancers did not start in flat areas. What about the patient with ulcerative colitis who eventually gets a cancer that is not in a polyp?

Dr. Ward: I left that completely out of the discussion because it was not pertinent to my subject. In ulcerative colitis, carcinomas occur more commonly in flat mucosa than in the so-called pseudopolypoid lesions. I did not get into that specific type of flat mucosal lesion.

Dr. Goligher: You may find many pseudopolyps and if there is cancer, it will not necessarily be in those polyps.

Moderator: I think the problem was that Dr. Ward was so emphatic about the fact that cancer does not arise de novo from flat colonic mucosa that somebody wanted to point out that it does occasionally start without polyps in other settings.

Dr. Goligher, how much does that Russian rectal stapling gun cost in England?

Dr. Goligher: I bought it for approximately $2000. I do not know what the price is now. The American instrument costs $1200 in England. So you can say that is an obvious argument for the American gun. The Russian gun comes with enough staples to do 120 cases but you have to load it with staples by hand, taking about three minutes to do so each time. The American gun has a disposable end containing the staples and knife, as Dr. Ravitch explained, each end costing $80. So that by the time you have done about 20 cases, you have spent enough money to buy the instrument over again. The other thing is that the Russian gun has four sizes of end, which you can vary, depending upon the size of the colon. But the American gun is very nice; I have used it also and like it very much indeed. I imagine that it is only a matter of time before alternative sizes of headpiece become available with it also.

Moderator: Dr. Goligher, do you always do a complementary colostomy with anterior or abdominosacral resections?

Dr. Goligher: I do it for any difficult low anastomosis, not for high easy anterior resections.

Moderator: How about the staple anastomoses?

Dr. Goligher: I do it for the low ones, especially the very low ones. It does not prevent the anastomosis from leaking. It may reduce the incidence a little. The main thing is that if they do leak, one is in a better position to deal with the situation. It is less serious and I sleep much better.

Moderator: When do you close it? Do you take a barium enema before you close it?

Dr. Goligher: The solution to closing colostomies is not to be in too great a hurry to get on with it. If you leave a colostomy for two months, all edematous swelling will be settled. Closing the colostomy then is like falling off a log. If you attempt to close it too soon, there is still much edema, which makes it a very difficult operation. Resecting the colostomy site and doing an end-to-end anastomosis is quite unnecessary, but I belive it is a frequent practice in the United States.

Moderator: Do you use the abdominosacral classic approach for villous tumors?

Dr. Goligher: If the villous tumor can be handled by low anterior resection, I would do that. Remember, when you are dealing with a villous tumor, the lower edge of which is quite soft, you do not need a 5 cm margin of clearance. You can divide the bowel almost at the villous tumor. Therefore, you have a greater range of choice for anterior resection by hand or with the gun in the management of villous tumors than of frank carcinomas. But if the tumor is low down, almost to the dentate line, anterior resection is clearly impracticable but there are available other methods of sphincter-saving excision if you think it is benign. A moderately popular plan at the moment in England for the latter tumors is to remove them by a local excision done either through the anal canal using a bivalve speculum or through an incision dividing the sphincters and levator posteriorly.

Moderator: This is confusing to some people now because the middle rectal lesion is being approached now by the stapler or by the transsacral technique and the like. What do you feel is the lowest you can go before you must say, "This must be abdominal perineal"?

Dr. Goligher: I would probably put it at about 7 cm. Some are quite happy with the 3 cm margin of clearance in resections for carcinoma. I like more than that, preferably 4 or 5 cm. I would accept a 7 cm lesion as the lowest on which I would normally do any sort of sphincter-saving rectal resection. If it were a very tiny lesion, however, I might do a local excision.

Moderator: Do you have any data to show the distance you must be distal to the lesion? Is this something we have just done by rote over the years?

Dr. Goligher: Yes, there are good data. I produced some myself!

Moderator: What are the data?

Dr. Goligher: Many years ago, research was done on this subject by Grinnell (1954) at Columbia Presbyterian Hospital in New York and by Garland and by Quen, Dahlin and Mayo (1953) at the Mayo Clinic. They showed that although most cancers were nicely circumscribed by a distal margin of about 2.0 or 2.5 cm, occasionally the margin would need to be a little more than that. They produced the magic figure of 4 to 5 cm as a good safe estimate.

Moderator: If actually you must cut closer than that, what sort of data do you have? If you have to cut closer and at the time of surgery have histology that shows the line of resection is negative, would you accept that?

Dr. Goligher: I do not know that you can do a really thorough investigation with frozen sections. I have not done that but it might be possible. Dr. DeCosse has something to say.

Dr. DeCosse: Much of the work was carried out, at least in this country, by Gilchrist, who established that a 2 cm margin in a formalin-fixed specimen was rarely associated with tumor at the suture line. The important thing to remember in looking at the data is that 2 cm in a formalin-fixed specimen is about 4 cm in your hand and is about 5 cm in vivo. That was, in part, how his numbers were developed.

Moderator: If you had an adequate frozen section, Dr. Ward, what would you do? Would you be willing to stick your neck out and state that a distal resection margin was free of tumor?

Dr. Ward: Yes.

Moderator: This is still commonly done here. No matter how far we go below the lesion, we usually ask the pathologist if he can tell us if our distal margin is free. Dr. Goligher, if you feel it is for you, would you be willing to accept that?

Dr. Goligher: I would like to ask the pathologist this question: How well can he do frozen section on a considerable range of tissue distal to the growth? The margin in cases with annular or nearly annular growths will also be circumferential. Are you getting frozen sections from all parts of that margin?

Dr. Ward: Our methods vary, depending upon the size of the lesion. When the lesion is small and close to the margin, we take sections perpendicular to the line of resection, often incorporating part of the lesion. When the lesion is large and circumferential, we prefer to do frozen sections parallel to the line of resection without necessarily incorporating the lesion.

Dr. Goligher: I am biased by the fact that Morson, who is a very influential pathologist in Britain in this field, is reluctant to do frozen sections. He feels he cannot make a good assessment of this sort of situation with them. There is another very practical point about the margin of clearance. If you set yourself to get a margin clearance of 5 cm, very frequently it is less than that when you get the specimen out. If you start out aiming for 3 cm, you may end up with a margin almost on the growth. So it is very important to look at the specimen as soon as you get it out, before you do the anastomosis, to see what sort of margin you have and perhaps get frozen sections as well.

Moderator: I agree with that. Dr. Nivatvongs, how do you retrieve a polyp that has now fallen free in the colon?

Dr. Nivatvongs: Do you mean doing colonoscopy?

Moderator: Yes.

Dr. Nivatvongs: The best and most practical way is to use suction on the scope. Most of the time you can get by that way. If not, we use tap water or saline washing. If the polyp is so big that it is heavy and drops down all the time, then we use biopsy forceps to grasp the base of the polyp and gently withdraw the scope.

Moderator: Dr. Nivatvongs, have you any experience with the 60-cm flexible sigmoidoscope?

Dr. Nivatvongs: If you know how to use the long scope, I do not think this has any place. For people who do not do colonoscopy, it has been shown in the past few years that it has a much better yield than the proctoscopy. No one will argue about that. But it is a compromising examination.

Moderator: Why do you say that?

Dr. Nivatvongs: Because this scope would reach only to the sigmoid colon most of the time. That means you would miss about 30% to 40% of the polyps.

Moderator: Admittedly, you could not do as well as with the colonoscope. If Dr. Gilbertsen's picture is correct, about 70% of your lesions are within about 60 cm.

Dr. Nivatvongs: If the indication, for example, is positive Hemoccult ®, you would need total colonoscopy. For a screening test, it is far more practical to use Hemoccult ® and then do a total colonoscopy when it is positive. That is my feeling. A 60-cm flexible sigmoidoscope, however, is useful to remove sigmoid polyps beyond reach of the rigid sigmoidoscope.

Moderator: You mentioned that only one day of preparation is necessary for colonoscopy. Please tell us how you prepare your patients for colonoscopy.

Dr. Nivatvongs: We use, one, two or three days, depending on the time available. For most of the inhospital cases, we use only one day. Citrate of magnesia and Dulcolax ® on the same day, tap water enemas on that night and clear liquid on that day. I think with this kind of prep it is safe enough to do a snaring of polyp. It has been shown by Michael Levitt and John Bond that with good mechanical bowel prep and a 12 to 24 hour clear liquid diet, there is negligible amount of explosive gases.

Moderator: This is a very important point because he has taken out some 800 polyps and he has not had an explosion yet.

Dr. Gilbertsen, what percentage of carcinomas of the colon were found by positive Hemoccult tests?

Dr. Gilbertsen: The percentage that were found in the series I presented was 100%. We do not have the answer as to how many were missed by the guaiac.

Moderator: What about air contrast barium enema?

Dr. Gilbertsen: I think that is possible but air contrast is much more work and is more expensive and the radiologists at least in this institution are reluctant to do it as a regular procedure.

Moderator: Dr. Gilbertsen, be specific on how the Hemoccult is taken. You get six specimens from three consecutive stools. How does the patient out on the small farm in northern Minnesota send you six specimens?

Dr. Gilbertsen: Specifically, the people take three successive stools and take two little samples on a little stick from each stool, put them on the Hemoccult paper and mail them to the laboratory. The only real difficulty in a place out in rural Minnesota is with the participant who has an outside lavatory. It is very difficult to reach down to get these specimens.

Moderator: You really need a long stick. Dr. Gilbertsen, what do you think the cost of finding each cancer was?

Dr. Gilbertsen: So far, based on these incomplete data, it is very encouraging. We are finding about 10% of these people with fecal blood have cancer and the cost of the diagnostic work-up is something like $600 to $800. That means $60,000 for each cancer found. Most of the cancers are curable, in contrast with the usual experience. It looks like that is going to come out quite favorably. People estimate it may be $15,000 or $20,000 for the usual cost of treatment of people with cancer of the colon and rectum, including supportive, palliative and terminal care. It is very encouraging so far.

Moderator: I think it is one of the most exciting studies around. I think some of us in this audience, who are approaching the age of 30 plus, would not have to have a proctosigmoidoscopic exam, maybe if we did a Hemoccult as described. I think this is a very important thing and may prevent the need for a proctosigmoidoscopic exam. Would you agree with that, Dr. Gilbertsen?

Dr. Gilbertsen: I would like to emphasize that the biggest disadvantage I think of the proctosigmoidoscopic exam is that it costs money. But for physicians, who should be aware of the virtue of the proctosigmoidoscopic exam and presumably the fiscal part would not be very pertinent, it is a tragic shame for any physician who gets a cancer of the rectum and lets it go to an incurable stage. I have regular proctosigmoidoscopic exams and I am sure that most of you do, too.

Moderator: Would those of you who get regular proctosigmoidoscopic examinations please raise your hand? Regular yearly proctosigmoidoscopic exams? We are looking, Dr. Gilbertsen, at about 10% of the audience. I agree with you, Dr. Gilbertsen. In a group of patients followed over 25 years with yearly proctosigmoidoscopic exam and removal of polyps at the cancer detection center only 12 cancers developed; 11 of these were Duke's A. In the same age group, the predicted number of cancers should have been about 70 or 80. If ever there was a statistic that should indicate to us the importance of proctological examinations, that is it.

Dr. DeCosse: I also think that is one of the most compelling bits of circumstantial evidence that adenomas become cancer.

Moderator: Adenomas do become cancer. That is true.

Dr. Goligher, with the stapled anastomosis low down, do you get continence in everybody?

Dr. Goligher: No, with any low anastomosis by whatever technique, within about 4 or 4.5 cm from the anal verge, you are going to have very frequent calls to stool and some incontinence for quite a while. In my experience, some of those patients are only just continent after some months. Then, if they get a bit of diarrhea, they are not completely master of the situation. Some of the people who write about these operations have rather glossed over this aspect of the results. On the other hand, I used to believe that it was virtually impossible for a patient with an anorectal stump of less than 6 cm from the anal verge to regain full continence, and I now know that that opinion is untenable for I have quite a number of patients with anastomoses of 4 to 4.5 cm who have recovered full control.

Moderator: In our department we look at their socks to see how continent they really are. Any patient who has had this much rectum removed does not have the storage area any more. As a result they find that they have very frequent movements and sometimes interpret this as being lack of continence. They have to go rather rapidly because they do not have the storage capacity. For up to three to six months, I have seen this occur but by one year they are usually reasonable.

How about urinary continence, Dr. Goligher? Do they have urinary problems with the low anastomosis? Retention?

Dr. Goligher: No, not any more than with ordinary abdominoperineal excision or anterior resection.

Moderator: Dr. DeCosse, if you did a local excision of a low lesion and it turned out that rather than an A it looked like it was a B, going through the wall of the rectum, would you then go further and do an abdominoperineal?

Dr. DeCosse: It would depend somewhat upon the patient's particular circumstances. The point I was trying to make is this: Here, you are relying very substantially on your pathologist. You are saying, "We can take this out. If it is totally excised, we can watch the patient. If it is not totally excised, then we are obligated to do something more." Again, it depends upon individual circumstances. One might consider a sleeve resection with a posterior approach or an abdominoperineal resection.

Dr. Goligher: In connection with the local treatment of cancers, as Dr. DeCosse mentioned, a very popular way is fulguration. Of course, it is technically much easier than doing a local excision. You may ask, "Why do local excision?" The great advantage of the local excision, if you can get out a disc of rectal wall, is that a good pathologist can examine the specimen and tell you whether you are doing the right thing. If he says, "No, although the original biopsy suggested this was well differentiated, in fact it is not well differentiated," or if he says, "This lesion is right through the wall," then you can change your tactics right away in favor of a rectal excision without waiting for weeks or months to see if the patient gets recurrence.

Miscellaneous

Gastrointestinal Surgical Emergencies in the Newborn

T. Baesl, M.D., R. H. Rich, M.D., K. Okinaga, M.D. and A. S. Leonard, M.D., Ph.D., F.A.C.S.

Objectives

The physician in attendance at delivery should be familiar with ten gastrointestinal surgical emergencies, which may be recognized by 13 danger signals, and which should be corrected whenever possible within the first 72 hours of birth.

Introduction

Although pediatric surgery has developed substantially in the last ten years, infant mortality in the United States is far from ideal. Ten years ago the United States ranked 14th in the world with an infant mortality of 22 in 1,000 live births in children under 1 year of age. Although this has improved somewhat, this figure still can be reduced significantly. Infant mortality varies not only within the United States, but also among cities. Mortality is partially dependent upon prenatal care and delivery mechanics, but it also relates to the ability of the physician in attendance, at the time of delivery or shortly thereafter, to recognize neonatal emergencies. Prematurity, multiple birth defects and severe congenital heart disease predispose to neonatal deaths. Early recognition of defects, prevention of the deterioration phase and the treatment of shock, hypothermia and respiratory distress will decrease infant mortality.

T. Baesl, M.D., R. H. Rich, M.D., and K. Okinaga, M.D., Research Fellows, Department of Surgery and A. S. Leonard, M.D., Ph.D., F.A.C.S., Professor of Surgery; Head, Pediatric Surgery, University of Minnesota Medical School, Minneapolis.

Early recognition of a number of signs and symptoms will alert the physician to congenital anomalies of the gastrointestinal tract. This will allow prompt investigation and accurate diagnosis concurrent with stabilization. The following danger signals should alert the physician to possible gastrointestinal anomalies:

1. Rapid respirations (over 40/min)
2. Difficulty with respirations (retraction, nasal flaring)
3. Cyanosis
4. Excess salivation
5. Abdominal distention
6. Abdominal mass
7. Scaphoid abdomen
8. Bile emesis
9. Failure to pass meconium within 24 hours
10. Inability to void (poor stream or inadequate stream)
11. Seizure
12. Jaundice
13. Lethargy (poor feeding, diminished reflexes, paralysis)

It is important to note that the earlier these anomalies are identified and operated upon, the better the prognosis. Newborns are well hydrated, have good nutritional stores in the form of glycogen, high serum steroid levels, a high level of inherited maternal antibodies and a high threshold for pain. All of these factors are advantages for early surgical correction. Within 72 hours of birth, these factors begin to decay. This delayed deterioration phase is one contributing cause of infant mortality.

It is important to recognize the altered intestinal physiology in neonatal GI emergencies. Ten to fifteen percent of the blood volume may be sequestered in the intestine or abdominal cavity. Gram negative sepsis may develop from gangrene or intestinal perforation. Because of changing metabolic rate and fluid shifts, hypovolemia and shock develop rapidly and may be complicated by hypothermia and metabolic acidosis. All of these factors increase infant mortality.

One must reverse the hypovolemia, acidosis and hypothermia. Hydration of these infants consists of flushing solutions of 0.2% normal saline at 360 cc/M^2 for 45 minutes. Plasma equivalent at 5 cc/lb should be given over a two-hour period as a loading volume. A nasogastric tube is placed for decompression. Fluid losses are replaced with 1/3 normal saline + 20 mEq KCI. Attention must be paid to electrolyte balance, urine output, central venous pressure and other monitoring systems [1]. After resuscitation the infant is now prepared for diagnostic investigation and surgical intervention.

Intestinal Obstruction

One of the most common surgical problems in the newborn period is intestinal obstruction. Polyhydramnios in the mother may offer a prenatal clue to intestinal obstruction. Radioactive absorption studies have demonstrated that amniotic fluid is absorbed and turned over in the intestinal tract several times per day. The higher the obstruction in the GI tract, the more likely the chance of hydramnios.

It is important to recognize in these infants the altered intestinal physiology present. As distention of the bowel wall occurs, venous return becomes compromised. Between 10% and 15% of the infant's blood volume may become trapped in the intestinal tract as a result of decreased absorption from the intestinal lumen, congestion of the bowel wall and transudation of the fluid from the serosa to the peritoneal cavity. Further distention or torsion of the vascular supply may result in infarction of the involved bowel, intestinal perforation and gram negative sepsis.

Intestinal atresias account for a large number of infant small bowel obstruction. Duodenal atresia is caused in the fetus by failure of vacuolization to reestablish a lumen. Jejunal and ileal atresias result from vascular accidents with resultant bowel infarction. These infants present with poor feeding, vomiting of bile, lack of passage of meconium and dehydration. Abdominal distention may or may not be present, depending upon the level of obstruction. Early infusion of plasma and electrolyte solution is mandatory. Nasogastric suction should be instituted early. An abdominal x-ray showing intestinal loops greater than thumb size indicates that an obstruction is present. The gas pattern may differentiate between a high and low obstruction. A barium enema performed with a Foley catheter and 3 cc balloon (10 to 15 cc barium injected) can serve to differentiate between microcolon, malrotation and Hirschsprung's disease.

Once the patient is in good fluid and electrolyte balance, he is taken to the operating room and the atresia repaired. Atresias occur in the ileum, duodenum and jejunum, in that order of frequency. Multiple atresias may be present. For duodenal atresia a duodenojejunostomy bypass is usually performed. It is important to run the bowel to check for intestinal patency. Intestinal webs or the so-called windsock deformity may be present and go unrecognized until the postoperative period when the infant remains obstructed. Annular pancreas and malrotation are other causes of duodenal obstruction. In the jejunum and ileum, atresias are handled by first resecting dilated, bulbous intestinal loops which have poor peristalsis. Then an end-to-end anastomosis to the residual gut is performed. If the baby is in poor condition, a distal mucous fistula and proximal ileostomy or jejunostomy may be utilized. The patient is placed on hyperalimentation and the intestinal tract is reconstructed at a later date [2-4].

Duplication of the intestinal tract occurs because of a double vacuolization process and must be recognized as distinct from Meckel's diverticulum or other diverticula. This duplication may result in partial or complete intestinal obstruction, perforation of the duplicated segment or bleeding. It is important to recognize duplication because in the formation of the duplicated intestine, a common blood supply resides in the intestinal wall between the duplicated segments. One must excise the entire area of duplication because of the common blood supply. Treatment of this defect is simple resection, and the diagnosis is usually made by contrast x-ray examination.

Meconium Ileus

Meconium ileus occurs because of a basic defect in the mucopolysaccharide secretion from the pancreas and is part of the mucoviscidosis syndrome. The intestinal tract is obstructed usually in the distal ileum due to inspissation of the intestinal contents. The respiratory tract is also involved with inspissated secretions and indeed may be the most important prognostic factor in these infants. Diagnosis is suspected by distention and bile emesis with a dilated gas pattern throughout the entire intestine up to the colon. Barium enema demonstrates a microcolon with inspissated meconium pellets in the colon and ileum. The diagnosis is confirmed by sweat chlorides which are greater than 50 mEq/L. Gastrographin with 10% acetylcysteine can sometimes relieve the intestinal obstruction by delivering a hyperosmotic load to the intestine and thus to loosen the secretions. Operative intervention requires resection of the distal ileum. Both limbs of the intestine must be irrigated with acetylcysteine to remove inspissated secretions. The intestine can be reconstituted with an end-to-end anastomosis.

If the baby is in poor condition, an ileostomy and mucous fistula may be created and final reconstruction performed at a later date. Whether the obstruction is relieved operatively or nonoperatively, pancreatic enzyme supplementation must be used to prevent future inspissation. In the postoperative period, strict attention must be paid to the potential respiratory problems. Humidification, bronchopulmonary drainage and Mucomyst should be used to prevent atelectasis and pneumonia [5,6].

Imperforate Anus

The diagnosis and treatment of imperforate anus is dependent upon understanding the embryology and anatomy of the distal end of the GI tract. Embryologically, the cloacal membrane divides the allantosis from the hind gut. The membrane gradually migrates to the anal area. If progress stops anywhere along its developmental pathway, a high or low imperforate anus occurs. The most complete form of imperforate anus is that of exstrophy of the cloaca where the urogenital sinus and the rectum nerves separate. One then has an imperforate anus, exstrophy of the bladder, omphalocele, meningomyelocele and an epispadius.

The next level of complexity is that of a high imperforate anus. This occurs above the puborectalis sling [7]. Eighty percent of high imperforate anus patients have fistulas to the urogenital sinus area. In the male, this is the prostatic urethra and, in the female, the distal third of the vagina. High fistulas must be recognized because the puborectalis sling is the rectal sphincter mechanism that will produce continence after repair. Initially, a colostomy is performed. At approximately 20 to 25 lb, or 2 years of age, the definitive repair is done. This can be through an abdominal, sacral or perineal approach. The colon is brought through the puborectalis sling. These infants do not have an internal sphincter so they will be unable to differentiate between gas and liquid stool during periods of diarrhea. In most instances, fair bowel habits can be established. It is important to remember that no imperforate anus should be repaired unless one is absolutely familiar with the anatomical variation that is present.

In the low imperforate anus the fistula enters below the puborectalis sling. The fistula enters the posterior vagina at the level of the fourchette in the female. In the male, the fistula can enter behind the scrotum at the skin level. These can be repaired immediately at birth with good later continence. Stenosis of the rectum requires simple dilatation [8]. There is a high association between imperforate anus and urinary tract anomalies. The anatomy of the urinary tract should be investigated before these infants are discharged from the hospital.

Malrotation

The diagnosis of malrotation of the intestinal tract may be suspected from intermittent mild episodes of regurgitation of bile-stained emesis and malabsorption. In the most severe form of volvulus, one sees bile emesis, abdominal distention and progressive shock from gram negative sepsis due to infarction of the intestines. Malrotation must be differentiated from upper intestinal obstruction due to annular pancreas and duodenal atresia or stenosis. Barium enema may demonstrate the cecum in the right upper quadrant or out of position, suggesting malrotation. Early recognition and operative intervention is important to prevent volvulus and resultant intestinal infarction.

In the sixth to eighth week of embryologic development the intestines move outside the celomic cavity. The intestines gradually return, rotating in a counterclockwise direction until the large bowel adheses in the ascending and descending positions. Failure of rotation results in malrotation with ensuing obstruction and possible volvulus. The lengthened mesentery is a factor predisposing to volvulus. In the repair of this condition, one must not only derotate the intestine, but also cut the adhesive bands which have formed as attempts to fix the intestine in a retroperitoneal position. An appendectomy should also be performed. These adhesions usually cross the duodenum, creating a fulcrum mechanism around which the lengthened mesentery can twist into a volvulus. If volvulus occurs, infarction in the distribution of the superior mesenteric artery follows with loss of the intestine from the ligament of Treitz to the midtransverse colon. In this situation, the infant is hypoxic, acidotic and in shock. Rapid fluid replacement, antibiotics and prompt surgical intervention are essential. After surgery, prolonged hyperalimentation is necessary until intestinal adaptation can occur [9].

Omphalocele and Gastroschisis

Omphalocele is a condition where the intestines remain outside the omphalomesenteric pathway and do not return to the abdomen. It usually has a membraneous covering over the defect, and the umbilical cord protrudes from the center of this membraneous covering.

Gastroschisis results from a somatic defect of the abdominal wall. The defect is usually superior and lateral to the umbilicus. A normal umbilicus is present. The intestinal contents protrude through the defect. There is no membraneous covering, and thus the intestines are bathed in amniotic fluid for the entire period in utero. Both conditions predispose the infant to hypothermia, hypovolemia and sepsis because the intestines are outside the celomic cavity and present a large exposed surface area.

These defects are obvious at birth. It is imperative that the attending physician institute immediate care. Nasogastric intubation is performed because these infants frequently have partial or complete intestinal obstruction. Saline dressings are applied to prevent drying of the membrane or the exposed intestines and to help decrease heat and fluid losses. These infants should be kept in a warm environment. Intravenous fluid replacement is begun at birth. Combination antibiotics are initiated because of the risk of infection. Prior to surgical intervention, strict adherence to fluid replacement, maintenance of normothermia and aseptic techniques will significantly increase survival. If the omphalocele is small, it can be repaired primarily as can gastroschisis. In all instances these defects are accompanied by malrotation, which must also be corrected. If the defect is large, a ventral abdominal hernia is formed by mobilizing skin and closing it over the intestine. Thus the intestines can adapt gradually to the celomic cavity. The hernia is repaired at a later date. A gastrostomy is used in these infants until they can take fluids orally.

In gastroschisis, where the intestine is coated with an exudate, oral feeding may take a month or two and hyperalimentation is required during this period. If the omphalocele or gastroschisis is very large, precluding skin coverage, a Silastic covering can be used to protect the intestines from the environment. This Silastic bag, or chimney, is then gradually reduced in size until the abdominal cavity completely accepts the intestines. In our institution, we have backed the Silastic with Marlex mesh which seems to stimulate peritoneal growth across the defect. When the apparatus is removed, no immediate surgery is necessary because the defect is covered. Several months later, the ventral hernia is closed.

One must not be too anxious to return the intestinal contents to the abdomen because done prematurely this causes increased abdominal pressure that can compromise venous return to the heart and decrease pulmonary function by interfering with diaphragmatic excursion. Clinical judgment plays a large part in deciding on the timing and type of repair used for omphalocele and gastroschisis.

Hirschsprung's Disease

Hirschsprung's disease results from an absence of ganglion cells in the parasympathetic plexus in the distal colon and rectum. In rare instances, the absence of ganglion cells may include the entire bowel. Embryologically, the parasympathetic innervation to the intestines develops from mouth to the anus. As a consequence, there are rarely skip lesions in Hirschsprung's disease. The absence of innervation causes a physiologic obstruction resulting from decreased peristaltic activity in the segment with the neurogenic defect. Dilatation of the colon above this region results from partial or complete obstruction. In many instances this progresses to enterocolitis which is the complication usually causing infant mortality in this disease. It is rare that infants die of diarrhea alone, but severe enterocolitis results in gram negative sepsis, shock and death. Thus, Hirschsprung's disease should be suspected if diarrhea does not resolve on the usual treatment measures.

The barium enema usually suggests the diagnosis and a rectal biopsy is carried out. Ganglion cells are characteristically absent in the submucosa and muscular layers. Motility studies also aid in the evaluation. Once the diagnosis is made, a colostomy is performed. A pull-through procedure is performed when the patient reaches 20 to 25 lb. In our institution, the Soave pull-through procedure is performed. The site of the colostomy is usually in the area of the transverse colon, but it is imperative to obtain a biopsy of the colon at the site of the planned colostomy to insure that the colon has normal innervation.

In the Soave pull-through procedure, the mucosa is stripped off the muscular layer of the colon. The upper normal colon is then placed in the cored-out distal rectum. In this manner one does not interfere with the nervi erigentes in the sacrum and therefore does not risk impotence.

It is also important to recognize pseudo-Hirschsprung's disease, which may occur in infants and small children with psychologic dietary problems. In these infants rectal biopsy is diagnostic because they have normal ganglion cells. They do have a large colon with impacted feces. Treatment consists of day-to-day regimens of cold juice in the morning. This sets up a gastric colic reflex and then the patient is placed on the toilet. If the patient does not have a bowel movement, an enema is given. This daily pattern keeps the rectal vault clean and gradually the children learn to correct their bowel habits. A stool softener is also added to this regimen. This approach has been uniformly successful in our hands. One must warn the parents never to punish these children for poor bowel function, for this is one of the basic reasons that the condition occurs [10,11].

Tracheoesophageal Fistulas

Early recognition of tracheoesophageal fistulas and esophageal atresia is a challenge to the practitioner. Signs suggestive of tracheoesophageal fistula include excessive salivation, regurgitation of food and gaseous abdominal distention with crying, secondary to forceful filling of the stomach with air through the fistula between the trachea and the stomach. Frequent pneumonia may also be a sign of tracheoesophageal fistula (H-type).

These infants should not be ventilated with positive pressure. This will result in gastric distention and aspiration of gastric contents into the lung, causing respiratory impairment secondary to distention of the abdomen and aspiration pneumonia. The resultant pneumonia, atelectasis and sepsis can lead to rapid deterioration. The diagnosis is made by a PA and lateral x-ray. The air in the upper pouch may be seen on lateral view and gives an early clue to the presence of this anomaly. A small volume of contrast, 0.5 cc of either barium or gastrographin can be placed in the upper pouch and the PA and lateral x-ray taken in order to establish its length. If the pouch extends to T-3 or T-4, a primary repair usually can be accomplished. The other important diagnostic measure is to determine the site of the aortic arch. The fistula is usually on the side opposite the aortic arch. If one is in doubt, an echocardiogram may be performed. It also helps to determine the air pattern. If there is a pouch above and no air in the gastrointestinal tract, then the patient has atresia of the esophagus and a cervical esophagostomy and gastrostomy must be performed rather than an attempt at primary repair. Occasionally, bougienage will gain enough length for a primary repair.

Prior to operation, strict attention should be paid to pulmonary problems. They should be kept at a 45° angle to decrease the incidence of aspiration of gastric acid. A tube should be placed via the nose into the pouch for decompression. Wide spectrum antibiotic protection should be instituted for the possibility of aspiration pneumonia. The decision for operation depends upon the infant's size, his general condition, whether or not he is infected and acidotic. Prematurity, acidosis, hypothermia, shock and the presence of additional severe congenital anomalies would lead one to defer correction of this condition until a more stable situation can be attained. A gastrostomy alone may be performed under these circumstances. If respiratory distress is present, ligation of the fistula may be necessary because the lungs cannot be ventilated with a fistula present.

The most common type of tracheoesophageal fistula is the so-called C-type (Gross) with the upper pouch blind and the esophagus entering into the trachea near the bifurcation. This type is present in 80% of patients. When the infant is in good condition and the esophagus is long enough to permit a primary repair, the esophagus is approached through a retropleural dissection. The tracheoesophageal fistula is divided. The esophagus is mobilized to minimize tension on the anastomosis. A mucosa-to-mucosa anastomosis is performed. The use of the retropleural approach has significantly decreased mortality from this procedure. A gastrostomy is performed during the primary operation.

Postoperatively, these infants may require intermittent esophageal dilatation. When the esophagus precludes primary repair, bougienage or magnets have occasionally been successful in approximating the proximal and distal segments. In most cases, however, esophageal reconstruction will require interposed segments of intestine by staged reconstruction. In the first stage, a gastrostomy is placed, the tracheoesophageal fistula is divided and a cervical esophagostomy is created. In the second phase, a Roux-en-Y loop of jejunum is fashioned, placed in the subcutaneous presternal position and anastomosed either primarily or at a later date to the cervical esophagus. After an adequate swallowing mechanism has been established, the Roux-en-Y limb is connected to the stomach. The loop can be placed in the substernal position at 5 to 6 years of age. We prefer jejunum rather than colon because of better peristalsis, lack of later dilatation and the ease of the procedure.

The H-type tracheoesophageal fistula is the most uncommon and the most difficult to diagnose. It is usually identified after repeated episodes of pneumonia and respiratory distress. Diagnosis is by cine-esophagram. Surgical correction is generally through a cervical incision and consists in simple division.

Diaphragmatic Hernia

Congenital diaphragmatic hernia occurs with a frequency of 1 in 2,200 live births. Despite prompt surgical correction, where respiratory distress is persistent, the mortality may be as high as 75%. It was originally believed that survival was associated with correction of the diaphragmatic defect, return of the abdominal viscus to the celomic cavity and reexpansion of the compressed lung. This has proven not to be the case. We now know that the lungs are not simply atelectatic, but are hypoplastic as well. The total lung volume, lung weight and the ratio of lung weight to total body weight are all reduced. These reductions are more striking in the ipsilateral lung, but are also present in the contralateral lung.

It has been shown that the total number of small bronchi and alveolar units are decreased. In addition, the branching pattern of the pulmonary vascular tree is abnormal. The arteries are smaller than appropriate for the age of the child and smooth muscle is found in smaller than normal vessels. Hemodynamically, the one consistent finding in these infants is that they all have pulmonary hypertension. Accompanying the pulmonary hypertension is bidirectional shunting with a primary right-to-left shunt. This situation is akin to that found in infants with persistent fetal circulation. It is the combined effect of the alveolar hypoplasia and pulmonary hypertension that results in such high infant mortality.

The defect in congenital diaphragmatic hernia is secondary to failure to close the pleuroperitoneal canal, thus leaving communication between the pleural and peritoneal cavities. This defect occurs 80% of the time through the left diaphragm in the posterior lateral foramen of Bochdalek. The pleuroperitoneal canal normally closes during the sixth week of intrauterine life. During normal development, the intestines return to the abdominal cavity after undergoing extra celomic rotation in the tenth week of fetal life. At this time, if the pleuroperitoneal canal is still patent, an opportunity is present for potential herniation of the newly returned viscus into the thoracic cavity. Herniation causes compression of the ipsilateral lung, mediastinal shift and consequent compression of the contralateral lung. The degree of herniation and the precise time at which actual herniation occurs are the two determinants of the degree of hypoplasia. The earlier herniation occurs, the more serious is the resultant pulmonary hyperplasia.

At birth, infants with diaphragmatic hernia present with respiratory distress, cyanosis and a scaphoid abdomen. A simple chest x-ray demonstrates intestine in the thoracic cavity. After recognition of the defect, prompt surgical correction is necessary because of the danger of infarction of the herniated viscus. A nasogastric tube should always be placed to decompress the stomach, potentially increasing the amount of thoracic cavity available for expansion of the lung and decreasing the chance of intestinal infarction.

Positive pressure ventilation through the mouth should be avoided because of the resultant dilatation of the stomach. Endotracheal intubation is usually required for respiratory distress. One must avoid positive pressure as much as possible because the lungs are hypoplastic and are predisposed to develop pneumothorax. Surgery is carried out through an abdominal approach. The hernia is reduced, allowing the hypoplastic lung to expand. Creation of a ventral abdominal hernia is usually necessary because the celomic cavity is not completely developed and is usually inadequate to accept the herniated viscus without undue intra-abdominal pressure. One should also look for evidence of associated malrotation.

Postoperatively, these infants require careful management of respiratory dynamics. As was mentioned earlier, these infants frequently have pulmonary hypertension, with resultant bidirectional shunting and poor pulmonary perfusion. In the survivors this pulmonary hypertension gradually resolves over the course of the next several weeks.

In the laboratory, we are investigating the possibility of pharmacological manipulation of the pulmonary vasculature in an attempt to increase pulmonary blood flow and oxygenation of the infant. Altering the hemodynamics can buy time to allow the increased muscularity of the small pulmonary vessels to regress, thus decreasing vascular resistance. Occasionally, membrane oxygenator support will be necessary.

Neonatal Necrotizing Enterocolitis

Neonatal necrotizing enterocolitis is a disease unique to the newborn. It is characterized by diffuse intestinal necrosis, accompanied by sepsis, jaundice, disseminated intravascular coagulation and frequently death. Neonatal necrotizing enterocolitis is a disease occurring with increasing frequency in newborn intensive care units nationally. The explanation for this is the vastly improved success rate of the neonatologist in resuscitation of critically ill patients. Risk factors for development of necrotizing enterocolitis include (1) prematurity with a birth weight to less than 1,500 gm, (2) respiratory distress syndrome and (3) neonatal and perinatal distress syndromes, including toxemic pregnancy or premature rupture of the maternal membranes.

Ninety percent of these infants are between 1 and 10 days old. Characteristically, they have passed a normal meconium stool and subsequently develop progressive abdominal distention. Physical examination and abdominal x-rays are the cornerstone of diagnosis. Physical examination reveals abdominal distention and bloody diarrhea in 25% of the cases. Localized abdominal tenderness may be present.

Passage of a nasogastric tube will reveal retained gastric secretions and, later in the course of the disease, bile. X-ray examination usually shows dilated loops of bowel consistent with adynamic ileus. Pneumotosis intestinalis is present in 75% of the cases and is considered pathognomonic. Free intestinal air and portal vein air are late signs of the disease. Sepsis, jaundice or disseminated intravascular coagulation may develop at any time. Blood cultures are positive for intestinal organisms in between 20% and 70% of the cases.

With aggressive medical management, surgery may be avoided in a substantial number of cases. This requires careful reevaluation of the infant every six hours with physical examination and abdominal x-rays. Therapeutically, a nasogastric tube is placed, intravenous fluids are started and intravenous antibiotics (ampicillin and gentamicin) are administered. Some authors advocate the instillation of antibiotics down the nasogastric tube to help sterilize the gastrointestinal tract. Since the nutritional support of these infants is paramount, peripheral or central hyperalimentation should be instituted.

Indications for surgical intervention include persistent shock, hypothermia, acidosis, resistant disseminated intravascular coagulation and a rising potassium. On physical examination, a localized mass or cellulitis of the abdominal wall may be present. X-rays demonstrating pneumoperitoneum or localized distended loops of bowel with pneumotosis, ascites and portal vein gas lead one toward a surgical approach. The operative approach consists of careful abdominal exploration, looking for perforation and abscess formation. The ileum and ascending colon are the most frequently involved areas. The pathologic findings include a distended, friable, hemorrhagic and sometimes necrotic bowel. The mucosa is frequently completely ulcerated. Some vascular engorgement is usually present. Intestinal perforation may be seen in areas of frank necrosis. Resection of all nonviable intestine, debridement of exudative material and exteriorization of the divided intestine are essential. Reconstruction of the intestine may be performed when the infant has completely recovered. At that time, further bowel resection may be necessary because of stricture formation. Using this combined medical and surgical approach, infant survival has been significantly increased [12,13].

Summary

One must pay strict attention to the signs and symptoms that occur at birth to recognize the types of congenital anomalies that exist in the gastrointestinal tract. These various problems result in both cardiac and respiratory compromise. Immediate institution of gastrointestinal drainage by nasogastric tubes is important in all instances. The x-ray pattern is usually helpful especially contrast study of the colon demonstrating malrotation, microcolon or Hirschsprung's disease.

If one recognizes these conditions early, institutes proper fluid and electrolyte management and prepares for early surgical intervention, the infant mortality should be significantly reduced. It is also incumbent upon the physician to evaluate other systems for congenital anomalies before the infant leaves the hospital.

References

1. Weintraub, W.H., Cuderman, B.S., Hunt, C.E. et al: Computer monitoring of cardiodynamics in the newborn. J. Ped. Surg. 6:372-380, 1971.
2. Moore, K.: The Developing Human Clinically Oriented Embryology. Philadelphia:W.B. Saunders Company, 1973, pp. 175-196.
3. Benson, C.D. and Lloyd, R.: *In* Mustard, W.: Pediatric Surgery. Chicago:Year Book Medical Publishers, 1969, pp. 841-851.
4. Raffensberger, J., Seeler, R. and Moncada, R.: The Acute Abdomen of Infancy and Childhood. Philadelphia:J.B. Lippincott Company, 1970, pp. 1-20.

5. Mustard, W., Ravitch, M. et al: Pediatric Surgery. Chicago:Year Book Medical Publishers, 1969, pp. 851-859.
6. Raffensberger, J., Seeler, R. and Moncada, R.: The Acute Abdomen of Infancy and Childhood. Philadelphia:J.B. Lippincott Company, 1970, pp. 1-20.
7. Santulli, T.: *In* Mustard, W.: Pediatric Surgery. Chicago:Year Book Medical Publishers, 1969, pp. 983-1007.
8. Stevens, F.D. and Smith, E.D.: Ano-Rectal Malformations in Children. Chicago:Year Book Medical Publishers, 1971.
9. Snyder, W. and Chaffin, L.: *In* Mustard, W.: Pediatric Surgery. Chicago:Year Book Medical Publishers, 1969, pp. 808-817.
10. Sieber, W. and Soave, F.: Hirschsprung's Disease in Current Problems of Surgery. Chicago:Year Book Medical Publishers, 1978, vol. XV, No. 6.
11. Schnaufer, L.: *In* Hendren, W.H. (ed.): Surgical Clinics of North America. Philadelphia:W.B. Saunders Company, 1976, vol. 56, pp. 349-360.
12. Touloukian, R.: *In* Hendren, W.H. (ed.): Surgical Clinics of North America. Philadelphia:W.B. Saunders Company, 1976, vol. 56, pp. 281-298.
13. Roback, S.A., Foker, J., Frantz, I.F. et al: Necrotizing enterocolitis. Arch. Surg. 109:314-319, 1974.

Self-Evaluation Quiz

1. How did the United States rank in 1968 among other nations re infant mortality?
   a) 5th
   b) 11th
   c) 14th
   d) 18th
2. To decrease infant mortality, one must quickly recognize and treat:
   a) Shock only
   b) Hypothermia only
   c) Shock, glucosuria and respiratory distress
   d) Respiratory distress, hypothermia and shock
3. Danger signals that alert one to GI anomalies include:
   a) Respiration rate over 30/min
   b) Hyperactivity and overfeeding
   c) Nasal flaring
   d) Failure to pass meconium within 24 hours
4. A common surgical problem during the newborn period is
   a) Polyhydramnios
   b) Intestinal obstruction except duodenal atresias

c) Intestinal obstruction including atresias
d) Monopulmonary distress

5. Meconium ileus is due to a:
   a) Basic defect in mucopolysaccharide synthesis
   b) Basic defect in mucopolysaccharide secretion from the liver
   c) Twisted colonic segment
   d) Basic defect in mucopolysaccharide secretion from the pancreas
6. What percentage of patients with high imperforate anus have fistulas to the urogenital sinus region?
   a) 25%
   b) 60%
   c) 80%
   d) 92%
7. Repair of imperforate anus is done at:
   a) ½ year of age
   b) 1 year of age
   c) 2 years of age
   d) 3 years of age
8. Intermittent mild regurgitation of bile-stained emesis and malabsorption indicate:
   a) Malrotation of the intestinal tract
   b) Imperforate anus
   c) Meconium ileus
   d) Gastroschisis

Answers on page 721.

Gastrointestinal Emergencies in Childhood

John E. Foker, M.D., Ph.D.

Objectives

Many different kinds of gastrointestinal emergencies can occur in children. Only a few will be discussed in this paper. They were chosen because new information on pathophysiology, diagnostic measures or treatment has arisen that will be helpful in the management of these problems. Emphasis will be placed on the subject of rectal bleeding in childhood because it differs in causes, significance and treatment from the same problem in adults.

Introduction

Many different kinds of gastrointestinal emergencies can occur in children. There are too many to be discussed in a satisfactory way in a short presentation. Therefore, no effort will be made to be comprehensive and only a few topics will be selected for comment. These will be principally in areas where new information or techniques have arisen that may be helpful. The principal emphasis will be placed on the subject of rectal bleeding in childhood. This common problem differs from adult rectal bleeding in causes, significance and, consequently, in treatment.

The Acute Abdomen

A discussion of acute gastrointestinal problems must begin with the acute abdomen. The incomplete list presented includes

John E. Foker, M.D., Ph.D., Assistant Professor of Surgery, Department of Surgery, University of Minnesota Medical School, Minneapolis.

the common gastrointestinal causes of an acute abdomen with or without peritonitis in childhood (Fig. 1). There have been advances made in the understanding and treatment, both by antibiotics and surgery, of peritonitis; these will be presented elsewhere in this volume. Intussusception, too, will be the subject of an individual presentation. Only primary peritonitis and Yersinia enterocolitis will be discussed here.

Primary peritonitis can be a difficult diagnosis to make, short of laparotomy [1], but it should be suspected in children who have no apparent cause, such as a ruptured appendix, for peritonitis. In younger children it occurs more frequently in girls. Children with renal problems such as the nephrotic syndrome, or with liver disease or prior splenectomy are particularly susceptible. For some of these children, laparotomy would have significant risk. The diagnosis can be made, however, by a peritoneal tap. The presence of a single, nonenteric organism in the peritoneal fluid can avert a laparotomy. If pneumococci, streptococci or *H. influenza* is the organism present, the best treatment is appropriate antibiotics, fluid maintenance, nasogastric suction and close observation.

Yersinia enterocolitis has been receiving attention recently [2]. The incidence and role of this gram-negative organism as a cause of terminal ileitis are unknown at present. When exploration of a child's abdomen for presumed appendicitis reveals a normal appendix, ileal inflammation without fat wrapping and large mesenteric nodes, culture of these nodes or later culture of the stool may reveal *Yersinia enterocolitica* and

Acute Abdomen / Peritonitis

Appendicitis
Unknown origin
Meckel's diverticulitis
Intussusception
Mesenteric adenitis
Primary peritonitis
Yersinia enterocolitis
Volvulus
Strangulated hernia

FIG. 1. Acute gastrointestinal problems.

avoid the more ominous diagnosis of Crohn's disease. Simple antibiotic therapy, if necessary, should clear the enterocolitis.

Complex Gastrointestinal Problems

There is a series of complex primary gastrointestinal diseases which can present as emergencies in a variety of ways. Bleeding, obstruction, the appearance of bowel necrosis and toxic megacolon are among the complex gastrointestinal emergencies caused by ulcerative colitis, Crohn's disease, eosinophilic gastroenteritis and pseudomembranous colitis (Fig. 2). These problems, however, are more similar than dissimilar to those seen in adults and will not be discussed further.

In addition to being a site of primary inflammatory disease, the gastrointestinal tract is a vulnerable target for a variety of insults. The mechanisms involved in producing a secondary enterocolitis are not always clear, but certainly splanchnic vascular reactivity, primarily vasospasm, plays an important part in making the gastrointestinal tract a common site of difficulties following stress. Pheochromocytoma, hemolytic-uremic syndrome, post cardiopulmonary bypass and post resection of aortic coarctation are all examples of conditions that may provoke acute gastrointestinal problems secondary to periods of

Complex Problems

Primary Enterocolitis
- Ulcerative colitis
- Granulomatous disease
- Eosinophilic gastroenteritis
- Pseudomembranous (antibiotic therapy)

Secondary Enterocolitis
- Pheochromocytoma
- Hemolytic-uremic syndrome
- Post cardiopulmonary bypass
- Post repair of aortic coarctation
- Cancer chemotherapy
- Immunosuppression
- Cyclic neutropenia

FIG. 2. Acute gastrointestinal problems.

prolonged splanchnic vasoconstriction (Fig. 2). This may result from high circulating levels of catecholamines or be secondary to hypotension and low perfusion. Complications include bleeding, bowel necrosis and perforation.

An important consequence of ischemia is loss of the intestinal mucosa in the areas affected. Continuing ischemia leads to full thickness necrosis and perforation. A suggestion that such a mechanism is operating under these circumstances was seen in a patient who began passing what appeared to be large amounts of blood per rectum two days following open heart surgery. A smear of the material passed revealed sheets of intestinal mucosa cells with very few red cells. This identified the problem as a diffuse intestinal insult with mucosal slough rather than bleeding. Because of this information the bowel was placed at rest for ten days with nasogastric suction, and antibiotics were given to cover the intestinal flora that were presumably passing through the wall of the denuded areas. A satisfactory recovery followed.

An even more complex group of gastrointestinal problems has resulted from the increasing success in use of cancer chemotherapy and transplant immunosuppression (Fig. 3) [3]. The challenge of this group of problems is readily apparent (Fig. 4). More than half of the children receiving chemotherapy will have significant vomiting and abdominal pain at some time during the course of treatment. At least 10% of these children have what appears to be melena. The numbers vary greatly depending upon the agents used and the dose and duration of therapy. Despite these symptoms, few children have problems that would benefit by surgery. In fact, these patients are usually anemic, have low platelet counts, a coagulation system in

Enterocolitis
Abdominal abscess
Perirectal abscess
Intestinal obstruction
"Peptic" ulceration
Small bowel perforation
Cecal ulceration
Pancreatitis

FIG. 3. Consequences of chemotherapy.

disarray and liver malfunction. The risk of operation can be great.

A variety of surgical problems do occur, however, among the most common gastrointestinal complications reported (Fig. 3). Localized gangrene of the bowel seems to be the common denominator and if perforation occurs, peritonitis or abscess formation can result. Bowel obstruction can be another consequence of this process. Ulcers with bleeding seem to result from the patchy areas of necrosis. For reasons that are not entirely clear, the area of the intestine most susceptible seems to be in the region of the distal ileum and cecum. Cecal ulcers with either significant bleeding or perforation have been found in these patients.

The pathological mechanism again appears to be a loss of an effective mucosal barrier (Fig. 4). The antiproliferative effect of the chemotherapeutic or immunosuppressive agents on the rapidly dividing mucosal cells seems to be a major component of the problem. In addition, these agents suppress the availability of competent lymphocytes and neutrophils to help in maintaining a functional mucosal barrier. Evidence that the leukocytes are important in cleaning up the bacteria which penetrate the mucosal layer comes from immunodeficient patients. For example, cyclic neutropenic patients have developed severe localized enterocolitis with spontaneous perforation [4]. Because these patients may have multiple problems,

Loss of Effective Mucosal Barrier

Secondary to antiproliferative effect on dividing mucosal cells
Absence of immune cells
Prolonged vasoconstriction

Invasion of Bowel Wall

Bacterial, fungal, viral

Result

Erosion, necrosis, perforation

FIG. 4. Pathological mechanisms following chemotherapy.

stress may add a component of splanchnic vasoconstriction which, in turn, contributes to the damage.

With the cellular barrier of the intestinal tract compromised, invasion of bacteria or fungi can increase the damage. This presumably starts a vicious cycle of localized areas of sepsis within the bowel wall. Even viruses may contribute to the damage. In several transplant patients who developed cecal and other gastrointestinal ulcers, inclusion bodies typical of cytomegalovirus have been found in biopsies of the ulcers. This is a very intriguing finding, but the role of the activation of viruses in the production of gastrointestinal problems is unknown.

A plausible, but speculative discussion of the mechanisms involved is easily made, but the diagnosis of surgical versus nonsurgical conditions in these patients can be quite difficult. The most common presenting problem is a child with severe, diffuse abdominal pain, ileus and the passage of guaiac-positive material from the rectum. Because the majority of these patients have an enterocolitis, the question is which ones have a complication that would benefit from surgical intervention. Many of the usual signs, symptoms and laboratory results are altered in these patients. The value of a white blood cell count in a child made severely neutropenic by chemotherapy is negligble. Certain studies remain helpful; the presence of free air on abdominal x-ray indicates perforation has occurred. A peritoneal tap is often a helpful diagnostic measure. The presence of bowel flora in a smear of a spun sample of peritoneal fluid indicates that perforation has taken place and that the risk of surgery may be justified. If only white blood cells are seen, the problem is more likely to be uncomplicated enterocolitis. In a few patients who are actively bleeding from the rectum, arteriography may be helpful as it has been in the diagnosis of bleeding cecal ulcers.

Rectal Bleeding in Childhood

When significant rectal bleeding is the only major gastrointestinal symptom, there are a number of possibilities (Fig. 5) [5]. This list omits two of the most common causes of rectal bleeding in childhood — anal fissure and intussusception. Anal fissures typically add only a milliliter or two of bright red blood to the outside of a passed stool. The bleeding of intussuscep-

Polyps
Meckel's diverticulum
Peptic ulcers
Esophageal varices
Hemangiomas
Intestinal ulcers
Angioosteohypertrophy

FIG. 5. Significant rectal bleeding as the major symptom.

tion, although a common cause of this problem, is usually not the only symptom and blood is usually found mixed with ample quantities of mucus to form the typical currant-jelly stool. Only two of the more common causes of significant rectal bleeding in childhood will be discussed: Meckel's diverticulum and colonic polyps.

Meckel's diverticulum is a remnant of the yolk sac duct or vitelline duct. This vestige of the communication between embryonic midgut and the yolk sac is easily remembered as being present in about 2% of the people, about 2 inches long (although lengths of 1 to 100 cm have been described) and located about 2 feet from the ileal cecal valve. The incidence of problems arising from this diverticulum is unknown but it has been suggested the majority cause trouble [6]. A variety of problems may occur: bleeding, diverticulitis or obstruction. Obstruction develops in several ways: (a) a fibrous cord may remain attached from the umbilicus to the tip of the diverticulum and act as a pivot point for a volvulus; (b) the diverticulum may act as a lead point for an intussusception; (c) a fibrous remnant of a vitelline artery may act as a constricting band if a loop of bowel herniates beneath it; (d) inflammation of the diverticulum may also produce obstructive signs; (e) the diverticulum may become incarcerated in an inguinal hernia (Littre's hernia). Another uncommon clinical symptom among this constellation of problems is a draining umbilical sinus. This occurs when the vitelline duct remains open, but this is rarely an emergency situation.

The incidence of complications of Meckel's diverticulum shown in Figure 6 is compiled from two series in the literature [6, 7]. Several points should be noted. Hemorrhage is the most common single complication of Meckel's diverticulum.

	Number	Deaths
Hemorrhage	84	1
Intestinal obstruction		
Intussusception	24	0
Bands and torsion	23	9
Littre's hernia	2	0
Diverticulitis		
Without perforation	30	0
With perforation	10	2
	193	12 (6%)

FIG. 6. Complications of Meckel's diverticulum.

It is typically intermittent in occurrence with several months often elapsing between episodes of bleeding. The bleeding is often quite massive, although exsanguination is unusual. Most of the mortality from a complicated Meckel's diverticulum comes from peritonitis, bowel necrosis and/or perforation. The mortality from these complications is high.

The problems of bleeding and diverticulitis are usually the consequence of ectopic gastric tissue within the diverticulum. In one representative series, gastric mucosa was found in only about half the specimens, but was present in all but one case in which rectal bleeding was the major symptom (Fig. 7) [7]. Acid secretion by the gastric mucosa results in ulcers in the adjacent normal small intestinal mucosa. Because the intestinal contents are alkaline, the secretion of the ectopic mucosa is quickly

Tissue	Number	Hemorrhage
Gastric	44	34
Gastric and pancreatic	5	3
Pancreatic	2	–
Duodenal	1	–
Ileum	45	1
	97	38

FIG. 7. Ectopic mucosa in Meckel's diverticulum. From Benson [7].

neutralized and the ulcers are usually found close to the gastric mucosa. Other ectopic tissue including pancreatic and duodenal mucosa is also occasionally found in a Meckel's diverticulum.

The diagnosis of a Meckel's diverticulum as the source of rectal bleeding is often difficult to make preoperatively. Neither an upper gastrointestinal series nor a barium enema is useful. Angiography is of help only at the time of active bleeding and is relatively difficult to do in a small child. But because of the likelihood that ectopic gastric mucosa is present, an additional diagnostic measure exists. Technetium (in the form of sodium pertechnetate) is concentrated by gastric mucosal cells. The isotope, Technetium 99m, has been used to identify ectopic gastric mucosa by radioisotope scan. Technetium scanning appears to be the best method of diagnosing a bleeding Meckel's diverticulum preoperatively, whether or not it is actively bleeding at the time of study, and appears to be effective about 50% to 75% of the time [8, 9]. This is a disappointingly low figure; the reasons for failure are not clear, but the scan is easy to do and the yield is better than any other preoperative diagnostic technique. It can be quite helpful in the preoperative assessment and surgical planning for the problem of rectal bleeding.

Colon polyps are probably the most common cause of rectal bleeding with an identifiable source in childhood. The vast majority of these polyps are of the juvenile or retention type (Fig. 8) [10]. Juvenile polyps are thought by some to be inflammatory in origin. Histologically they are quite distinct from the adenomatous polyps common in adults. Marked glandular dilatation, edematous and inflamed stroma and normal appearing, if often denuded, epithelial covering are all characteristic of the juvenile polyp.

Bright red, intermittent rectal bleeding is the hallmark of symptomatic juvenile polyps [11]. Typically, the bleeding is not severe and less than 10% of the patients will have a hemoglobin below 10 gm%. Colicky pain, of short duration and variable intensity, seems to be a relatively common phenomenon. Various series have reported intermittent abdominal pain to be present in 20% to 50% of these patients. The cause of this pain is unknown, but it has been proposed to be the result of the polyp producing a brief, local intussusception. The inci-

	Solitary	Multiple
Neoplastic		
Adenoma	3	1
Polyposis	–	2
Carcinoma	2	–
Hamartomatous		
Juvenile	220	22
Juvenile polyposis	–	3
Peutz-Jeghers	–	2
Inflammatory		
Parasitic/lymphoid	3	7

FIG. 8. Large bowel polyps in children. Adapted from Louw [10].

dence of juvenile polyps producing a definite intussusception is very low. Occasionally, the polyps prolapse through the rectum and are visible. Autoamputation has been noted by both patients and parents. Finally, diarrhea has occasionally been attributed to the presence of polyps and is more likely to be a problem when multiple polyps are present.

Most solitary juvenile polyps are located within reach of the sigmoidoscope. In several series, almost 70% were located within the rectum or rectosigmoid area and that figure reaches about 80% when the remainder of the sigmoid colon is included [10, 11].

Most juvenile polyps are found in children between the ages of 2 and 8 years of age. They are found with decreasing frequency through the early teenage years, although retention polyps have been found in patients 20 years old. In the child under 10, the chance of carcinoma or even an adenomatous polyp being present is exceedingly small.

When planning treatment of juvenile polyps several considerations should be kept in mind. The symptoms caused by juvenile polyps are usually mild. Although rectal bleeding is often an alarming sign to parents, the bleeding is rarely of a significant amount. The fate of these polyps is apparently to autoamputate. Despite the relatively low reported rate of autoamputation these polyps are so rare after the teenage years it seems likely that virtually all spontaneously slough. Juvenile polyps are very rarely the cause of an intussusception. This probably relates to the common location of juvenile polyps in the distal colon where the dynamics of intussusception are not favored.

As nearly as can be determined, the cancer potential of single or multiple juvenile polyps is nil. Even the diffuse blanketing of the juvenile polyposis syndrome apparently has no cancer potential. It should be noted, however, that some potential for malignant degeneration may exist in the Peutz-Jeghers syndrome and the Cronkhite-Canada syndrome. The incidence and origin of the carcinogenic risk from juvenile polyps is zero. Furthermore, there is no apparent overlap in the occurrence of juvenile and adenomatous polyps in patients. The simultaneous presence of a juvenile and an adenomatous polyp of the colon has not yet been reported to this author's knowledge. This must be due, at least in part, to the fact that juvenile polyps tend to occur in the first decade while adenomatous polyps begin to make their appearance later in the second decade. In a patient with two polyps, one of which is accessible and the other inaccessible, if removal of the first reveals a juvenile polyp the second can be safely followed if it does not produce sufficient symptoms to warrant its removal. There is little justification for removing juvenile polyps as a prophylactic measure.

With the previous considerations in mind an approach to the treatment of juvenile polyps can be formulated. In the case of a symptomatic polyp, removal by proctoscopy and snaring is recommended. There is a small risk of perforation and bleeding with this procedure, however. Colonoscopy can be used if the polyps are beyond the reach of the proctoscope. In skilled hands, this seems to be a better technique for detecting polyps than the barium enema. Based on the benign nature of juvenile polyps, it would seem that the risks of laparotomy and colotomy are rarely justified. Published series have indicated a 15% complication rate for the transabdominal removal of these polyps [11]. This rate ignores the possibility of late complications such as bowel obstruction secondary to adhesions. Colotomy, then, should be reserved for the very symptomatic patient. Occasionally, however, children with multiple polyps or diffuse polyposis experience significant bleeding or frequent recurrences of abdominal pain and may benefit from an operation. In the case of diffuse polyposis a partial colectomy may be needed.

Management of Rectal Bleeding in Childhood

When the rectal bleeding is limited in amount and duration, the evaluation should concentrate heavily on the history and physical exam (Fig. 9). Clues should be sought from the child and parents that might suggest the cause. Physical examination may reveal the source. Rectal exam often reveals the two most common defined causes: anal fissures and juvenile polyps. The remainder of the physical examination may produce other clues such as cutaneous hemangiomas, petechiae, melanin spots or purpuric lesions. The presence of cutaneous hemangiomas and calcifications which resemble phleboliths on abdominal x-ray very strongly suggests that the rectal bleeding may be due to intestinal hemangiomas. Hematological examination is necessary to determine if anemia is present, the platelet levels are adequate and to eliminate the possibility of leukemia. Similarly,

Limited Bleeding

- History
  - cough, epistaxis, vomiting, iron
- Family history
- Physical exam
  - hemangiomas, petechiae, melanin spots, purpura
- Rectal exam
  - fissures, polyps
- Blood studies (if indicated)
  - anemia, platelets, leukemias
- Coagulation studies (if indicated)
- Proctoscopy (may be limited)
- Follow

FIG. 9. Management of rectal bleeding in childhood.

if a systemic bleeding problem is suspected, a coagulation evaluation should be done. Proctoscopy should be done if possible. In the smaller child often only a limited proctoscopy can be accomplished without general anesthesia, but this may be enough to reveal the presence of a juvenile polyp. If these measures fail, it is justified to follow these patients. Rectal bleeding is almost always from a benign source in childhood and does not have the ominous significance that it does in adults. Most often no cause will be found and the problem will disappear. The explanation usually given is that small, self-healing abrasions in the mucosa are the source.

If the rectal bleeding is significant and/or continues, a more extensive work-up is indicated (Fig. 10). Nasogastric intubation should be done in children as in adults to help eliminate the possibility that the bleeding is from the esophagus, stomach or duodenum. If the previous attempt at proctoscopy was unsuccessful, it should be done under general anesthesia. Radiological studies may be helpful and a barium enema, and possibly an upper gastrointestinal series, should be considered. Colonoscopy, as mentioned, can be very useful in the diagnosis and treatment of polyps and in the diagnosis of other discrete conditions such as hemangiomas. Depending upon the previous findings, a Technetium scan or even arteriography may be indicated. Finally, if all else fails, an exploratory laparotomy may be justified. Diagnostic measures should be pursued vigorously

Recurrent Significant Bleeding

- Nasogastric intubation
- Barium enema
- Upper GI series
- Colonoscopy
- Technetium (99 Tc) scan (if indicated)
- Arteriogram (if indicated)
- Exploration (if warranted)

FIG. 10. Diagnosis of rectal bleeding in childhood.

prior to this step, however, because laparotomy has a high rate of failure. The unsuccessful, exploring surgeon becomes eligible for Willis Potts' S.O.B. Club, the Surgeons of Bleeders Club, and membership in this group is not altogether desirable [12].

References

1. Bose, B., Keir, W.R. and Godberson, C.V.: Primary pneumococcal peritonitis. Can. Med. Assoc. J. 110:305, 1974.
2. Rodgers, B. and Karn, G.: Yersinia enterocolitis. J. Pediatr. Surg. 10:497, 1975.
3. Kuffer, F., Fortner, J. and Murphy, M.L.: Surgical complications in children undergoing cancer therapy. Ann. Surg. 167:215, 1968.
4. Spencer, R.: Gastrointestinal hemorrhage in infancy and childhood: 476 cases. Surgery 55:718, 1964.
5. Geelhold, G.W., Kane, M.A., Dale, D.C. and Wells, S.A.: Colon ulceration and perforation in cyclic neutropenia. J. Pediatr. Surg. 8:379, 1973.
6. Rutherford, R.B. and Akers, D.R.: Meckel's diverticulum: A review of 148 pediatric patients. Surgery 59:618, 1966.
7. Benson, C.D.: Surgical Implications of Meckel's Diverticulum in Pediatric Surgery. (Mustard, W.T. et al [eds.]). Chicago:Yearbook, 1969, pp. 864-868.
8. Kilpatrick, Z.M. and Aseron, C.A. Jr.: Radioisotope detection of Meckel's diverticulum causing acute rectal hemorrhage. N. Engl. J. Med. 287:653, 1972.
9. Kilpatrick, A.M.: Scanning in diagnosis of Meckel's diverticulum. Hosp. Pract., p. 131, 1974.
10. Louw, J.H.: Polypoid lesions of the large bowel in children. S. Afr. Med. J. 46:1347, 1972.
11. Holgersen, L.O., Miller, R.E. and Zintel, H.A.: Juvenile polyps of the colon. Surgery 69:288, 1971.
12. Potts, W.J.: The Surgeon and the Child. Philadelphia:W.B. Saunders Co., 1959, p. 219.

Self-Evaluation Quiz

1. Which of the following conditions increases the likelihood a child will develop primary peritonitis?
   a) Prior splenectomy
   b) Nephrotic syndrome
   c) Cirrhosis
   d) All of the above
2. The presence of many pneumococci in a peritoneal tap of a child with a diffusely tender abdomen is against a diagnosis of primary peritonitis.

a) True
b) False
3. A self-limited form of terminal ileitis has been attributed to:
a) *Staphylococcus aureus*
b) *Escherichia coli*
c) *Yersinia enterocolitica*
d) *Diplococcus pneumoniae*
4. An important mechanism in producing intestinal damage seems to be:
a) Hepatic blood flow
b) Splanchnic vasoconstriction
c) Serosal hyperemia
d) Peristaltic activity
5. Integrity of the intestinal barrier depends upon:
a) Proliferation of mucosa cells
b) Presence of immune and inflammatory cells in the intestinal wall
c) Adequate intestinal blood flow
d) All of the above
6. Peritoneal tap can be useful in the diagnosis of bowel perforation.
a) True
b) False
7. Following stress of various kinds bleeding ulcers can occur in the:
a) Stomach
b) Duodenum
c) Cecum
d) All of the above
8. Rectal bleeding in childhood, as in adults, often indicates the presence of cancer, and the diagnosis should be vigorously sought.
a) True
b) False
9. Bleeding from a Meckel's diverticulum usually results from the secretion of:
a) Ectopic pancreatic tissue
b) Ectopic duodenal mucosa
c) Islet cells
d) Ectopic gastric mucosa

10. Bleeding from a Meckel's diverticulum is usually:
    a) Intermittent and often severe but very rarely exsanguinating
    b) A continuous trickle
    c) Fatal
    d) Accompanied by perforation

Answers on page 721.

Neuroendocrine Tumors of the Gastrointestinal Tract

Stanley R. Friesen, M.D.

Objectives

1. To present the underlying basic cytochemical and embryologic characteristics which are embodied in the APUD concept of endocrinopathies.
2. To correlate the function of neuroendocrine cells with their target (exocrine) cells by means of circulating hormones and their specific receptors.
3. To briefly describe and clarify the clinical pictures of the endocrine syndromes which emanate from the gastroenteropancreatic (GEP) system.

Introduction

There has been a proliferation of discoveries regarding functioning (hormone-secreting) tumors of the gastroentero-pancreatic (GEP) system. Some of the tumors which were considered to produce symptoms only by their physical or mechanical effects, such as by obstruction or by mucosal blood loss, now have been shown to cause systemic manifestations of bizarre endocrinopathies. Furthermore, the once typical carcinoid syndrome is now but a part of a spectrum of syndromes which result from excessive elaboration of newly identified polypeptide and amine hormones. The biochemical break-through of identification and synthesis of at least the active portions of polypeptide hormones has led to diagnostic differentiation of the hormone-producing tumor syndromes and

---

Stanley R. Friesen, M.D., Professor of Surgery, University of Kansas Medical Center College of Health Sciences, Kansas City, Kansas.

This research was aided by Grant RR-828 from the General Clinical Research Centers Program of the National Institutes of Health, and by the Morales-Foley Research Fund.

has provided a marker of tumor activity. An understanding of the myriad of hormones, tumors and the associated clinical pictures is best accomplished by a review of basic concepts of the cytochemistry and embryology of the reconstituted neuroendocrine system; such fundamental considerations are encompassed in what has recently been termed the APUD concept.

The APUD Concept

The acronym, APUD, identifies some of the common cytochemical characteristics of neuroendocrine cells: Amine-Precursor-Uptake and Decarboxylation, which means that the cells of this diffusely expansive system have the innate ability to take up precursor amines and decarboxylate them to store, synthesize and secrete amines and, in turn, polypeptides. These cells also have other common functions such as esterase activity, thus linking neural and humoral functions at the cellular level. The reason these cells, which are present both centrally (hypothalamus, pituitary, etc.) and peripherally (GEP system), share so many common characteristics is that they also share common embryologic origins from the neuroectoderm, including the neural crest, placodal extensions from the neuroectoderm, or by cellular migration to the entodermal layers. Thus two of the three general classes of humoral products of endocrine cells emanate from APUD cells; only the steroid hormones are secreted from cells and organs that arise from mesodermal derivations (adrenal cortex and gonads). APUD cells contain secretory granules.

The dimensions of the neuroendocrine system extend from the rapidly acting amine hormones and neurotransmitters (acetylcholine, catecholamines, serotonins and thyroxines) to the very slowly acting steroid hormones (cortisol, estrogens, androgens, aldosterones, etc.). The largest middle segment of hormones — the polypeptides, central and peripheral — are important in maintaining functional homeostasis; these include the trophic and inhibiting hormones and thyrocalcitonin and parathyrin, centrally, as well as the peripheral diffuse paracrine hormones of gastrin, secretin, glucagon, insulin, somatostatin, cholecystokinin, motilin, neurotensin and other peptides.

The normal ability of APUD cells and their secretory products to provide homeostatic balance within the numerous functions of the body is best illustrated by an elucidation of the antithetical capabilities of pairs of hormones; such examples include the opposing influences on carbohydrate metabolism by insulin and glucagon; on calcium metabolism by thyrocalcitonin and parathyrin; on acid-base secretion by gastrin and secretin; on growth by growth hormone (somatotrophin) and somatostatin (somatotrophin inhibiting hormone), etc. These and other polypeptides and amines are synthesized, stored and secreted (S-S-S) by the APUD cells in response to cellular stimulation or suppression (S-S), being influenced by physical, chemical, neural or humoral factors. Such modifications of function by stimulation or suppression form the basis of diagnostic tests for endocrinopathies. With few exceptions, hyperplasias of APUD cells respond in normal fashion to normal influences while autonomous neoplasias are usually not influenced by such factors.

When APUD cells become histologically abnormal and functionally hyperactive, for whatever reasons, genetic or environment, this homeostatic balance is lost and an excessive elaboration of a humoral product(s) produces a biologically abnormal endocrinopathy or syndrome. The clinical picture arising from such humoral hypersecretion depends upon the effect of that hormone on the target cell organ and its biologic (exocrine) activity. The target cell possesses membrane receptors which are specifically responsive to specific peptide hormones; these receptors, when coupled with their inciting hormones, set in motion an intracellular activation of cAMP (the second messenger) and a kinase instigation of its specific exocrine function. A gastric parietal cell for instance, with receptors for acetylcholine, histamine and gastrin, if unblocked, will respond to carry out its only biologic activity, releasing hydrogen ion as gastric hydrochloric acid. The histamine-2 receptor can be pharmacologically blocked, or the gastrin receptor can be occupied by CCK or the neural release of acetylcholine at the vagal ending can be inhibited at the parietal cell; these interceptions result in decreased gastric production.

Each endocrine cell and each exocrine cell, then, normally performs one primary function depending upon the influences acting on it. The excessive elaboration of single hormones in patients is indicative of a sporadic autonomous tumor (usually benign, such as an insulinoma or parathyroid adenoma). The secretion of multiple amine or peptide hormones connotes either a genetic abnormality of the multiple endocrine adenopathy type with excessive secretion from several endocrine organs or may, on the other hand, signal ectopic elaboration of multiple hormones from a single malignant tumor.

The genetic instigation of cellular abnormalities with hyperfunction in several predictable endocrine systems is said to be due to an abnormal pleiotropic gene which reacts with those cells having common embryologic origins (APUD cells). Thus all of the cells of the pancreatic islets, pituitary and parathyroid glands (P-P-P) may become hyperplastic or neoplastic in a patient and also in his siblings in a dominant fashion. Even more characteristic genetically are the syndromes in which there is an association of the charter members of the APUD family with the medullary malignancies of the thyroid and the adrenal glands (diffuse medullary carcinoma of the thyroid [MCT], and bilateral pheochromocytomas).

The phenomenon of ectopia, for many years a completely unexplainable clinical set of aberrations, is now more rationally clarified because of the acceptance of the APUD concept and the concept of de-repression of precursor hormones. At first it was not realized that the Zollinger-Ellison Ulcerogenic syndrome of pancreatic gastrinoma might be an ectopic manifestation. It is now known that the polypeptide antral hormone, gastrin, is not a native product of the normal cells of the adult pancreatic islets (gastrin, however, is present in the islets of the fetal human pancreas). Thus, an ulcerogenic islet cell gastrinoma of the pancreas is an example of an ectopic phenomenon. Other relatively common examples of ectopia are carcinoid tumors of the foregut and bronchopulmonary tumors (carcinoid and oat cell carcinomas). There are many other examples of rare malignant tumors which release unexpected hormones. It must be realized that most of these so-called ectopic sites are really normal locations of APUD cells which have undergone malignant change; these cells include the ubiquitous enterochromaffin (EC) cells which reside all through the extent of the entodermal tract from the pituitary to the proctodeum. Even malignant tumors of organs that are not usually considered endocrine in function may on occasion exhibit a humoral manifestation.

Well-differentiated malignant cells, particularly endocrine ones, have been found to produce within their cytoplasm common precursor hormone molecules of larger than normal size. A failure of enzyme activity to convert large molecular precursor hormone to small molecular hormone may be due to a process of de-repression in malignant cells. In the normal cell all primitive functions are repressed except its single biologic action; in these malignant cells this repression is lost and the cells revert (de-repress) to a primitively functioning state. Antibodies to these large molecular precursor hormones have been shown to react to several peptide hormones, demonstrating a polypotentiality of hormone function. Thus, a malignant tumor with its precursor hormone may elaborate any of the APUD cell prohormones in a seemingly ectopic fashion. The multiple and varied combinations of such amine and peptide elaborations can produce in this way a kaleidoscopic array of clinical syndromes of ectopic origin.

Clinical Considerations

Functioning tumors of the GEP system produce recognizable syndromes, most of which are briefly described here.

The Carcinoid Syndromes

The *classic carcinoid syndrome* is associated with carcinoid tumors of the *midgut* (ileum) which have metastasized to the liver, from which are liberated the amine, 5-hydroxytryptamine (5-HT, serotonin) and the enzyme kallikrein, which forms bradykinin in the plasma. The action of these substances which have escaped the metabolism of the liver and lungs is directed to the smooth muscles of the blood vessels and the intestine and to the right-sided endocardium. The cutaneous vasodilation produces episodic flushing of the head, neck and upper trunk; the spasm and hypermotility of the intestine produces crampy pain, borborygmi and nonbloody diarrhea due to tumor secretion of 5-HT and motilin, a polypeptide product of EC cells. Longstanding exposure of the right heart endocardium to these substances may cause tricuspid and pulmonary valvular abnormalities with heart failure.

Bronchial and ovarian carcinoid tumors liberate the amines into the systemic circulation, bypassing the liver. *Foregut* carcinoid tumors, including the bronchial tumors, may differ from the midgut tumors by their hypersecretion of 5-hydroxytryptophan (5-HTP) instead of 5-HT because they often lack the enzyme 5-HTP decarboxylase; consequently, 5-hydroxyindole acetic acid (5-HIAA) will not be elevated in the urine, but 5-HTP, 5-HT and histamine will be high. This *atypical carcinoid syndrome* displays a more prolonged and brighter red skin flush and may be accompanied by facial edema and lacrimation. Furthermore, the greatest distinction of foregut carcinoid tumors lies in more frequent associated elaboration of histamine and of polypeptides other than motilin, such as corticotrophin, insulin, gastrin and glucagon, which then modify the clinical picture of the atypical carcinoid syndrome by masking it with the biologic effects of those specific polypeptides. These tumors of the lung, stomach, duodenum and pancreas, benign or malignant, are sometimes called islet-carcinoid tumors. *Hindgut* carcinoid tumors usually do not produce symptoms due to hyperfunction, but when they do, the clinical picture is more likely to resemble the foregut than the midgut variety.

The Hypoglycemic Syndrome of Hyperinsulinism

Increased elaboration of insulin, a polypeptide of 51 amino acid residues, occurs most commonly from a single pancreatic adenoma, a Beta cell insulinoma. Organic hyperinsulinism is less frequently caused by multiple adenomatosis, by islet cell hyperplasia, by metastatic carcinoma, and rarely by "ectopic" tumors. The biologic action of insulin on carbohydrate metabolism is anabolic, stimulating glucose conversion to glycogen and promoting the uptake of amino acids for protein synthesis, thus storing energy and reducing the circulating level of glucose in the blood. The symptoms of hyperinsulinism occur in the fasting state, usually in early mornings, and are prompted by glucose levels under 45 mg%. The hypoglycemia provokes a compensatory release of epinephrine which, together with cerebral glucose deprivation (neuroglucopenia), produces the symptomatology in this syndrome. The rapid release of catecholamines causes symptoms of tremor, sweating, pallor, palpitation and a feeling of panic; the cerebral neuroglucopenia leads to anxiety, hunger, mental confusion, inappropriate behavior, stupor or coma. The endocrine response to hypoglycemia may reverse the symptoms, but usually the administration of glucose is necessary for rapid restoration to normal and is a diagnostic feature of organic hyperinsulinism.

The Hyperglycemic (Cutaneous) Syndrome of Hyperglucagonism

Glucagon is a polypeptide of 29 amino acid residues, released from the Alpha cells of the pancreatic islets, which when secreted in excess, usually by carcinoma with metastases, produces a hyperglycemia not unlike that seen in diabetes mellitus. With respect to carbohydrate metabolism, its action is catabolic and is a physiological antithesis of the action of insulin in that it promotes hepatic glycogenolysis and gluconeogenesis. The actions of glucagon include an increase in splanchnic blood flow, a chronotrophic tachycardia, an inotropic increase in cardiac output, an inhibition of intestinal motility and a decrease in gastric volume. There is usually, but not always, a characteristic clinical picture of migrating necrotizing skin lesions in a patient with hyperglycemia, associated with a slow-growing, metastatic non-Beta cell carcinoma (or rarely islet cell hyperplasia). There may also be associated ascites and ileus. An abnormal glucose tolerance curve is usually present. When exogenous glucagon is administered intravenously to a patient with endogenous hyperglucagonemia, there will be little effect on the blood glucose and insulin levels (a blunted, flat glucose curve) as contrasted to the increased glucose level in normal patients. Radioimmunoassay of serum for glucagon may confirm the presence of a glucagon-secreting APUD cell tumor. Excision of the tumor before hepatic metastases occur will occasionally result in cure.

The Ulcerogenic (Zollinger-Ellison) Syndrome of Hypergastrinism

Increased serum content of gastrin, a 17 amino acid residue polypeptide, measurable by bioassay and radioimmunoassay, is classically seen in patients having pancreatic islet cell malignancies, adenomas or hyperplasias or duodenal adenomas with marked acid hypersecretion and ulceration in the typical Zollinger-Ellison syndrome. Hypergastrinemia may also be due to increased release of gastrin from G cell hyperplasia of the gastric antrum. This results in acid hypersecretion and ulceration similar to but different from the typical Z-E syndrome. The antral type of the ulcerogenic syndrome is probably an intermediate stage between the duodenal ulcer diathesis and the classical pancreatic Zollinger-Ellison syndrome. Hypergastrinemia may result also from gastrin elaboration from other ectopic sites (mesodermal tumors, thyroid parafollicular cell tumors and parathyroid adenomas which have been found to contain and secrete gastrin). Finally, increased levels of circulating gastrin are sometimes found in association with achlorhydria, pernicious anemia, acromegaly, hyperparathyroidism and renal failure.

The symptoms of the ulcerogenic syndrome due to hypergastrinism, often over 1000 pg/ml, are referable primarily to the marked hypersecretion of gastric acids which exceeds a volume of 1 liter in 12 hours containing more than 100 mEq hydrochloric acid in that period. This maximal secretion is not increased significantly by histalog or insulin stimulation. The large volume causes acid-peptic ulceration of the duodenal bulb and areas more distal in the duodenum and jejunum. Diarrhea (steatorrhea due to acid neutralization of the duodenal alkaline activation of fat-splitting enzymes of the pancreas) is a common finding. Persistence of these symptoms after otherwise adequate medical and surgical treatment for duodenal ulcer is frequent. The parietal cells become markedly hyperplastic, presumably due to the trophic effect of the constant gastrin stimulation; thus gastric hyperrugation, gastric hypersecretion and intestinal hypermotility are radiographic findings. Immunochemical assays of serum for gastrin usually reveal levels in excess of 1000 pg/ml; if the values are only moderately elevated to levels of 400 to 600 pg/ml in a patient with duodenal ulcer, a diagnosis of the antral type (G cell hyperplasia) should be considered. In a patient with the usual duodenal ulcer diathesis the serum gastrin values will be normal or less than normal (50 to 125 pg/ml). In patients with circulating serum gastrin levels in the mid range of 400 to 600 pg/ml, the stimulation tests using secretin or calcium are required to differentiate between the pancreatic and the antral (intermediary) types. Secretin and calcium will not elevate the serum gastrin levels further in the antral (mucosal) G cell hyperplasia entity; if a rise to over 1000 pg/ml occurs, the instigating lesion is probably in or near the pancreas. If it is confirmed histologically that the patient has a non-Beta islet cell tumor or a tumor in the area of the pancreas and duodenum compatible with APUD cell neoplasia and/or hyperplasia, a total gastrectomy, in addition to excision of resectable tumor, is the treatment of choice; excision of the tumor alone is usually not beneficial because the tumors are often multiple or metastatic or there is an associated hyperplasia. Palliation by means of tumor excision in addition to the use of the receptor blocker, cimetidine, now is possible. If it is shown that the patient has only antral G cell hyperplasia without other lesions, a vagotomy and antrectomy will lead to normal serum gastrin levels. In some patients total gastrectomy has been followed by regression of metastatic deposits, for unknown reasons. There is a high incidence (20% to 40%) of associated multiple endocrinopathies and familial associations, which require repeated and prolonged follow-up studies.

The Diarrheogenic Syndrome (Verner-Morrison Syndrome, Watery Diarrhea, Hypokalemia and Hypo- or Achlorhydria [WDHA] Syndrome, Pancreatic Cholera Syndrome with Vasoactive Intestinal Polypeptide [VIP] Secretion)

This syndrome, at first thought to be a variant of the Zollinger-Ellison syndrome, is characterized by the prominent symptoms of explosive, episodic, watery diarrhea (over 2 liters/day) without acid-peptic ulceration or gastric hypersecretion. The non-Beta islet cell tumor is usually in the pancreas but has been reported in patients with sympathetic nerve tumors. About half the tumors are malignant. Stimulated acid secretory tests usually show hypochlorhydria or achlorhydria; if the former is present, the excessive polypeptide is probably VIP, while if histamine-fast achlorhydria is present, the likely polypeptide may be another secretin-like hormone such as gastric-inhibitory-polypeptide (GIP). Hypokalemia is common; there is occasional hypercalcemia. The rare occurrence of facial flushing suggests an associated secretion of the amine 5-HT. Assays of elevated appropriate polypeptides are diagnostic. These return to normal after successful excision of the vipoma.

The Inhibitory Syndrome of Somatostatinoma

Somatostatin, an inhibitory hormone, found both in the hypothalamus and in the pancreatic islet D cells, inhibits the release of gastrin, insulin, glucagon, cholecystokinin (CCK) and growth hormone. It has been found to be present in islet cell tumors and elevated in the blood of two patients exhibiting steatorrhea, abdominal cramps, hyperglycemia and hypochlorhydria. No elevations of gastrin, insulin, glucagon or vasoactive intestinal polypeptide have been reported in these patients. Resection is the treatment of choice.

Wermer's Syndrome (MEA I)

A combination of multiple endocrinopathies which occur synchronously or more commonly in a metachronous fashion involving the pancreas, pituitary and the parathyroids is often designated as the MEA type I syndrome and was first described by Cushing. Although it may rarely occur sporadically, Wermer emphasized the familial autosomal dominant nature of the syndrome. The clinical picture usually points to the pancreas, with hypergastrinism or hyperinsulinism, but hyperparathyroidism may predominate with acute hypercalcemic crises; the onset of pituitary acromegaly may be insidious. Adrenal cortical hypersecretion of cortisol (Cushing's syndrome), thyroid adenomas and multiple lipomas are not infrequent.

Sippel's Syndrome (MEA II)

A less frequent but well-documented syndrome, commonly known also as multiple endocrine neoplasia (MEN) type II, and sometimes occurring in families, consists of medullary carcinoma of the thyroid, pheochromocytoma in one or both of the adrenal medullas, and sometimes hyperparathyroidism. The latter is probably a secondary compensatory phenomenon in response to the hypercalcitoninism from the C cell thyroid malignancy. The hormones, thyrocalcitonin from the thyroid medullary carcinoma and the amines from pheochromocytoma, in MEA II are classic, being traditional members of the APUD system. Occasionally, in MEN, type IIb, there are associated submucosal neuromas and rarely, autonomic ganglioneuromatosis and Marfan's syndrome. This type of MEA is most virulent.

Ectopic Syndromes

These run the gamut of humoral manifestations but the more common hormones which are elaborated in them are gastrin, corticotrophin, parathyrin and VIP from the pancreas, lungs, liver, breast and kidney.

The hormone human pancreatic polypeptide (HPP), having normal functions relating to digestion of food, has not yet found its niche in clinical endocrinology. At this time it has been found to be reduced or absent in cystic fibrosis of the pancreas and to be elevated after eating. It has been reported further as a marker in some patients with pancreatic gastrinomas, vipomas, insulinomas and glucagonomas. Such universality suggests an origin in the associated hyperplasias of islet and interstitial cells of the pancreas.

Summary

The diagnosis of the endocrinopathies arising in the gastroenteropancreatic (GEP) system involves (1) an awareness of the possibility of a systemic response to tumor hormones; (2) an elimination of the more usual (nonhumoral) causes in the differential diagnoses; (3) radioimmunoassay measurement of the suspect amine and polypeptides, and (4) observation of associated exocrine and biologic effects of the target organs.

If an endocrinopathy is thus identified, the offending tumor may be further localized by angiography and by computerized axial tomography. Surgical excision of the functioning tumors or hyperplasias is usually indicated: nonresectable functioning metastases are sometimes treated by chemotherapy, using streptozotocin. In the future the use of inhibitory hormones such as somatostatin, and receptor modifiers such as cimetidine, will be more prevalent and, hopefully, more beneficial.

Bibliography

Bloom, S.R., Polak, J.M. and Pearse, A.G.E.: Vasoactive intestinal peptide and watery-diarrhoea syndrome. Lancet 2:14, 1973.

Bolande, R.P.: The neurocristopathies, a unifying concept of disease arising in neural crest maldevelopment. Hum. Pathol. 5:409, 1974.

Elias, E., Bloom, S.R., Welbourn, R.B. et al: Pancreatic cholera due to production of gastric inhibitory polypeptide. Lancet 2:791, 1972.

Friesen, S.R.: APUD tumors of the gastrointestinal tract. *In* Hickey, R.C. (ed.): Current Problems in Cancer. Chicago:Year Book Medical Publishers, Inc., 1976, Vol. 1, No. 4.

Friesen, S.R.: Surgical Endocrinology: Clinical Syndromes. Philadelphia: J.B. Lippincott Company, 1978.

Ganda, O.P. et al: "Somatostatinoma." A somatostatin-containing tumor of the endocrine pancreas. N. Engl. J. Med. 296:963, 1977.

Kahn, C.R., Levy, A.G., Gardner, J.D. et al: Pancreatic cholera: Beneficial effects of treatment with streptozotocin. N. Engl. J. Med. 292:941, 1975.

Kaplan, E.L., Jaffe, B.M. and Peskin, G.W.: A new provocative test for the diagnosis of the carcinoid syndrome. Am. J. Surg. 123:173, 1972.

Khairi, M.R.A. et al: Mucosal neuroma, pheochromocytoma, and medullary thyroid carcinoma: Multiple endocrine neoplasia type III. Medicine 54:89, 1975.

Larsson, L.I., Ljungberg, O., Sundler, F. et al: Antro-pyloric gastrinoma associated with pancreatic nesidioblastosis and proliferation of islets. Virchows. Arch. (Pathol. Anat.) 360:305, 1973.

Larsson, L.I. et al: Pancreatic somatostatinoma. Clinical features and physiological implications. Lancet 1:666, 1977.

Mallinson, C.N., Bloom, S.R., Warin, A.P. et al: A glucagonoma syndrome. Lancet 2:7871, 1974.

Pearse, A.G.E. and Polak, J.M.: Neural crest origin of the endocrine polypeptide (APUD) cells of the gastrointestinal tract and pancreas. Gut 12:783, 1971.

Polak, J.M., Adrian, T.W., Bryant, M.G. et al: Pancreatic polypeptide in insulinomas, gastrinomas, vipomas, and glucagonomas. Lancet 1:328, 1976.

Schein, P.S., DeLellis, R.A., Kahn, C.R. et al: Islet cell tumors, current concepts and management. Ann. Intern. Med. 79:293, 1973.

Self-Evaluation Quiz

1. The APUD system of endocrine cells is capable of secreting which of the following types of humoral substances: (1) amines; (2) steroids; (3) polypeptides; (4) prostaglandins?
   a) 1, 2 & 3
   b) 1 & 3
   c) 2 & 4
   d) 4 only
   e) All four
2. The acronym APUD denotes which of the following common cytochemical characteristics: (1) amine precursor uptake; (2) amine degradation; (3) decarboxylation; (4) amine polypeptide uptake?

a) 1, 2 & 3
b) 1 & 3
c) 2 & 4
d) 4 only
e) All four

3. The characteristics of the endocrine system include: (1) cells contain secretory granules; (2) cells are capable of being stimulated and inhibited; (3) cells are contiguous with vascular capillaries; (4) cells communicate with exocrine cells via ducts:
   a) 1, 2 & 3
   b) 1 & 3
   c) 2 & 4
   d) 4 only
   e) All four
4. The features of the classical type of the carcinoid syndrome include (1) a foregut tumor; (2) hepatic metastases; (3) elaboration of polypeptides; (4) secretion of serotonin:
   a) 1, 2 & 3
   b) 1 & 3
   c) 2 & 4
   d) 4 only
   e) All four
5. The clinical feature(s) associated with an insulinoma include (1) fasting hyperglycemia; (2) paroxysmal hypertension; (3) a cutaneous rash; (4) fasting hypoglycemia:
   a) 1, 2 & 3
   b) 1 & 3
   c) 2 & 4
   d) 4 only
   e) All four
6. An example of a tumor producing an ectopic endocrinopathy is which one of the following:
   a) Pancreatic insulinoma
   b) Pancreatic glucagonoma
   c) Pancreatic somatostatinoma
   d) Pancreatic gastrinoma
   e) Pancreatic carcinoid tumor
7. Pancreatic islet cell tumors may have causal relationship to all except:

a) Hyperglycemia
b) Mental deterioration
c) Refractory duodenal ulcer
d) Curling's ulcer
e) Episodic hypoglycemia

8. The Zollinger-Ellison syndrome is characterized by:
   a) Recurrent ulceration in the intestinal tract
   b) Marked hyperacidity
   c) Both
   d) Neither
9. Which of the following polypeptide hormones is *not* native to the human adult pancreas?
   a) Insulin
   b) Gastrin
   c) Glucagon
   d) Human pancreatic polypeptide
   e) Somatostatin
10. A patient presents with clinical findings of reduced serum potassium due to explosive, voluminous, tea-colored diarrhea, hypochlorhydria, increased cAMP activity and prostaglandin levels. The most likely humoral substance in excess is:
    a) Gastrin
    b) Serotonin
    c) Gastric inhibitory peptide
    d) Vasoactive intestinal polypeptide
    e) Glucagon

Answers on page 721.

The Peritoneum and Peritonitis

David H. Ahrenholz, M.D., Toni Hau, M.D.
and Richard L. Simmons, M.D.

Objectives

The purpose of this discussion is to briefly review the anatomy of the peritoneal cavity and the mechanisms by which the body deals with infections in this area. The role of adjuvant substances and of synergistic bacterial interactions is discussed. A rationale for radical peritoneal debridement and lavage with antibiotic solutions is presented.

Introduction

A number of unfounded fears related to the need to localize peritoneal infections are based on the practice (in a previous era) of nonoperative treatment. Our increasing knowledge of the mechanisms of peritoneal clearance of bacteria after the visceral leak is controlled by operative treatment has changed our outlook on the pathogenesis and treatment of peritonitis. We no longer fear dissemination of bacteria during exploration and feel semi-Fowler's position probably does little to localize infection in the pelvis. Vigorous peritoneal lavage and radical peritoneal debridement are two modalities which appear to have sound physiologic basis in the treatment of peritonitis. One overriding factor has become apparent; if the organisms can be cleared from the peritoneal cavity or killed in situ, the patient will recover. If the organisms remain, especially in the presence of adjuvant substances, the likelihood of recurrent infections increases. Therefore, the main problems in peritonitis are the removal of the vast majority of bacteria present in the

---

David H. Ahrenholz, M.D., Toni Hau, M.D. and Richard L. Simmons, M.D., Department of Surgery, University of Minnesota Medical School, Minneapolis.

abdominal cavity at the time of operation and the facilitation of the clearance of the remaining organisms by normal defenses.

Basic Concepts

Bacteria introduced into the peritoneal cavity are either killed in situ or physically removed from the cavity. The peritoneum has specific anatomical modifications of its surface to aid in this removal. Histologically the peritoneum consists of a monolayer of mesothelial cells resting on a basement membrane with underlying lymphatics and blood vessels. Although all serosal surfaces may participate in fluid exchange, the subdiaphragmatic lymphatics are specifically modified for the removal of particulate matter. Bacteria can be evacuated from the peritoneal cavity only through these lymphatics. The mesothelial cells overlying the lymphatics have intercellular gaps (stomata), 4 to 8 μ in diameter, which appear to directly communicate with diaphragmatic lymphatic vessels (Fig. 1).

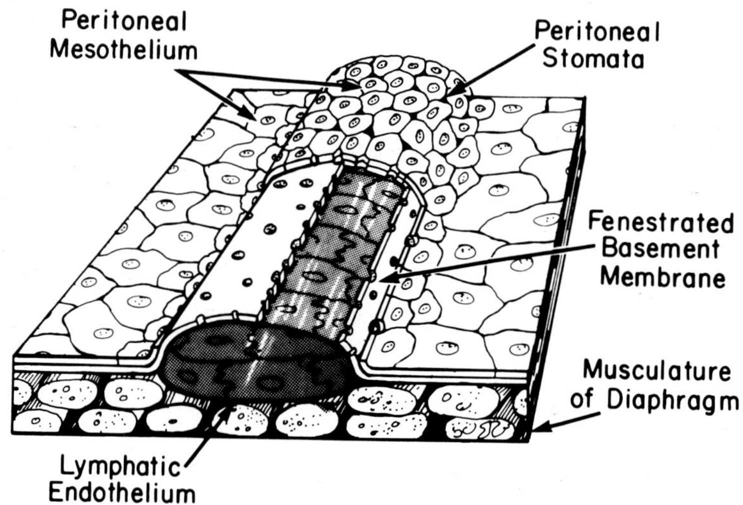

FIG. 1. Diagram of the lymphatics of the peritoneal surface of the diaphragm. The mesothelial cells are flattened except over the lymphatics, where they are smaller with stomata between the cells. The lymphatic endothelium lines the lymphatic channel and probably communicates with the peritoneal cavity through the stomata. (Modified from Allen, 1936.)

During respiration, fluid and particulate matter are sucked from the peritoneal cavity. Valves within lymphatic vessels prevent retrograde flow. This fluid traverses the retrosternal and anterior mediastinal lymphatics and is returned to the systemic circulation. The upward circulation of intraperitoneal fluid generated by this process accounts for the high incidence of subdiaphragmatic abscesses in patients with intraperitoneal infections. In the past surgeons have felt that the semi-Fowler's position would prevent subphrenic abscesses and localize infections in the pelvis where they could be drained more easily. But experiments in our lab have shown a higher mortality for rats maintained in the 45° head-up versus head-down position for only four hours after induction of E. coli peritonitis (Table 1). Experimentally the head-up position delays clearance of the bacteria from the peritoneal cavity; if the rapid removal of bacteria is important for recovery, the semi-Fowler's position appears to be disadvantageous.

The Role of Adjuvant Substances in Peritonitis

Although bacteria are the most important factor in peritonitis, a number of substances, including hemoglobin, bile salts, gastric mucin and feces increase the lethality of a bacterial inoculum. Hemoglobin has been intensively studied. Data from our lab suggest it not only delays the removal of bacteria from the peritoneal cavity but also delays the influx of neutrophils and their ability to phagocytose bacteria. For example, when *E. coli* and hemoglobin are injected into the peritoneal cavity, the bacteria multiply rapidly. The animal becomes septic and remains septic until death (Table 2). When bacteria are injected without hemoglobin, blood cultures are positive for the first several hours but become negative as the numbers of bacteria in the peritoneal cavity decrease. In vitro testing of bacterial

Table 1. Mortality as a Function of Body Position Maintained for Four Hours After *E. Coli*-Hb Peritonitis

Head up	Restrained	36/40 (90%)
Flat	Restrained	34/40 (85%)
Head down	Restrained	25/40 (62.5%)
Unrestrained	Unrestrained	26/34 (76%)

Table 2. Bacterial Counts in Blood and Peritoneum During Peritonitis

Time (Hr)	*E. Coli Plus Hgb*		*E. Coli*	
	Peritoneum	*Blood*	*Peritoneum*	*Blood*
0	1×10^{11}	–	1×10^{11}	–
1	1×10^{9}	+	7×10^{7}	+
2	3×10^{9}	+	2×10^{7}	+
4	6×10^{9}	+	8×10^{6}	+
22	1×10^{9}	+	1×10^{2}	–

phagocytosis in our lab has shown that hemoglobin inhibits this process as well.

But even large volumes of saline act as an adjuvant; if *E. coli* are suspended in saline and injected into the peritoneal cavity of rats, mortality increases with larger volumes (Table 3). Since there is a maximum rate of absorption of isotonic fluids from the peritoneal cavity, a portion of the bacteria remains suspended in the intraperitoneal fluid. They are able to multiply and consequently kill the test animals. Although saline causes a rapid influx of neutrophils, their ability to kill bacteria in situ is markedly decreased, because phagocytosis is not efficient in a free solution.

The mechanisms involved with other adjuvant substances are not well delineated. With particulate matter such as feces, the neutrophils may expend their intracellular digestive enzymes by trying to engulf noninfectious particles. Since an individual neutrophil can ingest only a limited amount of particulate material, much larger numbers may be required to effectively sterilize the peritoneal cavity.

It is our hypothesis that fibrin may be the single most important adjuvant substance in the peritoneal cavity. Hudspeth

Table 3. Mortality After Injection of *E. Coli* and Normal Saline in Rats

Volume	*2 × 10^7 E. Coli*	*2 × 10^8 E. Coli*
0.4 cc	7%	72%
2.0 cc	40%	100%
10.0 cc	100%	100%

has reported a series of 92 cases of intra-abdominal infection treated by radical peritoneal debridement in which all visible fibrin peel is removed from the serosal surfaces, in addition to the usual operative procedures. He reported no deaths and no reoperations for recurrent infections in these patients. We have experimental evidence that preventing fibrin deposition can decrease the mortality in canine peritonitis. Twenty-four hours after ligation of the blood supply to an isolated ileal segment, the dogs were opened and the necrotic ileum excised. The animals received no antibiotics but were given one dose of heparin subcutaneously or intraperitoneally. Thirteen of the 16 dogs treated with heparin survived with no evidence of infection compared to only two of eight control animals (Table 4). The risk of postoperative bleeding must be weighed in the clinical application of this modality, however.

Bacteriologic Considerations

The most common organisms isolated from bacterial peritonitis are gram negative coliform bacteria, the enterococcus (*Streptococcus faecalis*) and anaerobes, especially *Bacteroides fragilis.* Onderdonk et al have shown that facultative organisms and anaerobes act synergistically to produce intra-abdominal infections. Several mechanisms have been implicated. The facultative organisms are able to lower the oxygen concentration within the peritoneal cavity, allowing the growth of anaerobic organisms. *Bacteroides fragilis* and some other anaerobes have a glycoprotein capsule which prevents phagocytosis of most bacteria by neutrophils. *Bacteroides* species also

Table 4. Effect of Heparin (100 μ/kg) on Survival of Dogs With Fibrinopurulent Peritonitis

Group	*No. of Dogs*	*Died of Peritonitis*	*Survived With Peritoneal Infection*	*Survived Without IP Infection*
Control	8	5	2	1
Heparin IP	8	2	–	6*
Heparin SC	8	1	–	7†

*$p \leq 0.05$ compared with the control group.
†$p \leq 0.02$ compared with the control group.

elaborate nucleases, proteases and collagenases which contribute to their virulence.

Weinstein et al have studied selective antibiotic therapy for these organisms. In rats they found that of the antibiotic combinations tested, an aminoglycoside combined with clindamycin yielded the fewest abscesses and greatest number of surviving animals. Because enterococci are so frequently isolated from intraperitoneal infections, the combination of clindamycin, an aminoglycoside and ampicillin would cover the organisms expected to be present in acute peritonitis. Alternatively chloramphenicol or carbenicillin may be used rather than clindamycin. The culture and sensitivity reports obtained after operation are used to modify the choice of antibiotics in the postoperative period.

Therapeutic Considerations

In acute secondary bacterial peritonitis an operation is indicated to remove the bacteria and adjuvant substances and to close any leak in the GI, biliary, pancreatic or genitourinary tracts. Radical peritoneal debridement appears the most successful method of removing fibrin deposits, which act as adjuvants in peritonitis. Saline irrigation is very effective in lowering the total bacterial counts and increasing the survival of animals in experimental peritonitis. Adding antibiotics to the irrigation solution increases the efficacy of the process, and cephalothin and kanamycin have been approved by the FDA for clinical use in irrigation of the peritoneal cavity. Residual fluid contains antibiotic which is active locally and systemically against any remaining bacteria. Since fluid acts to inhibit the clearance of bacteria, excess fluid should be thoroughly aspirated.

Conclusions

Peritonitis remains a lethal disease, especially when it occurs as a complication of operation. In addition to the traditional modalities of therapy, we believe a number of newer concepts are important. These include the mechanical removal of bacteria by irrigation, killing the bacteria in situ with intraperitoneal as well as systemic antibiotics and the removal of adjuvant substances such as fibrin by means of radical peritoneal debridement. The appropriate choice of antibiotics to cover the expected spectrum of bacteria may also decrease the morbidity and mortality of this disease. Attempts to drain the peritoneal cavity, if these principles are followed, should rarely be necessary.

Bibliography

Allen, L.: The peritoneal stomata. Anat. Rec., 1936.

Hau, T., Ahrenholz, D.H. and Simmons, R.L.: Secondary Bacterial Peritonitis: The Biologic Basis of Treatment. Current Problems in Surgery. (In press.)

Hau, T., Hoffman, R. and Simmons, R.L.: Mechanisms of the adjuvant action of hemoglobin in experimental peritonitis. I. *In vivo* inhibition of peritoneal leukocytosis. Surgery 83:223, 1978.

Hudspeth, A.S.: Radical surgical debridement in the treatment of advanced generalized bacterial peritonitis. Arch. Surg. 110:1233, 1975.

Onderdonk, A., Bartlett, J., Louie, T. et al: Microbial synergy in experimental intraabdominal abscesses. Infect. Immun. 13:22, 1976.

Weinstein, W.M., Onderdonk, A.B., Bartlett, J.G. et al: Antimicrobial therapy of experimental intraabdominal sepsis. J. Infect. Dis. 132:282, 1975.

Self-Evaluation Quiz

1. Bacteria are removed from the peritoneal cavity via:
   a) The general peritoneal surface
   b) The visceral peritoneal surface
   c) The lymphatics of the diaphragm exclusively
2. Which of the following substances have been shown to have an adjuvant effect in experimental peritonitis?
   a) Fibrin
   b) Feces
   c) Hemoglobin
   d) All of the above
3. Intraperitoneal saline in experimental peritonitis:
   a) Has no effect
   b) Increases the mortality
   c) Decreases the mortality
4. Heparin in experimental peritonitis:
   a) Increases the mortality
   b) Decreases the mortality
   c) Has no effect

5. What two classes of organisms have been found to act synergistically in intraabdominal infections?
   a) Aerobic and facultative organisms
   b) Anaerobic and facultative organisms
   c) Aerobic and anaerobic organisms
   d) None of the above
6. Which antibiotic(s) would be effective against the expected bacteria in bacterial peritonitis?
   a) Clindamycin
   b) Ampicillin
   c) Tobramycin
   d) All of the above
7. The high incidence of postoperative subdiaphragmatic abscesses after peritonitis probably results from:
   a) Spread of bacteria by the surgeon
   b) The normal upward circulation of peritoneal fluid
   c) Failure to use Fowler's position
8. Fowler's position in the treatment of experimental peritonitis in rats:
   a) Increases mortality
   b) Has no effect on mortality
   c) Decreases mortality
9. The structures through which bacteria apparently are absorbed from the peritoneal cavity are called:
   a) Pinocytotic vesicles
   b) Stomata
   c) Endophagosomes
   d) Canaliculi
10. What antibiotics have been approved by the FDA for irrigation of the peritoneal cavity?
    a) Kanamycin
    b) Cephalothin
    c) Amikacin
    d) a and b

Answers on page 721.

Newer Uses of the Stapler and Some Complications

Mark M. Ravitch, M.D.

Objectives

To be informed about indications for the use of stapling instruments, their limitations, 12 possible reasons for anastomotic leaks when using staples and reports of adverse effects.

We have now had 20 years of experience with the use of stapling instruments in surgery of the gastrointestinal tract and in pulmonary surgery. In any operation involving transection or anastomosis or closure of the gastrointestinal tract, transection of lung substance, or bronchus and pulmonary vessels, we have come to expect that the first line of recourse will be a stapling transection and closure, or anastomosis, the use of manual suturing being reserved for special indications: (a) places difficult or mechanically awkward to reach with the instruments or (b) extremely edematous or thickened tissues which would have to be inordinately compressed, with the risk of subsequent necrosis.

The American manufacturers have recently provided an instrument for performing an inverting, circular, end-to-end anastomosis with the familiar double row of staggered staples. Our experiments ten years ago with the Russian prototype — a significantly less convenient instrument which has the disadvantages, among others, that it places only one row of staples and that the knife, not being replaceable, soon becomes dull — convinced us that an instrument of this kind would fill a real need. The two obvious applications are (1) low ileorectal or

---

Mark M. Ravitch, M.D., Professor and Head, Department of Surgery, Montefiore Hospital, Pittsburgh, Pa.

colorectal anastomoses in which the instrument is inserted through the anus and (2) esophagogastric or esophagojejunal anastomoses after esophagogastrectomy. We have also employed it for the Billroth I reconstruction. The same instrument has already been used, by insertion through a gastrotomy, to resect and staple an esophagogastric collar in the treatment of bleeding esophageal varices.

An additional technique for controlling variceal bleeding with the use of the staplers involves inserting the GIA without the knife blade through a small gastrotomy, high on the lesser curvature, applying it once transversely with one blade inside and one outside the posterior wall, then applying it the same way on the anterior wall.

We use the vascular staple regularly for the hepatic end of the portal vein in end-to-side portocaval anastomoses. The stapler has occasionally been used for stapling the aorta in special situations.

The stapling instruments do not transform an incompetent surgeon into a virtuoso, nor are the instruments foolproof. The instruments must always be properly assembled and loaded. In the TA instruments, the pin must always be driven home, lest tissues escape beyond the staple line, or the jaws not be perfectly aligned so that the staples are malformed and insecure. In the end-to-end instrument, the purse-string sutures must be tied tightly around the stem of the instrument to be sure the staples join the two ends a full 360 degrees. Anastomotic leaks, which occur no more commonly than with manual sutures, may be due to any of the following possibilities: (1) stapling ischemic tissue, (2) stapling diseased tissue, (3) in transecting bowel, failing to insure that the entire width of the bowel (for the EEA-circumference) is in the instrument, (4) in the mucosa-to-mucosa closure of the opening made for insertion of the GIA, failure to be absolutely certain that the lips of the opening are completely beyond the jaws of the TA instrument for the full circumference of the opening, (5) failure to set the pin in the TA instruments, (6) use of the wrong anvil (in the TA 30), (7) use of an expended cartridge, (8) failure to squeeze the handle and drive the staples in, (9) failure to use an anvil (we have seen all of the last three) and (10) inappropriate application of the GIA, (a) allowing two of the pusher rods to slide into one slot in the cartridge, (b) forcing the pusher when it will not yield (this almost always means incorrect mating of the instrument) and (c) failure to check that both halves of the GIA come from the same instrument when there is more than one set in the OR (the halves of the instrument are numbered).

We have never seen bleeding into the peritoneal cavity from TA suture lines, but it has been reported. A spurting bleeder in the edge should be sutured. Bleeding from the lumen side of a GIA anastomosis occasionally occurs; for that reason, the anastomosis should always be inspected before the GIA opening is closed and a fine catgut stitch placed in the occasional situation in which a spurter is present.

The TA and GIA instruments for anastomosis can be said to do at least as well as conventional manual techniques in terms of leaks and dehiscence. Early reports with the EEA (end-to-end anastomosis) instrument suggest that it accomplishes low rectal anastomoses more safely than manual sutures.

There has been one report of formation of stones on the staples in an ileal urinary diversion loop. We have not seen this in a series approaching 200 cases.

Self-Evaluation Quiz

1. Manual suturing is reserved for:
   a) Easily reached places
   b) Nonedematous tissue
   c) Extremely thickened tissues
   d) Places that can be inordinately compressed with risk of necrosis
2. The American stapler described in this paper does a:
   a) Semilunar end-to-end anastomosis
   b) Circular end-to-end anastomosis
   c) Circular anastomosis except end-to-end ones
   d) Closure with a single row of staggered staples
3. The stapler has been used for:
   a) High ileorectal anastomosis
   b) Low ileorectal anastomosis
   c) Colorectal anastomosis
   d) Esophagojejunal anastomosis
4. The vascular stapler has been used for:
   a) The hepatic end of the portal vein in end-to-end portocaval anastomosis

b) The aorta
c) Controlling variceal bleeding
d) All of the above

5. Anastomotic leaks cannot be caused by:
   a) Stapling diseased or ischemic tissues
   b) Failure to insure that the entire width of bowel (for EEA-circumference) is in the stapler
   c) Failure to set the pin in the TA instruments or failure to use an anvil
   d) None of the above
6. Anastomosis leaks can be caused by the use of expended cartridges.
   a) True
   b) False
7. Anastomosis leaks can be caused by allowing two of the pusher rods to slide into one slot in the cartridge.
   a) True
   b) False
8. Anastomosis leaks can be caused by forcing the pusher when it will not yield, which indicates:
   a) Empty cartridge
   b) Wrong anvil
   c) Ischemic tissue
   d) Incorrect mating of the instrument

Answers on page 721.

Gastrointestinal Anastomoses: Facts and Fiction

Daniel H. Dunn, M.D. and Henry Buchwald, M.D., Ph.D.

Objectives

The purpose of this review was to evaluate and compare various anastomotic techniques. The everted technique is compared to the inverted technique with respect to dehiscence rate and postoperative morbidity. Experiments using the stapling instruments are discussed. A comparison of the one-layer and two-layer anastomosis is made. An evaluation of catgut and the newer synthetic absorbables, along with Prolene® and nylon, the monofilament non-absorbables, is presented. Finally, basic principles for anastomosis success are reviewed and analyzed.

Introduction

In an address to the Association of Military Surgeons of the National Guard of the United States in 1893, Nicholas Senn stated: "The history of intestinal suture is replete with stupendous ignorance, clever mechanical ingenuity, patient experimental research, and the careful application of pathological knowledge to the treatment of injuries and diseases of the intestinal canal." He went on to prophesy: "We have reason to believe that the technique of intestinal suturing remains an unfinished chapter, and that the ideal method of uniting intestinal wounds has yet to be devised" [1]. These statements could have been made as well yesterday as 85 years ago.

A brief history of the origins and innovations of intestinal suturing techniques will be presented, along with an evaluation and comparison of anastomotic techniques, suture material and the properties of intestinal wound repair.

Daniel H. Dunn, M.D. and Henry Buchwald, M.D., Ph.D., Department of Surgery, University of Minnesota Medical School, Minneapolis.

Historical Overview

The earliest accounts of suturing of the intestine were those of Hippocrates (460 B.C.), Celsus (30 B.C.) and Galen (130 A.D.). Their general admonition was that suturing of the small intestine was always fatal and that only occasionally large intestinal wounds could be sutured to the abdominal wall successfully, thereby creating a permanent cutaneous fistula [1,2]. Few surgical advances were made until Abulkasim (963) introduced the ant-head closure technique in which ants were allowed to bite the everted bowel edge and were then decapitated [2]. Abulkasim was also the first to describe the use of "catgut" suture from sheep intestine. These primitive methods were used for several centuries.

In the 11th century, the practice of surgery became recognized with the teachings of two different groups from Salerno — the so-called four masters and the four monks. They introduced the internal intestinal stent made of various materials to prevent the dreaded complication of intestinal obstruction following intestinal repair. Since spontaneous healing of intestinal wounds occurred occasionally, and most attempts at operative intervention for intestinal trauma failed miserably, conservative treatment for intestinal wounds was recommended for the next several hundred years. Except for an occasional new intestinal stent and variations on telescoping bowel ends into each other, there was little progress in intestinal suturing techniques until the beginning of the 19th century, when Benjamin Travers wrote in 1812 in "An Inquiry Into the Process of Nature in Repairing Injuries of the Intestines" that healing of intestinal wounds was by agglutination of the visceral peritoneum [3]. He was the first to demonstrate experimentally that intestinal wounds would heal without being attached to the abdominal wall.

The concept of healing intestine demonstrated by Travers was used by Lembert in 1826 when he introduced a surgical anastomotic technique which has been utilized to the present day. Lembert is regarded by many as the founder of modern intestinal surgery. At about the same time, Denans used the first mechanical non-suture closure of intestine using a stent and two metal rings to create an inverted non-sutured closure [2]. Several mechanical closures were developed over the next 50 years, including the Murphy button in 1892. Kerr attributes the popularization of intestinal surgery to Murphy: "The necessity of intestinal resection had no terrors for the surgeon who had a button handy" [3].

With the introduction of ether by Long in 1842, elective surgery became feasible [2]. There was a surge of technical advances, the most important of which was the work of Halsted who conclusively demonstrated the importance and strength of the intestinal submucosal layer [4]. The incorporation of the submucosa in an anastomosis for adequate healing has been unchallenged as a basic surgical principle. He also confirmed the prior observations of Travers and Lembert regarding the necessity for coaptation of serosal surfaces for optimal healing. Halsted was a most vociferous proponent of the one-layer anastomosis, which not everyone before or since has agreed with. As there were many variations of the one-layer closure, so too were there multiple techniques for two-layer closures, but the basic principles Halsted demonstrated were applicable to both.

Improvements in anastomotic techniques in the early 1900s centered on attempts to perform intestinal closures aseptically. Ingenious closed anastomotic techniques were developed by Parker and Kerr [5] and by others [2]. Not until after the general use of antibiotics was there a gradual return to the open anastomosis. Side-to-side, end-to-side and variations of end-to-end anastomoses were also introduced in the early 1900s.

Simple intestinal clamps were devised to help the surgeon perform various anastomoses. Changes in bowel clamps led, eventually, to the development of the mechanical stapling devices. Hutl (1914), Von Petz (1924), and recently Ravitch successfully utilized stapling instruments for intestinal anastomoses [2]. Currently, there is an upsurge in the stapling machines available to the surgeon and there is promise of newer and better instruments in the future.

Although there have been alterations in anastomotic techniques over the past several decades, the basic principles taught by Travers, Lembert and Halsted are still sound: (1) incorporation of the submucosal layer in the anastomosis; (2) inversion to provide serosa to serosa healing; (3) performance of anastomosis with as little contamination and trauma as possible; (4)

maintenance of a good blood supply; and (5) avoidance of tension across the anastomosis. If these principles are observed, adequate and rapid healing can be expected.

Evaluation of Anastomotic Techniques

Eversion Vs. Inversion

Anastomotic techniques employing eversion have been advocated including the ant-head closure of Abulkasim [2], the metal clip of Henroz [2] and the gastrointestinal stapling instruments employed by Ravitch [6]. The most avid proponent of the clinical use of the everted technique has been L.C. Getzen [2,7-9]. He has reported clinical results to show that the everted technique can be performed with a low dehiscence rate (1%) and low mortality (0.25%) [9]. His experimental data indicate less anastomotic edema, greater tensile strength and a lower incidence of anastomotic obstruction with an everted as compared to an inverted anastomosis [7].

Few other studies support Getzen's results with an everted technique. In experimental trials comparing the everted with one-layer and two-layer inverted techniques, McAdams et al [10], Mellish [11], Canalis et al [12], Irvin et al [13] and Hamilton [14] have all found a greater spontaneous anastomotic dehiscence rate with the everted technique (Table 1). Experimentally stressing an anastomosis by wrapping with polyethylene plastic accentuates the disparity between the security of the inverted anastomosis as compared to the everted [12,15].

Table 1. Experimental Comparison of the Everted and Inverted Anastomosis

Author	*No. of Animals*	*Dehiscence %*	
		Everted	*Inverted*
McAdams	125	25%	8%
Mellish	79	7%	3%
Ravitch	12/36	17%	3%
Irvin	31/62	54%	4%
Hamilton	25/70	12%	11%

Although Getzen found greater tensile strength with an everted anastomosis, Loeb [16], McAdams [10], Hamilton [14] and Irvin [13] found the opposite to be true. In addition, Ravitch [17] and Abramowitz et al [18] have found delayed mucosal union in the everted anastomosis. Abramowitz et al [18] demonstrated no cross circulation across the everted anastomosis at six weeks but clearly visible vascular communications across the inverted anastomosis at one week.

Perianastomotic colon collagen content measured by Getzen [7] and Irvin [13] were found to be identical with the two types of anastomoses. Since colon collagen content is a sum of the synthesis of new collagen and destruction of old collagen, and the rate of collagen synthesis is affected by inflammation and infection in the area of the anastomosis, it is difficult to understand why the greater amount of inflammation with inverted anastomoses, as seen by Ravitch [17] and Getzen [9], does not retard healing and collagen synthesis.

The coup-de-grace for the everted colon anastomosis was administered by Goligher et al [19]. In a prospective clinical trial comparing the everted and the two-layer inverted techniques, 43% of everted colonic anastomoses (15 of 35) dehisced and were complicated by overt fecal fistulas, while 8.6% (3 of 35) inverted colonic anastomoses were associated with fecal fistulas. Their original trial was to include 100 patients but the trial was discontinued after 70 patients because of the gross disparity between the two techniques. The authors concluded that the everted technique for the large intestine should not be used in clinical practice. The available data show little to recommend the everted anastomosis in any gastrointestinal anastomosis anywhere in the gut.

Inversion Vs. Stapling

Stapled gastrointestinal anastomoses have become popular and well accepted in the past decade, primarily through the work of Ravitch et al [6,20]. Although the stapling instruments have been utilized for practically every conceivable gastrointestinal anastomosis, they have not been subjected to the same scrutiny as have the other anastomotic techniques. Many surgeons are awaiting reports from their colleagues on dehiscence rates with the use of these instruments before employing them. Others are reticent to use the instruments because of the partial eversion of mucosa which they require.

In Dr. J. P. Delaney's laboratory, we (DHD) have tested the thoraco-abdominal (T-A) stapling instrument (U.S. Surgical Corporation) in common use today for end-to-end triangular gastrointestinal anastomoses. Colon anastomosis using the T-A instrument was compared to the one-layer inverted colonic anastomosis in 12 dogs. Both anastomoses were performed in the same dog, in either the left or the right colon, with alternate proximal and distal positioning. Both anastomoses were "stressed" by wrapping circumferentially with a 5-cm-wide strip of polyethylene sheet secured in position with sutures. No antibiotics were used. Six of the 12 everted stapled anastomoses dehisced; none of the inverted hand-sutured anastomoses leaked ($p < .05$) (Table 2). Three of the stapled anastomoses which dehisced had fistulas at the junction of the everted and inverted staple lines. In one stapled anastomosis, the everted staple lines had completely separated while the inverted staple line was intact.

To answer the question whether the staples or the mucosal eversion caused the breakdown, we compared the stapled anastomosis with the hand-sutured everted anastomosis. The experimental protocol with "stressing" was the same. Nine of ten hand-sewn everted suture lines dehisced, while two stapled anastomoses leaked (Table 3). Thus, once again, the predisposition of the everted anastomosis to break down, especially if stressed, was demonstrated. The reason for the lower rate of dehiscence of the paired stapled anastomoses in the second experiment could well have been due to the rapidity of

Table 2. Dehiscence Rate of Stapled and Sutured Wrapped Colon Anastomoses

Position	*Everted Stapled*	*Inverted Sutured*
Proximal	4	0
Distal	2	0
Total	6/12	0/12

Table 3. Dehiscence Rate of Stapled and Sutured Wrapped Colon Anastomoses

	Everted	
Position	*Stapled*	*Sutured*
Proximal	1	4
Distal	1	5
Total	2/10	9/10

breakdown of the hand-sutured anastomoses, affording insufficient time to demonstrate a leak in the stapled anastomoses.

The fact that the everting stapler has been used with such success when experimental data would predict that it would fail is probably due to several factors. First, any anastomotic technique will work most of the time if basic surgical principles are followed. Second, although there is often bleeding through the staple line after the staples have been placed indicating a noncrushing application by the stapler, the mucosa may be injured and crushed enough so that it sloughs and the anastomosis becomes, in essence, an end-on instead of an everted anastomosis.

The new End-to-End Anastomoses (EEA) Stapling Instrument (U.S. Surgical Corporation) incorporates the use of the staples in a circumferential fashion with an inverted serosa-to-serosa closure. This instrument has been used primarily for low rectal anastomoses. In early clinical reports, this instrument promises to be useful [21]. We (DHD) tested this instrument against the one-layer hand-sewn inverted anastomosis in ten dogs, using the same protocol as for the other experiments. Since this instrument must be used intraluminally, we passed the instrument through a colotomy, completed the stapled anastomosis and then used the colotomy for our sutured anastomosis. One stapled anastomosis leaked and one hand-sewn suture line leaked. It was concluded that the inverting stapler produces an anastomosis which is widely patent, uniform and secure.

One-Layer Vs. Two-Layer

Halsted recommended a one-layer intestinal closure based on experimental data and felt that a two-layer closure was less secure and more dangerous. Despite his admonitions, the two-layer closure for gastrointestinal surgery has become firmly entrenched. A survey of members of the Southern Surgical Association in 1966 revealed an overwhelming preference for a two-layer closure of both stomach and colon [22]. Recent experimental and clinical experience with the Gambee [23], one-layer inverted (Halsted) [24] and two-layer [25] intestinal closures indicates that surgeons could well reappraise their reasons for their anastomotic preferences.

Several authors (Abramowitz et al [18], Hamilton [14], McAdams et al [10], Irvin et al [13], Canalis et al [12] and Loeb [16]) have shown no difference in the experimental dehiscence rate of Gambee, one-layer or two-layer intestinal closures (Table 4). These authors, as well as Sako and Wangensteen [26], have demonstrated equal, or a slightly increased, anastomotic bursting pressure of the two-layer technique when compared to the other techniques. Collagen content [24], microvascularity [18] and adhesion formation [14] were also found to be similar with all three techniques. Anastomotic stenosis, edema and inflammation were increased after two-layer closure, compared to the one-layer (Halsted) and Gambee anastomoses. The Gambee technique was associated with very little inversion of tissue and thus minimal stenosis. Healing, as judged by intestinal continuity at the anastomosis, was most rapid with an end-on technique (Gambee), followed by the Halsted. Slower resorption of the two-layer inverted cuff was usually observed; but the cuff was barely detectable at 30 days [26].

Table 4. Experimental Comparison of the One-Layer, Two-Layer and Gambee Suture Techniques

Author	*No. of Animals*	*Dehiscence %*		
		One-Layer	*Two-Layer*	*Gambee*
Hamilton	70	14	17	10
McAdams	103	–	15	23
Irvin	78	4	4	–
Canalis	36	0	0	–
Loeb*	28	0	0*	0

*Anastomotic bursting pressure tested and found two-layer technique to be the strongest.

Thus, experimental results indicate no dehiscence, or leak rate, advantage of the two-layer anastomosis over one-layer or end-on techniques. Microscopically, the one-layer or Gambee has less edema and inflammation, as well as faster resorption of inverted cuff and less anastomotic stenosis than the two-layer technique.

Irvin et al [24] conducted the first prospective randomized clinical trial comparing single-layer with two-layer intestinal closure (Table 5). They found no difference in dehiscence rates between the two methods. Everett [25] conducted a similar study but included only colorectal anastomoses: 17% of one-layer "high" (H) colon anastomoses leaked, compared to 16% for two-layer. There was a significantly lower dehiscence rate with a one-layer low (L) rectal anastomosis (9%), compared with the two-layer (50%). Bronwell et al [22] found comparable colonic dehiscence rates with both techniques. Matheson and Irving [27] had a 6% dehiscence rate of one-layer colorectal anastomoses in 52 consecutive patients with only one of 15 low rectal anastomoses showing demonstrable dehiscence. Gambee et al [23], after 163 colon anastomoses, had an 8.6% dehiscence rate. Beling [28] performed 60 single-layer intestinal closures with no leaks and Heifetz [29] showed no difference between one- and two-layer colon anastomoses in complications or mortality.

Several authors have shown less morbidity in terms of postoperative ileus following one-layer anastomosis compared to two-layer. In Bronwell's series [22] 72% of patients with

Table 5. Clinical Evaluation of One- and Two-Layer Intestinal Anastomoses

Authors	*No. of Patients*	*% Dehiscence One-Layer*	*% Dehiscence Two-Layer*
Goligher	60	17	16
Everett	(H) 67	17	16
	(L) 25	9	50
Bronwell	95/41*	0	10
Matheson	52	6	–
Gambee	163	8	–
Beling	60	0	–

*Ninety-five one-layer, 41 two-layer closures.

one-layer colon anastomoses had passed flatus and stool by the fourth postoperative day, in comparison to only 35% after two-layer. Forty-two percent of patients could be fed on the third postoperative day after single layer closure, as opposed to 10% after two-layer.

Similar extensive studies have not been performed on the small bowel or esophagus. However, Collis [30] has found the one-layer esophageal anastomosis to be very satisfactory, with no leaks in 100 consecutive esophageal anastomoses.

To summarize, there are extensive experimental and clinical data to support the use of a one-layer intestinal closure. The dehiscence rate for intestinal anastomoses, other than low rectal, are similar for the one- and two-layer closures. There may be less postoperative morbidity with the one-layer. For the low rectal anastomosis, there is a significantly lower leak rate with a single layer closure when compared to a two-layer.

On the other hand, for an even-handed appraisal, one must state that the experienced surgeon can perform as meticulous a two-layer as a one-layer anastomosis, and the two-layer closure has the advantage of visual assurance of hemostasis, which is absent in the closed one-layer techniques. We have seen serious anastomotic bleeds after closed one-layer anastomoses but, it must be added, this is a rarity.

Suture Materials

Absorbable: Synthetic and Catgut

"Gut" suture was first used by Abulkasim in 963 A.D. This suture material has remained popular for gastrointestinal operations through the years. Recently, synthetic absorbable suture materials have been developed which appear to be superior to catgut in tensile strength, tissue reaction, uniformity of dissolution and resistance to proteolytic degradation. Devaney and Way [31] measured the dissolution of plain and chromic catgut, Dexon® (Davis and Geck) and Vicryl® (Ethicon), in vivo and in vitro. There was no dissolution of Dexon® or Vicryl® in 17 days in solutions of pepsin, acid or gastric juice, while plain catgut lasted 3 to 29 hours and chromic catgut dissolved in one to nine days. With in vivo studies early and unpredictable absorption of both plain and chromic catgut sutures in stomach, small intestine and colon was demonstrated. The synthetic absorbables did not dissolve for three to four weeks in any portion of the gastrointestinal tract. Craig et al [32] reported uniform absorption of both Dexon® and Vicryl®, with 100% of the suture material remaining at 40 days and complete dissolution at 90 and 120 days, respectively.

The reason for the differences between catgut and the synthetic absorbable materials can be explained by their biochemical make-up. Catgut is an animal protein that dissolves by action of proteolytic enzymes. Polyglycolic acid (Dexon®) is a polyester of glycolic acid and Polyglactin 910 (Vicryl®) is a co-polymer of glycolide and lactide. These synthetic materials are not affected by proteolytic enzymes but dissolve by hydrolysis, which occurs at the same rate in all tissues. Because of this difference in biochemical structure, the dissolution of catgut is associated with more inflammation than Dexon® or Vicryl®.

The initial tensile strength of Dexon® and Vicryl® are comparable [32]. After 14 days tensile strength for both is reduced by 50%. Polyglycolic acid suture is considerably stronger than silk, polypropylene, merseline or chromic catgut [33]. Herman [34] and Howes [35] found that the synthetic absorbable suture is superior to catgut in knot security and wet tensile strength. Laufman and Rubel [36], in an extensive review, found the synthetics to be superior to catgut not only in tensile strength but in lack of tissue reactivity and resistance to infection.

The clinical use of synthetic absorbable suture material has increased and synthetics are now being used extensively to replace catgut and in some situations even in place of nonabsorbable suture. Clark et al [37] found a significantly lower rate of colonic anastomotic dehiscence with a polyglycolic acid suture compared to catgut for the inner row of a two-layer anastomosis. Certain plastic, orthopedic, gynecologic, ophthalmic and urologic surgeons have been favorably impressed with the clinical use of the synthetic absorbable sutures [36].

An additional factor that should be considered in the choice of catgut suture is the type of sterilization used in processing the catgut. Ethicon irradiates catgut, which is the least traumatic to the protein content. Other processes, such as heat sterilization or ethylene oxide impregnation, have adverse effects on catgut [38].

Can anything be said in favor of catgut? It is smoother than the synthetics and passes through tissue with greater ease. Thus, in the first part of a Parker-Kerr type closure, the "slippery" quality of catgut is preferable to the tearing or tissue resistance offered by the synthetics.

Nonabsorbable: Silk, Polypropylene, Nylon

Silk has been the standard nonabsorbable suture to which others have been compared. Most surgeons who use silk feel that it has a special "feel" or "handle." There is no question that immeasurable subjective qualities of suture material are important to the surgeon. Many are willing to accept more tissue inflammatory reaction, less tensile strength, stitch abscesses and delayed sinus tract formation in order to be a "silk" surgeon. Postlethwait [39] demonstrated that silk lost 50% of its original tensile strength by one year and had very little strength at two years. To be fair, there are certain advantages to silk. It slides through tissue easily and ties securely with two to three knots; whereas, some of the monofilament sutures require up to six to eight throws to prevent knot slippage.

Polypropylene (Prolene®) and nylon are very similar, synthetic, nonabsorbable, inert suture materials. Although tensile strength is not as great as some of the other nonabsorbable materials, they cause very little tissue reaction. They are recommended for both routine use and in contaminated wounds because of their resistance to infection [40]. Morphologic studies of the use of Prolene® in large intestine show no submucosal distortion and almost no inflammatory reaction [41] (Fig. 1). Some surgeons hesitate to use these materials because of knot slippage. Five to seven throws are usually necessary to be assured of a secure knot. The properties of Prolene® are similar if not identical with monofilament nylon. Several authors have suggested that it is the monofilament structure of the suture rather than the specific synthetic nature of the material that is most important. Braided or twisted suture material provides interstices for bacteria, fibrin deposition and resultant infection [42] (Fig. 2).

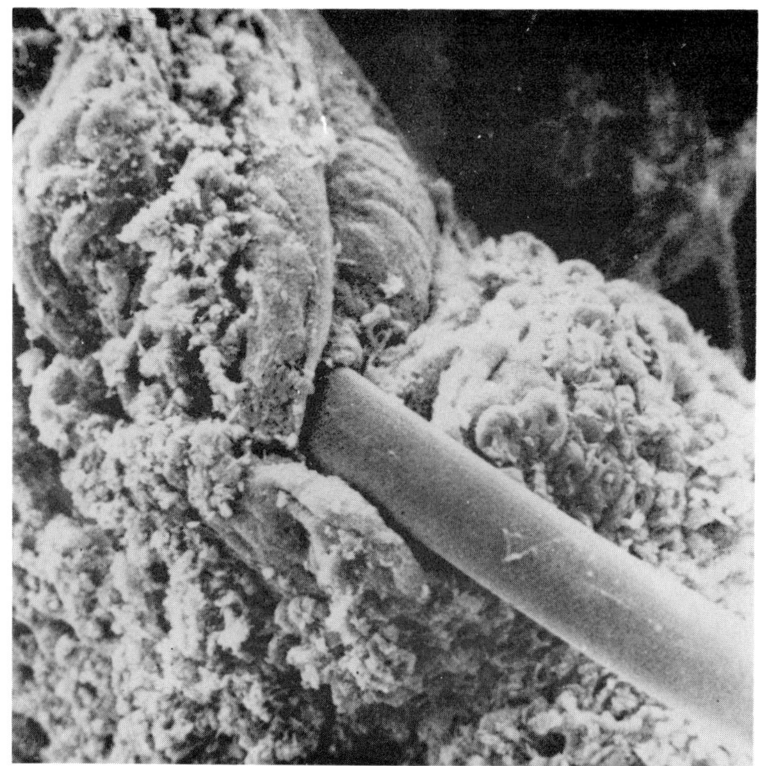

FIG. 1. Electron micrograph of Prolene® suture through colonic submucosa. (From Lord et al [41].)

Properties of Intestinal Wound Repair

Collagen is the basis for intestinal wound repair and anastomotic tensile strength. Healing is the summation of collagen lysis and synthesis. It is the balance of these critical processes which determines the resistance of an anastomosis to dehiscence. Hunt and Hawley [43] have reported several factors which may influence the rate of collagen synthesis and lysis. Malnutrition has been shown to decrease the tensile strength of wounds in experimental animals [44]. Infection and inflammation increase collagen lysis in experimental skin wounds and, probably, in anastomoses [45]. Steroids have a profound effect on collagen cross-linkage in all parts of the body and have a demonstrable effect on anastomotic healing [43,44]. Trauma,

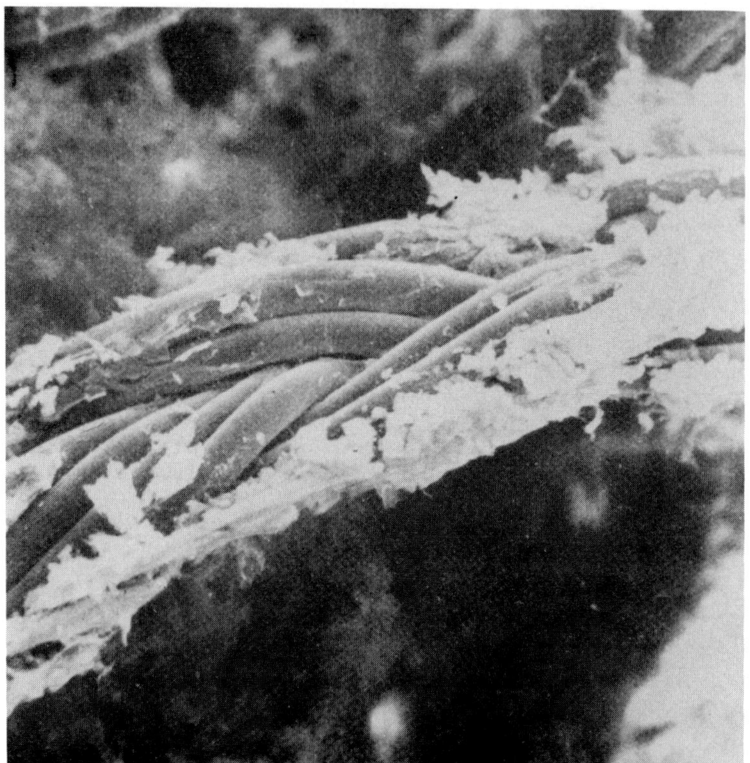

FIG. 2. Braided suture material providing interstices for bacterial growth and fibrin deposition. (From Lord et al [41].)

both local and distant, has been related to decreased tissue tensile strength [46-48]. Interstitial edema has been demonstrated to decrease the healing properties of wounds, irrespective of the hypoproteinemia which often accompanies an edematous state [49].

To understand why collagen is so important in wound healing a basic understanding of wound repair is necessary. Several investigators have divided normal wound healing into three phases [50,51]. The first phase is the latent or lag phase. In the colon this usually lasts three to four days after injury. During this period debris, infected material and necrotic tissue are cleared from the area. Collagenase is released from the bowel wall and also from colonic bacteria [52]. Collagen lysis begins almost immediately after injury. Collagenase activity is not restricted to the wound but extends more than 3 cm from the cut edge [53]. If collagen lysis is stimulated excessively by various factors, such as infection or inflammation, then the homeostatic mechanism for providing adequate tissue strength will be impaired. The collagenolytic response to injury is more important in the colon than in the rest of the gastrointestinal tract because the collagenase enzyme is present in the greatest concentration in the colon [52]. For this reason, perhaps, colonic anastomoses are more prone to disrupt.

While old collagen is being lysed, new collagen is being synthesized. Previously, the synthesis of collagen was believed to start on the third day following injury [53]. Now, by use of more sophisticated techniques collagen synthesis has been shown to begin almost immediately after injury [54]. The net effect of this synthesis is that total collagen stays the same, or decreases only slightly, through the first three days after injury. It then increases dramatically until at 14 days the collagen content stabilizes [54]. If the period (five to ten days) for rapid increase in collagen content is delayed, the anastomosis is susceptible to disruption. Any process which delays the "lag" phase of healing will increase the chances for anastomotic dehiscence. The sutures are the only thing holding the bowel together during this period.

The second phase of healing is characterized by fibroplasia, vascular ingrowth, capillary endothelial proliferation and deposition of collagen exceeding collagen lysis. During this period there is a rapid increase in the tensile strength of the anastomosis. When this phase begins is a function of the lag phase; however, day three to five is average. By the end of the second phase, the bowel wall will burst before the anastomosis with the application of high intraluminal pressures.

The final phase of intestinal healing is the remodeling phase, in which the collagen fibers are lined up in the lines of stress. Anastomotic edema is completely cleared and cicatrization plateaus. Tissue tensile strength continues to increase for three months to one year.

One of the major influences on intestinal healing is, of course, the blood supply to the injured tissue [43]. Contrary to popular belief, Delaney and Custer [55] have shown a greater

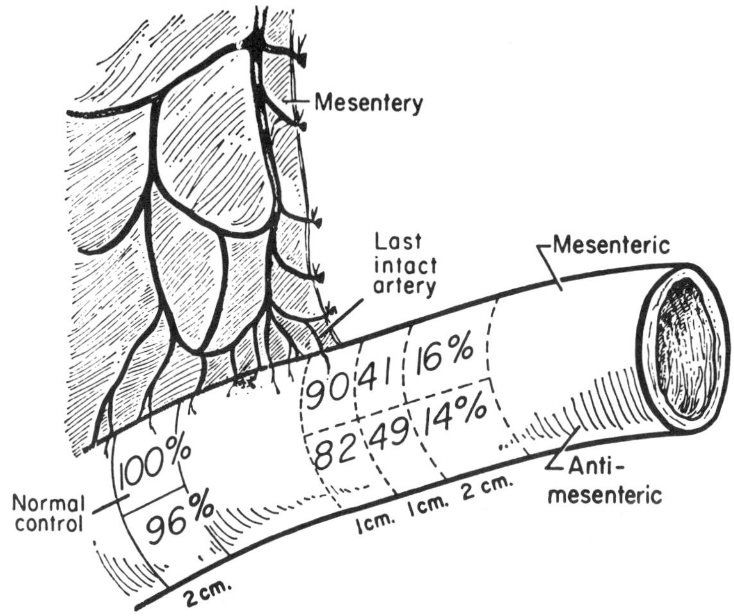

FIG. 3. Blood flow to a devascularized segment of canine small bowel demonstrating equal blood flow to mesenteric and antimesenteric border. (From Delaney and Grim [56].)

blood flow (per gram of tissue) to the colon than to the small intestine in the dog, indicating that decreased colonic blood supply is not the critical factor contributing to the higher incidence of colonic dehiscence in comparison to small bowel disruptions. They also demonstrated that the antimesenteric border receives the same percentage of blood flow as the mesteric [56] (Fig. 3).

In summary, anastomotic healing is affected by many factors, the most important of which are trauma, infection, inflammation, tension across the anastomosis and failure to maintain good blood supply to the healing tissue. If these factors are avoided or minimized, normal healing should occur.

References

1. Senn, N.: Enterorraphy: Its history, technique and present status. JAMA 21:215, 1893.

2. Getzen, L.C.: Intestinal Suturing. I. The development of intestinal sutures. Curr. Probl. Surg., August 1969.
3. Kerr, H.H.: The development of intestinal surgery. JAMA 81:641, 1923.
4. Halsted, W.S.: Circular suture of the intestine — an experimental study. Am. J. Med. Sci. 94:436, 1887.
5. Parker, E.M. and Kerr, H.: Intestinal anastomosis without open incisions by means of basting stitches. Bull. Johns Hopkins Hosp. 19:132, 1908.
6. Ravitch, M.M. and Steichen, F.M.: Technics of staple suturing in the gastrointestinal tract. Ann. Surg. 175:815, 1972.
7. Getzen, L.C. and Holloway, C.K.: Comparative study of intestinal anastomotic healing in inverted and everted closures. Surg. Gynecol. Obstet. 123:1219, 1966.
8. Getzen, L.C.: Clinical use of everted intestinal anastomoses. Surg. Gynecol. Obstet. 123:1027, 1966.
9. Getzen, L.C.: Intestinal suturing. II. Inverting and everting intestinal sutures. Curr. Probl. Surg., September 1969.
10. McAdams, A.J., Merkle, G. and Medina, R.: An experimental comparison of inversion and eversion colonic anastomoses. Dis. Colon Rectum 12:1, 1969.
11. Mellish, R.W.: Inverting or everting sutures for bowel anastomoses. An experimental study. J. Ped. Surg. 1:260, 1966.
12. Canalis, F. and Ravitch, M.: Study of healing of inverting and everting intestinal anastomoses. Surg. Gynecol. Obstet. 127:109, 1968.
13. Irvin, T.T. and Edwards, J.P.: Comparison of single layer inverting, two-layer inverting, and everting anastomoses in the rabbit colon. J. Surg. 60:453, 1973.
14. Hamilton, J.E.: Reappraisal of open intestinal anastomoses. Ann. Surg. 165:917, 1967.
15. Rusca, J.A., Bornside, G.H. and Cohn, I.: Everting versus inverting gastrointestinal anastomoses: Bacterial leakage and anastomotic disruption. Ann. Surg. 169:727, 1969.
16. Loeb, M.J.: Comparative strength of inverted, everted, and end-on intestinal anastomoses. Surg. Gynecol. Obstet. 125:301, 1967.
17. Ravitch, M.: Observations on the healing of wounds of the intestines. Surgery 77:665, 1975.
18. Abramowitz, H.B. and McAlister, W.H.: A comparative study of small bowel anastomoses by angiography and microangiography. Surgery 66:564, 1969.
19. Goligher, J.C., Morris, C., McAdam, A.F. et al: A controlled trial of inverting vs. everting intestinal suture in clinical large-bowel surgery. Br. J. Surg. 57:817, 1970.
20. Ravitch, M., Lane, R., Cornell, W.P. et al: Closure of duodenal, gastric, and intestinal stumps with wire staples: Experimental and clinical studies. Ann. Surg. 163:573, 1966.
21. Fain, S.N., Patin, C.S. and Morgenstern, L.: Use of a mechanical suturing apparatus in low colorectal anastomosis. Arch. Surg. 110:1079, 1975.

22. Bronwell, A.W., Rutlege, R. and Dalton, M.L.: Single layer open gastrointestinal anastomosis. Ann. Surg. 165:925, 1967.
23. Gambee, L.P., Gannjobst, W. and Hardwick, C.: Ten years' experience with a single layer anastomosis in colon surgery. Am. J. Surg. 92:222, 1956.
24. Irvin, T.T., Goligher, J.C. and Johnston, D.: A randomized prospective clinical trial of single-layer and two-layer inverting intestinal anastomoses. Br. J. Surg. 60:457, 1973.
25. Everett, W.G.: A comparison of one-layer and two-layer techniques for colorectal anastomosis. Br. J. Surg. 62:135, 1975.
26. Sako, Y. and Wangensteen, O.H.: Experimental studies on gastrointestinal anastomoses. Surg. Forum 3:117, 1952.
27. Matheson, N.A. and Irving, A.D.: Single layer anastomosis after rectosigmoid resection. Br. J. Surg. 62:239, 1975.
28. Beling, C.A.: Single layer end-to-end intestinal anastomosis. Am. J. Gast. 27:374, 1957.
29. Heifetz, C.J.: Technique of single layer end-to-end intestinal anastomosis by triangulation. Surg. Clin. North Am. 46:223, 1966.
30. Collis, J.L.: Surgical treatment of carcinoma of the esophagus and cardia. Br. J. Surg. 58:801, 1971.
31. Devaney, K.E. and Way, L.W.: Effect of different absorbable sutures on healing of gastrointestinal anastomoses. Am. J. Surg. 133:86, 1977.
32. Craig, P.H., William, J.A., Davis, K.W. et al: A biological comparison of polyglactin 910 and polyglycolic acid synthetic absorbable sutures. Surg. Gynecol. Obstet. 141:1, 1975.
33. Marchant, L., Knapp, S., Braun, H. and Apter, J.T.: Effect of elongation rate or the percentage elongation of surgical suture materials. Surg. Gynecol. Obstet. 139:389, 1974.
34. Herman, J.B.: Tensile strength and knot security of surgical suture materials. Am. Surg. 37:209, 1971.
35. Howes, E.L.: Strength studies of polyglycolic acid versus catgut sutures of the same size. Surg. Gynecol. Obstet. 137:15, 1973.
36. Laufman, H. and Rubel, T.: Synthetic absorbable sutures. Surg. Gynecol. Obstet. 145:597, 1977.
37. Clark, C.G., Harris, J., Elmasni, S. et al: Polyglycolic acid sutures and catgut in colonic anastomoses. Lancet 2:1006, 1972.
38. VanWinkle, W. and Hastings, J.C.: Considerations in the choice of suture material for various tissues. Surg. Gynecol. Obstet. 135:113, 1972.
39. Postlethwait, E.W.: Long-term comparative study of nonabsorbable sutures. Ann. Surg. 171:892, 1970.
40. Usher, F.C., Allen, J.E., Crosthwart, R.W. and Cogen, J.E.: Polypropylene monofilament, a new biologically inert suture for closing contaminated wounds. JAMA 179:780, 1962.
41. Lord, M.G., Broughton, A.C. and Williams, H.T.G.: A morphologic study on the effect of suturing the submucosa of the large intestine. Surg. Gynecol. Obstet. 146:211, 1978.

42. Everett, W.G.: Suture materials in general surgery. Progr. Surg. 8:14, 1970.
43. Hunt, T.K. and Hawley, P.R.: Surgical judgment and colonic anastomoses. Dis. Colon Rectum 12:167, 1969.
44. Findlay, C.W. and Howes, E.L.: Combined effect of cortisone and partial protein depletion on wound healing. N. Engl. J. Med. 246:597, 1952.
45. Smith, M. and Enquist, I.F.: A quantitative study of impaired healing resulting from infection. Surg. Gynecol. Obstet. 125:965, 1967.
46. Dunphy, J.E.: The effect of local trauma on repair by connective tissue. Bull. Soc. Int. Chir. 22:121, 1963.
47. Irvin, T.T. and Hunt, T.K.: The effect of trauma on colonic healing. Br. J. Surg. 61:430, 1974.
48. Irvin, T.T. and Hunt, T.K.: Pathogenesis and prevention of disruption of colonic anastomoses in traumatized rats. Br. J. Surg. 61:437, 1974.
49. Rhoades, J.E., Fliegelman, M.T. and Panzer, L.M.: The mechanism of delayed wound healing in the presence of hypoproteinemia. JAMA 118:21, 1942.
50. Carrel, A.: Cicatrization of wounds. XII. Factors initiating regeneration. J. Exp. Med. 34:425, 1921.
51. Edwards, L.C. and Dunphy, J.E.: Wound healing. I. Injury and normal repair. N. Engl. J. Med. 259:224, 1958.
52. Hawley, P.R., Faulk, W.P., Hunt, T.K. and Dunphy, J.E.: Collagenase activity in the gastrointestinal tract. Br. J. Surg. 57:896, 1970.
53. Cronin, K., Jackson, D.S. and Dunphy, J.E.: Changing bursting strength and collagen content of the healing colon. Surg. Gynecol. Obstet. 126:747, 1968.
54. Irvin, T.T. and Hunt, T.K.: Reappraisal of the healing process of anastomosis of the colon. Surg. Gynecol. Obstet. 138:741, 1974.
55. Delaney, J.P. and Custer, J.: Gastrointestinal blood flow in the dog. Circ. Res. 17:394, 1965.
56. Delaney, J.P. and Grim, E.: Collateral blood flow to a devascularized segment of the small intestine. Surg. Gynecol. Obstet. 116:494, 1963.

Self-Evaluation Quiz

1. Most experiments demonstrate the everted anastomotic technique to be superior to the inverted.
   a) True
   b) False
2. Chromic catgut is similar to Dexon® and Vicryl® in breaking strength.
   a) True
   b) False
3. Everett has shown the one-layer inverting technique to have a lower dehiscence rate than the two-layer inverted for low rectal anastomoses.

a) True
b) False

4. Dexon® and Vicryl®:
   a) Dissolve by hydrolysis
   b) Are not dissolved by pancreatic enzymes
   c) Are stronger than several nonabsorbable sutures
   d) All of the above
5. Arrange the anastomotic techniques according to their resistance to leakage — (a) one-layer inverted; (b) one-layer everted; (c) everted stapled:
   a) a, b, c
   b) a, c, b,
   c) c, b, a
   d) c, a, b
6. The clinical success of the T-A stapling instrument may be due to the fact that it creates an end-on anastomosis.
   a) True
   b) False
7. Halstead established the submucosa as the single strongest layer of the intestine.
   a) True
   b) False

Answers on page 721.

Current Status of Carcinoembryonic Antigen (CEA) in Gastrointestinal Malignancy

Donald R. Lannin, M.D. and Charles F. McKhann, M.D.

Objectives

After completion of this paper, the reader should be able to objectively assess in which situations, if any, a carcinoembryonic antigen determination can influence clinical patient care. The initial optimism and subsequent disappointing development of carcinoembryonic antigen will be reviewed briefly. A few situations where CEA may still have clinical usefulness will be discussed.

Introduction

Carcinoembryonic antigen (CEA) was described in 1965 by Gold and Freedman as a cell differentiation antigen which is present in the embryonic gastrointestinal tract, disappears in normal adult tissue but then reappears because of dedifferentiation in some colonic tumors [1-4]. It was characterized as a glycoprotein with a molecular weight of about 200,000. Because its presence in the adult was initially felt to be associated only with colorectal carcinoma, it was widely heralded as a "tumor specific" antigen and it was optimistically hoped that CEA would be useful as a screening test for cancer. Since the development of a sensitive radioimmunoassay by Thomson in 1969, and particularly since the licensing of a commercial test kit by Hoffman-La Roche Company in 1973, the test has been widely applied both in the United States and abroad. Unfortunately, greater experience has failed to confirm the initial reports of specific association with colorectal

---

Donald R. Lannin, M.D. and Charles F. McKhann, M.D., Department of Surgery, University of Minnesota Hospital, Minneapolis.

carcinoma and we now know that the test has neither sufficient sensitivity nor sufficient specificity to be generally useful as a screening test for cancer.

Table 1 has been compiled from several large series [1,5], including two major multicenter cooperative studies, and summarizes the best information to date regarding the incidence of elevated CEA in various conditions. Several points are noteworthy: (1) The level of CEA in normal people depends strongly upon smoking history. Whereas the incidence of elevated CEA in nonsmokers is only 3%, the incidence in heavy smokers is 19% and the incidence in a population unselected for smoking history is 11%. (2) CEA is elevated in a wide variety of nonmalignant diseases and in many different types of cancers. Therefore, elevated CEA is not at all specific for colon carcinoma. (3) Elevated CEA in colon cancer is related to the stage of the disease. Therefore, although the overall incidence of elevated CEA in colorectal cancer is 72% to 81%, the incidence in a Duke's A lesion is only 38% to 44%. Unfortunately, to be useful as a screening test it is exactly these early lesions that one would hope to detect. The reason the early studies on CEA showed such high sensitivity for colon cancer was because the cases consisted mostly of advanced metastatic disease. Thus we can see from Table 1 that if the CEA test were to be used as a screening test for colorectal cancer, the overall number of false-negatives would be 20% to 30%. The number of false-positives would be about 10% in healthy patients, under ideal circumstances, but much higher if the patients had concomitant disease. The test is therefore not applicable as a routine screening test.

The question now is, does the test have any clinical usefulness at all? The ultimate role of CEA in evaluating clinical disease is not yet clear. After the disappointing realization that it is not suitable for screening, investigators are now trying to assess objectively whether it might have other benefits. Four possible uses are described.

Diagnostic Adjunct

Although the CEA test is not useful for routine screening of asymptomatic patients, it has been suggested that it may help make the diagnosis in patients where cancer is already sus-

Table 1. Circulating CEA Levels in Various Conditions*

Clinical Status	% Elevated CEA
Normal	
Healthy, unselected	11
Healthy, nonsmokers	3
Healthy, smokers	19
Healthy, pregnant	3
Nonmalignant diseases	
Alcoholic cirrhosis of liver	70
Alcohol addiction	65
Pulmonary emphysema	57
Kidney transplant	56
Pancreatitis	53
Granulomatous colitis	47
Pneumonia	46
Gastric ulcer	45
Ulcerative colitis	31
Malignant diseases	
Colorectum, all stages	72–81
Dukes' A	38–44
Dukes' B	60–76
Dukes' C	60–75
Metastasized	80–89
Stomach	61
Pancreas	91
Breast	47
Lung	76
Prostate	40
Bladder	42
Gynecologic	65
Lymphomas	35
Acute and chronic leukemias	37

*Compiled from results in Hansen et al (1974), Reynoso et al (1972), Laurence et al (1972), LoGerfo et al (1971), Hall et al (1973), Laurence and Neville (1972), Khoo (1974) and Martin et al (1976). (From Goldenberg [1].)

pected. If we assume a false-positive rate of 20% and a false-negative rate of 30% and apply the test to a selected population where the prevalence of colorectal cancer is 50%, that is, where each patient has a 50-50 chance of having cancer, the numbers work out such that those patients with a positive CEA have a 77% incidence of cancer whereas those patients with a negative CEA have only a 27% incidence of cancer. Therefore, the test does give diagnostic information. However, it must be stressed that a negative CEA in no way rules out cancer and a positive CEA does not make the diagnosis. Therefore, in any situation where carcinoma is strongly suspected the clinician will probably use every other diagnostic aid available; it remains to be seen whether CEA will give any additional useful information.

It is not yet clear in which specific clinical situations CEA may provide helpful diagnostic information. One example that has been suggested is pancreatic carcinoma. We see from Table 1 that pancreatic carcinoma has a very high incidence of elevated CEA — over 90%. This disease is notoriously difficult to diagnose and is rarely recognized early. In one study [6] CEA was more frequently positive than any other diagnostic tests including upper gastrointestinal series, hypotonic duodenography, celiac arteriography, and percutaneous transhepatic cholangiography. However, it should also be noted that the incidence of CEA elevation is also very high (about 50%) in pancreatitis and other benign diseases. It is clear that additional studies are necessary before we can determine whether CEA will have any ultimate role as a diagnostic adjunct.

Prognosis

Another suggested use for CEA is that it may provide information regarding the prognosis of a patient undergoing resection for colorectal carcinoma. We can see from Table 1 that the incidence of elevated CEA preoperatively correlates well with the Duke's Stage of the tumor. Therefore, the more advanced tumors do have a higher percentage of elevated CEA. Herrera et al [7] correlated the preoperative CEA levels with the chance of ultimate recurrence. Figure 1 shows his results. Forty-six patients who underwent a curative resection for colorectal cancer were followed and 23 of them developed a

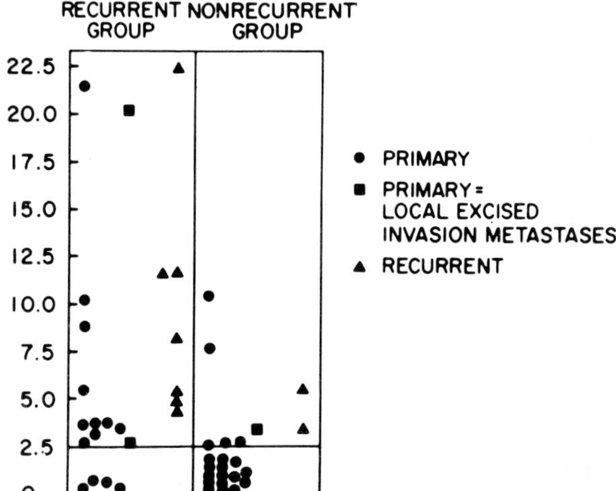

FIG. 1. Nineteen of 23 patients who developed recurrence had CEA values above 2.5 ng/ml as opposed to 8 among the 23 control patients. (From Herrera [7].)

recurrence. Of the 23 who recurred, 19 had elevated preoperative CEA levels, whereas of the 23 who did not recur, only 8 had elevated CEA. Furthermore, an initial CEA value greater than 4.5 ng/ml predicted a greater than 80% chance of recurrence within 18 months of resection. Therefore, it appears that the initial CEA level is about as good as pathological staging in predicting the likelihood of recurrence. It has been proposed that as successful adjuvant chemotherapy programs are developed, CEA may be a good indicator of which patients would most benefit from adjuvant chemotherapy.

The initial postoperative CEA level also may indicate prognosis. Several studies have suggested that a return of the CEA to the normal range correlates with the completeness of surgical resection. Figure 2 shows the results of Mach et al [8]. Patients who had metastases or an incomplete surgical resection usually had no change in postoperative CEA levels. When the surgeon felt the resection was macroscopically complete, however, 40 out of 45 patients had a fall of CEA levels to normal limits. The five patients whose values did not return to normal were all found later to have tumor recurrence. Thus the failure of CEA levels to drop postoperatively to the normal

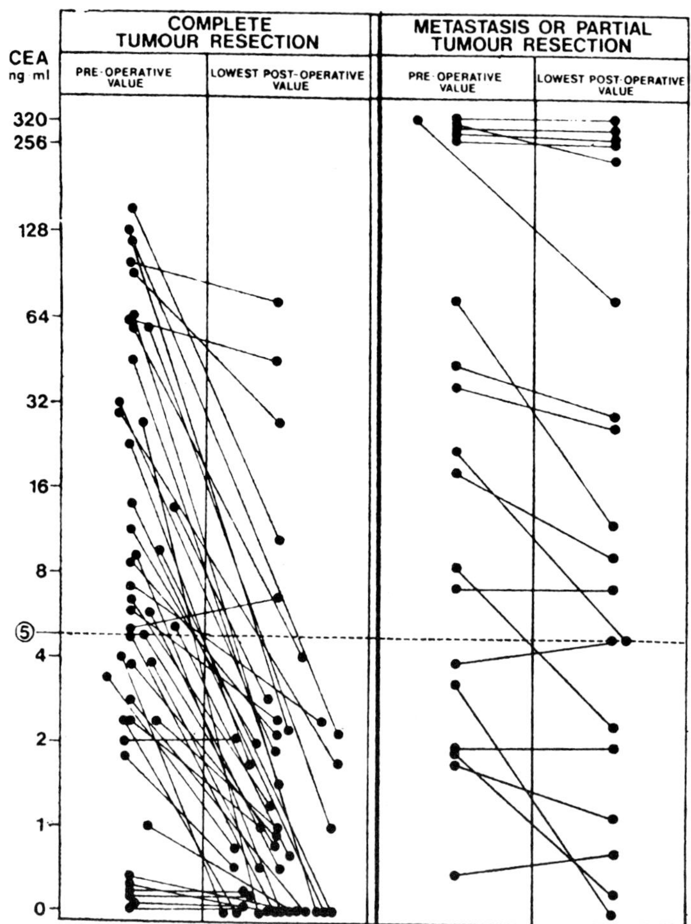

FIG. 2. Change in CEA levels before and after surgery. On the left, CEA levels in 45 patients for whom a macroscopically complete tumor resection was reported. The five patients whose CEA level did not fall below 5 ng/ml showed a subsequent rise in CEA level and tumor relapse. On the right, CEA levels in 19 patients with either distant metastases or a macroscopically partial tumor resection. (From Mach [8].)

range was felt to indicate residual microscopic disease and a poor prognosis. This has not been a universal finding, however, as some authors [9] have found that patients may have an elevated postoperative CEA for other reasons and that if the level is stable and not rising, it does not necessarily predict recurrence. More experience will be required to resolve this issue.

Detection of Postoperative Recurrence

Perhaps the most useful ultimate role of CEA will be to detect early recurrence in patients who have undergone a curative resection for colorectal carcinoma. Several studies suggest that serial CEA determinations following surgery may detect early recurrence in patients whose CEA was elevated preoperatively and then fell to normal or at least stabilized at a lower level postoperatively. The results of several series are compiled in Table 2 [7-13]. A total of 200 patients had recurrences following resection and of these 157 or 78% had a rise in CEA level associated with the recurrence. More important, in 114 or 57% the rising CEA level *preceded* any objective clinical signs of disease. Thus it appears that in some cases rising CEA level may be the first indication of cancer recurrence. It must also be noted, however, that in 43 patients, or 22%, the CEA level never rose despite obvious clinical recurrence. This percentage can be decreased somewhat if we exclude patients who did not have elevated CEA levels preoperatively, but nevertheless it is clear that a normal CEA cannot be used to rule out recurrence. A total of 334 patients in the series did not have recurrence and of these, 294 or 88% had unchanged CEA levels. Forty patients who did not recur had at least transient rises in CEA, some of which later returned to normal. Since the follow-up in some of these series was quite short, it is possible that some of the patients in this group may develop later recurrence. However, there do seem to be at least a few cases of false-positive CEA elevations.

If CEA is to ultimately be a useful addition, the critical question is its ability to detect recurrence *before* other methods. Figure 3 is taken from the series by Mach et al [8] and shows serial CEA levels of eight individual patients who

Table 2. Detection of Postoperative Recurrence by Serial CEA Levels Following Resection for Cure

Series	No Recurrence		Recurrences		
	Unchanged CEA	Rising CEA	Unchanged CEA	Rising Simultaneously With Clinical Detection	Rising Before Objective Clinical Detection
Mackay, 1974	150	17	17	10	26
Mach, 1974	8	6	-	-	8
Booth, 1974	96	7	19	26	37
Sugarbaker, 1976	20 (a)	1	4	1	7
Herrera, 1976	17	6 (b)	3	6	14
Martin, 1977	3	3	(c)	(c)	22
Totals	294 (88%)	40 (12%)	43 (21%)	43 (21%)	114 (58%)

(a) 12 patients had elevated but stable CEA levels.

(b) 2 of these had other diseases accounting for elevated CEA, and the remainder later returned to normal.

(c) This series was detected by 2nd look surgery so very few were operated on without some sign of recurrence.

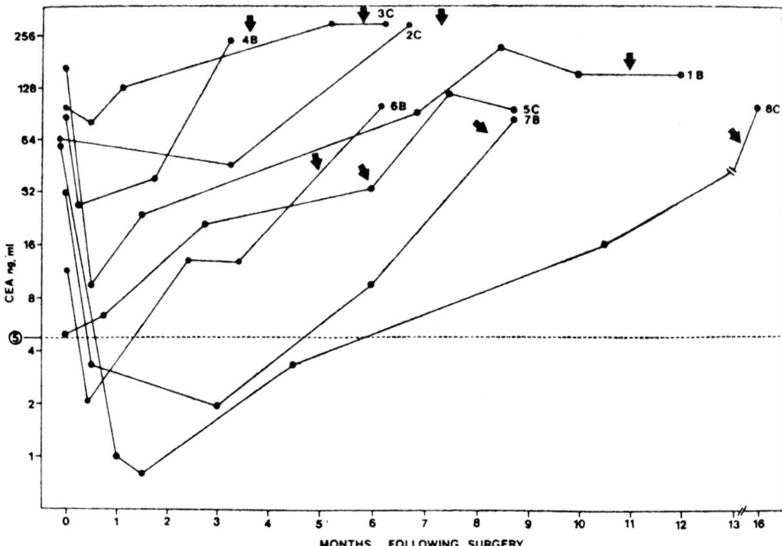

FIG. 3. Variations of CEA level in eight patients who showed a relapse of their carcinoma after what was considered as a macroscopically complete tumor resection. (From Mach [8].)

developed recurrence following resection of colon carcinoma. All of the levels dropped following surgery and then gradually increased. The arrows indicate the point at which recurrence became clinically apparent and in all cases the CEA level rose two to ten months before detection of recurrence by other means. Figure 4 shows similar data of Herrera et al [7] expressed in a slightly different form. Fourteen of 23 patients demonstrated a rise in CEA more than three months before other evidence of recurrence. Sugarbaker et al [9] did a prospective study of 33 patients following curative resection of colon cancer and compared monthly CEA determinations to other methods of follow-up. Of 12 patients with recurrence, seven were detected first by serial CEA determinations. CEA seemed to be especially useful in detecting intrahepatic and retroperitoneal disease, which is difficult to pick up by other methods. Therefore, it appears that although CEA is not a substitute for careful clinical follow-up, it may be useful as an adjunct for detection of early recurrent cancer.

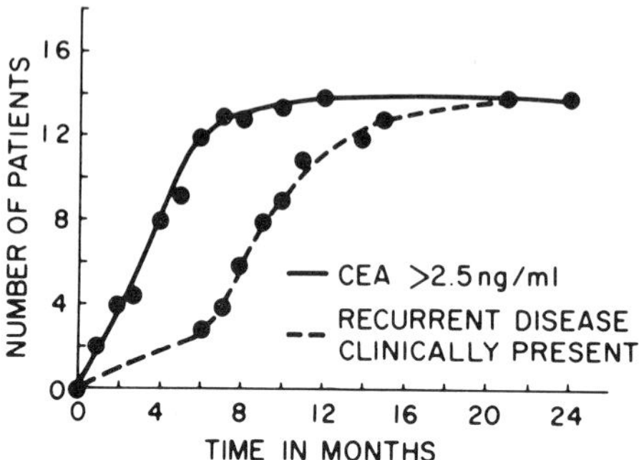

FIG. 4. Following curative resection 14 of 23 patients demonstrated a rise in CEA more than three months before recurrence was otherwise detected. (From Herrera [7].)

If CEA monitoring can detect early cancer recurrence, can we use this information in any way to base clinical decisions regarding therapy? Over 25 years ago Dr. Owen Wangensteen realized that colorectal carcinomas often recur within the abdominal cavity prior to the time of distant spread and instituted the "second-look" program. In this program patients with Duke's C carcinomas underwent systematic planned re-exploration six to nine months following primary resection even though they were asymptomatic. The program never gained widespread popularity because many patients underwent unnecessary negative explorations and because of the rather high morbidity and mortality associated with the procedure. Of 36 patients in whom recurrence was detected and removed at the time of second-look surgery, however, six were converted to long-term cures. Martin et al [12,14] have now reinstituted a "second-look" program based on rising CEA levels in the postoperative period. Figure 5 summarizes their results. They have now reoperated on 25 patients solely on the basis of rising CEA levels. None of these patients had any other objective evidence of cancer recurrence. Twenty-two of the 25 patients (88%) were found to have recurrent disease at laparotomy and in only 3 patients (12%) was the exploration negative. Of the 22 recurrences 16 had unresectable metastases and 6 had localized disease which could be resected. Of the six patients who had resection of localized disease, five are still free of tumor, one for over three years and four others for shorter periods. It appears

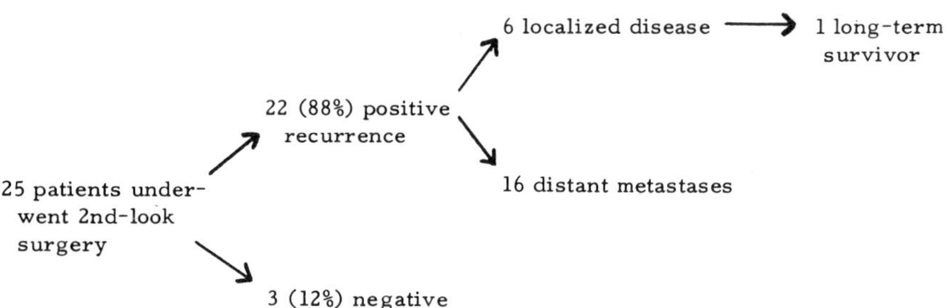

FIG. 5. Second-look surgery solely for rising CEA. (From Martin et al [12].)

hopeful that serial postoperative CEA determinations may detect recurrences early enough so that further trials of second-look surgery based on CEA monitoring may be worthwhile.

The protocol in Figure 6 was adopted from that recommended by Martin et al. It requires that each patient has a CEA determination preoperatively, secondly an initial baseline postoperatively, and finally serial CEA levels are recorded each month for the first year, every two months for the next two years, and every three months for two more years. If the CEA values show a definite rising trend which is confirmed by two or three independent determinations, the patient should undergo second-look operation. This protocol may permit real changes in patient management that may affect prognosis. Further prospective clinical trials appear warranted.

Monitoring Palliative Therapy

CEA levels may possibly be used to measure the effectiveness of palliative therapy in patients with advanced disease; ie, chemotherapy or radiotherapy, when effective, may cause a decrease in the CEA level. Ravry et al [15,16] from the Mayo Clinic correlated CEA levels with objective patient response to chemotherapy. Although the number of patients was small, 75% of those who showed objective improvement had reductions in CEA levels and 87% had either reduced or unchanged levels. Among those who showed objective progression, 65% had increased CEA levels and 80% had either increased or unchanged levels. Thus changes in CEA seemed to correlate with

·Draw preoperative CEA level

·Curative colon resection

·"Baseline" postoperative CEA level

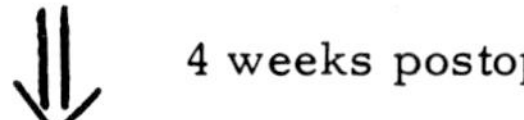

·Periodic CEA levels

- every month 1st year.
- every 2 months for 2 years.
- every 3 months for 2 years.

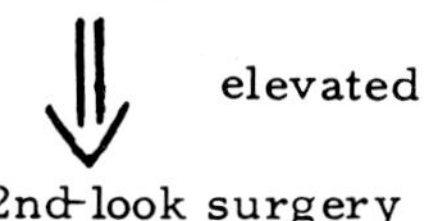

2nd-look surgery

resectable — Continued periodic CEA levels; If elevated third-look

non-resectable — Palliative therapy

FIG. 6. Recommended CEA protocol. (From Martin et al [12].)

clinical evidence of response to chemotherapy. Herrera et al [17] came to similar conclusions. Eighty percent of their patients who showed objective improvement had falling CEA levels. Furthermore, they noted that patients whose CEA values decreased with therapy had a slightly longer survival than those with rising levels even if they could not document an objective clinical response. Sugarbaker et al [18] had similar results. Figure 7 shows a patient from Sugarbaker's series who had metastatic rectal cancer. CEA levels rose initially with the onset of metastases but then decreased as the patient had an objective response to chemotherapy. When the level later increased again the authors concluded that a change in chemotherapy was indicated even though the patient had no evidence of a worsening clinical condition. The important question that must be answered is, can CEA levels indicate necessary changes in

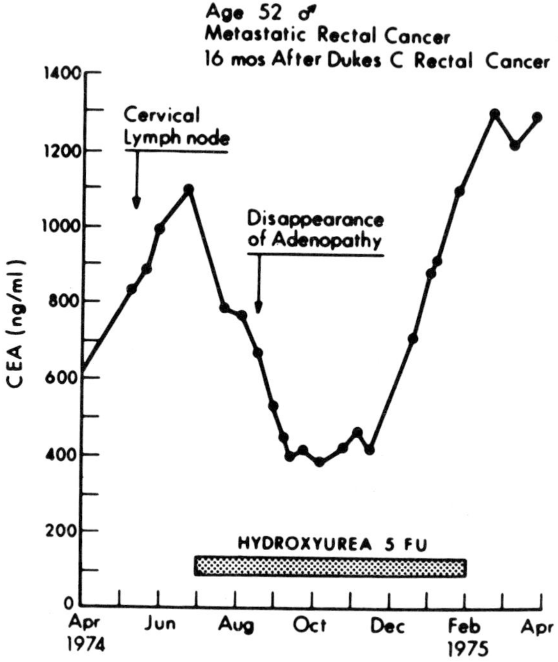

FIG. 7. Rapidly rising CEA in this 52-year-old man with metastatic rectal cancer signaled the need to change chemotherapy. (From Sugarbaker [18].)

therapy before other methods of monitoring? If CEA merely correlates with other parameters of clinical performance, it is of limited use as an addition to our current armamentarium. At present we do not have data to answer this question. However, scattered cases suggest that CEA may be useful for monitoring palliative therapy.

Summary

In summary, it is apparent that the story of CEA is not yet complete. After great initial enthusiasm investigators became generally discouraged when they realized that the assay was not sufficiently precise to be used for screening. There is now some renewed optimism that CEA may prove to be clinically useful in several areas. However, it is important that we accurately define specific clinical situations where CEA determinations can be used to make decisions regarding patient management. William Meeker recently reviewed the charts on 437 patients who had 1089 CEA determinations at the University of Kentucky Medical Center [19]. The test was ordered for a wide variety of indications; he could find only four instances where the test led to changes in patient management. Cost analysis revealed that the CEA test cost $5,047 per patient benefited. It is imperative, therefore, that further studies be performed before the test is indiscriminately applied.

The conclusions we can draw at this time are (1) CEA is not a useful screening test for cancer; (2) CEA will probably be most useful in detecting postoperative recurrence of carcinoma in cases where the level is elevated preoperatively and falls following curative resection. Prospective trials of "second-look" surgery are warranted: (3) CEA can give important prognostic information and may help determine which patients would most benefit from adjuvant chemotherapy. (4) CEA may be useful in monitoring palliative therapy or as a primary diagnostic adjunct but its ultimate role in specific clinical situations is still not clear.

References

1. Goldenberg, D.M.: Oncofetal and other tumor-associated antigens of the human digestive system. Curr. Top. Pathol. 63:289-342, 1976.
2. Holyoke, E.D. and Cooper, E.H.: CEA and tumor markers. Semin. Oncol. 3:377-385, 1976.
3. Martin, E.W., Jr., Kibbey, W.E., DiVecchia, L. et al: Carcinoembryonic antigen. Cancer 37:62-81, 1976.
4. Neville, A.M. and Cooper, E.H.: Biochemical monitoring of cancer. Ann. Clin. Biochem. 13:283-305, 1976.
5. Hansen, H.J., Snyder, J.J., Miller, E. et al: Carcinoembryonic antigen (CEA) assay. Hum. Pathol. 5:139-147, 1974.
6. Zamcheck, N.: Carcinoembryonic antigen. Adv. Int. Med. 19:413-433, 1974.
7. Herrera, M.A., Chu, T.M. and Holyoke, E.D.: Carcinoembryonic antigen (CEA) as a prognostic and monitoring test in clinically complete resection of colorectal carcinoma. Ann. Surg. 183:5-9, 1976.
8. Mach, J.P., Jaeger, P.H., Bertholet, M.M. et al: Detection of recurrence of large bowel carcinoma by radioimmunoassay of circulating carcinoembryonic antigen (CEA). Lancet 2:535-540, 1974.
9. Sugarbaker, P.H., Zamcheck, N. and Moore, F.D.: Assessment of serial carcinoembryonic antigen (CEA) assays in postoperative detection of recurrent colorectal cancer. Cancer 38:2310-2315, 1976.

10. Mackay, A.M., Patel, S., Carter, S. et al: Role of serial plasma C.E.A. assays in detection of recurrent and metastatic colorectal carcinomas. Br. J. Med. 4:382-385, 1974.
11. Booth, S.M., Jamieson, C.G., King, J.P.G. et al: Carcinoembryonic antigen in management of colorectal carcinoma. Br. Med. J. 4:183, 1974.
12. Martin, E.W., James, K.K., Hurtubise, P.E. et al: The use of CEA as an early indicator for gastrointestinal tumor recurrence and second-look procedure. Cancer 39:440-446, 1977.
13. Livingstone, A.S., Hampson, L.G., Shuster, J. et al: Carcinoembryonic antigen in the diagnosis and management of colorectal carcinoma. Arch. Surg. 109:259-264, 1974.
14. Balz, J.B., Martin, E.W., Jr. and Minton, J.P.: CEA as an early indicator for second-look procedure in colorectal carcinoma. Rev. Surg. 34:1-4, 1977.
15. Ravry, M., Moertel, C.G., Shutt, A.J. and Go, V.L.W.: Usefulness of serial serum carcinoembryonic antigen (CEA). Determinations during anticancer therapy or long-term followup of gastrointestinal carcinoma. Cancer 34:1230-1234, 1974.
16. Go, V.L.W.: Carcinoembryonic antigen. Cancer 37:562-566, 1976.
17. Herrera, M.A., Chu, T.M., Holyoke, E.D. and Mittelman, A.: CEA monitoring of palliative treatment for colorectal carcinoma. Ann. Surg. 185:23-30, 1977.
18. Sugarbaker, P.H., Skarin, A.T. and Zamcheck, N.: Patterns of serial CEA assays and their clinical use in management of colorectal cancer. J. Surg. Oncol. 8:523-537, 1976.
19. Meeker, W.R., Jr.: The use and abuse of CEA test in clinical practice. Cancer 41:854-862, 1978.

Self-Evaluation Quiz

1. The incidence of elevated CEA is *highest* in which of the following conditions?
   a) Normal, healthy smoker
   b) Duke's A colorectal carcinoma
   c) Alcoholic cirrhosis of the liver
   d) Malignant lymphoma
2. The incidence of elevated CEA is *highest* in which of the following population groups?
   a) Healthy, unselected
   b) Healthy, pregnant
   c) Healthy, nonsmoker
   d) Healthy, smoker
3. The incidence of elevated CEA in various stages of colorectal carcinoma can be ranked in the following order, starting with the highest:

a) Duke's A carcinoma/Duke's C carcinoma/metastatic carcinoma
b) Metastatic carcinoma/Duke's C carcinoma/Duke's A carcinoma
c) Duke's C carcinoma/Duke's A carcinoma/metastatic carcinoma
d) Duke's C carcinoma/metastatic carcinoma/Duke's A carcinoma
e) The incidence of elevated CEA is approximately equal in all stages of colorectal carcinoma

4. In the authors' opinion, which of the following possible clinical applications of CEA is felt to be the most useful at the present time?
a) Mass screening of large populations for cancer
b) Diagnostic adjunct in cases where carcinoma is suspected
c) Early detection of postoperative recurrence in patients who have undergone a curative resection for colorectal carcinoma
d) Monitoring of chemotherapy in cases of metastatic colorectal carcinoma
e) There is no clinical usefulness for CEA

5. A 67-year-old man presents with a four-week history of mild abdominal cramping and occasional melena. Upper and lower GI series are nondiagnostic but of poor quality due to an inadequate prep. A CEA determination has been obtained. Depending upon the results of the CEA test, the following conclusion can be drawn:
a) An elevated CEA makes the diagnosis of colorectal carcinoma
b) If the CEA is elevated, colonic carcinoma or some other GI malignancy is by far the most likely diagnosis and the possibility of gastric ulcer or ulcerative colitis is very remote
c) If the CEA is negative, the possibility of colorectal cancer is ruled out, but further elective workup should be obtained since ulcerative colitis, gastric ulcer, or other benign conditions are still possibilities
d) A negative CEA rules out ulcerative colitis, gastric ulcer and GI malignancy

   e) Regardless of the CEA value, this patient should receive further workup because colonic carcinoma, gastric ulcer and ulcerative colitis are still possibilities

6. Which statement concerning CEA is true?
   a) An elevated CEA level can diagnose primary gastrointestinal malignancy and a normal level can rule out malignancy
   b) An elevated CEA level can diagnose primary gastrointestinal malignancy but a normal level cannot rule out malignancy
   c) An elevated CEA level cannot diagnose primary gastrointestinal malignancy but a normal level can rule out malignancy
   d) CEA determination alone can neither diagnose nor rule out primary gastrointestinal malignancy
7. A 55-year-old man undergoes a curative resection for colorectal carcinoma. His preoperative CEA level is markedly elevated but the surgeon feels that all macroscopic tumor has been removed. The following statements may be made about this patient's prognosis:
   a) This patient has a greater chance of recurrence than a similar patient with a normal preoperative CEA level; the chance of recurrence may be as high as 80% within 18 months
   b) This patient has the same chance of recurrence as any other patient with macroscopically complete resection of a primary colorectal tumor
   c) The high CEA indicates metastatic disease and all such patients will eventually have recurrences
   d) The chance of recurrence in this patient cannot be predicted without knowing the Duke's classification of the resected specimen
8. The patient from question 7 is now four weeks following his curative resection for colorectal carcinoma. A postoperative baseline CEA level has been established. All of the following statements are true *except*:
   a) Most but not all patients with a macroscopically complete resection will have a fall in the postoperative CEA levels to normal

b) Those patients whose CEA values do not return to normal are probably likely to develop recurrent carcinoma, although a few authors note that the value can stabilize at an elevated level for reasons apparently unrelated to the carcinoma
c) If the postoperative CEA level returns to normal this indicates a "cure" and there is very little chance of cancer recurrence
d) If multiple liver metastases had been found at the time of surgery, the postoperative CEA level would almost certainly remain elevated

9. The CEA level in the patient from question 8 has returned to normal following his curative resection. It is decided to monitor his progress with monthly CEA determinations. The following statement is true:
a) If the CEA level remains normal, there is almost no chance of cancer recurrence
b) If the CEA level becomes elevated, this absolutely diagnoses cancer recurrence
c) If the patient develops recurrent cancer, the CEA level will probably rise, but it will seldom rise before the recurrence is obvious by other conventional clinical and diagnostic methods
d) If the CEA level rises to abnormal levels and is confirmed by a repeat determination, this indicates a strong likelihood of recurrent cancer even though all other diagnostic tests are negative. A "second look" operation should be considered

10. The patient in question 9 develops elevated CEA and undergoes exploration at which time unresectable hepatic metastases are discovered. After recovery from surgery he is placed on chemotherapy. The following statement is true:
a) CEA levels will no longer be useful, since the CEA will remain elevated until the patient's death
b) The CEA level will gradually decline as the patient's condition deteriorates, but it will not correlate with clinical status
c) CEA levels will drop if the chemotherapy reduces the patient's tumor burden and will rise again as the tumor

growth increases, but it is not yet known whether a rise in CEA may precede clinically obvious tumor recurrence

d) It has been shown conclusively that a rising CEA will be the first indicator of tumor progression and is therefore an indication to change chemotherapy

Answers on page 721.

Answers to Self-Evaluation Quizzes

Page 10: 1 (b); 2 (c); 3 (d); 4 (c); 5 (b); 6 (b); 7 (a).

Page 23: 1 (b); 2 (a); 3 (b); 4 (e); 5 (b); 6 (b); 7 (b); 8 (e); 9 (c); 10 (a).

Page 34: 1 (a); 2 (b); 3 (b); 4 (a); 5 (b); 6 (b); 7 (b); 8 (c); 9 (a); 10 (b); 11 (b); 12 (b).

Page 43: 1(b); 2(b); 3(a); 4(a); 5(b); 6(a); 7(a).

Page 52: 1 (a); 2 (a); 3 (b); 4 (c); 5 (a); 6 (b); 7 (a); 8 (a); 9 (b); 10 (b).

Page 68: 1 (d); 2 (c); 3 (b); 4 (a); 5 (b); 6 (c); 7 (a); 8 (a).

Page 84: 1 (c); 2 (d); 3 (b); 4 (b); 5 (b); 6 (a); 7 (b); 8 (b).

Page 105: 1 (d); 2 (d); 3 (c); 4 (c); 5 (a); 6 (b); 7 (a); 8 (b).

Page 115: 1 (b); 2 (a); 3 (a); 4 (a); 5 (a); 6 (d); 7 (d); 8 (b).

Page 140: 1 (c); 2 (b); 3 (b); 4 (a); 5 (d); 6 (b); 7 (b).

Page 152: 1 (a); 2 (b); 3 (b); 4 (e); 5 (a); 6 (a); 7 (b); 8 (d).

Page 163: 1 (c); 2 (a); 3 (a); 4 (a); 5 (a); 6 (c); 7 (a); 8 (e); 9 (c).

Page 184: 1 (c); 2 (b); 3 (b); 4 (a); 5 (c,d); 6(b); 7 (d); 8 (a).

Page 193: 1 (d); 2 (a); 3 (b); 4 (c); 5 (a).

Page 203: 1 (a); 2 (c); 3 (c); 4 (a,d); 5 (b); 6 (b); 7 (b): 8 (a); 9 (a).

Page 214: 1 (a,b,c); 2 (b); 3 (c); 4 (b); 5 (b); 6 (d); 7 (c); 8 (b); 9 (a).

Page 224: 1 (a); 2 (b); 3 (c); 4 (b); 5 (c); 6 (e); 7 (b); 8 (b); 9 (a); 10 (a).

Page 231: 1 (b); 2 (c); 3 (a); 4 (b); 5 (a); 6 (a); 7 (b); 8 (a).

Page 237: 1 (c); 2 (b); 3 (d); 4 (a); 5 (a); 6 (b); 7 (b); 8 (a); 9 (d).

Page 245: 1 (a); 2 (a); 3 (b); 4 (b); 5 (c).

Page 273: 1 (d); 2 (d); 3 (b); 4 (c); 5 (b); 6 (b); 7 (b); 8 (c).

Page 279: 1 (c); 2 (a); 3 (d); 4 (b); 5 (d); 6 (b); 7 (d); 8 (a).

Page 288: 1 (d); 2 (c); 3 (d); 4 (c); 5 (e); 6 (a); 7 (c); 8 (a).

Page 299: 1 (a); 2 (b); 3 (a); 4 (b); 5 (a); 6 (c); 7 (b); 8 (a); 9 (b).

Page 314: 1 (a); 2 (a); 3 (a); 4 (b); 5 (a); 6 (b); 7 (b,d,e); 8 (a,d,e).

Page 337: 1 (b); 2 (b); 3 (a); 4 (a); 5 (b); 6 (b); 7 (a); 8 (b); 9 (a); 10 (b).

Page 376: 1 (c); 2 (a); 3 (a); 4 (a); 5 (a); 6 (b); 7 (c); 8 (b).

Page 388: 1 (b); 2 (b); 3 (b); 4 (a); 5 (a); 6 (b); 7 (a); 8 (b); 9 (c).

Page 400: 1 (c); 2 (b); 3 (b); 4 (a); 5 (b); 6 (c); 7 (b); 8 (a).

Page 410: 1 (d); 2 (a); 3 (a); 4 (b); 5 (a); 6 (c); 7 (b); 8 (a); 9 (d).

Page 419: 1 (d); 2 (c); 3 (c); 4 (c); 5 (e).

Page 426: 1 (c); 2 (d); 3 (b); 4 (c); 5 (b).

Page 453: 1 (b); 2 (a); 3 (d); 4 (a); 5 (b); 6 (a); 7 (b); 8 (d).

Page 458: 1 (b); 2 (a); 3 (a); 4 (c); 5 (b); 6 (b); 7 (b); 8 (b); 9 (b).

Page 470: 1 (a); 2 (a); 3 (b); 4 (b); 5 (b); 6 (b); 7 (a); 8 (a).

Page 478: 1 (a); 2 (d); 3 (a); 4 (e); 5 (e); 6 (d): 7 (c); 8 (d); 9 (i).

Page 497: 1 (c); 2 (a); 3 (d); 4 (c); 5 (e).

Page 512: 1 (c); 2 (b); 3 (a); 4 (b); 5 (a); 6 (a); 7 (c); 8 (b); 9 (a); 10 (b).

Page 519: 1 (b); 2 (d); 3 (d); 4 (b); 5 (a); 6 (d); 7 (c); 8 (a); 9 (d); 10 (c).

Page 527: 1 (a); 2 (d); 3 (c); 4 (a); 5 (a); 6 (a); 7 (b); 8 (a); 9 (c); 10 (a).

Page 540: 1 (c); 2 (b); 3 (d); 4 (d); 5 (d); 6 (d); 7 (c); 8 (c); 9 (d); 10 (d).

Page 561: 1 (b); 2 (a); 3 (e); 4 (b); 5 (a); 6 (a); 7 (b).

Page 574: 1 (b); 2 (b); 3 (b); 4 (b); 5 (a); 6 (d); 7 (b); 8 (e); 9 (d); 10 (e).

Page 585: 1(a); 2(b); 3(b); 4(c); 5(d).

Page 591: 1(c); 2(d); 3(a,b); 4(c); 5(d); 6(d); 7(b); 8(c).

Page 599: 1(a); 2(c); 3(a); 4(b); 5(d).

Page 606: 1 (c); 2 (b); 3 (b).

Page 636: 1(c); 2(d); 3(d); 4(c); 5(d); 6(c); 7(c); 8(a).

Page 652: 1 (d); 2 (b); 3 (c); 4 (b); 5 (d); 6 (a); 7 (d); 8 (b); 9 (d); 10 (a).

Page 666: 1 (b); 2 (b); 3 (a); 4 (c); 5 (d); 6 (d); 7 (d); 8 (c); 9 (b); 10 (d).

Page 675: 1(c); 2(d); 3(b); 4(b); 5(b); 6(d); 7(b); 8(a); 9(b); 10(d).

Page 679: 1 (c); 2 (b); 3 (b,c,d); 4 (d); 5 (d); 6 (a); 7 (a); 8 (d).

Page 699: 1(b); 2(b); 3(a); 4(d); 5(b); 6(a); 7(a).

Page 715: 1 (c); 2 (d); 3 (b); 4 (c); 5 (e); 6 (d); 7 (a); 8 (c); 9 (d); 10 (c).

Subject Index